Medical Imaging Techniques and Applications

Medical Imaging Techniques and Applications

Editor: Marcus Lewis

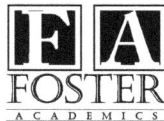

FOSTER
ACADEMICS

www.fosteracademics.com

www.fosteracademics.com

FA FOSTER ACADEMICS

Cataloging-in-Publication Data

Medical imaging techniques and applications / edited by Marcus Lewis.
    p. cm.
Includes bibliographical references and index.
ISBN 978-1-63242-494-5
1. Imaging systems in medicine. 2. Imaging systems in medicine--Equipment and supplies.
3. Medical instruments and apparatus. I. Lewis, Marcus.
R857.O6 M43 2017
616.075 4--dc23

© Foster Academics, 2017

Foster Academics,
118-35 Queens Blvd., Suite 400,
Forest Hills, NY 11375, USA

ISBN 978-1-63242-494-5 (Hardback)

Printed and bound in the United States of America.

Contents

Preface

Medical imaging encompasses the techniques and methods for the visual representation of the anatomy as well as processes of the body. It is primarily used for medical diagnosis. Some of the most widely implemented medical imaging techniques include ultrasound, positron emission tomography, magnetic resonance imaging, etc. This book presents the complex subject of medical imaging in the most comprehensible and easy to understand language. The aim of this text is to present researches that have transformed this discipline and aided its advancement. From theories to research to practical applications, case studies related to all contemporary topics of relevance to this field have been included in this book. The topics covered herein offer the readers new insights in the field of medical imaging.

This book is a result of research of several months to collate the most relevant data in the field.

When I was approached with the idea of this book and the proposal to edit it, I was overwhelmed. It gave me an opportunity to reach out to all those who share a common interest with me in this field. I had 3 main parameters for editing this text:

1. Accuracy – The data and information provided in this book should be up-to-date and valuable to the readers.

2. Structure – The data must be presented in a structured format for easy understanding and better grasping of the readers.

3. Universal Approach – This book not only targets students but also experts and innovators in the field, thus my aim was to present topics which are of use to all.

Thus, it took me a couple of months to finish the editing of this book.

I would like to make a special mention of my publisher who considered me worthy of this opportunity and also supported me throughout the editing process. I would also like to thank the editing team at the back-end who extended their help whenever required.

Editor

A Novel Technique of Contrast-Enhanced Optical Coherence Tomography Imaging in Evaluation of Clearance of Lipids in Human Tears

Pietro Emanuele Napoli*, Franco Coronella, Giovanni Maria Satta, Maurizio Fossarello

Department of Surgical Sciences, Eye Clinic, University of Cagliari, Cagliari, Italy

Abstract

Purpose: The aim of this work was to gather preliminary data in different conditions of healthy eyes, aqueous tear deficient dry eyes, obstructive meibomian gland disease (MGD) and non-obvious obstructive MGD (NOMGD) individuals, using a new, contrast-enhanced optical coherence tomography (OCT) imaging method to evaluate the clearance of lipids in human tears.

Methods: Eighty-two adult patients presenting with complaints of ocular irritation were studied for abnormalities of the ocular surface and classified as healthy (n = 21), aqueous tear deficient dry eyes (n = 20), obstructive MGD (n = 15) and NOMGD (n = 26) individuals. A lipid-based tracer, containing an oil-in-water emulsion, was used to obtain an enhanced OCT imaging of the lower tear meniscus. After instillation, a dramatic initial increase of reflectivity of the lower tear meniscus was detected by OCT, followed by a decay back to baseline values over time. Based on this finding, the clearance of lipids was measured in real-time by Fourier-domain anterior segment OCT.

Results: The differences in the clearance of lipids among the four groups as well as the correlations between symptom questionnaire score, standardized visual scale test, fluorescein break-up time, ocular surface fluorescein staining score, Schirmer I test scores were found to be statistically significant. The individual areas under the curve of the clearance of lipids calculated by the receiver operating characteristic curve technique ranged from 0.66 to 0.98, suggesting reliable sensitivity and specificity of lipid-enhanced OCT imaging.

Conclusions: This new technique of contrast-enhanced OCT imaging of the tear film following lipid-based tracer instillation provides a measure of the clearance of lipids. The quantitative values found are in agreement with other methods of evaluation of the lacrimal system. An improvement of the clinician's ability in the diagnosis and understanding of abnormalities of the ocular surface may be achieved by this simple approach.

Editor: Christof Markus Aegerter, University of Zurich, Switzerland

Funding: The authors have no support or funding to report.

Competing Interests: The authors have declared that no competing interests exist.

* Email: pietronapoli@ymail.com

Introduction

The current model of the precorneal tear film consists of a thick aqueous-mucin layer covered by a thin lipid layer. The lipid layer is the most anterior layer of the tear film, composed of meibomian lipids that limit tear evaporation and stabilize the tear film. [1] In case of absence or altered integrity of the lipid layer, the evaporation rate of tears increases, and produces tear-film instability. [2,3] In fact, the lipid layer measured by interferometry has been reported to correlate with tear-film evaporation, tear-film break-up time, and clinical symptoms. [4,5]

In various pathological conditions, such as meibomian gland dysfunction (MGD), the appearance of the lipid layer may change. A meibomian lipid deficiency due to obstructive MGD is an area of growing clinical interest since it is now recognized to be the most common cause of evaporative dry eye. [6,7] The latest clinical classification of the ocular surface disorders includes a type

of obstructive MGD that is obvious upon examination, and a non-obvious obstructive meibomian gland dysfunction (NOMGD). [8] NOMGD is potentially considered the most common form of obstructive MGD, but it is frequently missed during clinical examination, since it starts with minimal signs and symptoms, requiring clinical evaluation of meibomian gland expressibility for its diagnosis.

Although several studies have assessed the flow of the aqueous layer by means of the clearance of fluorescein sodium, the turnover or clearance of lipids (CoL) in the tears of patients with abnormalities of the ocular surface has not been yet documented in literature. [9–18] Since fluorescein sodium is highly water-soluble at physiologic pH, its clearance is essentially an index of the aqueous tear turnover. However, the elimination rate of other tear components does not parallel the aqueous tear clearance. [19]

Recently, optical coherence tomography (OCT) has been used to obtain detailed cross-sectional images of anterior tissues of the eye and to assess the tear film. [20–24] OCT imaging may potentially permit observation of fine details of the ocular surface and understanding new aspects about the behavior of human tears in vivo.

In the present study, we used Fourier-domain anterior segment OCT to analyze the dynamic distribution of lipids in the lower tear meniscus and to determine the CoL in humans. For this purpose, we administered a lipid-based tracer to enhance the visibility of lipids and to track their flow in the lower tear meniscus with OCT. In this way, we evaluated the correlation between the CoL and aqueous tear turnover as well as classical tear tests, and the diagnostic validity of this new technique of contrast-enhanced OCT imaging, in healthy subjects and in patients with aqueous tear deficiency (ATD), obstructive MGD and NOMGD.

Materials and Methods

1. Subjects and procedure

Adult patients presenting with complaints of ocular irritation were evaluated at the Eye Clinic, Department of Surgical Sciences and Odontostomatology, University of Cagliari, School of Ophthalmology. Written informed consent for participation was obtained from all subjects, after ethics approval obtained from the Office of Research Ethics, University of Cagliari. The study complied with the guidelines in the Declaration of Helsinki for research involving human subjects.

All examinations were conducted in the same conditions of temperature (within a range of 15°C to 25°C), humidity (within a range of 30% to 50%) and time of the day (between 3 PM to 5 PM) in a dimly lit consulting room.

All subjects completed a symptom questionnaire (OSDI = Ocular Surface Disease Index) [25] consisting of a set of questions assessing the level of discomfort and the functional impact of their irritation symptoms.

On the day before OCT imaging, a standard clinical assessment was performed on all subjects in the same sequence. It included: clinical history, fluorescein break-up time (FBUT), fluorescein staining of the cornea and conjunctiva graded according to the Oxford system, [26] standardized visual scale test (SVST), Schirmer I test, and a slit lamp examination of the lid margins and meibomian glands.

Since it is good practice to work from the least invasive to the most invasive test, [26] OCT imaging was carried out a day after the clinical assessment, in order to avoid one tear test interfering with the CoL, as well as to prevent manipulation disrupting the tear film/ocular surface.

Based on the results of these tests, patients were classified into one of four groups based on the following inclusion criteria:

1.1. Aqueous tear deficiency. If the subject exhibited all of the following characteristics: significant subjective symptoms (OSDI score ≥13), a FBUT <10 seconds, a significant vital staining of the ocular surface (Oxford scheme ≥2 or panel B) and a Schirmer I test ≤5 mm.

1.2. Obvious Obstructive meibomian gland disease. It was considered to be present when the patient exhibited Schirmer I test>5 mm and all of the following three signs/findings: [27]

• Chronic ocular discomfort (OSDI score ≥13).
• Anatomic abnormalities around the meibomian gland orifices (presence of one or more of the following is positive):

a. irregularity of the lid margin;

b. vascular engorgement;
c. anterior or posterior displacement of the mucocutaneous junction.

• Obstruction of the meibomian glands (presence of both is considered positive):

a. decreased meibum expression by moderate digital pressure;
b. obstructive findings of the gland orifices by slit lamp biomicroscopy (pouting, plugging, or ridge).

1.3. Non-obvious obstructive meibomian gland disease. It was diagnosed only after gland expression [8] (gland orifices failing to yield any secretion on expression), in patients with asymptomatic dysfunction or occasional symptoms (OSDI < 12), Schirmer I test>10 mm and normal lid margin features.

1.4. Healthy. Subjects with no history of use of eyedrops, no significant symptoms of ocular irritation (OSDI <12), FBUT>10 seconds, Oxford scheme ≤ panel A, and a Schirmer I test score more than 10 mm were considered as healthy.

Subjects with other *abnormalities* of the ocular surface or of the tear film, other eye diseases in the previous 6 months, excessive meibomian lipid secretion (meibomian seborrhea) or any evidence of abnormal blinking, history of contact lenses wear or of eye surgery, were excluded from the study.

2. FBUT and fluorescein ocular surface staining

In order to enhance the observation of dry spots in the fluorescent tear film, over the entire cornea, and the conjunctival staining, the ocular surface was examined with a biomicroscope and the ×10 objective under both blue-light illumination and Kodak Wratten 12 yellow filter, within 10–30 seconds (for FBUT) and after 2 minutes (for grading staining) of fluorescein sodium instillation (t = 0). Three evaluations of FBUT were conducted, and the mean value was taken for data analysis. Staining of the ocular surface was graded according to the Oxford system as follows: 1 = panel A, 2 = panel B, 3 = panel C, 4 = panel D, 5 = panel E, 6 = panel>E.

3. Standardized Visual Scale Test (tear fluorescein clearance)

The SVST was performed as previously reported. [28] Briefly, the color of the tear meniscus in the third lateral of the lower lid was visually compared with one of the colors of the standardized visual scale. If the color of the tear meniscus was judged to be between two of the six standard scale colors, then the score was graded between these two standard colors.

After the SVST, Schirmer I test and the slit lamp examination of the lid margins and meibomian glands were performed.

4. Lipid-based tracer

The castor oil is a vegetable oil containing a mixture of lipids (approximately 90 percent of fatty acid chains are ricinoleate), which mimics the oily lipid secretions produced by meibomian glands, i.e. the natural lipids in the tear film. In fact, for this reason it is contained in some lipid-based artificial tears. The lipid-based tracer was obtained in the following way: a castor oil emulsion (0.50%) was prepared in sterile 0.067 M phosphate-buffered saline, pH 7.4, with Tween 80.

A preliminary experiment was performed to test the association between OCT reflectivity and the amount of lipids. Immediately after instillation of 35 μl of tracer containing various concentrations of castor oil (0.5%, 0.25%, 0.125%, 0.06%) or saline solution

(35 µl, Blu Sal, Sooft, Italy) into five subjects' eyes was performed OCT imaging. Thus, a positive correlation between OCT reflectivity and lipids concentration was revealed (fig 1). Castor oil concentration of 0.50% offered the greatest clarity of details and, therefore, was used as tracer. Accordingly, the tracer (castor oil 0.5%) was detected by OCT as a dramatic initial increase of reflectivity in the lower tear meniscus, followed by a decay back to baseline values over time (fig 2). In this way, we obtained a lipid-enhanced OCT imaging. No signs of inflammation or damage were detected either immediately or after 24h.

To test the stability of the tracer in the absence of tear clearance (in order to obtain a *control* sequence of contrast-enhanced OCT imaging), a drop of the lipid emulsion (35 µl, castor oil 0.5%) was placed on a glass slide and its reflectivity was evaluated at instillation, at 5 minutes, at 10 minutes and at 15 minutes (i.e., at the same time-points of OCT examination, as described below). As expected, the tracer remained hyper-reflective for all the time of the test (fig 3).

5. OCT measurements and scoring

The lower tear meniscus of one randomly chosen eye in each patient was imaged by vertical scans on the vertical axis passing across the corneal apex. OCT scans were performed by using Cirrus[TM] HD-OCT 4000 (Carl Zeiss Meditec Inc., Dublin, California, USA). This system is a Fourier-domain OCT platform that works at a wavelength of 840 nm, takes 27,000 axial scans per second and has a 5 µm axial resolution. The cross-sectional ocular surface images were acquired using the Anterior Segment 5 Line Raster scanning protocol. The mode acquires a set of five parallel lines of equal length at 3 mm. Each scan line comprised 4096 A-scans with the overall 5 Line Raster scan taking approximately 0.75 seconds to complete. For our purposes, the scan lines were orientated vertically and each separated horizontally by 250 µm. After image capture, the individual line with greatest clarity of detail was selected for our analysis. The subject was asked to blink normally during the examination period. Before each scan, patients were instructed to look straight ahead. The lower tear meniscus was imaged 2 seconds after a blink. The axial distance of patients was adjusted so that the lower tear meniscus was within the middle third of the scan. [20]

The evaluation of the CoL in human tears was performed by analyzing the clearance of the lipid-based tracer (35 µl) in the lower tear meniscus.

The OCT scans were performed at baseline and after the instillation of the tracer in four serial scans: immediately (within 30 seconds), at the 5th, at the 10th and at the 15th minute. Thus, we have classified the tear clearance of lipids, with respect to the apparent reflectivity, according to the following grading scale: grade 1 or excellent (black = absence of reflectivity), grade 2 or good (from black to blue = low reflectivity), grade 3 or fair (from blue to green = moderate reflectivity), grade 4 or poor (from green to yellow/red = high/intense reflectivity).

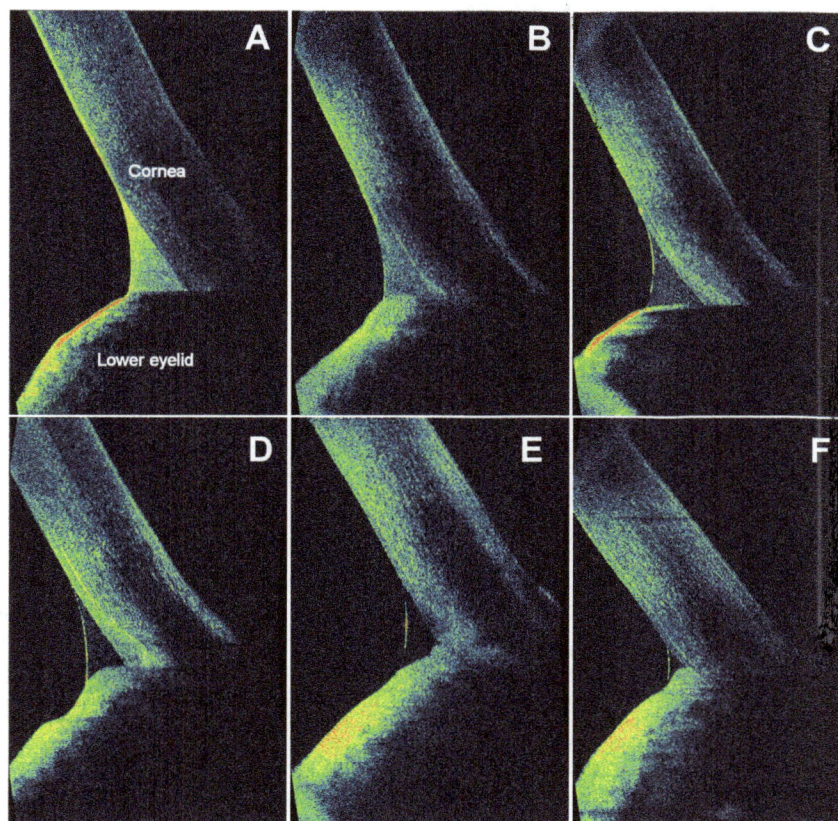

Figure 1. Association between OCT reflectivity and amount of lipids. Vertical, 3-mm OCT scans of the lower tear meniscus. The lipid-based tracer containing different concentrations of castor oil (0.5%, 0.25%, 0.125%, and 0.06%) or saline solution were instilled in five subjects (A, B, C, D, and E, respectively). OCT imaging revealed a positive correlation between the signal intensity detected by OCT and lipids concentration. At baseline (F), the reflectivity in the lower tear meniscus was nearly undetectable.

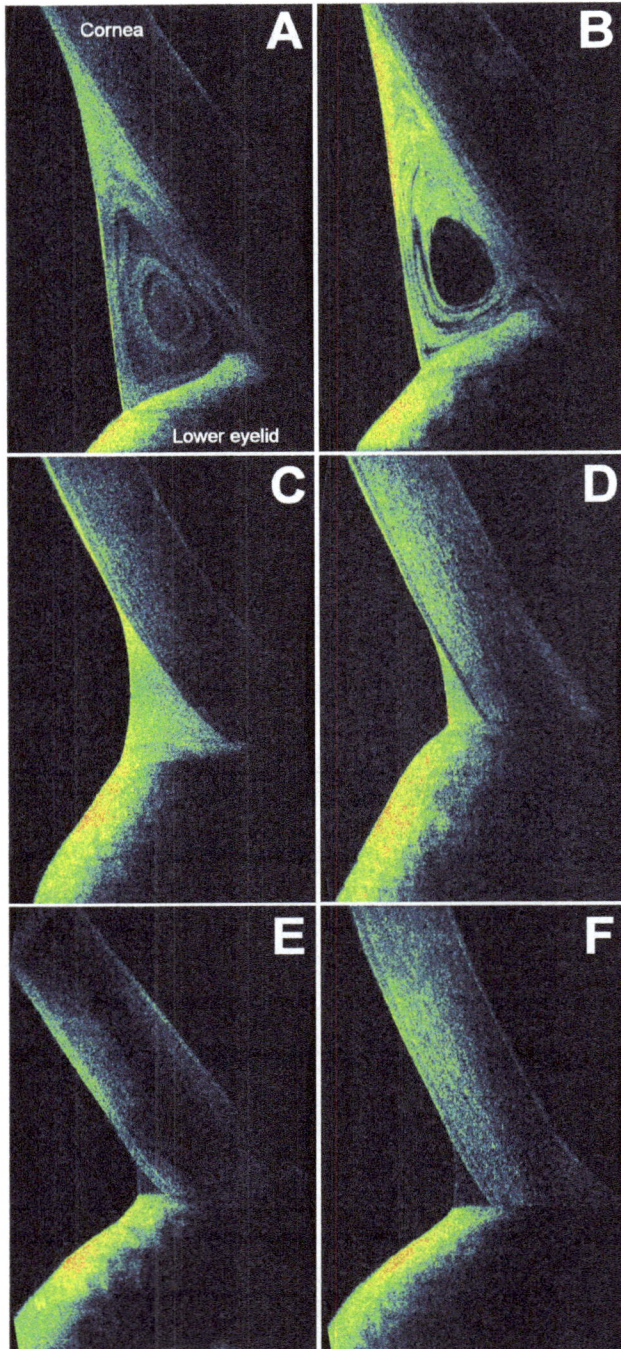

Figure 2. OCT images of the different patterns of the lower tear meniscus. Vertical, 3-mm OCT scans. The cross-sectional ocular surface images were acquired during normal blinks and evaluated in real-time. A dramatic initial increase of reflectivity in the lower tear meniscus was detected by OCT after instillation of the lipid-based tracer, followed by a decay back to baseline values over time. The reflectivity of the lower tear meniscus at the 15th minute was considered an index of turnover of tear lipids. The tracer was distributed in the lower tear meniscus according to the two morphological patterns: a vortex type (A and B), which shows areas of high/moderate reflectivity distributed concentrically around a central area of low/absent reflectivity, and a homogeneous type (C, D, E and F), which shows areas of similar reflectivity in the whole lower tear meniscus, classified according to the reflectivity grading scale. At instillation (C and D), the reflectivity was high/intense

in all patients. At baseline (E and F), the reflectivity detected by OCT in the lower tear meniscus was nearly undetectable.

The reflectivity of the lower tear meniscus at the 15th minute was considered an index of turnover of tear lipids.

The dynamic distribution of the tracer was also classified according to the morphological pattern in two different categories (fig. 2): a homogeneous type (areas of similar reflectivity in the whole lower tear meniscus, classified according the previous grading scale) and a vortex type (areas of high/moderate reflectivity distributed concentrically around a central area of low/absent reflectivity).

All information were recorded anonymously, so that subjects could not be identified, directly or through identifiers linked to the subjects.

6. Index of Lipid/Aqueous dysfunction

To improve the sensitivity of our test in differentiating the impact of a lipid alteration from an aqueous deficiency, the following tear dysfunction index (TDI) was introduced: TDI = CoL grade/Schirmer I test grade

The lipid turnover at the 15th minute was graded as follows: 1 = excellent, 2 = good, 3 = fair, 4 = poor. Since the Schirmer test score is also a discrete variable, [6] as wetting length values are taken as the nearest integer or half integer rather than as continuous fractions of a millimeter, it was evaluated, considering the severity of the aqueous deficiency, [6] in four ranks: 1 = normal (score >10 mm), 2 = borderline (score between 6 mm and 10 mm), 3 = abnormal (score between 5 mm and 3 mm), 4 = abnormal with considerable severity (score ≤ 2 mm).

The TDI has a precise rationale: to compare the influence of a lipid alteration with respect to an aqueous deficiency. Therefore, the TDI does not aim to differentiate a normal subject from a dry eye patient, which is the role assigned to tear tests. The best cutoff point (y) for the TDI was calculated by analyzing the receiver operating characteristic curves (ROCs). Thus, the TDI score was considered as follows: predominant lipid alteration (TDI score > y), predominant aqueous deficiency (TDI score < y).

7. Statistical analysis

Statistical analysis was performed using Statistical Package for Social Science SPSS version 21.0. Numeric data were summarized as mean ± standard deviation (SD) for parametric data, as median and mode ± average absolute deviation for ordinal data, while nominal data were summarized as percentage.

Data were analyzed by Shapiro-Wilk test and Lilliefors test for normality. If data were normally distributed, then parametric statistical tests were used, otherwise nonparametric tests were used. Particularly, the difference in age among the four groups was studied by means of one-way analysis of variance, and Bonferroni correction for the *post-hoc* analysis. The difference in gender, OSDI, FBUT, fluorescein staining of the ocular surface, SVST, Schirmer I test, CoL and TDI, among the four groups was studied using the Kruskal-Wallis test, followed by *post-hoc* Mann–Whitney U tests with Bonferroni correction to identify specific differences between each group.

Diagnostic results for dry eye were analyzed by receiver operating characteristics (ROC) curve, and the area under the ROC curve (AUC) was calculated. Other specific statistical tests are described as they are encountered in the article. P-values less than 0.05 were considered significant.

A Novel Technique of Contrast-Enhanced Optical Coherence Tomography Imaging in Evaluation of Clearance...

5

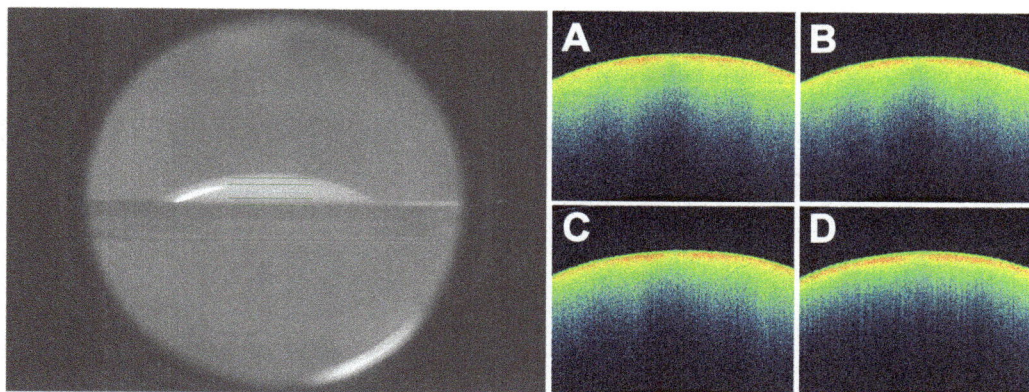

Figure 3. OCT serial images of a calibrated drop of the lipid-based tracer (35 μl, castor oil 0.5%) on a glass slide. Infrared image (left), and horizontal, 3-mm OCT scans (right). The OCT scans were performed at instillation, at the 5th, at the 10th and at the 15th minute (A, B, C and D, respectively). No changes in reflectivity of the tracer were observed in this *control* sequence of contrasted-enhanced OCT imaging.

Results

1. Differences in CoL among the four groups

No significant differences in age and gender were found between control participants (n = 21; age: 45.89±15.14 years, 90.5% female), patients with ATD (n = 20; age: 45.10±13.95 years, 90% female), patients with obstructive MGD (n = 15; age: 49.13±19.50 years, 86.7% female), and patients with NOMGD (n = 26; age: 46.88±16.82 years, 88.5% female). Descriptive statistics for diagnostic tests, as well as the statistically significant differences among the four studied groups are provided in Table 1 and 2.

The differences in CoL among the four groups were found to be statistically significant (Kruskal–Wallis statistic, 65.8; $p<0.001$; Table 1). However, no significant differences in CoL were found between ATD and obstructive MGD (*post-hoc* Mann–Whitney U test with Bonferroni correction, 120.0; $p = 0.07$; Table 1).

2. TDI

The cutoff value, derived from the ROC curve, is the point with an *optimal relationship* between sensitivity and specificity. The best cutoff point (y) for TDI was calculated to be 1.35. By applying the y for TDI, the differences among the four groups were raised significantly (Kruskal–Wallis statistic, 57.30; $p<0.001$; Table 1). Interestingly, no significant differences in TDI were found between obstructive MGD and NOMGD (*post-hoc* Mann–Whitney U test with Bonferroni correction, 192.0; $p = 0.92$; Table 1) since both MGDs (obstructive MGD or NOMGD) are involved in determining a lipid alteration.

Gender did not influence the results (Kruskal–Wallis statistic, 0.009; $p = 0.92$).

3. Dynamic variations of the tear film and of the ocular surface

The vortex-pattern was observed only at the 5th minute (14.3%) and 10th minute (14.3%) in healthy subjects; in all other cases, the homogeneous pattern was detected (see Table 2). The results of correlation analyses are presented in Table 3.

The differences over time of CoL and SVST are provided in Table 2 and 4. In all groups, the CoL has been slower than the aqueous flow, as assessed by SVST. Interestingly, a biphasic decay of the reflectivity elicited by the tracer was observed in some cases: after a dramatic initial dilution of tracer, probably due to the reflex tearing, there was a slower washout of lipids, probably due to the progressive reduction of tear volume. However, in case of healthy individuals, a highly significant clearance of tracer was restored after the 10th minute.

4. Diagnostic validity of the novel OCT technique

We have considered the values of CoL as *abnormal* when they were fair or poor, and *normal* when values were excellent or good, or when it was present a vortex pattern. The individual AUCs of CoL calculated by the ROC technique ranged from 0.66 to 0.98, suggesting reliable sensitivity and specificity of lipid-enhanced OCT imaging (Tables 5 and 6). Particularly, the AUC of CoL in the differential diagnosis between healthy subjects and patients with both abnormalities of the ocular surface (ATD + MGDs), was 0.98 ($p<0.001$), asymptotic 95% confidence interval (0.0, 1.0). Again, the TDI showed a promising ability in differentiating ATD patients than patients with lipid deficiency due to MGDs, AUC = 1.00 ($p<0.001$), asymptotic 95% confidence interval (0.0, 1.0).

The sensitivity of the CoL in diagnosing healthy (only in this case, healthy subject = positive diagnosis), obstructive MGD, NOMGD, ATD, was 93.6%, 100%, 51.1%, 48.7%, respectively. The specificity was 100%, 33.8%, 84%, 36.2%, respectively. The diagnostic accuracy was 97.5%, 43.9%, 52.4%, 50%, respectively. Moreover, the positive predictive value (PPV) was 100%, 26.7%, 84.6%, 35%, respectively, and the negative predictive value (NPV) was 84%, 100%, 37.5%, 100%, respectively.

By applying the TDI (cut-off point at 1.35), the sensitivity of lipid-enhanced OCT imaging in diagnosing ATD or MGDs was raised to 100%.

The sensitivity, specificity, accuracy, PPV and NPV of the vortex-pattern (at the 5th and 10th minute) in diagnosing healthy patients (in this case, healthy = positive diagnosis) was 14.2%, 100%, 96.3%, 100%, 77.2%, respectively.

Discussion

The lipids found in human tears are numerous and exert several functions. [29] The meibomian gland secretes a complex mixture comprising families of non-polar lipids, polar lipids, and proteins. Although over one hundred major compounds have been identified, Tiffany estimated that there could be thousands yet undiscovered. [30,31] In the outer layer of the tear film – the lipid layer – there is a polar phase, which has surfactant properties, and

Table 1. Statistical Comparison of four Groups: Healthy, Aqueous Tear Deficiency (ATD), obvious obstructive Meibomian Gland Dysfunction (MGD), and Non-obvious Obstructive MGD (NOMGD) Patients.

Group	OSDI†	FBUT*	FSOS grade†	SVST grade†	Schirmer 1 test*	CoL grade (15th minute)†	TDI*
Healthy persons (n=21)	4.2±3.3	10.7±4.2	1±0.0	1±0.1	23.6±10.7	1±0.9	1.3±0.4
ATD patients (n=20)	47.4±16.7	5.1±2.9	3.(4)±0.1	6±0.8	1.9±1.5	4±0.5	0.9±0.1
Obstructive MGD patients (n=15)	25.2±3.1	5.1±1.3	2±0.0	4±0.6	11.9±7.3	4±0.0	2.8±1.0
NOMGD patients (n=26)	6.5±4.1	8±1.1	1±0.0	4±0.1	17.7±11.4	3±0.0	3.0±0.0
Differences among the four groups	K=65.3 $p<0.001$	K=45.7 $p<0.001$	K=51.0 $p<0.001$	K=61.2 $p<0.001$	K=52.9 $p<0.001$	K=65.8 $p<0.001$	K=57.3 $p<0.001$
Differences between healthy and ATD	U=0.0 $p<0.001$	U=37.0 $p<0.001$	U=63.0 $p<0.001$	U=0.0 $p<0.001$	U=0.0 $p<0.001$	U=0.0 $p<0.001$	U=123.5 $p=0.009$
Differences<between healthy<and<MGD	U=0.0 $p<0.001$	U=0.0 $p<0.001$	U=21.0 $p<0.001$	U=16.0 $p<0.001$	U=60.0 $p=0.002$	U=0.0 $p<0.001$	U=36.0 $p<0.001$
Differences<between healthy<and<NOMGD	U=181.0 $p=0.04$	U=188.0 n.s.	U=273.0 n.s.	U=155.0 $p=0.007$	U=156.0 $p=0.01$	U=16 $p<0.001$	U=32.0 $p<0.001$
Differences<between MGD<and<NOMGD	U=0.0 $p<0.001$	U=10.0 $p<0.001$	U=26.0 $p<0.001$	U=56.0 $p<0.001$	U=110.0 $p=0.02$	U=30 $p<0.001$	U=192.0 n.s.
Differences<between ATD<and<MGD	U=7.5 $p<0.001$	U=135 n.s.	U=104.0 n.s.	U=21.0 $p<0.001$	U=0.0 $p<0.001$	U=120 n.s.	U=0.0 $p<0.001$
Differences<between ATD<and<NOMGD	U=0.0 $p<0.001$	U=76 $p<0.001$	U=78.0 $p<0.001$	U=0.0 $p<0.001$	U=0.0 $p<0.001$	U=84 $p<0.001$	U=0.0 $p<0.001$
Differences<between healthy<and<both†	U=181.0 $p<0.001$	U=225 $p<0.001$	U=357.0 $p<0.001$	U=171 $p<0.001$	U=216.0 $p<0.001$	U=16 $p<0.001$	U=364.5 $p=0.002$

* Average ± standard deviation.

†Median (mode) ± Average Absolute deviation. Mode was added if different from the median.

OSDI = Ocular Surface Disease ndex; FBUT = fluorescein break-up time; FSOS = fluorescein staining of the ocular surface; SVST = standardized visual scale test; CoL = clearance/turnover of lipids in human tears; TDI= tear dysfunction index; Obstructive MGD = (obvious) obstructive meibomian gland dysfunction; U = post-hoc Mann–Whitney U tests with Bonferroni correction; K= Kruskal–Wallis statistic; n.s. = not significant;

Table 2. Percentage Distributions of the lipid-based tracer at the 5th, 10th and 15th minute.

	Homogeneous type at the 5th minute*				*Vortex* type at the 5th minute*
	Excellent	Good	Fair	Poor	
Healthy	0%	9.5%	76.2%	0%	14.3%
ATD	0%	0%	0%	100%	0%
MGD	0%	0%	0%	100%	0%
NOMGD	0%	15.4%	46.1%	38.5%	0%
	Homogeneous type at the 10th minute				*Vortex* type at the 10th minute
	Excellent	Good	Fair	Poor	
Healthy	9.5%	28.6%	47.6%	0%	14.3%
ATD	0%	0%	10%	90%	0%
MGD	0%	0%	0%	100%	0%
NOMGD	0%	23.1%	61.5%	15.4%	0%
	Homogeneous type at the 15th minute				*Vortex* type at the 15th minute
	Excellent	Good	Fair	Poor	
Healthy	61.9%	38.1%	0%	0%	0%
ATD	0%	0%	20%	80%	0%
MGD	0%	0%	0%	100%	0%
NOMGD	0%	15.4%	69.2%	15.4%	0%

* Immediately after tracer instillation (within 30 seconds), the reflectivity of the lower tear meniscus was high/intense (grade 4 or poor, homogeneous pattern) in all cases (100%).
ATD = aqueous tear deficiency; MGD = obvious obstructive meibomian gland disease; NOMGD = non-obvious meibomian gland obstruction.

a non-polar phase, which retards water vapor transmission. Although considerable importance has been given to the study of lipid component of tears in the understanding of dry eye, the degree of washing out of the lipids in ATD, obstructive MGD, NOMGD patients, remains unknown.

In the present study, we have used an oil-in-water emulsion as an OCT tracer for analyzing the dynamic distribution of lipids in human tears. The degree of washing out of tracer, graded according to the OCT reflectivity, was considered an index of turnover of tear lipids. Since the lower tear meniscus shows a reflectivity absent (or nearly undetectable) at baseline, the signal intensity detected by OCT, after instillation of tracer, is directly dependent on its amount on the ocular surface. Thus, our method

Table 3. Correlation Coefficients and Statistical Significance (*p*) between Clearance of lipids in human tears, and Ocular Surface Disease Index, Fluorescein Break-up time, grade of Fluorescein Staining of the ocular surface, grade of Standardized Visual Scale Test, Schirmer I Test, and age.

All participants	Clearance of lipids (CoL) in human tears
OSDI	$r_s = 0.79$
	$p < 0.001$
FBUT	$r_s = -0.68$
	$p < 0.001$
Fluorescein Staining of the ocular surface (grade)	$r_s = 0.58$
	$p < 0.001$
Standardized Visual Scale test (grade)	$r_s = 0.68$
	$p < 0.001$
Schirmer I Test	$r_s = -0.5$
	$p < 0.001$
Age	$r_s = -0.43$
	n.s.

Correlation coefficients (r_s = Spearman correlation coefficient). OSDI = Ocular Surface Disease Index; FBUT = fluorescein break-up time; SVST = standardized visual scale test; *n.s.* = not significant.

Table 4. Statistical Differences for Clearance of lipids (CoL) in human tears and Standardized Visual Scale Test (SVST) within and between the four Groups: Healthy Persons, Aqueous Tear Deficiency (ATD), obvious obstructive Meibomian gland Dysfunction (MGD) and non-obvious obstructive Meibomian gland Dysfunction (NOMGD) Patients.

Intervals (minute)	Differences of CoL				Overall change (%)	Friedman test and Wilcoxon Signs Ranks test	Statistical Significance (p)
	Grade variations (percentage points)						
	Excellent*	Good	Fair	Poor			
ALL patients[†]							
t = 0 and the 5th	+3.7	+7.3	+34.1	−45.1	−14.9%	$\chi_F = 37.0$	<0.001
the 5th and the 10th	+2.4	+7.3	0	−9.8	−6.4%	$\chi_F = 16.0$	<0.001
the 10th and the 15th	+9.8	0	−7.3	−2.4	−6.8%	$\chi_F = 14.2$	<0.001
t = 0 and the 15th	+15.9	+14.6	+26.8	−57.3	−25.9%	$\chi_F = 47.0$	<0.001
HEALTHY subjects [†]							
t = 0 and the 5th	+14.3	+9.5	+76.2	−100	−34.5%	$Z = -4.2$	<0.001
the 5th and the 10th	+9.5	+19.1	−28.6	0	−14.5%	$Z = -2.2$	=0.02
the 10th and the 15th	+38.1	+9.5	−47.6	0	−38.2%	$Z = -3.8$	<0.001
t = 0 and the 15th	+61.9	+38.1	0	−100	−65.4%	$Z = -4.1$	<0.001
ATD patients[†]							
t = 0 and the 5th	-	-	-	0	0%	$Z = 0.0$	n.s.
the 5th and the 10th	-	-	+10	−10	−2.5%	$Z = -1.4$	n.s.
the 10th and the 15th	-	-	+10	−10	−2.5%	$Z = -1.4$	n.s.
t = 0 and the 15th	-	-	+20	−20	−2.5%	$Z = -2.0$	<0.04
MGD patients[†]							
t = 0 and the 5th	-	-	-	0	0%	$Z = 0.0$	n.s.
the 5th and the 10th	-	-	-	0	0%	$Z = 0.0$	n.s.
the 10th and the 15th	-	-	-	0	0%	$Z = 0.0$	n.s.
t = 0 and the 15th	-	-	-	0	0%	$Z = 0.0$	n.s.
NOMGD patients[†]							
t = 0 and the 5th	-	+16	+44	−60	−19%	$Z = -3.5$	<0.001
the 5th and the 10th	-	+16	+16	−44	−9.8%	$Z = -2.8$	=0.005
the 10th and the 15th	-	0	+8	0	−3.4%	$Z = -0.6$	n.s.
t = 0 and the 15th	-	+16	+68	−84	−25%	$Z = -4.2$	<0.001

Intervals (minute)	Differences of SVST			Differences between CoL-SVST
	Overall change (%)	Friedman test and Wilcoxon Signs Ranks test	Statistical Significance (p)	Cochran's test and McNemar's test
ALL patients[†]				
t = 0 and the 15th	−46.69%	$\chi_F = 76.0$	<0.001	$\chi_C = 7.6$ =0.006
HEALTHY subjects [†]				
t = 0 and the 15th	−72.1%	$Z = -4.1$	<0.00	χ_M[††] n.s.
ATD patients[†]				
t = 0 and the 15th	−14.2%	$Z = -3.3$	=0.001	χ_M[††] <0.001
MGD patients[†]				
t = 0 and the 15th	−36.1%	$Z = -3.5$	<0.001	χ_M[††] =0.002
NOMGD patients[†]				
t = 0 and the 15th	−57.7%	$Z = -4.4$	<0.001	χ_M[††] n.s.

* = Excellent or Vortex-pattern;
[†] = Immediately after tracer instillation (t = 0), the reflectivity of the lower tear meniscus was high/intense (grade 4 or poor, homogeneous pattern) in all cases (100%); - = Absent in the two scans performed at different times (subsequent serial scans or performed at t = 0 and the 15th).
[††] = Binomial distribution use; CoL = clearance of tear lipids; SVST = standardized visual scale test; *n.s.* = not significant; Z = Wilcoxon Signs Ranks test; χ_F = Friedman test; χ_C = Cochran's test; χ_M = McNemar's test.

has allowed us to study in vivo the behavior of lipids and their role in the complex dynamics of fluids of the lacrimal system.

Although lipids are distributed in the outer layer of the precorneal tear film, it has been possible to document their distribution in the tear meniscus, which appears as a vortex pattern. For its dynamic characteristics, the tear meniscus may function both as reserve and as scavenger for lipids. In fact, the vortex pattern has allowed highlighting the presence of centrifugal forces that push the tears outside, toward the lid skin. It is, therefore, possible to hypothesize that the mechanism of excretion of tear lipids toward the lid skin occurs following these centrifugal forces (and not only for an overflow due to a large tear volume). [1,12] This condition has been well evident in the case of high fluid dynamics, which has occurred only in healthy patients. Since the turnover of lipids in tears has been slower than the clearance of aqueous tear (SVST) in all groups, and because of water is non-reflective whereas lipids are hyper-reflective, the hypo-reflective substances at the center of the vortex, rinsed faster, are clearly those of the aqueous layer. In case of abnormality of the ocular surface, we observed a less dynamic distribution of lipids in the meniscus and a slower washout of lipids (CoL). For all these reasons, we believe that there are different routes of lipid excretion from tears. Probably, the biochemical interactions between lipids and proteins in the aqueous layer (e.g., lipocalin) may have a role in the mechanism of excretion, [13,14,32–34] and transfer some lipids in the aqueous flow, at the center of the vortex.

Although previous studies have documented the importance of tear lipids, our work revealed a prolonged retention time of tear lipids in abnormal eyes. Since tear lipids can easily coalesce to form droplets because of their thermodynamic instability, it follows that the slower the CoL, the greater the alteration of their stability and their functions.

Moreover, the results of our research indicate the existence of a correlation between the turnover of aqueous tear, as assessed by SVST, and the CoL. In fact, patients with high aqueous flow tend to have a faster washout of lipids and, conversely, patients with slow aqueous tear turnover (e.g., ATD) have more difficulty in excretion of lipids from tears. Again, a slower CoL has also been found in individuals with MGDs. Probably, alterations of lipids induce an increase of evaporation such as to reduce the dynamics of fluids of the ocular surface. In fact, several abnormalities of tear lipids in MGD patients have been found. For instance, variations in the conformation of lipids due to the changes of amount of lipid saturation governing lipid-lipid strength, or an increased viscosity due to an increase in protein and others compositional differences of *meibum* (also known as "meibomian gland secretions"). It is

interesting to note that patients with NOMGD, despite the minimal signs of their dysfunction, already show a slower CoL.

A significant correlation with others traditional tests and a promising diagnostic validity of turnover of tear lipids (CoL) has been revealed in our work. The CoL can be used in the differential diagnosis between healthy and ATD/MGDs individuals, and may be useful in providing a permanent record, which permits masking of scoring and therefore provides greater objectivity. Such records can be handled at a reading center, to provide improved standardization in clinical trials. By applying the TDI, it is also possible to clarify the impact of a lipids alteration or an aqueous deficiency, and even differentiate the two forms. Therefore, based on the clinical results and statistical significance of specificity, sensibility, PPV, NPV and accuracy, we believe that CoL can be considered a useful test for the diagnosis and follow-up of dry eye patients.

Although the fluorophotometric measurement using fluorescein sodium as a tracer has been the gold standard to quantify tear flow, [13,14,35] since the report of Mishima et al, [11] the analysis of lipids turnover by using OCT (compared to the fluorometer) has several advantages: it allows a morphological evaluation of the dynamic distribution of lipids; it does not require fluorescein sodium, which destabilizes the tear film, can penetrate through the cornea, and may create staining and pseudo-staining of the ocular surface; it provides final results that are not influenced by the autofluorescence of the cornea; lipid-enhanced OCT imaging is easier to perform because it is more practical to obtain a drop (~35 µl) of tracer that 5 µl of fluorescein sodium with a micropipette; it provides an objective and permanent record, important for the patient follow-up and the analysis among multiple examiners.

The current study shows that the lipids contribute largely to the increase of OCT reflectivity of the tear meniscus, which is otherwise non-reflective (or nearly undetectable). To the best of our knowledge, our study is the first that describes the use of a tracer to enhance the reflectivity of OCT images and to obtain an increase in the contrast and visibility of scanned structures. This finding could be of clinical relevance in the interpretation of OCT images and may be used for the construction of new contrast media for OCT technologies.

There are potential limitations when interpreting the results of the present study. The turnover of the tracer used in our work can be considered a surrogate measure of the tear lipids washout. In fact, in the future, when all the tear lipids will be known, a tracer most similar to the lipid layer (with all compounds, in physiological proportions) could be built and used to obtain a new *non-specific*

Table 5. The diagnostic validity of the clearance of lipids (CoL) in human tears, considering the values abnormal when fair or poor, and normal when excellent or good (for the homogeneous type) or in case of the vortex pattern.

	Sensitivity	Specificity	Accuracy	PPV	NPV
Healthy[†]	93.6%	100%	97.5%	100%	84%
ATD	48.7%	32.2%	50%	35%	100%
Obstructive MGD	100%	33.8%	43.9%	26.7%	100%
NOMGD	51.1%	84%	52.4%	84.6%	37.5%
Vortex pattern[†] (at the 5th and 10th minute)	14.2%	100%	96.3%	100%	77.2%

[†]In this case, no abnormalities of the ocular surface (ATD, MGD/NOMGD) = positive diagnosis.
PPV = positive predictive value; NPV = negative predictive value; ATD = aqueous tear deficiency; obstructive MGD = (obvious) obstructive meibomian gland dysfunction; NOMGD = non-obvious obstructive meibomian gland dysfunction.

Table 6. The AUCs (areas under the curves) analyzed by receiver operating characteristics (ROC) curves.

Diagnosis (or Differential Diagnosis)	Area under the ROC curve (AUC)	Statistical Significance (p)	Asymptotic 95% Confidence Interval	
			Lower Bound	Upper Bound
DD:. Healthy or abnormalities of the ocular surface†	0.98	$P<0.001$	0.00	1.00
ATD	0.78	$p<0.001$	0.68	0.88
MGDs	0.66	$p=0.013$	0.53	0.78
DD:. ATD or MGDs	0.67	$p=0.025$	0.54	0.81
By applying the TDI (cutoff = 1.35) in the *DD* between ATD from MGDs	1.00	$p<0.001$	1.00	1.00

†In this case, no abnormalities of the ocular surface (ATD + MGDs) = positive diagnosis.
DD = differential diagnosis. ATD = aqueous tear deficiency; obstructive MGD = (obvious) obstructive meibomian gland dysfunction; NOMGD = non-obvious obstructive meibomian gland dysfunction; MGDs = obstructive MGD or NOMGD; ROC curves = (receiver operating characteristics) curves.

index of CoL. On the other hand, further studies could evaluate the different routes of excretion using different *specific* tracers for *each lipid*. Moreover, a more comprehensive database of normal individuals must be created to analyze possible age- and sex-dependent variations.

Conclusion

In conclusion, lipid-enhanced OCT imaging is a promising method to detect changes of the tear film and of the ocular surface. Assessment of the dynamic distribution of the tear lipids may improve the clinician's ability in achieving significant information regarding the complex fluid dynamics of human tears and in correctly classifying the dry eye syndrome. Moreover, this technique should facilitate the widespread use of the clearance of tear lipids for diagnosis and could be useful for the identification and follow-up of patients with specific abnormalities of the ocular surface, in particular with NOMGD.

Author Contributions

Conceived and designed the experiments: PEN. Performed the experiments: PEN GMS FC. Analyzed the data: PEN. Contributed reagents/materials/analysis tools: PEN MF. Wrote the paper: PEN MF.

References

1. Bron AJ, Tiffany JM, Gouveia SM, Yokoi N, Voon LW (2004) Functional aspects of the tear film lipid layer. Exp Eye Res 78: 347–360.
2. Foulks GN (2007) The correlation between the tear film lipid layer and dry eye disease. Surv Ophthalmol 52: 369–74.
3. Breustedt DA, Schonfeld DL, Skerra A (2006) Comparative ligand binding analysis of ten human lipocalins. Biochim Biophys Acta 1764: 161–73.
4. Craig JP, Tomlinson A (1997) Importance of the lipid layer in human tear film stability and evaporation. Optom Vis Sci 74: 8–13.
5. Nichols JJ, Nichols KK, Puent B, Saracino M, Mitchell GL (2002) Evaluation for tear film interference patterns and measures of tear break-up time. Optom Vis Sci 79: 363–399.
6. (2007) Methodologies to diagnose and monitor dry eye disease: Report of the Diagnostic Methodology Subcommittee of the International Dry Eye Workshop. Ocul Surf 5(2): 108–152.
7. Tomlinson A, Bron AJ, Korb DR, Amano S, Paugh JR, et al. (2011) The International Workshop on Meibomian Gland Dysfunction: Report of the Diagnosis Subcommittee. Invest Ophthalmol Vis Sci 52(4): 2006–2049.
8. Blackie CA, Korb DR, Knop E, Bedi R, Knop N, et al. (2010) Nonobvious obstructive meibomian gland dysfunction. Cornea 29(12): 1333–1345.
9. Gobbels M, Goebels G, Breitbach R, Spitznas M (1992). Tear secretion in dry eyes as assessed by objective fluorophotometry. Ger J Ophthalmol 1: 350–353.
10. Kuppens EV, Stolwijk TR, de Keizer RJ, Van Best JA (1992) Basal tear turnover and topical timolol in glaucoma patients and healthy controls by Fluorophotometry. Invest Ophthalmol Vis Sci 33: 3442–3448.
11. Mishima S (1965) Some physiological aspects of the precorneal tear film. Arch Ophthalmol: 73, 233–241.
12. Mishima S, Gasset A, Klyce SD, Baum JL (1966) Determination of tear volume and tear flow. Invest Ophthalmol Vis Sci 5: 264–275.
13. Mathers WD, Thomas ED (1996) Tear flow and evaporation in patients with and without dry eye. Ophthalmology 103: 664–9.
14. Mathers WD, Lane J, Zimmerman M (1996) Tear film changes associated with normal aging. Cornea 15: 229–334.
15. Mathers WD (2004) Evaporation from the ocular surface. Exp Eye Res 78: 389–394.
16. Van Best JA, del Castillo Benitez JM, Coulangeon LM (1995) Measurement of basal tear turnover using a standardized protocol. Graefes Arch Clin Exp Ophthalmol 233: 1–7.
17. McNamara NA, Polse KA, Bonanno JA (1998) Fluorometry in contact lens research: The next step. Optom. Vis Sci 75: 316–322.
18. Pearce EI, Keenan BP, McRory C (2001) An improved fluorophotometric method for tear turnover assessment. Optom Vis Sci 78: 30–36.
19. Mochizuki H, Yamada M, Hato S, Nishida T (2008) Fluorophotometric measurement of the precorneal residence time of topically applied hyaluronic acid. Br J Ophthalmol 92(1): 108–111.
20. Napoli PE, Zucca I, Fossarello M (2014) A qualitative and quantitative analysis of filtering blebs with optical coherence tomography in patients after primary trabeculectomy. Can J Ophthalmology 49: 210–216.
21. Napoli PE, Coronella F, Satta GM, Zucca IA, Fossarello M (2014) A novel OCT technique to measure in vivo the corneal adhesiveness for sodium carboxymethylcellulose in humans and its validity in the diagnosis of dry eye. Invest Ophthalmol Vis Sci 55(5): 3179–3185.
22. Napoli PE, Satta GM, Coronella F, Fossarello M (2014) Spectral-domain optical coherence tomography study on dynamic changes of human tears after instillation of artificial tears. Invest Ophthalmol Vis Sci 55(7): 4533–4540.
23. Wang J, Aquavella J, Palakuru J, Chung S, Feng C (2006). Relationships between Central Tear Film Thickness and Tear Menisci of the Upper and Lower Eyelids. Invest Ophthalmol Vis Sci 47: 4349–4355.
24. Wang J, Aquavella J, Palakuru J, Chung S (2006) Repeated Measurements of Dynamic Tear Distribution on the Ocular Surface after Instillation of Artificial Tears. Invest Ophthalmol Vis Sci 47: 3325–3329.
25. Walt JG, Rowe MM, Stern KL (1997) Evaluating the functional impact of dry eye: the Ocular Surface Disease Index. Drug Inf J 31: 1436.
26. Bron AJ, Evans VE, Smith JA (2003) Grading of corneal and conjunctival staining in the context of other dry eye tests. Cornea 22: 640–50.
27. Amano S (2010) MGD Working Group: Definition and diagnostic criteria for meibomian gland dysfunction. J Eye (Atarashii Ganka) 27: 627–631.
28. Macri A, Rolando M, Pflugfelder S (2000) A standardized visual scale for evaluation of tear fluorescein clearance. Ophthalmology 107(7): 1338–1343.
29. Butovich IA (2008) Understanding and analyzing meibomian lipid-a review. Curr Eye Res 33: 405–420.
30. Tiffany JM (1987) The lipid secretion of the meibomian glands. Adv Lipid Res 22: 1–62.
31. De La Lágrima TS (2006) Surface tension in tears. Arch Soc Esp Oftalmol 81: 365–366.

32. Gasymov OK, Abduragimov AR, Prasher P, Yusifov TN, Glasgow BJ (2005) Tear lipocalin: evidence for a scavenging function to remove lipids from the human corneal surface. Invest Ophthalmol Vis Sci 46: 3589–3596.

33. Glasgow BJ, Marshall G, Gasymov OK, Abduragimov AR, Yusifov TN, et al. (1999) Tear Lipocalins Potential Lipid Scavengers for the Corneal Surface. Invest Ophthalmol Vis Sci 40: 3100–3107.

34. Redl B (2000) Human tear lipocalin. Biochim Biophys Acta 1482: 241–248.

35. Lemp MA (1992) Basic principles and classification of dry eye disorders. In:The Dry EyeSpringer Berlin Heildelbergpp101–131.

2

Retinal Thickness Measurement Obtained with Spectral Domain Optical Coherence Tomography Assisted Optical Biopsy Accurately Correlates with *Ex Vivo* Histology

Lee R. Ferguson[1], Sandeep Grover[1], James M. Dominguez II[2], Sankarathi Balaiya[1], Kakarla V. Chalam[1]*

1 Department of Ophthalmology, University of Florida College of Medicine, Jacksonville, Florida, United States of America, 2 Department of Pharmacology and Therapeutics, University of Florida College of Medicine, Gainesville, Florida, United States of America

Abstract

Background: This study determines 'correlation constants' between the gold standard histological measurement of retinal thickness and the newer spectral-domain optical coherence tomography (SD-OCT) technology in adult C57BL/6 mice.

Methods: Forty-eight eyes from adult mice underwent SD-OCT imaging and then were histologically prepared for frozen sectioning with H&E staining. Retinal thickness was measured via 10x light microscopy. SD-OCT images and histological sections were standardized to three anatomical sites relative to the optic nerve head (ONH) location. The ratios between SD-OCT to histological thickness for total retinal thickness (TRT) and six sublayers were defined as 'correlation constants'.

Results: Mean ($\pm$ SE) TRT for SD-OCT and histological sections was 210.95 µm (± 1.09) and 219.58 µm (± 2.67), respectively. The mean 'correlation constant' for TRT between the SD-OCT and histological sections was 0.96. The retinal thickness for all sublayers measured by SD-OCT vs. histology were also similar, the 'correlation constant' values ranged from 0.70 to 1.17. All SD-OCT and histological measurements demonstrated highly significant ($p < 0.01$) strong positive correlations.

Conclusion: This study establishes conversion factors for the translation of *ex vivo* data into *in vivo* information; thus enhancing the applicability of SD-OCT in translational research.

Editor: Knut Stieger, Justus-Liebig-University Giessen, Germany

Funding: The Department of Ophthalmology Jacksonville, Jacksonville, Florida provided all financial support for this study. The funders had no role in study design, data collection and analysis, decision to publish, or preparation of the manuscript.

Competing Interests: The authors have declared that no competing interests exist.

* Email: Kakarla.Chalam@jax.ufl.edu

Introduction

Spectral-domain optical coherence tomography (SD-OCT) is an important imaging modality, in clinical ophthalmology and animal research, for characterizing morphology and understanding pathophysiological changes in the retina. The rapid, high resolution, non-invasive cross sectional images produced by SD-OCT is an important tool in diagnosing posterior segment pathology and monitoring it longitudinally [1,2]. Although SD-OCT provides non-invasive histological–grade sections of the rodent posterior segment, image acquisition is technologically cumbersome as human devices are retrofitted for animal use.

Histological evaluation of retinal tissue in animal models has traditionally been the primary method for investigating the microstructure of the retina. Retinal tissue histology has contributed to our understanding of retinal cellular mechanisms and disease pathophysiology. With advancements in OCT technology, the *ex vivo* histological methodology is being replaced with the more innovative SD-OCT *in vivo* 'optical biopsy' [3]. SD-OCT avoids the inherent limitations of the time-consuming, destructive, and cumbersome histological procedures. Moreover, high resolu-

tion detailed images comparable to mid- to high-range microscope objective lens is attained with newer generation OCT technology [4]. Additionally, volumetric data can be generated which would provide more insight into structural changes at the microscopic level than visualizing two-dimensional anatomical sections [5].

In this study, we measured retinal thickness non-invasively with SD-OCT optical biopsy and compared it to measurements obtained with histological sections from the same eye and similar anatomical location after sacrificing the animals. We established a correlation constant between SD-OCT retinal thickness and histological retinal thickness. Such a constant can then be applied to estimate the retinal thickness as well as volume in a variety of diseases longitudinally.

Methods

Animals

Healthy adult C57BL/6 mice (Jackson Laboratory, Bar Harbor, ME), between the ages of 3 to 5 months, were used for the study. All mice were maintained under a 12-hour light/dark schedule with unrestricted access to food and water at the University of

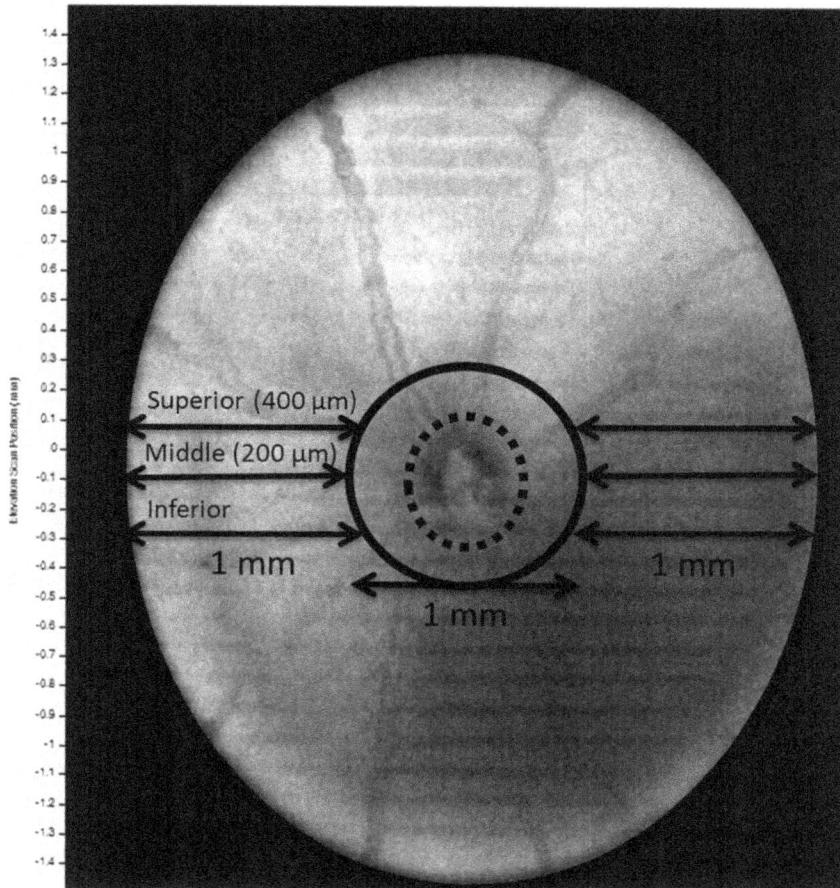

Figure 1. C57BL/6 mouse retina showing the reference points for SD-OCT and histological measurements. Dotted circle – optic nerve head (ONH); black solid circle – 1 mm diameter central area surrounding the ONH; inferior, middle and superior reference points, each 200 μm apart, both to the left and the right of the ONH.

Florida animal care services (ACS) facility. All procedures performed on the mice were implemented in an ACS-authorized location with study approval acquired from the University of Florida institutional animal care and use committee. In addition, the guidelines set by the Association for Research in Vision and Ophthalmology Statement for the Use of Animals in Ophthalmic and Vision Research were followed during experimentation on animal subjects.

SD-OCT Imaging and Analysis

SD-OCT imaging was performed on the right eye of all animals. The Bioptigen spectral-domain ophthalmic imaging system (Bioptigen, Inc., Durham, NC) was used to capture SD-OCT images. The mice were secured and scanned with the use of the animal imaging mount and rodent alignment stage apparatus [6]. This device allowed for multi-axial manipulation of the animal in order to properly align the mouse eye with the SD-OCT probe. As a result, rapid and reproducible acquisition of the retinal scans, centered at the optic nerve head (ONH), was possible. Mice were anesthetized with an intraperitoneal mixture of ketamine (Keta-ject; 80 mg/kg; Webster Veterinary, Devens, MA) and xylazine (Ana Sed; 10 mg/kg; Webster Veterinary; Devens, MA). Topical tropicamide (1%; Akorn Inc.; Lake Forest, IL) was used to dilate the pupils. Corneal desiccation was prevented by applying topical

Systane Ultra lubricant eye drop (Alcon, Fort Worth, TX) every minute during the procedure.

SD-OCT images were obtained with the InVivoVue Clinic software (Bioptigen, Inc., Durham, NC). Briefly, a 3×3 mm perimeter scanning protocol was used to obtain an imaging sequence comprising of 100 B-scans, with each B-scan consisting of 1000 A-scans, through a 50-degree field of view from the mouse lens. Once the ONH was centered within the InVivoVue Clinic imaging application, three scanning sequences were acquired. Measurements were restricted to retinal regions outside a radius of 500 μm from the center of the ONH. Retinal layer measurements were performed via the automated segmentation software provided by the instrument manufacturer (Bioptigen, Inc., Durham, NC). All layers were measured except for the retinal pigment epithelial layer because of the extensive artifactual changes associated with histological preparation and the limited depth penetrance associated with the SD-OCT 4.5 μm axial resolution. Total retinal thickness (TRT) represented the summation of all retinal layers spanning from the retinal nerve fiber layer (RNFL) to the outer segment of photoreceptors/inner segment of photoreceptors/external limiting membrane (OS/IS/ELM) region. Retinal sublayer measurements consisted of the OS/IS/ELM, outer nuclear layer (ONL), outer plexiform layer (OPL), inner nuclear layer (INL), inner plexiform layer/ganglion cell

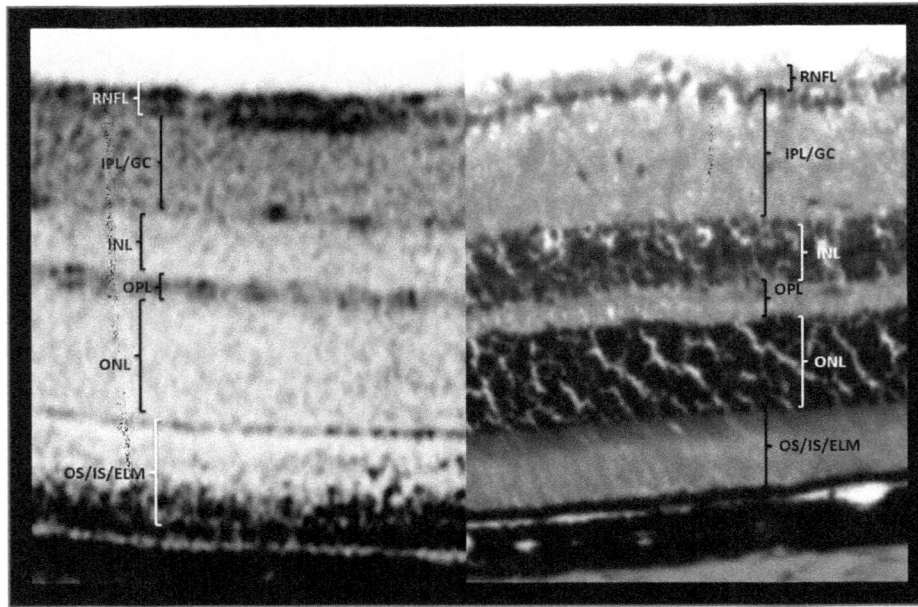

Figure 2. Cross-sectional views of the C57BL/6 mouse retina by SD-OCT (left) and histology (right). OS/IS/ELM, outer segment/inner segment/external limiting membrane; ONL, outer nuclear layer; OPL, outer plexiform layer; INL, inner nuclear layer; IPL/GC, inner plexiform layer/ganglion cell; RNFL, retinal nerve fiber layer.

(IPL/GC), and the RNFL. In order to standardize retinal thickness measurements from SD-OCT scans and histology sections, three arbitrary points were selected. The "inferior point" was the reference point that passed through the inferior margin of the ONH. The "middle point" was designated as the B-scan 200 μm above the "inferior point". Lastly, the "superior point" was comprised of the B-scan that measured 400 μm above the "inferior point". To determine the overall total retinal and sublayer thickness for each study eye, measurements were made at each of these reference points to both the left and right of the ONH (Fig 1). These six measurements were then averaged together to acquire final retinal thickness values.

Histological Evaluation

Animals were euthanized with CO_2 inhalation followed by cervical dislocation. The same eyes that had SD-OCT scans were enucleated and then punctured with a 30-gauge needle and submerged into 4% paraformaldehyde (PFA) for 2–4 hours. This was followed by a series of submersions into phosphate buffered saline (PBS) with increasing concentrations of sucrose in the following manner: PBS with 5% sucrose (6 hrs), PBS with 10% sucrose (10 hrs), and PBS with 20% sucrose (10 hrs). Samples were then removed from the PBS with sucrose solution and solidified into optimal cutting temperature compound in a container with dry ice and 2-methylbutane. A cryostat microtome was used to produce sample slices of 10 μm per section. Every twentieth section was selected for tissue staining. The samples were then stained with H&E using standard laboratory protocols. The Zeiss Axioskop 2 Mot Plus (Carl Zeiss MicroImaging, Inc., Thornwood, NY) microscope, with 10x objective lens, was used to evaluate histological sections. All sections selected for light microscopy evaluation contained optic nerve tissue landmarks. The histological section that first demonstrated the appearance of the ONH was considered the histological 'inferior point'. As illustrated in Figures 1 and 2, histological measurements of retinal sublayers were similarly performed as mentioned for SD-OCT scan

thickness measurements. The manual caliper instrument, from the Axiovision 4.8 (Carl Zeiss MicroImaging, Inc., Thornwood, NY) imaging software, was used to measure histological sublayer retinal thickness. TRT was derived from the sum of all measured histological layers up to but not including the retinal pigment epithelium.

Statistical Analysis

Mean retinal thickness values, for each study eye, were acquired by averaging the thickness values obtained from the retinal layers left and right of the ONH corresponding to the zero point, 200 μm, and 400 μm locations. Overall mean and standard error of the mean ($\pm$ SE) for the retinal layers were calculated from the sample observations for thickness values for each retinal layer obtained from the eight animals evaluated (n = 48). Correlation analysis (GraphPad Software Inc., La Jolla, CA) was used to assess the association between thickness measurements from histology and SD-OCT images. The statistical significance of correlations for the TRT and retinal sublayers was achieved if the p-values were less than 0.05.

Results

The mean thickness of each retinal sublayer and TRT in each animal measured by SD-OCT and histology is depicted in Table 1. The overall mean retinal thickness of individual sublayers and TRT when measured by the two methods is displayed in Table 2. The overall TRT by SD-OCT evaluation was 210.95 ± 1.09 μm while TRT measurement from histology was 219.58 ± 2.67 μm.

Table 2 also exhibits the correlation constants for retinal thickness (TRT and individual sublayers) as the ratio of measurements from SD-OCT scan sections to histological sections. The mean 'correlation constant' for TRT, when comparing mean SD-OCT TRT to mean histology is 0.96. The

Table 1. Mean SD-OCT and histology retinal thickness (in μm) for each study animal.

Animals	OS/IS/ELM	ONL	OPL	INL	IPL/GC	RNFL	TRT
SD-OCT							
Animal 1	42.33	59.08	15.92	26.83	51.28	15.20	210.65
Animal 2	41.38	60.05	13.95	25.48	52.58	13.17	206.62
Animal 3	43.72	57.80	14.87	24.23	53.60	15.82	210.03
Animal 4	41.77	64.50	15.88	23.62	55.28	15.52	216.57
Animal 5	38.55	63.78	16.63	23.47	51.70	16.65	210.78
Animal 6	39.87	58.05	16.87	25.13	52.27	16.17	208.35
Animal 7	40.23	61.65	16.82	23.95	52.43	15.77	210.85
Animal 8	44.55	61.10	15.45	25.52	51.40	15.78	213.80
Histology							
Animal 1	48.33	53.33	20.00	31.67	66.67	15.00	225.00
Animal 2	41.67	53.33	18.33	35.00	63.33	13.33	210.00
Animal 3	48.33	55.00	20.00	36.67	71.67	16.67	216.67
Animal 4	38.33	51.67	15.00	33.33	65.00	11.67	211.67
Animal 5	45.00	58.33	16.67	38.33	68.33	11.67	223.33
Animal 6	60.00	51.67	18.33	35.00	58.33	11.67	228.33
Animal 7	38.33	51.67	18.33	36.67	70.00	16.67	213.33
Animal 8	55.00	51.67	20.00	38.33	61.67	11.67	228.33

(n = 48).
SD-OCT, spectral domain optical coherence tomography; OS/IS/ELM, outer segment/inner segment/external limiting membrane; ONL, outer nuclear layer; OPL, outer plexiform layer; INL, inner nuclear layer; IPL/GC, inner plexiform layer/ganglion cell; RNFL, retinal nerve fiber layer; TRT, total retinal thickness.

Table 2. Mean (± SE) SD-OCT/histology retinal thickness and calculated 'correlation constant' for each retinal sublayer.

Layer	SD-OCT (μm)	Histology (μm)	SD-OCT/Histology
Outer Segment/Inner Segment/External Limiting Membrane/	41.55 (±0.60)	46.88 (±1.43)	0.91
Outer Nuclear Layer	60.75 (±0.70)	53.33 (±0.75)	1.14
Outer Plexiform Layer	15.80 (±0.36)	18.33 (±0.54)	0.87
Inner Nuclear Layer	24.78 (±0.60)	35.63 (±0.72)	0.70
Inner Plexiform Layer/Ganglion Cell	52.57 (±0.67)	65.63 (±1.26)	0.80
Retinal Nerve Fiber Layer	15.51 (±0.43)	13.54 (±.70)	1.17
Total Retinal Thickness	210.95 (±1.09)	219.58 (±2.67)	0.96

SD-OCT, spectral domain optical coherence tomography.

variance (± SD = 0.04) in the mean TRT measurement ratio was small (Table 3).

Sublayer analyses showed that the 'correlation constant' of SD-OCT to histology thickness was greater than one for the ONL (1.14) and RNFL (1.17) and was less than one for the OS/IS/ELM (0.91), OPL (0.87), INL (0.7), and IPL/GC (0.8) layers (Tables 2&3). In general, thickness measurement comparisons between SD-OCT and histology demonstrated significant correlations. The ONL and RNFL, with 'correlation constants' greater than one, showed a highly significant strong correlation ($r^2 = 0.98$, $p<0.01$) [Figure 3]. Similarly, for the layers with 'correlation constants' less than one, the relationship exhibited between SD-OCT and histological measurements was also significantly correlated ($r^2 = 0.99$, $p<0.01$) [Figure 4].

Discussion

In retinal diseases, ocular histology is still considered to be the gold standard for assessing structural morphology. Histology provides a snapshot view of the microstructural environment of the retina by staining and tissue preservation techniques. The drawback of histology in humans is that it is difficult to conduct longitudinal studies to describe the course of a disease process. However, in animal studies, the animals can be sacrificed sequentially to get longitudinal data to improve our understanding of many retinal disorders.

Technological innovation in ophthalmic imaging has led to *in vivo* OCT, possibly replacing histology for assessing retinal morphology. Over time, OCT technology has advanced from the time-domain (TD-OCT) capability of the Stratus (Carl Zeiss Meditec) to the SD-OCT features of the Cirrus (Carl Zeiss Meditec) and Spectralis (Heidelberg Engineering, Inc.), with better speed and resolution. The advent of higher bandwidth SD-OCT imaging devices has allowed for single digit micrometer resolution potentials, which show comparable anatomical delineation as histology [7].

With the possible shift from histological biopsies to optical biopsies with OCT, several studies have reported normative data for macular retinal thickness using TD-OCT [8] and the SD-OCT [9] devices. Furthermore, there have been some reports comparing OCT retinal thickness measurements to histological measurements. In one study the authors used TD-OCT to 'qualitatively' correlate macular retinal thickness scans to histology in three patients with exenterated cancerous orbits [10]. They reported some level of association between high magnification light microscopic histologic images to lower resolution TD-OCT scans, but no 'quantitative' measurements were made [10]. Similarly, another study utilized *ex vivo* SD-OCT macular scans of donor

eyes, prior to histological processing, to determine the extent of volumetric changes associated with histology [11]. They reported a median tissue shrinkage of 14.5% overall with 29% in the foveal area. In yet another maturation study of the human retina, SD-OCT morphology and retinal layer thickness measurements from 22 premature infants, 30 term infants, 16 children and one adult were qualitatively contrasted with light microscopy histologic images from age-matched donors [12]. Their findings suggested that at all ages, SD-OCT images demonstrated high agreement with histology.

In animal studies too, although histological measurements are still the gold standard for retinal morphological evaluation, there has been a transition of retinal disease animal model research towards *in vivo* imaging [13–15]. Moreover, studies utilizing SD-OCT have provided useful information on longitudinal changes resulting from retinal disease pathophysiology [14,16]. The reproducibility, reliability, and non-invasive qualities of this technology make it ideal for use in clinical as well as research applications [17–19]. Since different histological fixation techniques can be used and also since different OCT instruments can be utilized in different studies, it is not advisable to compare absolute values of TRT or its sublayers. Instead, a ratio in the form of a 'conversion constant' would be more useful and accurate. There are no studies that establish a 'conversion constant' to show the relationship between OCT and histological retinal thickness measurements.

The present study demonstrated retinal thickness measurement correlations between SD-OCT assisted optical biopsy to histological methods in a C57BL/6 mouse model. Histological measurements for the total retinal thickness and its sublayers were compared to the SD-OCT measurements in the same eyes at similar locations to generate a 'conversion constant'. We determined that the mean and standard deviation conversion constant was approximately 0.96±0.04 for the TRT. We also determined the different retinal sub-layer 'conversion constants', where the ratio of retinal thickness by SD-OCT to histology ranged from 0.70 to 1.17 (Table 2). It seemed that the variation in this constant was less in outer retinal layers (0.87–1.14) as compared to inner retinal layers (0.70–1.17).

There are very few studies [14,15,20] that have compared the retinal thickness, as measured by histology vs. OCT, in C57BL/6 mice models (Table 4). Even those studies did not use an elaborate point-to-point methodology as the present study. Two of the three studies [14,20] were from the same lab. The third study [15], although performed on C57BL/6 mice, compared the retinal thickness by OCT and histology after artificially creating a retinal detachment.

Table 3. Correlation constant (SD-OCT/histology) for total and retinal sublayer thickness measurements in each animal.

Animals	OS/IS/ELM	ONL	OPL	INL	IPL/GC	RNFL	TRT
Animal 1	0.88	1.11	0.80	0.85	0.77	1.01	0.90
Animal 2	0.99	1.13	0.76	0.73	0.83	0.99	0.92
Animal 3	0.90	1.05	0.74	0.66	0.75	0.95	0.85
Animal 4	1.09	1.25	1.06	0.71	0.85	1.33	1.01
Animal 5	0.86	1.09	1.00	0.61	0.76	1.43	0.88
Animal 6	0.66	1.12	0.92	0.72	0.90	1.39	0.89
Animal 7	1.05	1.19	0.92	0.65	0.75	0.95	0.91
Animal 8	0.81	1.18	0.77	0.67	0.83	1.35	0.90
Average	0.91	1.14	0.87	0.70	0.80	1.17	0.96
Standard Dev.	0.14	0.06	0.12	0.07	0.06	0.22	0.04

SD-OCT, spectral domain optical coherence tomography; OS/IS/ELM, outer segment/inner segment/external limiting membrane; ONL, outer nuclear layer; OPL, outer plexiform layer; INL, inner nuclear layer; IPL/GC, inner plexiform layer/ganglion cell; RNFL, retinal nerve fiber layer; TRT, total retinal thickness.

The study by Fischer et al. [20] compared retinal thickness measurements by OCT and histology in the similar mice model as well as other retinal degeneration models. They utilized a third generation SD-OCT instrument (Heidelberg Engineering, Germany) for the measurements. It seems that nine data points were used (extrapolating from their Figure Two A [20]) but it is not clear whether these were nine points from different sites of the same animal or 9 different animals were used. They also do not mention whether they averaged measurements at each point or only one measurement was performed. Unlike the present study, the comparison of histology and OCT were not performed at similar sites. Nevertheless, they found a significant correlation coefficient of 0.89 for the total retinal thickness between the two methodologies. They also reported a close agreement between histology and OCT for the retinal sub-layers they measured (ILM-IPL, INL, OPL, ONL and IS/OS layers). Although quantitative measurements are not reported, extrapolating from their figure (Figure Two B [20]), it seems that the TRT was in the range of $\approx$245 µm by histology and $\approx$230 µm by SD-OCT, leading to a 'conversion constant' of $\approx$0.94. This is similar to the 'conversion constant' of 0.96 in the present study. The sub-layer analyses in the study were performed on five sublayers and were very similar to that in our study (Table 4). The tissue fixative used in this histological study was 2.5% gluteraldehyde as compared to PFA in our study.

The study by Huber et al. [14] utilized the HRA + SD-OCT (Heidelberg, Germany) device and investigated its efficacy to study mouse models of retinal degeneration as compared to the C57BL/6 mice (n = 37). Although the SD-OCT was done on 37 mice, only three of these animals were sacrificed to study their histological structure. The measurement of TRT was based on similar points of the retina. They reported a TRT of 237$\pm$2 µm by SD-OCT whereas they do not report the TRT by histology. However, extrapolating from their figure (Figure Six C [14]), it seems that the TRT was in the range of 225 µm by histology. That would calculate the approximate 'conversion constant' to be 1.05 (Table 4). They do report that they obtained a high correlation of TRT between SD-OCT and histology measurements ($R^2 = 0.897$). It is interesting to note that whereas the TRT in the present study was in the range of 210.95 µm by SD-OCT, it was reported to be 237 µm by Huber et al. This difference could possibly be due to the instrumentation – the Heidelberg SD-OCT measures the TRT, inclusive of the retinal pigment epithelium layer (RPE) whereas the Bioptigen SD-OCT (used in the present study) does not include the RPE sub-layer. In the sub-layer analyses, they also reported that the correlation coefficient was even higher for the outer retinal thickness ($R^2 = 0.978$). This was similar to what was observed in the present study. The fixative used in this study was also 2.5% gluteraldehyde as compared to PFA in our study.

The study by Cebulla et al. [15] reported longitudinal data on the SD-OCT measurements of the retinal thickness in a C57BL/6 model where retinal detachment was artificially created. In the same model, they also compared the TRT by SD-OCT and histology. They utilized a custom-made ultra high resolution imaging system and created retinal detachment in 17 mice. Although they do not report the TRT by SD-OCT or histology, extrapolation from their figures (Figures Five A and Five B [15]) show that the TRT by SD-OCT and histology were approximately 210 µm and 320 µm, respectively. This would calculate the conversion constant as approximately 0.66, much lower than found in the present study or the other studies [14,20]. However, they stated that the imaging system used measured the retinal thickness from nerve fiber layer to the base of the photoreceptor

Measurement Relationship Between Sub-Layers with Correlation Constants > 1

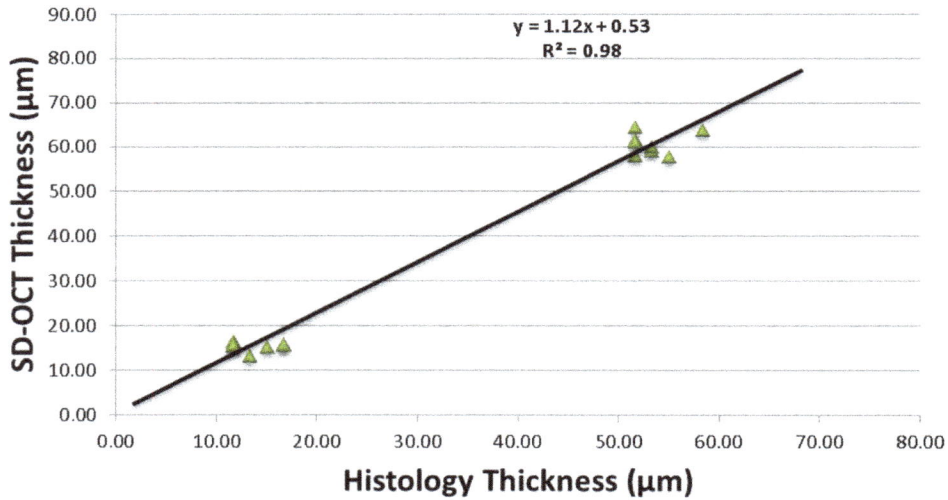

Figure 3. Association between mean SD-OCT and histological thickness with correlation constants >1. Scatter plot points refer to all observations for outer nuclear layer and retinal nerve fiber layer.

outer segment. Moreover, they used a retinal detachment model despite calculating the TRT in the attached part of the retina. They used the same fixative as our study (PFA).

The present study and some of the other studies in the past have shown a good correlation between the measurements obtained by optical section (SD-OCT) and histological sections. The observed small differences in values between the *ex vivo* and *in vivo* measurements could be due to multiple reasons. Histological

artifacts such as shrinkage, dehydration, and swelling can contribute to changes in the retinal structure as histological sections are prepared. This can be due to the choice of fixative which can also lead to artifacts. Also, when measuring retinal thickness by SD-OCT or histology with algorithms dependent on demarcating retinal layers, the precision of the measurement tool affects the reliability of the measurement [21]. In the present study, the caliper used for light microscopic measurement was

Measurement Relationship Between Sub-Layers with Correlation Constants < 1

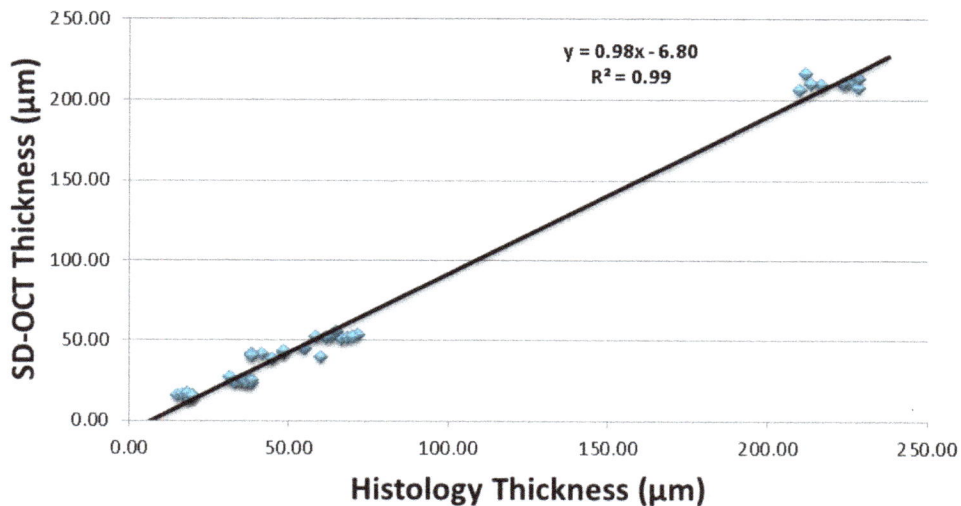

Figure 4. Association between mean SD-OCT and histological thickness with correlation constants <1. Scatter plot points refer to all observations for outer segment/inner segment/external limiting membrane, outer plexiform layer, inner nuclear layer, inner plexiform/ganglion cell layers, and total retinal thickness.

Table 4. Comparison of SD-OCT/histology 'correlation constant' between present and prior studies.

Layer	Ferguson et al.	Fischer et al.	Huber et al.	Cebulla et al.
Outer Segment/Inner Segment/External Limiting Membrane/	0.91	0.94	...	0.50
Outer Nuclear Layer	1.14	1.10	...	0.58
Outer Plexiform Layer	0.87	...	...	...
Inner Nuclear Layer	0.70	0.77	...	...
Inner Plexiform Layer/Ganglion Cell	0.80	0.88	...	...
Retinal Nerve Fiber Layer	1.17	...	...	...
Total Retinal Thickness	0.96	0.93*	1.05*	0.66*

*The correlation constants in all prior studies were not reported but calculated by 'extrapolating' from the data presented in those studies.

calibrated to a resolution limit of 10 μm. This could have hampered our ability to accurately measure thinner layers such as the RNFL. The resolution capability of the SD-OCT unit also plays a role when defining and measuring retinal thickness. The Bioptigen Envisu R 2200 SDOIS commercial unit used for this study has a tissue axial resolution of approximately 1.7 mm. This resolution power was not enough to accurately define deeper layers such as the RPE. Although RPE measurements were available in histological sections, corresponding measurements were not available for SD-OCT images. For this reason, as this was a comparative study, we did not include RPE measurements in our study, both in the histology as well as the SD-OCT measurements.

The present study has established a 'conversion constant' of 0.96 for the measurement of retinal layer thickness between high-resolution SD-OCT optical biopsies to that of light microscopy histology. This study suggests that for all practical purposes, the retinal thickness, as measured by SD-OCT is equivalent to gold standard histological biopsy measurements. SD-OCT is more convenient, inexpensive, and requires no animals to be sacrificed, as for histology. In the era of growing utilization of SD-OCT technology and continued improvement of its resolution, this study can influence the design of future vision science research with animal models when analyzing longitudinal disease pathology as well as in monitoring the effects of pharmacological interventions on retinal disease processes.

Author Contributions

Conceived and designed the experiments: LRF KVC SG. Performed the experiments: LRF SB JMD. Analyzed the data: LRF KVC SG. Contributed reagents/materials/analysis tools: LRF KVC JMD. Wrote the paper: LRF KVC SG.

References

1. Strouthidis NG, Fortune B, Yang H, Sigal IA, Burgoyne CF (2011) Longitudinal change detected by spectral domain optical coherence tomography in the optic nerve head and peripapillary retina in experimental glaucoma. Invest Ophthalmol Vis Sci. 52(3): 1206–1219.
2. Yehoshua Z, Rosenfeld PJ (2012) Strategies for following dry age-related macular degeneration. Ophthalmic Res. 48 Suppl 1: 6–10.
3. Brown NH, Koreishi AF, McCall M, Izatt JA, Rickman CB, et al. (2009) Developing SDOCT to assess donor human eyes prior to tissue sectioning for research. Graefes Arch Clin Exp Ophthalmol. 247(8): 1069–1080.
4. Gloesmann M, Hermann B, Schubert C, Sattmann H, Ahnelt PK, et al. (2003) Histologic correlation of pig retina radial stratification with ultrahigh-resolution optical coherence tomography. Invest Ophthalmol Vis Sci. 44(4): 1696–1703.
5. Strouthidis NG, Grimm J, Williams GA, Cull GA, Wilson DJ (2010) A comparison of optic nerve head morphology viewed by spectral domain optical coherence tomography and by serial histology. Invest Ophthalmol Vis Sci. 51(3): 1464–1474.
6. Ferguson LR, Balaiya S, Grover S, Chalam KV (2012) Modified protocol for in vivo imaging of wild-type mouse retina with customized miniature spectral domain optical coherence tomography (SD-OCT) device. Biol Proced Online. 14(1): 9.
7. Spaide RF, Curcio CA (2011) Anatomical correlates to the bands seen in the outer retina by optical coherence tomography: literature review and model. Retina. 31(8): 1609–1619.
8. Chan A, Duker JS, Ko TH, Fujimoto JG, Schuman JS (2006) Normal macular thickness measurements in healthy eyes using Stratus optical coherence tomography. Arch Ophthalmol. 124(2): 193–198.
9. Grover S, Murthy RK, Brar VS, Chalam KV (2009) Normative data for macular thickness by high-definition spectral-domain optical coherence tomography (spectralis). Am J Ophthalmol. 148(2): 266–271.
10. Chen TC, Cense B, Miller JW, Rubin PA, Deschler DG, et al. (2006) Histologic correlation of in vivo optical coherence tomography images of the human retina. Am J Ophthalmol. 141(6): 1165–1168.
11. Curcio CA, Messinger JD, Sloan KR, Mitra A, McGwin G, et al. (2011) Human chorioretinal layer thicknesses measured in macula-wide, high-resolution histologic sections. Invest Ophthalmol Vis Sci. 52(7): 3943–3954.
12. Vajzovic L, Hendrickson AE, O'Connell RV, Clark LA, Tran-Viet D, et al. (2012) Maturation of the human fovea: correlation of spectral-domain optical coherence tomography findings with histology. Am J Ophthalmol. 154(5): 779–789.
13. Ferguson LR, Dominguez Ii JM, Balaiya S, Grover S, Chalam KV (2013) Retinal Thickness Normative Data in Wild-Type Mice Using Customized Miniature SD-OCT. PLoS One. 27: 8.
14. Huber G, Beck SC, Grimm C, Sahaboglu-Tekgoz A, Paquet-Durand F, et al. (2009) Spectral domain optical coherence tomography in mouse models of retinal degeneration. Invest Ophthalmol Vis Sci. 50(12): 5888–5895.
15. Cebulla CM, Ruggeri M, Murray TG, Feuer WJ, Hernandez E (2010) Spectral domain optical coherence tomography in a murine retinal detachment model. Exp Eye Res. 90(4): 521–527.
16. Martin PM, Roon P, Van Ells TK, Ganapathy V, Smith SB (2004) Death of retinal neurons in streptozotocin-induced diabetic mice. Invest Ophthalmol Vis Sci. 45(9): 3330–3336.
17. Zhou X, Xie J, Shen M, Wang J, Jiang L, et al. (2008) Biometric measurement of the mouse eye using optical coherence tomography with focal plane advancement. Vision Res. 48(9): 1137–1143.
18. Gabriele ML, Ishikawa H, Schuman JS, Bilonick RA, Kim J, et al. (2010) Reproducibility of spectral-domain optical coherence tomography total retinal thickness measurements in mice. Invest Ophthalmol Vis Sci. 51(12): 6519–6523.
19. Ruggeri M, Wehbe H, Jiao S, Gregori G, Jockovich ME, et al. (2007) In vivo three-dimensional high-resolution imaging of rodent retina with spectral-domain optical coherence tomography. Invest Ophthalmol Vis Sci. 48(4): 1808–1814.
20. Fischer MD, Huber G, Beck SC, Tanimoto N, Muehlfriedel R, et al. (2009) Noninvasive, in vivo assessment of mouse retinal structure using optical coherence tomography. PLoS One. 4(10): e7507.
21. Giani A, Cigada M, Choudhry N, Deiro AP, Oldani M, et al. (2010) Reproducibility of retinal thickness measurements on normal and pathologic eyes by different optical coherence tomography instruments. Am J Ophthalmol. 150(6): 815–824.

3

A Phase 1 Study of ^{131}I-CLR1404 in Patients with Relapsed or Refractory Advanced Solid Tumors: Dosimetry, Biodistribution, Pharmacokinetics, and Safety

Joseph J. Grudzinski[1,2]*, Benjamin Titz[1,2], Kevin Kozak[1], William Clarke[1], Ernest Allen[1], LisaAnn Trembath[1], Michael Stabin[4], John Marshall[5], Steve Y. Cho[6], Terence Z. Wong[7], Joanne Mortimer[8], Jamey P. Weichert[1,3]

1 Cellectar Biosciences, Inc., Madison, WI, United States of America, 2 Department of Medical Physics, University of Wisconsin School of Medicine and Public Health, Madison, WI, United States of America, 3 Department of Radiology, University of Wisconsin, Madison, WI, United States of America, 4 Department of Radiology and Radiological Sciences, Vanderbilt University, Nashville, TN, United States of America, 5 Department of Medicine and Lombardi Comprehensive Cancer Center, Medstar Georgetown University Hospital, Washington, DC, United States of America, 6 Department of Radiology, Johns Hopkins Hospital, Baltimore, MD, United States of America, 7 Department of Radiology, Duke University Medical Center, Durham, NC, United States of America, 8 Department of Medical Oncology and Therapeutics Research, City of Hope, Duarte, CA, United States of America

Abstract

Introduction: ^{131}I-CLR1404 is a small molecule that combines a tumor-targeting moiety with a therapeutic radioisotope. The primary aim of this phase 1 study was to determine the administered radioactivity expected to deliver 400 mSv to the bone marrow. The secondary aims were to determine the pharmacokinetic (PK) and safety profiles of ^{131}I-CLR1404.

Methods: Eight subjects with refractory or relapsed advanced solid tumors were treated with a single injection of 370 MBq of ^{131}I-CLR1404. Whole body planar nuclear medicine scans were performed at 15–35 minutes, 4–6, 18–24, 48, 72, 144 hours, and 14 days post injection. Optional single photon emission computed tomography imaging was performed on two patients 6 days post injection. Clinical laboratory parameters were evaluated in blood and urine. Plasma PK was evaluated on [127]I-CLR1404 mass measurements. To evaluate renal clearance of ^{131}I-CLR1404, urine was collected for 14 days post injection. Absorbed dose estimates for target organs were determined using the RADAR method with OLINDA/EXM software.

Results: Single administrations of 370 MBq of ^{131}I-CLR1404 were well tolerated by all subjects. No severe adverse events were reported and no adverse event was dose-limiting. Plasma [127]I-CLR1404 concentrations declined in a bi-exponential manner with a mean $t_{1/2}$ value of 822 hours. Mean Cmax and AUC(0-t) values were 72.2 ng/mL and 15753 ng•hr/mL, respectively. An administered activity of approximately 740 MBq is predicted to deliver 400 mSv to marrow.

Conclusions: Preliminary data suggest that ^{131}I-CLR1404 is well tolerated and may have unique potential as an anti-cancer agent.

Trial Registration: ClinicalTrials.gov NCT00925275

Editor: T. Mark Doherty, Glaxo Smith Kline, Denmark

Funding: Cellectar Biosciences, Inc. funded the study and Cellectar Biosciences, Inc. personnel were responsible for study design, data collection and analysis, decision to publish, and manuscript preparation.

Competing Interests: Joseph Grudzinski, Benjamin Titz, and Kevin Kozak are employees of Cellectar Biosciences, Inc. William Clarke, Ernest Allen, and LisaAnn Trembath were past employees of Cellectar Biosciences, Inc. Jamey Weichert is the cofounder of Cellectar Biosciences, Inc. Michael Stabin is a paid consultant. Despite these potential competing interests.

* Email: grudzinski@wisc.edu

Introduction

In 2013, it was estimated that there were over 1.6 million new cases of cancer and 580,000 cancer-related deaths in the United States [1]. Worldwide, cancer of all types accounts for 3.5 million deaths annually. Treatment of neoplastic diseases represents a critical, unsatisfied medical need worldwide [2].

Tumor treatment with radioactive isotopes has been used as a fundamental cancer therapy for decades. Selective delivery of effective doses of radioactive isotopes that ablate tumor tissue and spare surrounding normal tissue remains a goal of targeted radiotherapies. CLR1404 is a novel radioiodinated therapeutic that takes advantage of the unique chemistry of alkylphosphocholine analogs (APCs) and their analogs that may achieve this goal [3].

Radioiodinated (^{124}I, ^{125}I, ^{131}I) CLR1404 has been evaluated in both xenograft and transgenic tumor models in mice and rats. Overall, these studies demonstrated specific uptake and retention in over 50 malignant tumor models [3], [4], [5], [6]. In addition, ^{131}I-CLR1404 potently inhibited tumor growth in nine murine tumor models (breast, prostate, lung, glioma, ovarian, renal, colorectal, pancreatic and melanoma) confirming it as a potential anti-cancer agent [6]. These promising preclinical results provided motivation for clinical translation of ^{131}I-CLR1404.

The primary endpoints of this study were to perform organ and total body dosimetry calculations and to determine the amount of radioactivity (megabecquerel (MBq)) expected to deliver 350-400 mSv to bone marrow – the initial administered radioactivity in subsequent maximum tolerated dose (MTD) phase I studies. The secondary endpoints of the study were to determine the pharmacokinetic (PK) and safety profiles of ^{131}I-CLR1404.

Materials and Methods

The protocol for this trial and supporting TREND checklist are available as supporting information; see Protocol S1 and Checklist S1, respectively.

Ethical Conduct of the Study

This study was conducted in accordance with International Conference on Harmonisation (ICH) guidance for good clinical practice (GCP) and all applicable regulatory requirements and ethical principles, including the Declaration of Helsinki. Written informed consent from each subject was obtained at screening, prior to the performance of any study-specific procedures.

This multi-center study (Georgetown University, Johns Hopkins University, Duke University, and City of Hope) evaluating dosimetry and safety (clinicaltrials.gov number, NCT00925275) was approved by each institution's Institutional Review Board (IRB).

Study Population

The study population consisted of eight patients (6 male and 2 female) with refractory or relapsed advance solid tumors who failed standard therapy or for whom no standard therapy existed. Primary tumors and metastatic sites for each patient are listed in Table 1. Subjects had a median age of 59 years (range of 46–71 years) and a median weight of 83.95 kg (range of 61.1–143.7 kg).

Study Design

Subjects were infused with 370 MBq of ^{131}I-CLR1404. All subjects received thyroid protection medication 24 hours prior to injection of the study drug and for 14 days afterwards. Whole body imaging for dosimetry calculations was performed at 15–35 minutes post infusion; 4–6, 18–24, 48, 72, and 144 hours post infusion and on days 6 and 14 post infusion. At the Investigator's discretion, optional single photon emission computed tomography (SPECT) imaging was obtained between day 3 and 14 to further characterize tumor uptake. Vital signs were monitored pre-infusion, 5, 15, 30 and 60 minutes as well as 4–6 hours post-infusion and at all study visits. ECGs were performed at screening, pre-infusion, 5 and 60 minutes post infusion, as well as 4–6 hours, 18–24 hours, day 6 and day 14 post infusion. Blood and urine were collected for clinical laboratory evaluation pre-infusion and on days 6, 14, 30 and 42. Blood was drawn for evaluation of lipids

pre-infusion and at 72 hours post infusion. Blood was collected for plasma PK analysis prior to infusion, and at 5, 15, 30, and 60 minutes; 4–6, 18–24, 48, and 72 hours; 6, 14, 30, and 42 days post infusion. To evaluate the radiological clearance of ^{131}I-CLR1404 from the renal system, subjects collected all of their urine for 14 days post infusion. This data was also used for radiation dosimetry calculations. Subjects were monitored at each visit for adverse events (AEs) and for the use of concomitant medications. The study design is presented in Figure 1 and the protocol deviations are listed in Table S1.

After all subjects completed the protocol, calculations were performed using Organ Level INternal Dose Assessment (OLINDA)-generated biodistribution curves to predict the administered ^{131}I-CLR1404 in MBq that would deliver a radiation absorbed dose of 350–400 mSv to total bone marrow [7]. This dose, as calculated with the OLINDA/EXM software, determined the starting dose for subsequent Phase 1 maximum tolerated dose (MTD) protocols. 350–400 mSv was chosen because it is one-fifth of the assumed tolerance dose of the bone marrow [7].

After reviewing the dosimetry and safety results of the first 8 subjects enrolled, a decision was made to terminate enrollment since analysis of the dosimetry data demonstrated minimal variance from subject to subject with regard to total body and organ dosimetry, specifically the bone marrow.

Treatments

^{131}I-CLR1404 Administration. ^{131}I-CLR1404 ($t_{1/2,phys}$ = 192 hours) was supplied as a ready-for-use radiopharmaceutical for intravenous dosing consisting of ^{131}I-CLR1404 (18-(p-[131I]iodophenyl)octadecyl phosphocholine) and ^{127}I-CLR1404 (18-(paraiodophenyl) octadecyl phosphocholine) in sodium chloride injection USP, ethanol USP/NF, polysorbate 20 NF, and sodium ascorbate USP. The study drug was packaged in a single-use glass vial and was passed through a 25 mm, 0.22 or 0.45 micron sterile filter prior to administration. The appropriate volume of study drug sufficient to give 370 MBq was diluted to 10 mL with normal saline and thoroughly mixed prior to administration via slow IV infusion.

Each subject received a single administration of 370 MBq ^{131}I-CLR1404 (0.26–0.43 mg mass dose) through a freely-running peripheral intravenous catheter over a period of at least 10 minutes. The selection of 370 MBq was based on organ and total body radiation dose estimates for ^{131}I-CLR1404 determined from dosimetry studies performed in mice. These studies indicated that 370 MBq of ^{131}I-CLR1404 provided an acceptable range of total body dosimetry, approximately 0.72 mSv/MBq.

To protect the thyroid from radioactive iodine uptake, thyroid protection was required. Thyroid protective agents were initiated at least 24 hours prior to, the day of, and for 14 days after administration of ^{131}I-CLR1404. Thyroid protective medications included either a saturated solution of potassium iodide (SSKI) 4 drops orally, Lugol's solution 20 drops orally three times daily, or potassium iodide tablets 130 mg orally once daily. The choice of thyroprotection was left to the discretion of individual study sites.

Dosimetry and Biodistribution

Assessment of radiological clearance. Study subjects were asked to collect all of their urine for the first 14 days of the study. The urine collection began at the first void after the 15–35 minute post-infusion scan. Urine was collected in the following incremental time points: 0–24 hours, 25–48 hours, 49–72 hours, 73–96 hours, Days 4–6, Days 6–10, and Days 10–14 post infusion.

Whole Body Imaging. Planar whole body nuclear medicine scans were obtained of each subject, from the anterior and

Table 1. Subject Information.

Subject	Center	Age	Gender	Race or Ethnicity	Primary Solid tumor	ECOG Status Screening	ECOG Status Day 42	Metastatic Sites	Prior Chemotherpy	Prior Hormonal, Immunological, Biological and Other Therapy
101	Georgetown	71	Female	White	Colon	0	1	Ovary	5-FU	bevacizumab
								Abdominal wall	leucovorin	
								Umbilicus	oxaliplatin	
102	Georgetown	46	Male	Black	Colon	1*	0	Lymph nodes	5-FU	bevacizumab
								Kidney	leucovorin	cetuximab
								Liver	oxaliplatin	
								Lung	irinotecan	
									capecitabine	
103	Georgetown	58	Male	White	Colon	0	0	Lymph nodes	5-FU	bevacizumab
									leucovorin	cetuximab
									irinotecan	
									capecitabine	
201	Johns Hopkins	69	Male	White	Esophageal	1	1	Lymph nodes	paclitaxel	
								Liver	cisplatin	
								Lung	irinotecan	
301	Duke	54	Male	White	Colon	1	1	Lung	5-FU	CEA(6D) VRP vaccine
									leucovorin	interferon alpha 2B
									oxaliplatin	bevacizumab
									irinotecan	
									capecitabine	
302	Duke	66	Male	White	Prostate	1	1	Bone	docetaxel	leuprolide
										bicalutamide
401	City of Hope	60	Female	Latino	Left Breast	0	0	Spleen		anastrazole
										fulvestrant
402	City of Hope	52	Male	White	Prostate	0	0	Lung		leuprolide (Ongoing)
								Bone		bicalutamide

Details about the subjects enrolled in the study.
*ECOG status is for Day 0.

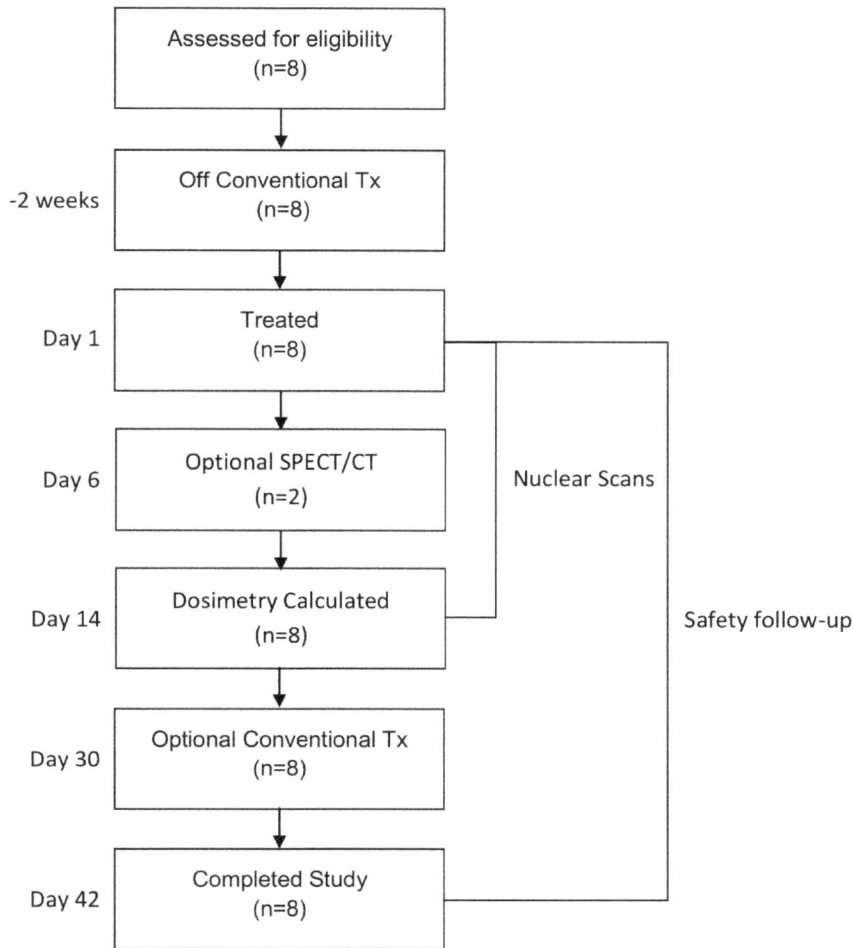

Figure 1. Consort diagram and clinical outcome of enrolled patients. Patients were taken off of conventional therapies from two weeks prior to and 30 days after treatment with ^{131}I-CLR1404. After treatment with ^{131}I-CLR1404, patients underwent nuclear medicine procedures for 14 days and were followed for safety for 42 days.

posterior projection, at the following times post injection: 15–35 minutes, 4–6 hours, 18–24 hours, 48±6 hours, 72±6 hours, 144±6 hours, and day 14±1. These images were acquired with a high energy parallel hole collimator, usingon a triple energy window (364 keV ±10%, 298 keV ±7.5%, 436 keV ±7.5%) and a minimum matrix size of 256×1024, for a speed of no faster than 10 cm/min. With the exception of the scan acquired 15 minutes post injection, each subject was asked to void their bladder prior to each imaging session. Using the MedDisplay software program, regionsRegions of interest (ROIs) were then drawn manually over identified geometrical structures in the body, including the liver, spleen, lungs, kidneys and the whole body. Data from the whole body were used to establish a time-activity pattern for activity not accounted for in the primary organs of uptake, with the net difference attributed to renal and/or gastrointestinal excretion. Body thickness in the various regions was estimated by evaluating attenuation as observed in Co-57 flood source scans, using attenuation coefficients determined at each participating site in experiments with [57]Co and ^{131}I sources [8].

Data in all regions were expressed as a percent of the initial activity in the total body from the early (e.g. 15 minute) whole body ROI. Data for subjects were fit to one or more exponential retention functions using the SAAM II software [9]. Time integrals

of activity were calculated from the SAAM II results and then expressed as normalized numbers of disintegrations (residence times) in the source organs [10]. Time integrals for urinary bladder were calculated using the data provided for activity excreted in urine and assuming that the bladder was emptied regularly every 4.8 hours. It is unknown whether radioactivity measured within the urine originated from ^{131}I-CLR1404, metabolites, or free [131]I. Organ time-activity integrals were entered into the OLINDA/ EXM software [11], using the adult male model. Integrals for major organs were calculated directly from the image data; values for remainder of body were calculated by inference (i.e. "whole body" minus the sum of all other organs).

Dosimetry calculation. Biodistribution data were analysed to produce time activity curves for each organ of interest that were integrated to calculate organ-specific residence times. These residence times were used in OLINDA/EXM to generate organ specific radiation absorbed doses from a 370 MBq injection of ^{131}I-CLR1404. This data, along with total urine collection for up to 14 days, was used to extrapolate and predict organ specific and total body radiation absorbed doses from projected therapeutic injections of ^{131}I-CLR1404.

Optional SPECT/CT. The protocol also permitted the acquisition of single-photon emission tomography (SPECT) or

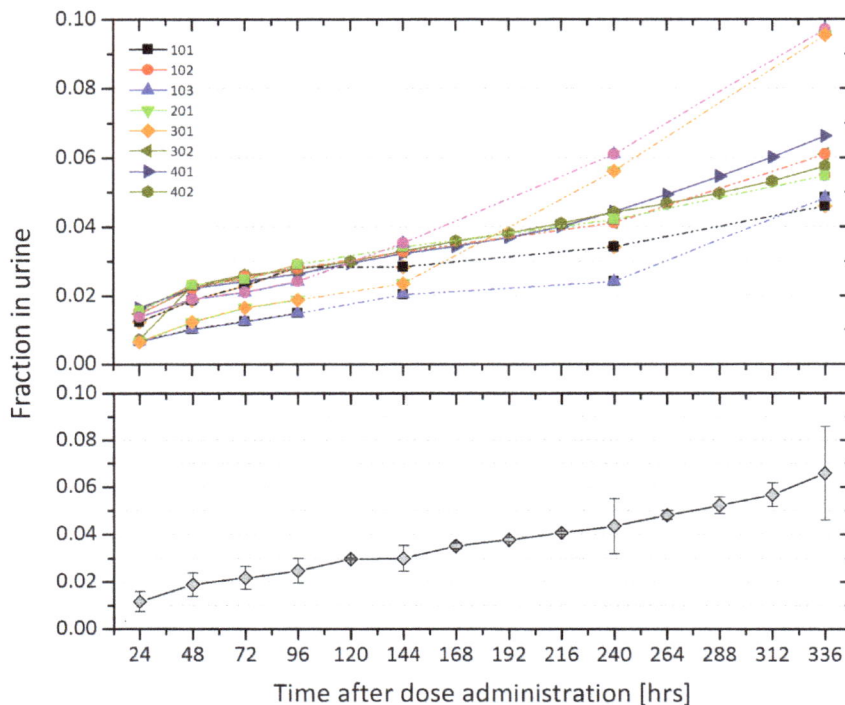

Figure 2. Renal clearance of ^{131}I-CLR1404. The cumulative fraction of ^{131}I-CLR1404 within the urine is shown following a single dose injection of 370 MBq of ^{131}I-CLR1404. The top graph shows each subject individually while the bottom graph shows the average of the group with the standard deviation represented with error bars. These data are used as input into OLINDA/EXM for dosimetry calculations.

SPECT with computed tomography (CT) attenuation (SPECT/CT) for the qualitative imaging of tumor uptake of ^{131}I-CLR1404 at the investigator's discretion in subjects with tumors amenable to imaging.

Two patients, 301 and 402, had tumors that were amenable to SPECT imaging. Their respective anatomical regions of interest, chest and pelvis, were imaged on the GE Infinia SPECT/CT camera using a high energy general purpose parallel-hole collimator with counts from the 15% energy window at 364 KeV. For patient 301, a total image of 120 projections was acquired over 360° with an acquisition time of 1 s/frame and an angular step of 3°. For patient 402, a total image of 60 projections was acquired over 360° with an acquisition time of 1 s/frame and angular step of 6°. After Each SPECT acquisition, both patients underwent a low-dose helical CT scan. The non-contrast CT, with acquisition parameters of 140 KeV and 5 mAs, was used for attenuation correction and anatomical conformation. The SPECT images from both patients were reconstructed with a conventional iterative algorithm, ordered subset expectation maximization (OSEM). A workstation providing multiplanar resampled images was used for image display and analysis (Amira; MA, U.S.A.).

Pharmacokinetics

Pharmacokinetic variables. Pharmacokinetic assessment of the plasma concentration of ^{127}I-CLR1404 was performed using a validated HPLC method with MS/MS detection (LLOQ 2.00 ng/mL) [12]. Plasma ^{127}I-CLR1404 concentration-time data were calculated using non-compartmental methods. The following parameters were defined: maximum plasma concentration (C_{max}), area under the concentration curve from 0 to 144 hours [$AUC_{(0-144hr)}$], area under the concentration curve from time 0 to time t (t is the time of last quantifiable concentration; t = 1008 hr) [$AUC_{(0-}$

$_{1008hr)}$], plasma half-life ($t_{1/2}$), apparent terminal phase rate constant (λz), clearance (CL), volume of distribution (Vd), and volume of distribution at steady-state (Vss).

Sampling procedure. For ^{127}I-CLR1404 mass measurements, blood was drawn pre-treatment and at 5, 15, 30, 60 minutes, 4–6, 18–24, 48, and 72 hours, 6, 14, 30 and 42 days post-infusion. Samples were frozen and stored until the radioactivity decayed to background levels (approximately 80 days) and then forwarded to Covance Laboratories (Madison, WI) for analysis. CLR1404 has previously been shown to be chemically stable under the storage conditions employed.

Analysis. Pharmacokinetic analysis of ^{127}I-CLR1404 mass measurements was performed by Covance Laboratories (Madison, WI), using WinNonlin Professional Edition (Pharsight Corporation, Version 5.2). A nominal dose level of 0.3 mg and actual sampling times were used for PK analysis. For PK calculation purposes, all times were normalized to the start of infusion.

Safety Assessments

Blood was drawn and urine was collected for evaluation of clinical laboratory parameters pre-infusion and on days 6, 14, 30 and 42. Baseline signs and symptoms were recorded. All adverse events (AEs) were recorded at each visit for the duration of the study. The severity of each AE was graded using the National Cancer Institute Common Toxicity Criteria for Adverse Events (NCI CTCAE) version 3.0.

Results

Dosimetry and Biodistribution

Assessment of bodily clearance. Figure 2 shows the fraction of ^{131}I-CLR1404 in the urine over time. ^{131}I-CLR1404 displayed very slow elimination. Most subjects had only about 5% elimination in the urine over the course of measurement, although two had clearances closer to 10% (Figure 2, top panel).

Whole Body Imaging. Figure 3 shows a representative series of whole-body planar images from patient 301 who had colorectal cancer with a lung metastasis. Qualitatively, most of the activity is cleared from the heart and liver within the first 24 hours after injection but is visible past 6 days in the extremities. After 14 days, there is very little activity left in the body.

Dosimetry calculation. Table 2 shows the dosimetry results for the eight patients who received 370 MBq of ^{131}I-CLR1404. The average red marrow dose for the eight subjects is 0.56 mSv/MBq (2.09 rem/mCi). Based on this, approximately 740 MBq (20 mCi) is predicted to deliver 400 mSv (40 rem) to marrow. Organs involved in metabolism of ^{131}I-CLR1404, namely the liver, kidneys, and spleen, exhibited higher doses of 1.09 mSv/MBq, 1.05 mSv/MBq, and 1.60 mSv/MBq, respectively.

Optional SPECT/CT. Two subjects had tumors that were amenable to SPECT/CT imaging: 301 and 402. Subject 301 had colorectal cancer that had metastasized to the left lung. The subject had undergone a partial left lower lobectomy for removal of metastatic tumor, but residual tumor remained which was surgically unresectable due to proximity to the pulmonary vein. At day 6 after the injection of 370 MBq of ^{131}I-CLR1404, a SPECT/CT was performed (Figure 4). The left, center, and right panels from Figure 4 show axial, coronal, and sagittal slices of the patient data, respectively. The top row shows the CT data and the bottom row shows SPECT overlaid onto the CT data. Residual tumor adherent to the left pulmonary vein and in close apposition to the aorta can be seen in the CT scan taken from the SPECT/CT data set. It should be noted that the tumor-to-muscle ratio (TMR), where the 'muscle' was defined as a region-of-interest within the healthy pectoral muscle, was as high as 7.6.

Subject 402 had metastatic prostate cancer. Images taken on day 6 after the injection of 370 MBq ^{131}I-CLR1404 are presented in Figure 4; accumulation of ^{131}I-CLR1404 in the involved areas identified on CT - the soft tissue and bony metastases - is seen in the images. It is also worth noting the relative lack of uptake in bone marrow.

Pharmacokinetics

After reaching C_{max}, plasma concentrations of ^{127}I-CLR1404 appeared to decline in a bi-exponential manner, with a mean ($\pm$ SD) t½ value of 822 ($\pm$101) hours (Table 3). The start of the apparent terminal elimination phase generally occurred between 67.5 and 333 hours post administration. Mean ($\pm$ SD) C_{max} and AUC(0-t) values were 72.2 ($\pm$11.5) ng/mL and 15753 ($\pm$3598) ng·hr/mL, respectively. The mean ($\pm$ SD) AUC_{0-144} and λz were 3420 ($\pm$574) ng·hr/mL and 0.000855 ($\pm$0.000112) hr^{-1}, respectively.

For all subjects except 101, C_{max} of ^{127}I-CLR1404 appeared at the first blood collection (5 minutes after infusion). In the case of 101, the 5 minute blood sample for plasma PK was drawn during the 10 minute infusion of the study drug, rather than 5 minutes after the end of the infusion as all of the other subjects' 5 minute samples were. The mean plasma concentration-time profile is shown in the bottom panel of Figure 5.

For individual subjects, the apparent elimination half-life ranged from 665 to 974 hours. The coefficient of variation (%CV) for C_{max} and area under the curve (AUC) values ranged from 16 to 23%, indicating that the inter-individual variation for exposure to ^{127}I-CLR1404 was generally low. The extrapolated portion of the $AUC_{0,\sqrt{-\infty}}$ was greater than 30% for all subjects; therefore, results for $AUC_{0-\infty}$ and the associated parameters (CL, Vd, and Vss) are subject to considerable uncertainty and are provided for completeness. shows the individual and mean pharmacokinetic parameters of ^{127}I-CLR1404.

Adverse Events

There were no, clinically significant changes over time in any hematology, clinical chemistry, or urinalysis parameter during the study. The adverse events (AEs) are listed in Table 4. There were no deaths or serious adverse effects AEs reported during the study. A total of 7 subjects reported 19 AEs during this study, 5 of which were considered related to study medication by the Investigator.

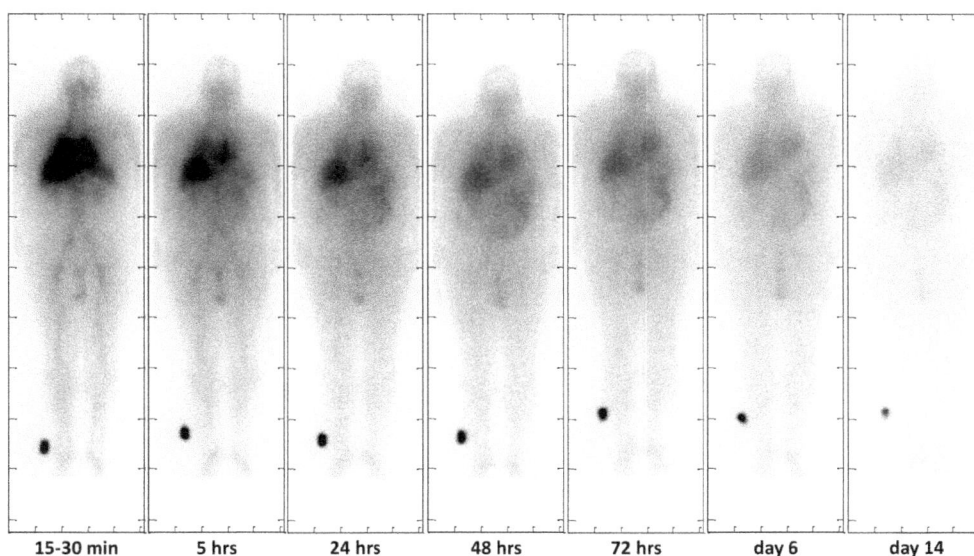

| 15-30 min | 5 hrs | 24 hrs | 48 hrs | 72 hrs | day 6 | day 14 |

Figure 3. Whole body conjugate-view planar images for subject 301. Images are shown for 15–30 minutes, 4, 24, 48, 72 hours, 6 and 14 days post injection, respectively. Because the agent is metabolized in the hepatobiliary system, there is evidence of ^{131}I-CLR1404 within the liver and intestines at relatively late time points.

Table 2. Dosimetry Results Calculated by OLINDA/EXM.

	Average		Std Dev		COV	95% CI (lower upper)			
	mSv/MBq	rem/mCi	mSv/MBq	rem/mCi		mSv/MBq	rem/mCi	mSv/MBq	rem/mCi
Adrenals	7.41E-01	2.74E+00	4.00E-02	1.47E-01	5.40%	7.13E-01	7.69E-01	2.64E+00	2.84E+00
Brain	5.86E-01	2.17E+00	3.38E-02	1.26E-01	5.80%	5.63E-01	6.09E-01	2.08E+00	2.26E+00
Breasts	5.61E-01	2.08E+00	2.93E-02	1.07E-01	5.20%	5.41E-01	5.81E-01	2.01E+00	2.15E+00
Gallbladder Wall	7.74E-01	2.86E+00	3.53E-02	1.29E-01	4.60%	7.50E-01	7.98E-01	2.77E+00	2.95E+00
LLI Wall	8.88E-01	3.28E+00	2.35E-01	8.64E-01	26.50%	7.25E-01	1.05E+00	2.68E+00	3.88E+00
Small Intestine	7.42E-01	2.75E+00	3.60E-02	1.32E-01	4.80%	7.17E-01	7.67E-01	2.66E+00	2.84E+00
Stomach Wall	7.11E-01	2.63E+00	3.50E-02	1.31E-01	4.90%	6.87E-01	7.35E-01	2.54E+00	2.72E+00
ULI Wall	7.81E-01	2.89E+00	7.91E-02	2.94E-01	10.10%	7.26E-01	8.36E-01	2.69E+00	3.09E+00
Heart Wall	7.11E-01	2.63E+00	3.49E-02	1.29E-01	4.90%	6.87E-01	7.35E-01	2.54E+00	2.72E+00
Kidneys (all subjects)	1.05E+00	3.90E+00	9.83E-01	3.65E+00	93.30%	3.69E-01	1.73E+00	1.37E+00	6.43E+00
Kidneys (excluding 301)	7.11E-01	2.63E+00	1.81E-01	6.71E-01	25.40%	5.77E-01	8.45E-01	2.13E+00	3.13E+00
Liver	1.09E+00	4.03E+00	3.29E-01	1.22E+00	30.30%	8.62E-01	1.32E+00	3.18E+00	4.88E+00
Lungs	9.28E-01	3.43E+00	4.48E-01	1.65E+00	48.30%	6.18E-01	1.24E+00	2.29E+00	4.57E+00
Muscle	6.29E-01	2.33E+00	3.26E-02	1.21E-01	5.20%	6.06E-01	6.52E-01	2.25E+00	2.41E+00
Ovaries	7.35E-01	2.72E+00	4.08E-02	1.52E-01	5.50%	7.07E-01	7.63E-01	2.61E+00	2.83E+00
Pancreas	7.72E-01	2.86E+00	4.17E-02	1.55E-01	5.40%	7.43E-01	8.01E-01	2.75E+00	2.97E+00
Red Marrow	5.63E-01	2.09E+00	2.80E-02	1.04E-01	5.00%	5.44E-01	5.82E-01	2.02E+00	2.16E+00
Osteogenic Cells	1.29E+00	4.77E+00	7.12E-02	2.63E-01	5.50%	1.24E+00	1.34E+00	4.59E+00	4.95E+00
Skin	5.33E-01	1.97E+00	2.90E-02	1.06E-01	5.40%	5.13E-01	5.53E-01	1.90E+00	2.04E+00
Spleen	1.60E+00	5.93E+00	8.52E-01	3.14E+00	53.10%	1.01E+00	2.19E+00	3.75E+00	8.11E+00
Testes	6.20E-01	2.30E+00	3.57E-02	1.34E-01	5.70%	5.95E-01	6.45E-01	2.21E+00	2.39E+00
Thymus	6.59E-01	2.44E+00	3.47E-02	1.27E-01	5.30%	6.35E-01	6.83E-01	2.35E+00	2.53E+00
Thyroid	6.52E-01	2.41E+00	3.68E-02	1.35E-01	5.70%	6.26E-01	6.78E-01	2.32E+00	2.50E+00
Urinary Bladder Wall	7.10E-01	2.63E+00	3.61E-02	1.35E-01	5.10%	6.85E-01	7.35E-01	2.54E+00	2.72E+00
Uterus	7.35E-01	2.72E+00	4.15E-02	1.54E-01	5.70%	7.06E-01	7.64E-01	2.61E+00	2.83E+00
Total Body	6.69E-01	2.47E+00	3.21E-02	1.18E-01	4.80%	6.47E-01	6.91E-01	2.39E+00	2.55E+00
Effective Dose	7.41E-01	2.74E+00	9.74E-02	3.59E-01	13.20%	6.74E-01	8.08E-01	2.49E+00	2.99E+00

The table shows the statistical summary of the eight subjects' dosimetry calculations.

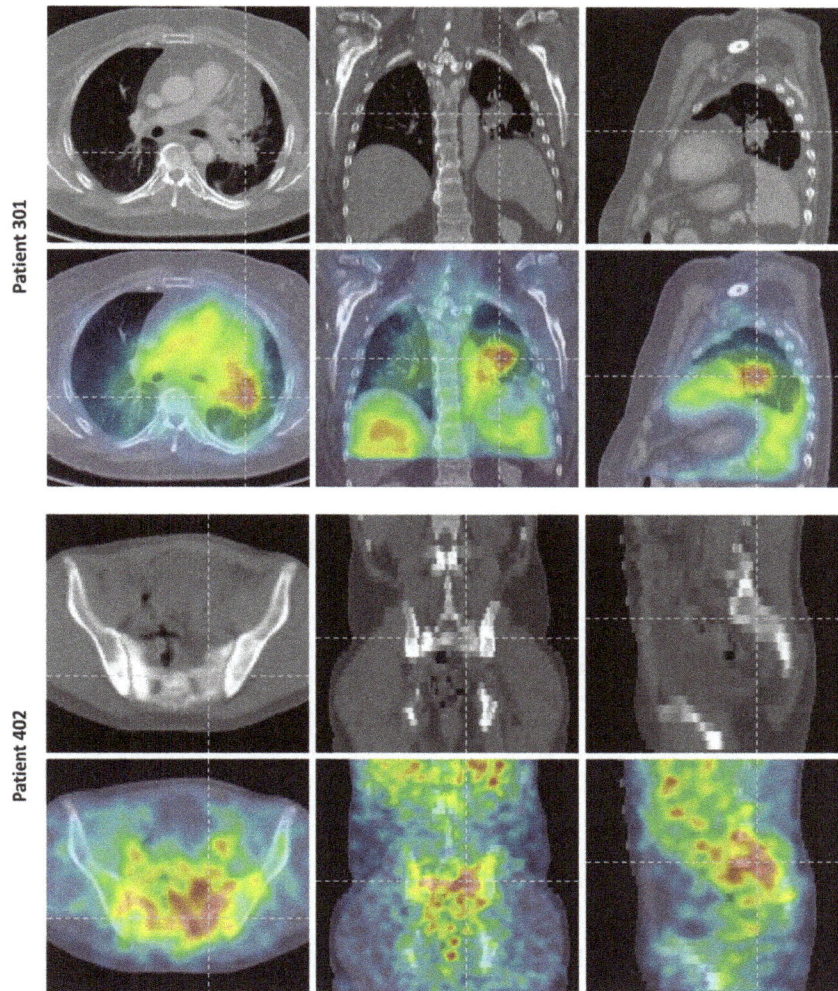

Figure 4. Imaging data from the optional SPECT/CT scans. Top: Day 6 SPECT/CT Images for a subject with colorectal cancer that metastasized to the lung (301). The three columns represent an axial, coronal, and sagittal slice, respectively. The top row shows the diagnostic quality CT alone while the bottom row shows the SPECT data overlayed onto the diagnostic CT. Bottom: Day 6 SPECT/CT Images for a subject with metastatic prostate cancer (402). The top row shows the low dose CT data alone while the bottom row shows the SPECT data overlayed onto the CT data. Note the increased uptake in the osteolytic lesion. The sagittal and coronal slices are of lower resolution compared to the axial plan because the CT was not of diagnostic quality; it was only used for attenuation correction of the SPECT data. A diagnostic quality CT of this subject was unavailable.

Three subjects had treatment-related AEs of CTCAE grade 1 fatigue, while one subject each had CTCAE grade 1 constipation and CTCAE grade 1 sialadenitis. AEs were mostly CTCAE grade 1 (n = 17); two AEs were CTCAE grade 2 neither of which was considered related to 131I-CLR1404. Two subjects had ongoing AEs at the completion of the study. Subject 102 had ongoing CTCAE grade 1 AEs of fatigue and constipation which were considered related to study medication administration in the opinion of the Investigator. Subject 201 had ongoing diarrhea (CTCAE grade 1) and back pain (CTCAE grade 2), which were considered unrelated to study medication by the Investigator.

Discussion

The activity administered (370 MBq) was sufficient to obtain good quality images. In almost all cases, radioactivity was still clearly seen in the blood pool at the latest imaging time (14 days). 131I-CLR1404 had very slow and minor elimination from the body, which is indicative of a long plasma half-life, $t_{1/2}$. Limited renal clearance was identified; generally only about 5% of the injected dose was cleared in urine. In a few cases, moderate gastrointestinal activity was seen; rough approximations were made of the uptake, and dose to the gastrointestinal organs was estimated. No thyroid uptake was visualized on any of the subject images.

There was generally high agreement with organ dose estimates between subjects. However, one subject (301) had a higher kidney uptake and radiation dose than the other subjects, so the analysis was repeated with the seven subjects that had agreement between the organ doses (Table 2). Note that renal clearance was not higher for 301 than for others (Figure 2, top panel). Based on the eight-subject calculated average red marrow dose of 0.56 mSv/MBq (2.09 rem/mCi), an administered activity of approximately 740 MBq (20 mCi) is predicted to deliver 400 mSv (40 rem) to marrow.

Table 3. Individual and Mean Pharmacokinetic Parameters following a Single Dose Infusion of 10 mCi of ^{131}I-CLR1404.

Subject Number	C_{max} (ng/mL)	AUC_{0-144} (ng hr/mL)	AUC_{0-1088} (ng hr/mL)	$AUC_{0-\infty}$ (ng hr/mL)	λz 1/hr	$t_{1/2}$ (hr)	CL (L/hr)	Vd (L)	Vss (L)
101	66.9	3848	22208	33565	0.000829	836	0.00894	10.8	11.0
102	54.6	2576	11059	16683	0.001	691	0.018	17.9	17.5
103	91.3	4019	16185	26452	0.00104	665	0.0113	10.9	10.8
201	73.5	3219	14255	25803	0.000791	877	0.0116	14.7	14.5
301	63.5	2599	11560	19851	0.000848	818	0.0151	17.8	17.5
302	70.1	3471	16129	29489	0.000793	874	0.0102	12.8	12.7
401	84	3916	18285	31216	0.00082	846	0.00961	11.7	11.3
402	73.8	3713	16347	30962	0.000712	974	0.00969	13.6	13.2
Mean	72.2	3420	15753	26753	0.000855	822	0.0118	13.8	13.6
SD	11.5	574	3598	5874	0.000112	101	0.0032	2.9	2.7
Min	54.6	2576	11059	16683	0.000712	665	0.00894	10.8	10.8
Median	71.8	3592	16157	27970	0.000825	841	0.0108	13.2	12.9
Max	91.3	4019	22208	33565	0.00104	974	0.018	17.9	17.5
CV%	16	17	23	22	13	12	27	21	20

Note: The extrapolated portion was greater than 30% for all subjects; therefore, results for $AUC_{0-\infty}$ and the associated parameters (CL, Vd, and Vss) were provided for informational purposes only.

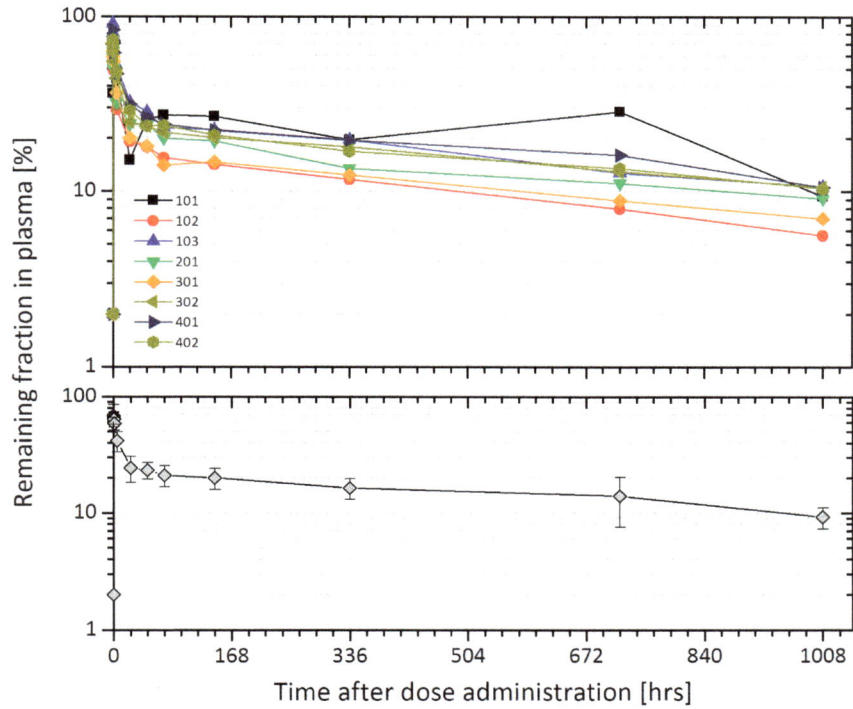

Figure 5. Plasma pharmacokinetics of ^{127}I-CLR1404. The remaining fraction of ^{127}I-CLR1404 within the plasma is plotted over time. The top graph shows each individual subject while the bottom graph shows the average of the group with the standard deviation represented with error bars.

Table 4. Adverse Events (AE).

Subject number	AE No.	Preferred Term	CTCAE Grade	Frequency*	Relationship†
101	1	Fatigue	1	2	1
102	1	Fatigue	1	2	1
	2	Constipation	1	1	1
103	None				
201	1	Sialadenitis	1	1	1
	2	Diarrhoea	1	1	2
	3	Back pain	2	1	2
	4	Blood pressure decreased	1	1	2
	5	Skin ulcer	1	3	2
	6	Skin ulcer	1	3	2
	7	Nasal congestion	1	2	2
	8	Gamma-glutamyltransferase increased	2	3	2
301	1	Fatigue	1	2	2
	2	Wheezing	1	2	2
302	1	Fatigue	1	2	1
	2	Hordeolum	1	2	2
401	1	Erythema	1	3	2
402	1	Oedema peripheral	1	3	2
	2	Erythema	1	3	2
	3	Erysipelas	1	3	2

The AE experienced during the study are listed.
*Frequency: 1 = Intermittent, 2 = Continuous, 3 = Single Episode.
†Relationship to Study Drug: 1 = Related, 2 = Not related.

Since OLINDA/EXM was designed to compute 'organ level' dosimetry of radiopharmaceuticals using a 'Standard Man' phantom, it only requires low resolution planar images for input. Hence, tumors in regions of high background signal are often difficult to delineate on planar whole body images and can sometimes incorrectly be included in lung dosimetry calculations within OLINDA/EXM. To avoid this problem, high resolution tomographic imaging such as SPECT/CT should always be used to not only better delineate tumors but also compute dosimetry for radiotherapeutic agents. The relatively low number of patients in this study with lesions amenable for SPECT may have been the result of lesions that were not visible via planar imaging.

370 MBq of ^{131}I-CLR1404 was well-tolerated by all subjects. There were no serious AEs or AEs that were CTCAE grade 3 or higher. Only 5 of the 19 AEs recorded in the study were considered related to study medication. All treatment related AEs were CTCAE grade 1. There were no identified changes in clinical laboratory evaluations, ECGs, vital signs, temperature, oxygen saturation, or physical examinations

The single time point non-quantitative SPECT/CT images, taken at day 6 after an administration of 370 MBq of ^{131}I-CLR1404, show that there is uptake of ^{131}I-CLR1404 in tumors. This uptake occurs in both visceral and bony metastases, shown in the two different malignancies. Conversely, the images also show the relative lack of uptake in adjacent normal tissue or bone marrow.

Estimating the potential tumor dosimetry of ^{131}I-CLR1404 will be helpful in understanding its potential as a therapeutic. To estimate the tumor dosimetry from therapeutic administrations of ^{131}I-CLR1404, further studies will include quantitative SPECT/CT imaging at multiple points in subjects in an ongoing phase 1b study.

Conclusion

The results obtained in this Phase 1 study demonstrated that ^{131}I-CLR1404 is well tolerated at a dose of 370 MBq and exhibited prolonged retention within solid tumors compared to normal tissues. An administered radioactivity of approximately 740 MBq (20 mCi) is predicted to deliver 400 mSv (40 rem) to the bone marrow, which is the dose limiting organ. This will serve as a reference dose in additional clinical investigations.

Supporting Information

Table S1   Protocol Deviations. Details are listed about each subject's deviations from the protocol.

Author Contributions

Conceived and designed the experiments: WC EA LT MS JW. Performed the experiments: JM SC TW JM. Analyzed the data: MS JG BT KK. Contributed reagents/materials/analysis tools: JW MS JG BT. Wrote the paper: JG BT KK WC EA LT MS JM SC TW JM JW. Provided medical assessment of study as a whole: KK. Oversaw patient care during trial: JM SC TW JM. Processed PK and imaging data: BT JG. Oversaw production of I-131 radioisotope: JW.

References

1. Siegel R, Naishadham D, Jemal A (2013) Cancer Statistics, 2013. CA Cancer J Clin 63: 11–30. doi:10.3322/caac.21166.
2. Ries LAG, Melbert D, Krapcho M, Stinchcomb DG, Howlander N, et al. (2008) SEER Cancer Statistics Review, 1975–2005. Available: http://seer.cancer.gov/csr/1975_2005/. Accessed 2014 Oct 21.
3. Pinchuk AN, Rampy MA, Longino MA, Skinner RW, Gross MD, et al. (2006) Synthesis and structure-activity relationship effects on the tumor avidity of radioiodinated phospholipid ether analogues. J Med Chem 49: 2155–2165. Available: http://www.ncbi.nlm.nih.gov/entrez/query.fcgi?cmd=Retrieve&db=PubMed&dopt=Citation&list_uids=16570911.
4. Deming DA, Leystra AA, Farhoud M, Nettekoven L, Clipson L, et al. (2013) mTOR inhibition elicits a dramatic response in PI3K-dependent colon cancers. PLoS One 8: e60709. Available: http://www.pubmedcentral.nih.gov/articlerender.fcgi?artid=3621889&tool=pmcentrez&rendertype=abstract. Accessed 14 November 2013.
5. Zasadny KR, Longino MA, Fisher SJ, Counsell RE, Wahl RL (1999) A Phospholipid Ether Agent for Tumor Imaging and Possible Therapy. J Nucl Med 40: 39.
6. Weichert JP, Clark PA, Kandela IK, Vaccaro AM, Clarke W, et al. (2014) Alkylphosphocholine Analogs for Broad-Spectrum Cancer Imaging and Therapy. Sci Transl Med 6: 240ra75–240ra75. Available: http://stm.sciencemag.org/cgi/doi/10.1126/scitranslmed.3007646. Accessed 12 June 2014.
7. Stabin MG, Siegel JA (2003) Physical Models and Dose Factors for Use in Internal Dose Assessment. Heal Phys 85: 294–310. Available: http://journals.

lww.com/health-physics/Fulltext/2003/09000/Physical_Models_and_Dose_Factors_for_Use_in.6.aspx.
8. Siegel JA, Thomas SR, Stubbs JB, Stabin MG, Hays MT, et al. (1999) MIRD pamphlet no. 16: Techniques for quantitative radiopharmaceutical biodistribution data acquisition and analysis for use in human radiation dose estimates. J Nucl Med 40: 37S–61S. Available: http://www.ncbi.nlm.nih.gov/entrez/query.fcgi?cmd=Retrieve&db=PubMed&dopt=Citation&list_uids=10025848.
9. Barrett PH, Bell BM, Cobelli C, Golde H, Schumitzky A, et al. (1998) SAAM II: Simulation, Analysis, and Modeling Software for tracer and pharmacokinetic studies. Metabolism 47: 484–492. Available: http://www.ncbi.nlm.nih.gov/pubmed/9550550.
10. Stabin MG, da Luz LC (2002) Decay data for internal and external dose assessment. Heal Phys 83: 471–475. Available: http://www.ncbi.nlm.nih.gov/entrez/query.fcgi?cmd=Retrieve&db=PubMed&dopt=Citation&list_uids=12240721.
11. Stabin MG, Sparks RB, Crowe E (2005) OLINDA/EXM: the second-generation personal computer software for internal dose assessment in nuclear medicine. J Nucl Med 46: 1023–1027. Available: http://www.ncbi.nlm.nih.gov/entrez/query.fcgi?cmd=Retrieve&db=PubMed&dopt=Citation&list_uids=15937315.
12. Jiang H, Cannon MJ, Banach M, Pinchuk AN, Ton GN, et al. (2010) Quantification of CLR1401, a novel alkylphosphocholine anticancer agent, in rat plasma by hydrophilic interaction liquid chromatography-tandem mass spectrometric detection. J Chromatogr B Analyt Technol Biomed Life Sci 878: 1513–1518. Available: http://www.ncbi.nlm.nih.gov/pubmed/20434411. Accessed 19 February 2014.

4

Factors Influencing Superimposition Error of 3D Cephalometric Landmarks by Plane Orientation Method Using 4 Reference Points: 4 Point Superimposition Error Regression Model

Jae Joon Hwang[1], Kee-Deog Kim[2], Hyok Park[1], Chang Seo Park[1], Ho-Gul Jeong[1]*

1 Department of Oral and Maxillofacial Radiology, Dental Hospital of Yonsei University of College of Dentistry, Seoul, Korea, 2 Department of General Dentistry, Dental Hospital of Yonsei University of College of Dentistry, Seoul, Korea

Abstract

Superimposition has been used as a method to evaluate the changes of orthodontic or orthopedic treatment in the dental field. With the introduction of cone beam CT (CBCT), evaluating 3 dimensional changes after treatment became possible by superimposition. 4 point plane orientation is one of the simplest ways to achieve superimposition of 3 dimensional images. To find factors influencing superimposition error of cephalometric landmarks by 4 point plane orientation method and to evaluate the reproducibility of cephalometric landmarks for analyzing superimposition error, 20 patients were analyzed who had normal skeletal and occlusal relationship and took CBCT for diagnosis of temporomandibular disorder. The nasion, sella turcica, basion and midpoint between the left and the right most posterior point of the lesser wing of sphenoidal bone were used to define a three-dimensional (3D) anatomical reference co-ordinate system. Another 15 reference cephalometric points were also determined three times in the same image. Reorientation error of each landmark could be explained substantially (23%) by linear regression model, which consists of 3 factors describing position of each landmark towards reference axes and locating error. 4 point plane orientation system may produce an amount of reorientation error that may vary according to the perpendicular distance between the landmark and the x-axis; the reorientation error also increases as the locating error and shift of reference axes viewed from each landmark increases. Therefore, in order to reduce the reorientation error, accuracy of all landmarks including the reference points is important. Construction of the regression model using reference points of greater precision is required for the clinical application of this model.

Editor: Francesco Cappello, University of Palermo, Italy

Funding: The authors have no support or funding to report.

Competing Interests: The authors have declared that no competing interests exist.

* Email: RARI98@yuhs.ac

Introduction

Inevitably, error due to the position change of patient occurs during every x-ray taking despite the patient alignment protocol such as the bite material. Therefore, superimposition has been used as a method to evaluate the changes of orthodontic or orthopedic treatment.

Two-dimensional (2D) cephalometric analysis, introduced by Hofrath [1] and Broadbent [2] in 1931, has been the gold standard for clinical measurement tool in orthodontics and craniofacial surgery for the last decades. In traditional analysis, superimposition using anterior cranial base is a method to show the changes due to the growth and due to orthodontic treatment. But superimposition of anatomic structures in 2D images has limitations such as difficulty in determining landmarks and overestimating changes in the superimposed direction [3,4].

With the introduction of cone beam CT (CBCT), evaluating changes three-dimensionally after orthodontic or orthopedic treatment became possible by superimposing images. [5–8] Newly

introduced methods of 3D superimposition include superimposing the landmarks of the bone surface, setting up a new plane orientation and superimposing a certain selected area.

Many studies reported high reliability of identifying cephalometric landmarks with CBCT, especially on multiplanar reconstruction (MPR) images compared to 3D surface models. [9,10] Because landmarks for superimposition should have high reproducibility, recent studies superimposed CBCT images by reorientation adopting widely used landmarks/planes as reference coordinates/planes on MPR images. [11,12] But there have not been any studies about statistical analysis and mathematical modelling on the factors influencing superimposition error. The purposes of this study were 1) to find the factors influencing 4 point plane reorientation error, and 2) to find whether the orthodontic landmarks had sufficient reproducibility as reference landmarks and as points for analyzing superimposition error.

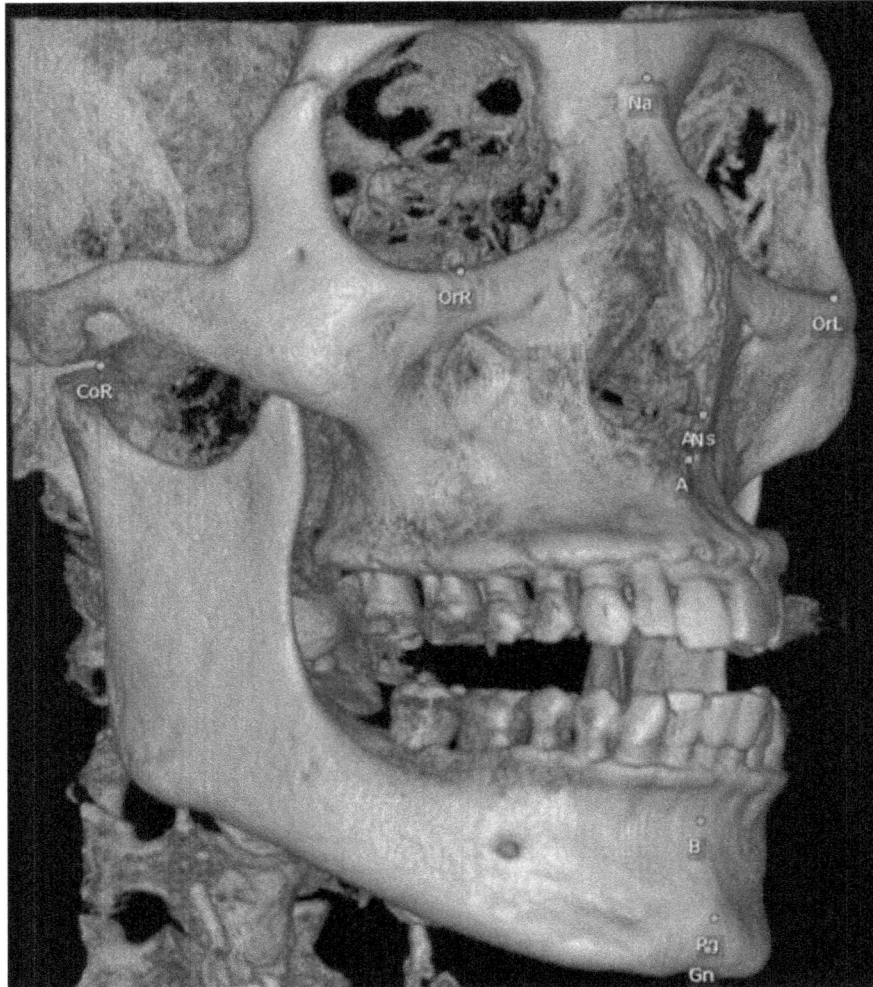

Figure 1. Landmarks before reorientation.

Materials and Methods

Ethics Statement

This study was approved by the IRB of Yonsei University Dental Hospital (Approval number: 13-0103(2-2013-0049)). A written or verbal informed consent was not obtained by any participants because this study was a non-interventional retrospective design and all data were analyzed anonymously. The IRB of Yonsei University Dental Hospital waived the need for individual informed consent.

Sample

In this study, the CBCT data of 20 patients (9 males and 11 females; ranging in age from 23 to 72 years, 53.6 mean age) who visited the hospital for temporomandibular joint evaluation and took CBCT for suspected condylar pathologic bone change were selected for analysis. CBCT volumetric data (Alphard3030, Alphard Roentgen Ind., Ltd., Kyoto, Japan) were taken at 80 kV, 5 mAs with scanning time of 17 s. These images were taken using 'P mode (154 mm×154 mm FOV)'. The voxel size was 0.30 mm. All CT images were stored using DICOM 3.0 as a medical image file format (512×512 pixel) into a Window 7-based graphics workstation (Intel Core i5 3570, 4 GByte, calibrated 21.3-

inch color monitor, resolution 1563×2048 pixel, NVIDIA Quadro 2000 graphic card) and subsequently transferred toward OnDemand 3D 3Dceph application (Cybermed, CA, USA). Sagittal, axial and coronal volumetric slices as well as the 3D image reconstruction were used to determine the landmark location.

Landmarks determination

19 landmarks were located manually by 'Tracing' function of the software on 3D MPR images. (Figure 1).

MLWS was defined as the midpoint between the most posterior points of bilateral lesser wings of sphenoid bone. The MLSW was selected as the center of reorientation because it was close to the sella turcica in the midsagittal plane and the bilateral lesser wings had sharp posterior points, which were thought to be highly precise. All landmarks except MLWS are commonly used craniofacial structures in orthodontics and can be located without difficulty [13]. Landmarks used in the present study are defined in Table 1. Landmarks were placed by using mouse firstly on the bone surface of reconstructed CBCT images and revised secondly on MPR images. After a radiologist located all 19 landmarks, at least 1 week apart, same radiologist repeated the procedure on the same images. During the procedures, the x, y, z coordinates were gained. Locating error was obtained by measuring the absolute

Table 1. Definition of the three spatial planes of the 19 points used in this study.

Point Name	Anatomical definition	Sagittal view	Coronal view	Axial view
Median point of bilateral lesser wings(MLWS)	midpoint between the most posterior point of bilateral lesser wing of sphenoid bone	most PP	MP	most PP + MP
Sella turcica(S)	APP MP pituitary fossa sphenoid bone	MP APP width	MP lateral width fossa, determined antero-posteriorly by the other two slices(2)	MP APP and lateral width fossa
Nasion(Na)	most AP frontonasal suture	most AP	MP	most AP+MP anterior contour
Basion(Ba)	most AP foramen magnum	most PP + LP	MP foramen, determined antero-posteriorly by the 2	most AP foramen
Anterior Nasal spine(Ans)	most AP and maxillary process nasal floor region	most AP	AP + MP	AP + MP
Point A(A)	most PP maxillar curvature, between anterior nasal spine and supradental point	most PP	MP determined antero-posteriorly by the 2	AP + MP
Posterior Nasal spine(Pns)	most PP and mid-point palatine bone contour	most PP	PP + MP	PP + MP
Pogonion(Pg)	most AP mandibular symphysis	most AP	MP	AP + MP
Menton(Me)	LP mandibular symphysis	LP	LP	LP + MP
Gnathion(Gn)	most ASP mandibular symphysis	MA + LP	MA + LP	AP, LP + MP
Point B(B)	most PP anterior surface mandibular symphysis	most PP	MP determined antero-posteriorly by the 2	AP + MP
Right and left orbitale (OrR, OrL)	most AUP infraorbital orbital	most AP	UP + MP	Most AP
Right and left Porion (PoR. PoL)	UP and MP external ridge roof auditory meatus	UP + MP	UP	MP determined supero –inferiorly by the 2
Right and left Condylion (CoR, CoL)	UP point head right condyle	UP + most PP	most UP + MP	most PP
Right and left Gonion (GoR, GoL)	most PP edge branch. Bisection tangents posterior edge branch and lower body	most PP	most PP + MP	most PP determined supero-inferioly by the 2

Anteroposterior point(APP), Midpoint(MP), Posterior point(PP), Lowest Point(LP), Upper point(UP), Anterior-lower Point(ALP), Anterior-upper Point(AUP), Posterior-lower Point(PLP), Highest Point(HP), Inner Point(IP).

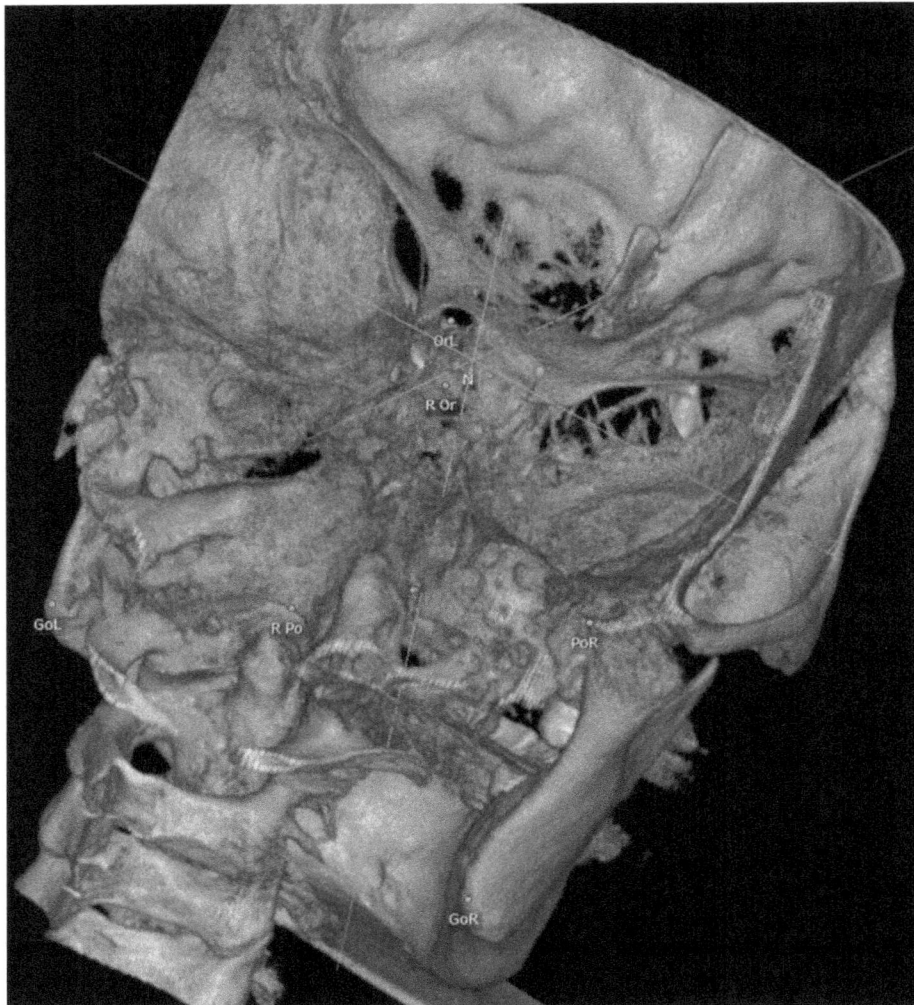

Figure 2. Landmarks after reorientation. N, ROr and RPo each refers to MLWS, S and Ba according to the initial setting of Ondemand 3Dceph module.

value of the coordinate difference and distance between the repeatedly marked landmarks.

Reorientation procedure and Measurement of reorientation error

After all 19 landmarks were defined (Figure 1), the reorientation procedure was accomplished 3 times by using 'Reorientation' function of the software (Figure 2).

Four reference landmarks out of total 19 landmarks were used to define a 3D reference co-ordinate system. Using four landmarks as the setting point is one of the simplest way of plane reorientation which can be readily applicable in the clinic. The nasion (Na), sella turcica (S) and basion (Ba) were selected for axes determination. The orientation of y (anteroposterior) axis was parallel to the line which passes through Na and S. Z (vertical) axis was parallel to the line which is orthogonal to y axis and passes through Ba. (Figure 3) Orientation of x(transverse) axis was orthogonal to the y and z axis. And MLWS was set to a new starting point of the reoriented Cartesian co-ordinate system.(Figure 4).

After plane orientation, the x, y, z coordinates were measured by the new starting point, and the vertical distance from the new x axis was measured for each point.

Reorientation error was defined as the distance of repeatedly marked landmarks after reorientation procedure.

Statistical analysis

Statistical analysis was carried out with SPSS 20.0 (SPSS Inc., Chicago, III). Intraclass correlation Coefficient (ICC) was obtained for all coordinates of 19 landmarks. Reoriented 15 commonly used orthodontic landmarks were analyzed by stepwise linear regression tests for finding statistically significant independent variables of reorientation error.

Results

ICC (Intra-examiner reliability) and Locating error

ICC for x, y and z coordinates for all landmarks were above 0.99. However, there were large average locating errors in the x coordinates of OrR (0.89 mm), OrL (0.68 mm) and PoR (0.61 mm) (Table 2, Figure 5). Standard deviation was large at

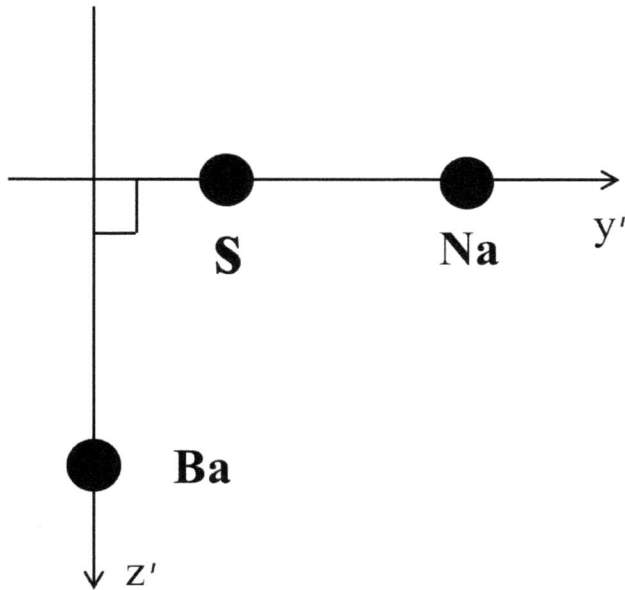

Figure 3. Reorientation axes. y and ź are lines parallel to y and z axis respectively.

the locating error of A (0.74), OrR (0.58), OrL (0.48), PoR (0.45), PoL (0.55), GoR (0.52) and GoL (0.49) in comparison to MLWS (0.22), Ba (0.28), Ans (0.28), CoR (0.32) and CoL (0.29) (Table 3).

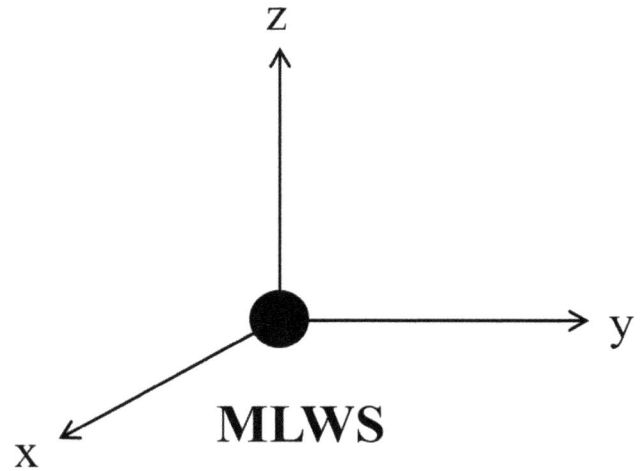

Figure 4. MLWS as a new starting point. x, y and z axis each represent reoriented transverse, anteroposterior and vertical axis.

Reorientation error

Reorientation error was greater than locating error on every landmarks (Table 3). In Table 3, when locating error, vertical distance from x axis, sum of angle errors from Na, S, Ba increases, reorientation error increased as well, but all three did not show proportional change.

Linear regression model for Reorientation error

According to the stepwise method, multiple linear regression model which explains reorientation error was found from a

Table 2. Locating error (coordinate).

Landmarks	Locating error		
	X	**Y**	**Z**
MLWS	0.19(0.18)	0.16(0.17)	0.14(0.13)
Na	0.32(0.26)	0.20(0.15)	0.31(0.40)
S	0.39(0.33)	0.31(0.26)	0.38(0.33)
Ba	0.30(0.22)	0.33(0.29)	0.20(0.15)
Ans	0.27(0.22)	0.26(0.21)	0.24(0.22)
A	0.24(0.18)	0.20(0.22)	0.79(0.77)
Pns	0.24(0.19)	0.25(0.21)	0.31(0.30)
Pg	0.50(0.37)	0.17(0.13)	0.58(0.40)
Me	0.53(0.36)	0.17(0.13)	0.27(0.21)
Gn	0.55(0.40)	0.24(0.22)	0.44(0.35)
B	0.33(0.25)	0.14(0.11)	0.68(0.47)
OrR	0.89(0.60)	0.38(0.37)	0.23(0.18)
OrL	0.68(0.50)	0.34(0.29)	0.30(0.24)
PoR	0.61(0.49)	0.46(0.32)	0.32(0.25)
PoL	0.56(0.50)	0.50(0.37)	0.38(0.28)
CoR	0.38(0.35)	0.25(0.19)	0.14(0.09)
CoL	0.29(0.25)	0.31(0.27)	0.12(0.10)
GoR	0.46(0.38)	0.56(0.35)	0.70(0.47)
GoL	0.45(0.35)	0.45(0.36)	0.63(0.42)

Table 3. Reorientation error (RE) and factors influencing RE.

Landmarks	Reorientation error (distance)			Locating error (distance)			Distance from reoriented X axis	Sum of angle errors from Na, S, Ba(°)
	Mean(SD)	Q1	Q3	Mean(SD)	Q1	Q3		
MLWS	0.00(0.00)	0.00	0.00	0.33(0.22)	0.18	0.38	0.00(0.00)	
Na	0.77(0.37)	0.49	0.98	0.57(0.40)	0.29	0.67	2.58(1.42)	
S	0.84(0.39)	0.55	1.06	0.73(0.38)	0.45	0.96	2.59(1.42)	
Ba	0.84(0.41)	0.54	1.11	0.56(0.28)	0.34	0.68	37.03(3.44)	
Ans	1.71(1.19)	0.90	2.17	0.51(0.28)	0.26	0.65	55.35(2.63)	1.10(0.39)
A	2.01(1.23)	1.08	2.85	0.92(0.74)	0.44	1.22	61.14(2.85)	1.04(0.37)
Pns	1.27(0.74)	0.70	1.56	0.54(0.32)	0.33	0.63	47.82(3.66)	1.60(0.57)
Pg	2.98(2.15)	1.34	3.61	0.88(0.38)	0.52	1.12	120.21(5.67)	0.66(0.22)
Me	3.08(2.16)	1.53	3.59	1.01(0.47)	0.71	1.33	126.63(6.25)	0.64(0.21)
Gn	3.01(2.33)	1.41	3.85	0.83(0.43)	0.54	1.04	124.70(6.14)	0.65(0.22)
B	2.64(1.84)	1.28	3.01	0.83(0.44)	0.47	1.09	105.81(4.73)	0.73(0.25)
OrR	1.77(1.07)	1.10	2.19	1.08(0.58)	0.70	1.49	47.01(2.93)	1.33(0.59)
OrL	1.54(0.93)	0.97	1.90	0.91(0.48)	0.56	1.10	45.90(2.77)	1.25(0.53)
PoR	1.58(1.21)	0.89	1.85	0.94(0.45)	0.64	1.17	50.14(6.09)	1.35(0.56)
PoL	1.72(1.13)	0.94	2.28	0.93(0.55)	0.61	1.13	54.43(5.41)	1.28(0.53)
CoR	1.42(0.98)	0.74	1.96	0.53(0.32)	0.34	0.65	57.98(3.06)	1.28(0.51)
CoL	1.57(1.27)	0.79	1.97	0.51(0.29)	0.31	0.68	58.80(3.74)	1.25(0.51)
GoR	2.27(1.39)	1.29	2.88	1.11(0.52)	0.80	1.45	95.37(8.04)	0.91(0.37)
GoL	2.08(1.24)	1.16	2.49	1.00(0.49)	0.62	1.26	95.14(8.12)	0.91(0.35)

Locating error(mm)

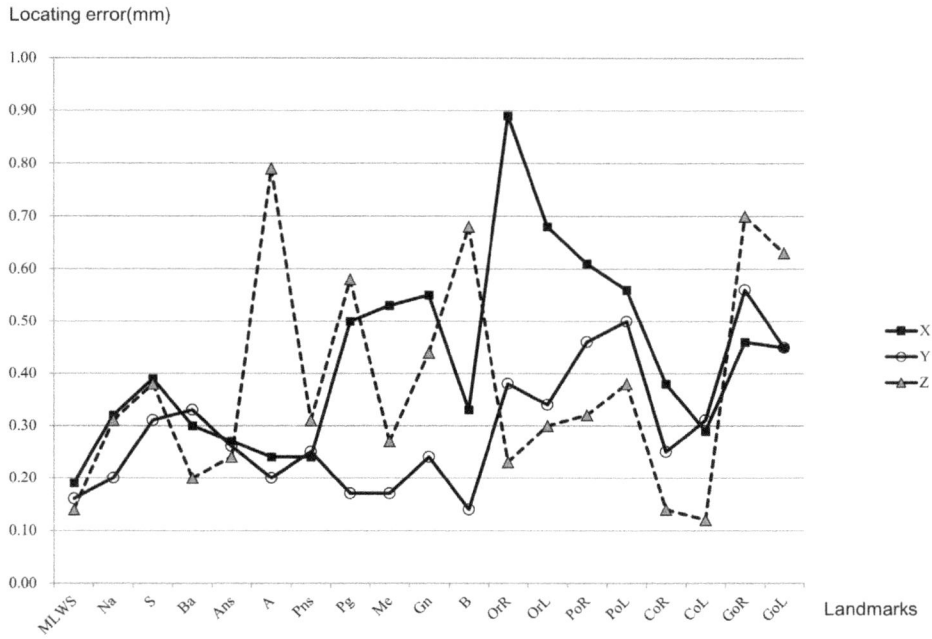

Figure 5. Locating error (coordinate).

viewpoint of each landmark, as follows.

$$Y = -0.665 + 0.758 * Db + 0.018 * DX + 0.545 * A3r \quad (1)$$

(Y = Reorientation error,
Db = Locating error before reorientation (Figure 6),
DX = vertical distance from reoriented x axis (Figure 7),
A3r ($\alpha+\beta+\gamma$) = sum of angle errors of reference points located twice (Figure 8),
All the coefficient are from multiple regression of total data).

Where a and b refer to the different measurement trial of the same image and $\overline{A}$ stands for the average coordinate of a landmark (A) between two trials (Figure 6, 7, 8).

The model shown in 1 was statistically significant (P = 0.000) for all T1–T2, T1–T3, T2–T3 and total analysis. The Adjusted R-square (r^2) was around 0.23 (Table 4).

Table 4 also shows that all 3 independent variables of tested model are all statistically significant (P<0.05), and multicollinearity does not exist between the independent variables (VIF≒1).

Discussion

3D reproducibility of cephalometric landmarks

Generally, marking on 2D cephalometry is quite straightforward, and 1 mm is traditionally accepted as the precise

measurement. Identifying the cephalometric landmarks in 3D CBCT was reported reliable in many studies, especially on MPR images. [9,13] But locating error is larger in 3D than 2D, and this seems to be the reason why 3D cephalometry is not widely used clinically [14].

Table 2 and 3 showed reproducibility of some widely used cephalometric points were not very high in 3D MPR images. The locating errors were about 1 mm on average. However, some points at the third quartile had 1.2–1.5 mm locating errors, and some of the locating errors were greater than 2 mm. This results correlates partially with the study of Zamora et al. [10] which reporting high errors in A, OrR, OrL, PoR, B and GoR. In addition, Hassan et al. [9] reported large locating errors (average 1.2~2.1 mm) in PoR, PoL and GoL. In Table 2 and figure 5,

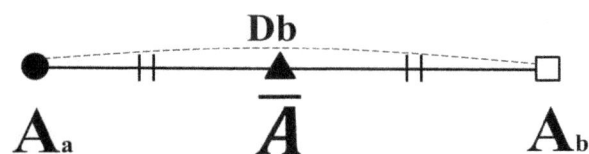

Figure 6. DB: Locating error (distance) of a landmark (A). $\overline{A}$ represents an averaged landmark of A.

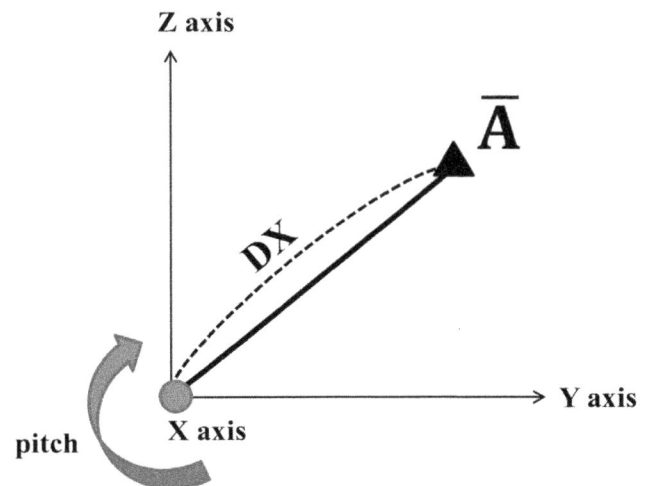

Figure 7. DX: Distance from X-axis to an averaged landmark.
($\overline{A}$) The rotated arrow around X axis represents pitch rotation

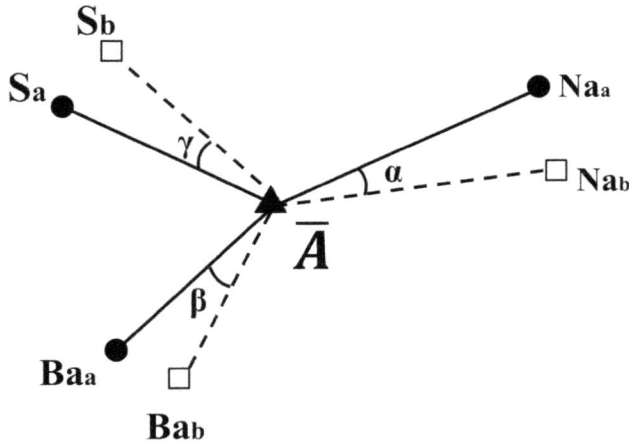

Figure 8. A3r: Sum of angle errors (S, Na, Ba) from an averaged landmark. $(\overline{A})$ α, β and γ represent angle errors viewed from an averaged landmark $(\overline{A})$ respectively.

most of the landmarks showed the largest locating errors on the x coordinates. These results can be assumed to have been produced due to defining of the cephalometric landmarks on lateral view without the consideration of the transversal plane.

Na, S, Ba used as reference landmarks generally showed good reproducibility.(Table 2 and 3) However, the S point tended to exhibit slightly higher locating error than Na and Ba. MLWS showed better reproducibility than Na, S, Ba in this study. The locating error of MLWS (mean 0.33, SD 0.22) was similar to the smallest locating error (mean 0.31, SD 0.19) of the upper left incisor in the study of Hassan et al. [9].

Plane orientation system for superimposition

Superimposition methods that use 3D anatomical landmarks or surface has recently become the focus of interest. [15,16] But when superimposition is made on bone surface landmarks or certain areas, the superimposition error increases as it gets further from the superimposition area or growth area.

Lagravère et al. [11] used 4 landmarks at the skull base, a stable structure, for carrying out plane orientation but a different superimposition method was used compared to this study. In this study, 4 landmarks were also used for plane orientation, but unlike the study above in which the new starting point was fixed on the new axes, the two were separated, making it a more flexible reorientation system.

If multiple landmarks are marked on the skull base, the results would be more accurate, but time consuming and clinically inefficient, making the reorientation system more complicated and harder to analyze statistically. So in this study, Na, S, Ba were used which have previously been used [17–19] or recommended [10] cephalometric landmarks in several studies, as reference points of axes set up. Also, the most accurate MLWS was used as the center of reorientation and made a plane reorientation system considering both efficiency and accuracy.

Reorientation error

Increased error after reorientation. After reorientating the landmarks which were positioned repeatedly at the same image in this study, reorientation error increased than locating error (Table 3). This is because every point, including the reference landmarks, differs whenever it is located, so the landmark at each trial is reoriented by different axes and origin.

Factors influencing reorientation error. In a previous study [11], factors influencing reorientation were mentioned as voxel size and locating error of the center point. This study showed voxel size imposes smallest measurement uncertainty (0.25 mm) that makes errors when determining reference points and planes. And those errors can produce up to 1 mm error after transformation in one axis of reference points. Ondemand 3D program could enlarge MPR images and measure up to second decimal number and therefore, was hardly influenced by voxel size.

Same study mentioned that as the errors which are imposed at origin increase, errors of reference points increase after transformation, but, in this study there was no further quantitative explanation except the increase is not directly proportional.

Until now, the factors that produce errors during reorientation using cephalometric landmarks have never been analyzed statistically. In this study, the plane orientation error was analyzed by multiple regression. When making this model, the understand-

Table 4. Variables included in multiple regression model.

	Independent variable	B	P value	VIF	Adjusted R-square
T1–T2	Db	0.412	0.000	1.013	0.230
	DX	0.015	0.000	1.436	
	A3r	0.242	0.038	1.447	
T1–T3	Db	0.677	0.000	1.024	0.153
	DX	0.018	0.000	1.507	
	A3r	0.614	0.002	1.485	
T2–T3	Db	0.866	0.000	1.022	0.297
	DX	0.022	0.000	1.342	
	A3r	0.657	0.000	1.322	
Total	Db	0.758	0.000	1.016	0.233
	DX	0.018	0.000	1.409	
	A3r	0.545	0.000	1.397	

Outliers outside 3 standard deviations are excluded in regression analysis, VIF: variance inflation factor.

ing of transformation was changed by analyzing axes change from a peripheral viewpoint (each landmark), rather than center perspective (origin and reference axes).

This linear regression model (1) could explain reorientation error (distance of a landmark after reorientation, Y) of this plane orientation system about 1/4 with 3 simple factors below.

First, Db stands for locating error of each landmark itself. As locating error before transformation (Db) increases 1 mm, reorientation error increases approximately 0.76 mm in this system. This explains that the locating error is reflected on the reorientation error up to approximately 76%.

Second, DX stands for vertical distance from reoriented x axis to each landmark. As DX increases 10 cm, reorientation error increases approximately 1.8 mm in this system. This means that mandibular chin area which is about 13 cm away from the newly set x axis can get approximately 2.3 mm reorientation error only due to its far location from reoriented x axis.

Third, A3r stands for shift of reference axes viewed from each landmark during two landmark determination trial. As one (1) degree of A3r from a point increases, reorientation error increases about 0.55 mm. This result shows that small axes shift can affect the reorientation error substantially.

This model shows that A3r with DX may have possibility to be 'position scalar' in a system which consists of limited number of points (eg. cephalometric analysis). A3r alone has the difficulty in explaining reorientation error. However, by analyzing A3r with DX, the approximate reorientation error can be predicted which is the outcome of vector transformation. This idea of 'position scalar' can be established because the locating error of reference landmarks is small enough to produce the unique value of A3r combine with DX.

Among the above values, if the accuracy of the landmarks including the reference could be improved, the Db & A3r value and the coefficient of DX would decrease, thereby reducing the reorientation error. However, in terms of the A3r value, assuming that Na, S, Ba are sufficiently accurate, the patient's anatomical structures are likely to have a greater impact than the locating error of those three points.

The hypothesis that the distance of each point from MLWS as well as the perpendicular distance from the reoriented y, z axes could have an effect on the amount of reorientation error has been denied through regression analysis.

Limitation of this study and works to be done

The selected Na, S, Ba points for the determination of the reorientation axes are positioned on the mid sagittal plane. Therefore, even though the location error of these points were relatively small, the pitch direction of the reoriented x axis will be the most greatly affected. This is the reason for the increase in reorientation error with increase in DX. In this model, the points with large DX can already be expected to have a large reorientation error; hence, accurate superimposition will be difficult to achieve. Thus, to promote clinical application, accurate setting of the reference landmarks will be required to reduce the value of the constant in front of DX, and further research will be needed to minimize the increase in reorientation error caused by DX.

As shown by the above data, a locating error of 1 mm on average may result in the increase of 0.76 mm in reorientation error. When the other two factors that affect the reorientation error are considered, further research necessitates the selection of accurate points with locating errors less than 1 mm.

The difference in adjusted R-square value between T1–T2, T1–T3 and T2–T3 can be explained by the low reproducibility of some of the landmarks that would have acted as outliers to weaken the explanation power of the regression model (table 4). This is another reason why this model can be considered limited yet for clinical application.

Future plane orientation exercises should utilize precise reference points rather than the well-known orthodontic landmarks. The highly precise reference points of this experiment include sharp points such as ANS and PNS, midpoints of two sharp points such as MLWS, as well as an end point of a protruding eminence such as Ba. Previous studies [11,20] indicate that center points of foramina are also highly precise points of reference. In further studies, regression models based on such precise reference points should be evaluated for its accuracy after CBCT image superimposition based on 4 point plane orientation.

Conclusions

In present study, 3D reproducibility of some widely used cephalometric points was not adequate for accurate evaluation of 4 point plane reorientation error. This model showed that locating error, vertical distance from reoriented x axis and shift of reference plane viewed from each landmark are important factors that explain the reorientation error.

Supporting Information

Table S1 Coordinates before and after reorientation (Sample Number 1).

Table S2 Coordinates before and after reorientation (Sample Number 2).

Table S3 Coordinates before and after reorientation (Sample Number 3).

Table S4 Coordinates before and after reorientation (Sample Number 4).

Table S5 Coordinates before and after reorientation (Sample Number 5).

Table S6 Coordinates before and after reorientation (Sample Number 6).

Table S7 Coordinates before and after reorientation (Sample Number 7).

Table S8 Coordinates before and after reorientation (Sample Number 8).

Table S9 Coordinates before and after reorientation (Sample Number 9).

Table S10 Coordinates before and after reorientation (Sample Number 10).

Table S11   Coordinates before and after reorientation (Sample Number 11).

Table S12   Coordinates before and after reorientation (Sample Number 12).

Table S13   Coordinates before and after reorientation (Sample Number 13).

Table S14   Coordinates before and after reorientation (Sample Number 14).

Table S15   Coordinates before and after reorientation (Sample Number 15).

Table S16   Coordinates before and after reorientation (Sample Number 16).

Table S17   Coordinates before and after reorientation (Sample Number 17).

Table S18   Coordinates before and after reorientation (Sample Number 18).

Table S19   Coordinates before and after reorientation (Sample Number 19).

Table S20   Coordinates before and after reorientation (Sample Number 20).

Acknowledgments

We are grateful to Dr. Jin Young Park, Yonsei University Dental Hospital for his helpful advice on the English grammar and graphical representation of this journal article.

Author Contributions

Conceived and designed the experiments: JJH. Performed the experiments: JJH. Analyzed the data: JJH HGJ HP CSP. Contributed reagents/materials/analysis tools: KDK HGJ HP CSP. Contributed to the writing of the manuscript: JJH HGJ KDK. Obtained ethics approval from the Institutional Review Board of Yonsei university dental hospital: JJH HGJ.

References

1. Hofrath H (1931) Importance of teleroentgenograms for diagnosis of maxillary abnormalities. J Orofac Orthop 1: 232–258.
2. Broadbent BH (1931) A new X-ray technique and its application to orthodontia. Angle Orthod 1: 45–66.
3. Gu Y, McNamara Jr JA (2008) Cephalometric superimpositions: A comparison of anatomical and metallic implant methods. Angle Orthod 78: 967–976.
4. Arat ZM, Rübendüz M, Akgül AA (2003) The displacement of craniofacial reference landmarks during puberty: A comparison of three superimposition methods. Angle Orthod 73: 374–380.
5. Berkowitz S (1999) A multicenter retrospective 3D study of serial complete unilateral cleft lip and palate and complete bilateral cleft lip and palate casts to evaluate treatment: Part 1 - The participating institutions and research aims. Cleft Palate Craniofac J 36: 413–424.
6. Seckel NG, Van der Tweel I, Elema GA, Specken TFJM (1995) Landmark positioning on maxilla of cleft lip and palate infant - A reality? Cleft Palate Craniofac J 32: 434–441.
7. Sachdeva R (2001) SureSmile technology in a patient-centered orthodontic practice. J Clin Orthod 35: 245–253.
8. Ashmore J, Kurland B, King G, Wheeler TT, Ghafari J, et al. (2002) A 3-dimensional analysis of molar movement during headgear treatment. Am J Orthod Dentofacial Orthop 121: 18–29.
9. Hassan B, Nijkamp P, Verheij H, Tairie J, Vink C, et al. (2013) Precision of identifying cephalometric landmarks with cone beam computed tomography in vivo. Eur J Orthod 35: 38–44.
10. Zamora N, Llamas JM, Cibrian R, Gandia JL, Paredes V (2012) A study on the reproducibility of cephalometric landmarks when undertaking a three-dimensional (3D) cephalometric analysis. Med Oral Patol Oral Cir Bucal 17: e678–688.
11. Lagravere MO, Major PW, Carey J (2010) Sensitivity analysis for plane orientation in three-dimensional cephalometric analysis based on superimposition of serial cone beam computed tomography images. Dentomaxillofac Radiol 39: 400–408.
12. Swennen G, Schutyser F, Barth E, De Groeve P, De Mey A (2006) A new method of 3-D cephalometry part I: The anatomic cartesian 3-D reference system. J Craniofac Surg 17: 314–325.
13. Zamora N, Llamas J, Cibrián R, Gandia J, Paredes V (2012) A study on the reproducibility of cephalometric landmarks when undertaking a three-dimensional (3D) cephalometric analysis. Med Oral Patol Oral Cir Bucal 17: e678-e688.
14. Lagravere MO, Low C, Flores-Mir C, Chung R, Carey JP, et al. (2010) Intraexaminer and interexaminer reliabilities of landmark identification on digitized lateral cephalograms and formatted 3-dimensional cone-beam computerized tomography images. Am J Orthod Dentofacial Orthop 137: 598–604.
15. Hoffmann J, Westendorff C, Leitner C, Bartz D, Reinert S (2005) Validation of 3D-laser surface registration for image-guided cranio-maxillofacial surgery. J Craniofac Surg 33: 13–18.
16. Kang SH, Kim MK, Kim JH, Park HK, Park W (2012) Marker-free registration for the accurate integration of CT images and the subject's anatomy during navigation surgery of the maxillary sinus. Dentomaxillofac Radiol 41: 679–685.
17. Maeda M, Katsumata A, Ariji Y, Muramatsu A, Yoshida K, et al. (2006) 3D–CT evaluation of facial asymmetry in patients with maxillofacial deformities. Oral Surg Oral Med Oral Pathol Oral Radiol Endod 102: 382–390.
18. Kitaura H, Yonetsu K, Kitamori H, Kobayashi K, Nakamura T (2000) Standardization of 3-D CT measurements for length and angles by matrix transformation in the 3-D coordinate system. Cleft Palate Craniofac J 37: 349–356.
19. Katsumata A, Fujishita M, Maeda M, Ariji Y, Ariji E, et al. (2005) 3D–CT evaluation of facial asymmetry. Oral Surg Oral Med Oral Pathol Oral Radiol Endod 99: 212–220.
20. Schlicher W, Nielsen I, Huang JC, Maki K, Hatcher DC, et al. (2012) Consistency and precision of landmark identification in three-dimensional cone beam computed tomography scans. Eur J Orthod 34: 263–275.

5

A Novel Mutation in the *RPE65* Gene Causing Leber Congenital Amaurosis and Its Transcriptional Expression *In Vitro*

Guoyan Mo[1], Qin Ding[2], Zhongshan Chen[2], Yunbo Li[3], Ming Yan[2], Lijing Bu[4], Yanping Song[2]*, Guohua Yin[5,6]*

1 China Key Laboratory of TCM Resource and Prescription, Hubei University of Chinese Medicine, Ministry of Education, Wuhan 430065, China, **2** Department of Ophthalmology, Wuhan General Hospital of Guangzhou Military Command, Wuhan 430070, China, **3** Beijing University of Chinese Medicine Third Affiliated Hospital, Beijing 100029, China, **4** Department of Biology, University of New Mexico, Albuquerque, NM, 87131, United States of America, **5** Department of Plant Biology and Pathology, Rutgers, The State University of New Jersey, New Brunswick, NJ, 08901, United States of America, **6** Wuhan Sheng Da An Biotech Service Co. Ltd., Wuhan, China

Abstract

The retinal pigment epithelium-specific 65 kDa protein is an isomerase encoded by the *RPE65* gene (MIM 180069) that is responsible for an essential enzymatic step required for the function of the visual cycle. Mutations in the *RPE65* gene cause not only subtype II of Leber congenital amaurosis (LCA) but also early-onset severe retinal dystrophy (EOSRD). This study aims to investigate a Chinese case diagnosed as EOSRD and to characterize the polymorphisms of the *RPE65* gene. A seven-year-old girl with clinical symptoms of EOSRD and her parents were recruited into this study. Ophthalmologic examinations, including best-corrected visual acuity, slit-lamp, Optical coherence tomography (OCT), and fundus examination with dilated pupils, were performed to determine the clinical characteristics of the whole family. We amplified and sequenced the entire coding region and adjacent intronic sequences of the coding regions of the *RPE65* gene for the whole family to explore the possible mutation. Our results demonstrate that the patient exhibited the typical clinically features of EOSRD. Her bilateral decimal visual acuity was 0.3 and 0.4 in the left and right eyes, respectively. Spectral-domain optical coherence tomography (SD-OCT) was used to assess the retinal stratification for the whole family. All together, we identified four mutations within the *RPE65* gene (c.1056G>A, c.1243+2T>A, c.1338+20A>C and c.1590C>A) in the patient. Among the four mutations, c.1056G>A and c.1338+20A>C had been reported previously and another two were found for the first time in this study. Her mother also carried the novel mutation (c.1243+2T>A). Either a single or a compound heterozygous or a homozygous one mutation is expected to cause EOSRD because mutations of *RPE65* gene usually cause an autosomal recessive disease. Therefore, we speculate that the c.1590C>A mutation together with the c.1243+2T>A mutation may cause the patient's phenotype.

Editor: Knut Stieger, Justus-Liebig-University Giessen, Germany

Funding: This research was funded by the National Science Foundation of Hubei Province of China [Grant No. 2013CFB069]. The funders had no role in study design, data collection and analysis, decision to publish, or preparation of the manuscript.

Competing Interests: Dr. Guohua Yin is employed as a research consultant by Wuhan Sheng Da An Biotech Service Co. Ltd.

* Email: songyanping@medmail.com.cn (YS); guohuayin1997@gmail.com (GY)

Introduction

Retinal pigment epithelium-specific 65 kDa protein (RPE65, GenBank accession No. NP000320.1) is an isomerase preferentially expressed in the retinal pigment epithelium (RPE) [1,2]. It is responsible for retinol isomerization and converts all-*trans* retinyl ester to 11-*cis* retinol in the visual cycle [3–5]. Previous research demonstrated that retinol isomerization was an essential enzymatic step required for functional vision [6,7]. RPE65 is a microsomal protein encoded by *RPE65* gene (MIM 180069), containing 14 coding exons and localizing in chromosome 1p31 [8]. Mutations in *RPE65* gene were primarily reported in patients with Leber congenital amaurosis (LCA, MIM204000). Now, 86 mutations have been identified in the *RPE65* gene in patients with LCA [9–33]; we summarize these mutations in Figure 1.

LCA, first described in 1869 by Leber T [34], is a severe congenital or early infant-onset form of inherited retinal dystrophy [35]. In general, LCA is defined as blindness within the first two years of life. Based on previous descriptions of patients with LCA, this disease has a wide spectrum of presentation such as early severe visual deficits in childhood, the oculo-digital sign (habitually rubbing or poking the eyes), refractive errors, heterogeneity in retinal appearance, macular atrophy, and optic nerve pallor [36]. In addition, congenital onset and amaurosis by the second year of life are features that define LCA. Early-onset severe retinal dystrophy (EOSRD) is one of phenotype of all *RPE65* mutations. Unlike LCA, EOSRD is characterized by an amaurosis in the second decade and later and leaves a vision of 0.3 at the two-year age. The EOSRD has several names: juvenile and early-onset retinitis pigmentosa, childhood-onset severe retinal dystrophy, and severe early childhood onset retinal dystrophy (SECORD) [37–40]. Many studies indicated that LCA was extremely genetically heterogeneous and was associated with more than 17 genes. Moreover, many mutations associated with the inheritance of

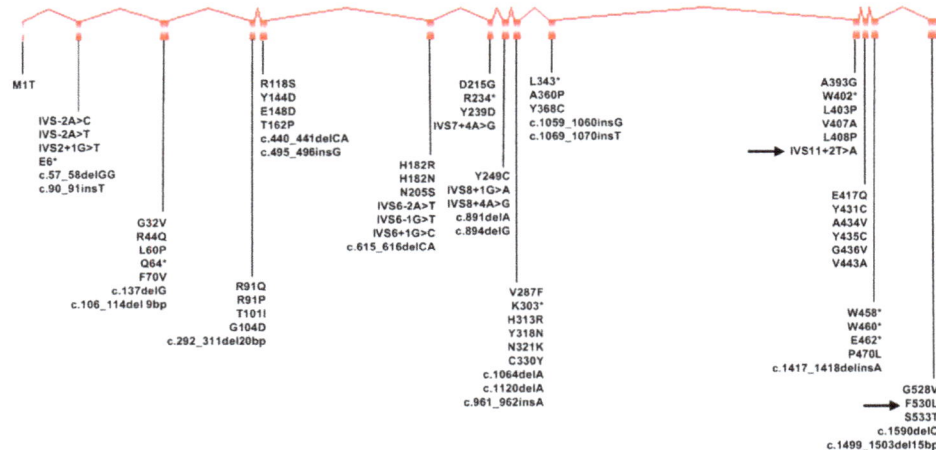

Figure 1. LCA related mutations in *RPE65* gene. The black arrow indicates the novel mutation discovered in this study.

LCA have been described and used to differentiate the subtypes of LCA1~15, for instance, *GUCY2D* (LCA1), *RPE65* (LCA2), *AIPL1* (LCA4), *RPGRIP1* (LCA6), *CRX* (LCA7), and *CRB1* (LCA8) (http://www.ncbi.nlm.nih.gov/omim). Among these known diseased-causing genes, *RPE65* mutations were first identified and their prevalence ranges from 1.7% to 16% in LCA cohorts in the United States, Canada, Saudi Arabia, Asia, and India [10,41,42]. To date, two cases of *RPE65* mutations with LCA have been reported in China [31,32], while most cases occur in Western populations. Notably, homozygous and compound heterozygous mutations in *RPE65* gene are associated with subtype II of LCA or EOSRD [37,43]. The description of EOSRD was coined for *RPE65* mutations.

In this study, we report the clinical examinations and genetic analysis of *RPE65* gene in a Chinese family. Sanger sequencing was used to analyze all the coding regions of the *RPE65* gene along with the adjacent intronic regions. Furthermore, we constructed the *RPE65* minigene containing the c.1243+2T>A mutation and investigated the effects of that mutation in *in vitro* splicing.

Materials and Methods

Clinical data and sample collection

This study was reviewed by the Department of Ophthalmology, Wuhan General Hospital of Guangzhou Military Command on Clinical Investigation and it conformed to the tenets of the Declaration of Helsinki. The seven-year-old girl and her family were referred to the Department of Ophthalmology, Wuhan General Hospital of Guangzhou Military Command on Clinical Investigation. After informed consent was obtained, all participants underwent six ophthalmologic examinations, including best-corrected visual acuity, slit-lamp, and fundus examination with dilated pupils to exclude infection or other diseases. Ophthamoscopic findings were recorded by color fundus photography. Optical coherence tomography (OCT, Topcon 3D-1000 Mark II, Tokyo Japan) was used to examine the retinal structure. Spectral-domain OCT (SD-OCT) recording with 3D macular protocol was performed with 6-mm single line scans over the fovea. In detail, the 3D macular protocol consists of a radial-scanning composed of 512×128 scan resolution covering an area of 6×6 mm in the macular region. The patient underwent fundus fluorescein angiography (FFA) and visual field examination. Clinical diagnosis

was based on the results of the above-mentioned ophthalmologic examinations.

Mutation identification

Blood samples were obtained by venipuncture and genomic DNA was extracted according to the manufacturer's protocol (TIANamp Blood DNA Kit, Tiangen) as described in our previous report [44]. For sequencing, the entire coding region and adjacent intronic sequences of 14 coding regions of the *RPE65* gene were amplified by PCR, using the primers in Table 1. PCR products were purified with the AxyPrep DNA Gel Extraction Kit (Axygen, CA, USA). All PCR products were bi-directionally sequenced with the dideoxy nucleotide chain terminator technique. Sequencing was performed on an automated sequencer – ABI 3730XL DNA Analyzer (ABI, USA). The results were assembled and analyzed using the Applied Biosystems Sequencing Analysis 5.2 software. Sequences were aligned with the published cDNA sequences of *RPE65* gene (GenBank accession no. NM_000329). We also assessed the potential functional consequences of nucleotide changes using multiple web servers for mutation analysis such as PolyPhen-2 (Polymorphism Phenotyping, http://genetics.bwh.harvard.edu/pph-2/) [45], SIFT (Sorting Intolerant From Tolerant, http://sift.jcvi.org/) [46], and Automated Splice Site and Exon Definition Analyses (http://splice.uwo.ca/) with default parameters.

Cell line and cell culture

The 293T cell line was purchased from the Type Culture Collection of the Chinese Academy of Sciences (Wuhan, China) and cultured in Dulbecco's modified Eagle's medium (DMEM, GIBCO) supplemented with 2 mM glutamine, 10% fetal calf serum (FBS, GIBCO), 100 UI/ml penicillin, and 100 μg/ml streptomycin sulfate. The Cells were maintained at 37°C in a 5% CO_2 incubator until confluent, then sub-cultured at 1:3 to 1:10 dilutions using trypsin-EDTA.

RPE65 minigene construction

RPE65 mutated minigenes (pCIneo-m65) were constructed by subcloning the c.1243+2T>A mutation from the patient into pCI-neo vector (Promega, Madison, WI). The wild-type minigene (pCIneo-65), without the c.1243+2T>A mutation, was generated by subcloning the genomic DNA of her father. PCR-amplified exons (11, 12, and 13) of the *RPE65* gene were inserted at the

Table 1. Primers used in the study.

Exons	Primers	Sequencing (5'→3')
2	RPE65–2F	GCAGGAGTGAACAGGCTTTG
	RPE65–2R	AGAGACGCCAAGGAATAGGAA
3	RPE65–3F	GAGGGCTGGAAATGAAAATC
	RPE65–3R	ACATTGTGAGAAGAAAGTGGGTA
4/5	RPE65–45F	GGTCACCCCAAGAAAGTGAG
	RPE65–45R	GGATTTGAAACTTAATGTGGCTC
6	RPE65–6F	AACTCAAGGTGAAAGAGGGTAGA
	RPE65–6R	AGAGAACTTGGACACTTGCTTTC
7–9	RPE65–789F	GGAGAAAATGAAAATAACCCCTC
	RPE65–789R	GAGTGCAGCAGCTCTGTAAAA
10	RPE65–10F	GAATAAAGAACAGGCAGGCACT
	RPE65–10R	TTGCTTTTGCTAAGTCACAGTAC
11–13	RPE65–1123F	CCTCCCTGCATGTTGACCT
	RPE65–1123R	GCTCCATCGTGACACCAAAT
14	RPE65–14F	ATGCCAGGTGGTACAAGAGTCA
	RPE65–14R	TGCTCAACTCAGTGCTTTCTGTA
	F1*	GTC**GAATTC**GTCACGCTCCCCAATACAAC
	R1*	GCA**GTCGAC**GATGGGTTCTGATGGGTATG
	F2*	CTCGTCAAGGAGAGATGATCTAGAGAAAACTTCACACGGGAG
	R2*	TCTCTAGATCATCTCTCCTTGACGAGGCCCTG

Notes: *denotes primers for amplification of the wild and mutant fragments of exons 11, 12, and 13 of RPE65 gene. Bold and underlined sequences are restriction enzyme sites.

*Eco*RI/*Sal*I restriction enzyme site in pCI-neo vector. Primers and conditions used in the PCR amplification of the inserts were listed in Table 1. The corresponding DNA inserts were confirmed by sequencing.

Transfection, RNA isolation, and RT-PCR

To analyze the effects of the c.1243+2T>A mutation on splicing *in vitro*, 293T cells were transfected with *RPE65* minigenes. Prior to transfection, cells were seeded with a density of 4.0×10^5 cells per well in a six-well plate and grown to approximately 80% confluence. *RPE65* minigene used in this study was transfected into cells with Lipofectamine 2000 reagent (Invitrogen) by using 2 μg of DNA per well. After 24 h transfection, cells were serum starved for another 24 h before harvest. Total RNA was extracted from cells using TRIzol reagent (Invitrogen) according to the manufacturer's instructions. DNase I (Promega) was used to treat the RNA extract to eliminate DNA contamination. 1.0 μg of treated RNA was used as a template for reverse transcription using the First Strand cDNA Synthesis Kit (TOYOBO). The exogenous *RPE65* minigene transcript was amplified using F1 and R1 primers (Table 1) and the fragment sizes of the wild and mutant PCR products were detected by 2% agarose gels electrophoresis and stained with ethidium bromide. To confirm the nucleotide sequences, the wild and mutant PCR products were purified from the gel and sent for sequencing.

Results

Clinical features

In this Chinese family, only the seven-year-old girl reported the typical characteristics of EOSRD. She was a primary school student. When she was three years old in 2008, her parents found she could not see toys in the dark, which meant her visual acuity was markedly decreased in dimmer conditions. Moreover, when she went inside from outdoor sunlight, her dark adaption took nearly two hours. In 2011, her eyesight problem made it difficult for her study at school. She was diagnosed as EOSRD by a full ophthalmologic examination in 2012. Her fundus examination demonstrated mildly attenuated retinal vessels, some whitish dots, and numerous grayish deposits in the mid-peripheral retina (Figure 2). However, no whitish dots or grayish deposits were observed on the fundi of her parents.

The SD-OCT scanning with 3D macular protocol was used to examine the retinal stratification. Compared with foveal SD-OCT scanning recordings of her parents' eyes, the patient's foveal SD-OCT images of both eyes showed several characteristics of alterd retinal stratification including extremely thinned outer nuclear layer (ONL), heavily thinned retinal pigment epithelial (RPE) layer, altered photoreceptor layers including external limiting membrane (ELM), inner segment (IS), outer segments (OS), and inner segment elipsoid (ISe) (Figure 3a and 3b). In her patients' grayscale SD-OCT recording (Figure 3 c-2, 3d-2, 3e-2, and 3f-2), the boundaries of the photoreceptor layers (ELM, IS, ISe, and OS) were not well demarcated. The enlargement of grayscale SD-OCT recordings at the fovea of her patients' eyes (Figure 3 c-3, 3d-1, 3e-3, and 3f-1) showed that the ELM, IS, ISe and OS layers were not continuous and could not be clearly identified, and the ISe layer previously named IS/OS junction could hardly be shown. In addition, the boundaries of OS/RPE and RPE-Bruch's membrane complex could not be discerned. But her parents' foveal SD-OCT recordings showed that the boundaries of the retinal layers were well demarcated and the retinal layers could be clearly identified

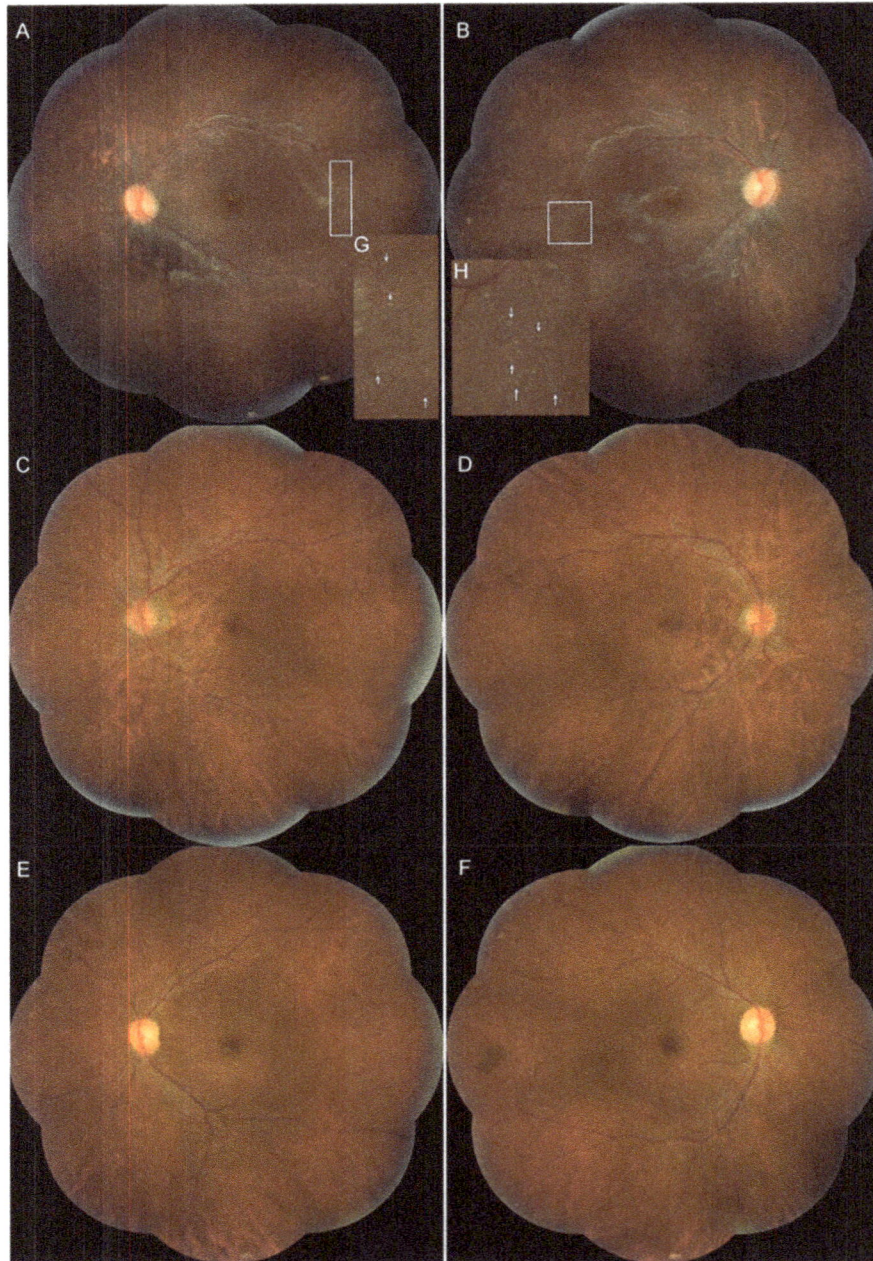

Figure 2. Fundus photographs of both eyes in the family. Color fundus photographs of both eyes (a: left eye; b: right eye) show mildly attenuated retinal vessels, some whitish dots, and numerous grayish deposits in the mid-peripheral retina of the patient. The inserted panels (g, h) show a magnification of the indicated areas. Whitish dots are marked by white arrowheads. Fundus photographs of her father (c, d) and her mother (e, f) show no whitish dots or grayish deposits in the mid-peripheral retina.

(Figure 3c-2, 3d-2, 3e-2, and 3f-2). The aforementioned abnormalities were not presented in her parents' grayscale foveal SD-OCT recordings (Figure 3 c-2, 3d-2, 3e-2, and 3f-2). Meanwhile, we also measured the thinkness of ISe, RPE, and RPE-choroid of the patient and her parents's right eyes (Figure 3g, 3h, and 3i). Her father/mother' results were 15 μm/15 μm (Figure 3h-2 and 3i-2), 16 μm/16 μm (Figure 3h-3 and 3i-3), and 40 μm/35 μm (Figure 3h-4 and 3i-4). Because the boundaries of IS, ISe, OS, and RPE are not clear, we cannot measure the thickness of ISe and RPE. Therefore, we measured the noncontiguous area of ISe

layer, RPE-choroid and ISe-choroid,and the results were 239 μm (Figure 3g-2), 24 μm (Figure 3g-3), and ISe-choroid (Figure 3g-4), respectively.

RPE65 gene mutation analysis

Based on the complete sequence analysis of the coding and adjacent intronic regions of *RPE65* gene, four mutations were detected in this family. These mutations included one missense, one silent, and two intronic changes. All mutations are listed in Table 2. All four mutations were present in the heterozygous state.

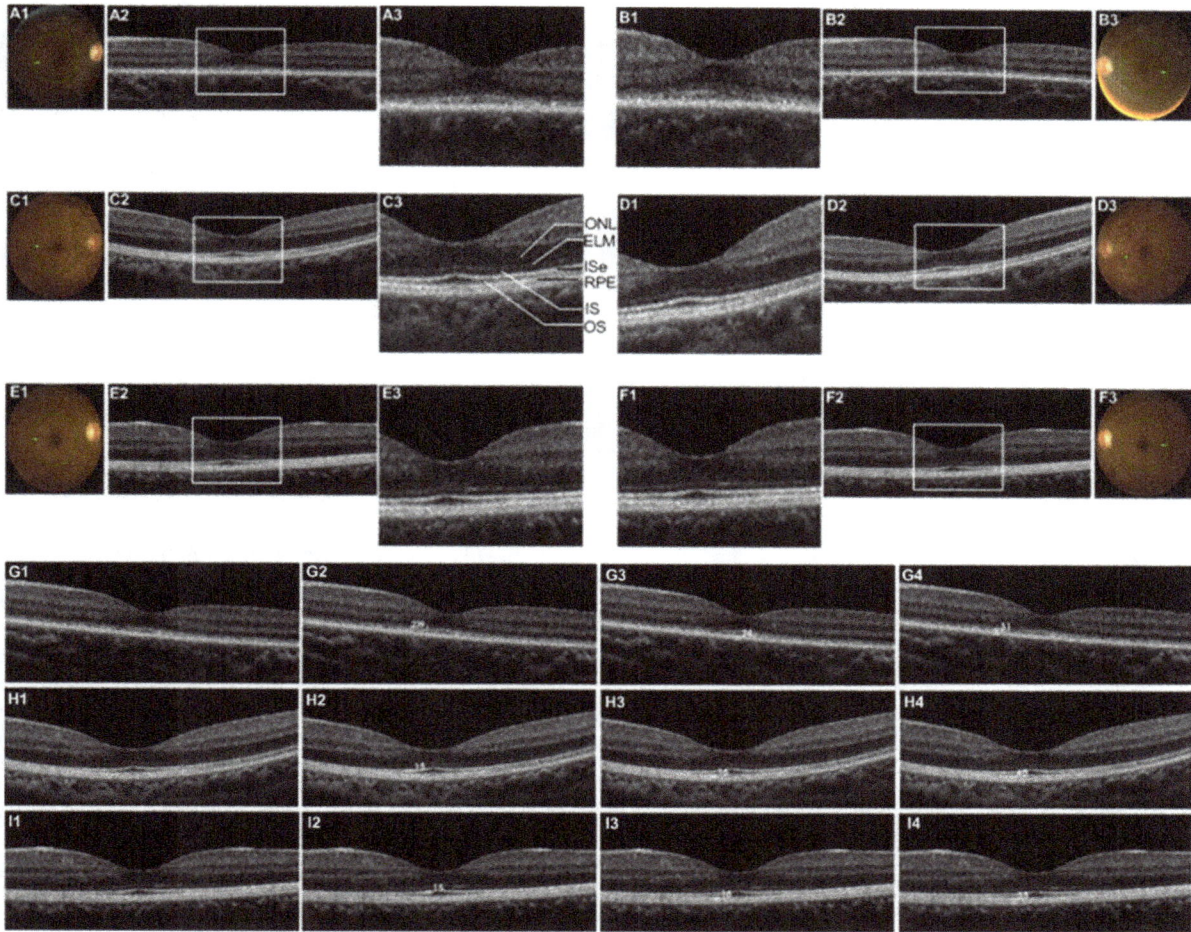

Figure 3. Foveal spectral-domain optical coherence tomography (SD-OCT) recordings of eyes in the whole family. The green circle in fundus photographies (a-1, b-3, c-1, d-3, e-1, and f-3) shows the scanning position of the presented SD-OCT recordings of the family using 3D macular protocol. Foveal SD-OCT pictures of the patients (a-2 and b-2) show abnormalities of retinal stratification including extremely thinned ONL (outer nuclear layer), heavily thinned RPE (retinal pigment epithelial) layer, altered photoreceptor layers (ELM, IS, ISe, and OS). The patient's grayscale SD-OCT recordings (a-2, and b-2) show that the boundaries of ELM, IS, ISe and OS layers are not well demarcated and the ISe layer could hardly be discerned. The white box in grayscale SD-recordings (a-2, b-2, c-2, d-2, e-2, and f-2) indicates the area of enlargement. The enlargement of grayscale SD-OCT recordings at the fovea of both eyes (a-3, and b-1) show that the ELM, IS, ISe and OS layers are not continuous. The abnormalities of retinal stratification are not present on the foveal SD-OCT recordings of her father (c and d) or mother (e and f). We measured the thickness of ISe, RPE, and RPE-choroid of the patient and her parents's right eyes (Figure 3g, 3h, and 3i). Her father/mother' results were 15 μm/15 μm (Figure 3h-2 and 3i-2), 16 μm/16 μm (Figure 3h-3 and 3i-3), and 40 μm/35 μm (Figure 3h-4 and 3i-4). Because the boundaries of IS, ISe, OS, and RPE are not clear, we measured the noncontiguous area of ISe layer, RPE-choroid and ISe-choroid,and the results were 239 μm (Figure 3g-2), 24 μm (Figure 3g-3), and ISe-choroid (Figure 3g-4), respectively.

The father carried only one point mutation (c.1338+20A>C, Figure 4), and the mother carried two point mutations (c.1243+2T>A and c.1338+20A>C, Figure 4). The daughter carried four mutant points: c.1338+20A>C (from her parents), c.1243+2T>A (from her mother), c.1056G>A, and c.1590C>A (Figure 4). Meanwhile, we also used mutiple web servers including PolyPhen, SIFT, and Automated Splice Site Analyses to perform the mutation analysis (Table 2). The loss of the splice site was predicted for the c.1243+2T>A mutation by Automated Splice Site Analyses; the c.1056G>A (rs12145904) mutation is predicted to be "benign" and "neutral" according to the results of PolyPhen and SIFT; the c.1590C>A (F530L) mutation is predicted to be "possibly damaging" and "deleterious" by PolyPhen and SIFT; the c.1338+20A>C (rs12564647) mutation cannot be evaluated by Polyphen and SIFT. The c.1338+20A>C (rs12564647) mutation

is listed in the SNP database of GenBank (http://www.ncbi.nlm.nih.gov/projects/SNP/snp_ref.cgi?rs=12564647).

Transcriptional expression of *RPE65* minigenes in 293T cells

To identify the effects of the c.1243+2T>A mutation in intron 11 of *RPE65* gene on splicing, we constructed two minigenes: the c.1243+2T>A mutation in *RPE65* gene (pCIneo-m65) and the wild type (pCIneo-65), and transfected them into 293T cell line. Total RNA was isolated from 293T cells transfected with the minigene constructs (Figure 5), and then used for RT-PCR to amplify the exons of 11, 12, and 13 of *RPE65* gene. PCR products indicating variations in splicing, were resolved and analyzed by a 2% agarose gel electrophoresis (Figure 6b). The RT-PCR product of the wild type showed a 264 bp DNA band, as the expected normal transcript (Figure 6a), but the mutant type produced a

Table 2. The *RPE65* gene mutations in the seven-year-old patient.

Variants Description				Computational Prediction		References or Annotations	Daughter or Parent
Nucleotide Change	Amino Acid Change	State	Conservation	PolyPhen/Splice Site	SIFT		
c.1056G>A	E352E	Hetero	No	benign	neutral	rs12145904, [33]	daughter
c.1243+2T>A	Splicing change	Hetero	N/A	Splicing site abolished	N/A	this study	daughter, mother
c.1338+20A>C	N/A	Hetero	N/A	N/A	N/A	rs12564647, [33]	daughter, mother, father
c.1590C>A	F530L	Hetero	Yes	possibly damaging	deleterious	this study	daughter

Abbreviation: Hetero - Heterozygous, N/A - Not applicable.

358 bp band (Figure 6a). It is 94 bp longer than the normal transcript of 264 bp (Figure 6b), indicating an insertion of the complete intron 11 (Figure 6a). Sequence analysis of the product revealed that 94 bp were indeed inserted at the 3′ end of exon 11. The sequence of the 94 bp insertion perfectly matched that of intron 11 in *RPE65* gene containing the c.1243+2T>A mutation. Interestingly, there was another smaller size DNA band (about 200 bp) in wild-type (Figure 6b) not present in mutant. This could be caused by mispriming. These results show that the novel mutation (c.1243+2T>A) may completely inactivate the original splice-donor site.

Conclusion and Discussion

In this study, we report the case of a girl clinically diagnosed as EOSRD in her family. This Chinese family were clinically and genetically characterized. The girl had obvious clinical characteristics of EOSRD; however, these characteristics were absent in the fundi of her parents. Clinically, OCT is an important auxiliary diagnosis method to provide in vivo visulization of intraretinal stratification. Disorders of retinal stratification is generally considered to be related with disease. Segmentation of retinal layers is important for diagnosis and analysis of desease [47,48]. In the grayscale foveal SD-OCT recordings, differences of retinal stratification were very extinct (Figure 3). Based on the method of retinal layers segmentation reported by Ehnes A *et al* [49], the patient's SD-OCT recordings at the foveal showed altered photoreceptor layers (ELM, IS, ISe, and OS). The boundaries of photoreceptor layers could not be clearly discerned (Figure 3a-2, 3a-3, 3b-1, and 3b-2), and the ELM, IS, ISe and OS layers were not continuous. The ISe, previously named IS/OS junction, could hardly be shown in the OCT. Therefore, we cannot measure the thickness of Ise and RPE; instead, we measured the noncontiguous area of Ise layer (Figure 3g-2), RPE-choroid (Figure 3g-3), and ISe-choroid (Figure 3g-4).

In addition, abnormalities of retinal stratification also included extremely thinned ONL and heavily thinned RPE layer (Figure 3a and 3b). These abnormalities proved the aforementioned relation of disease and retinal stratification disorder. But in her parents' foveal SD-OCT recordings, the retinal layers could be clearly identified (Figure 3c-2, 3c-3, 3d-1, 3d-2, 3e-2, 3e-3, 3f-1, and 3f-2), and meanwhile the thickness of ISe,RPE, and RPE-choroid could be measured (Figure 3h and 3i). This may be caused by autosomal recessive inheritance (Figure 4). It has been verified that the *RPE65* mutation causes EOSRD [9,37]. By analysis of mutations in *RPE65* gene in this case, we found that both the mother and the daughter have the mutation (c.1243+2T>A) at the consensus sequence of the splice donor. This mutation uniformly results in splicing errors [50] and is diseasing-causing. However, by ophthalmologic examination, only the daughter has obvious symptoms of EOSRD; we speculate that the daughter's phenotype may be associated with the combined effects of the c.1243+2T and c.1590C>A mutations.

The entire coding region and adjacent intronic regions of *RPE65* gene were sequenced. Four mutations were identified in the patient, two of which were found novel (c.1243+2T>A and c.1590C>A) and have not been reported before (Table 2). According to previous studies, mutations in *RPE65* gene could cause EOSRD. There are several mutant types in this study:- missense, nonsense, splicing site, deletion, insertion, and indel mutation. Eighty-six mutations of *RPE65* gene in patients with LCA have been reported in twenty-four published studies [9–32]. Two cases have been reported in 188 Chinese patients [31,32] containing nine point mutations were identified in *RPE65* gene.

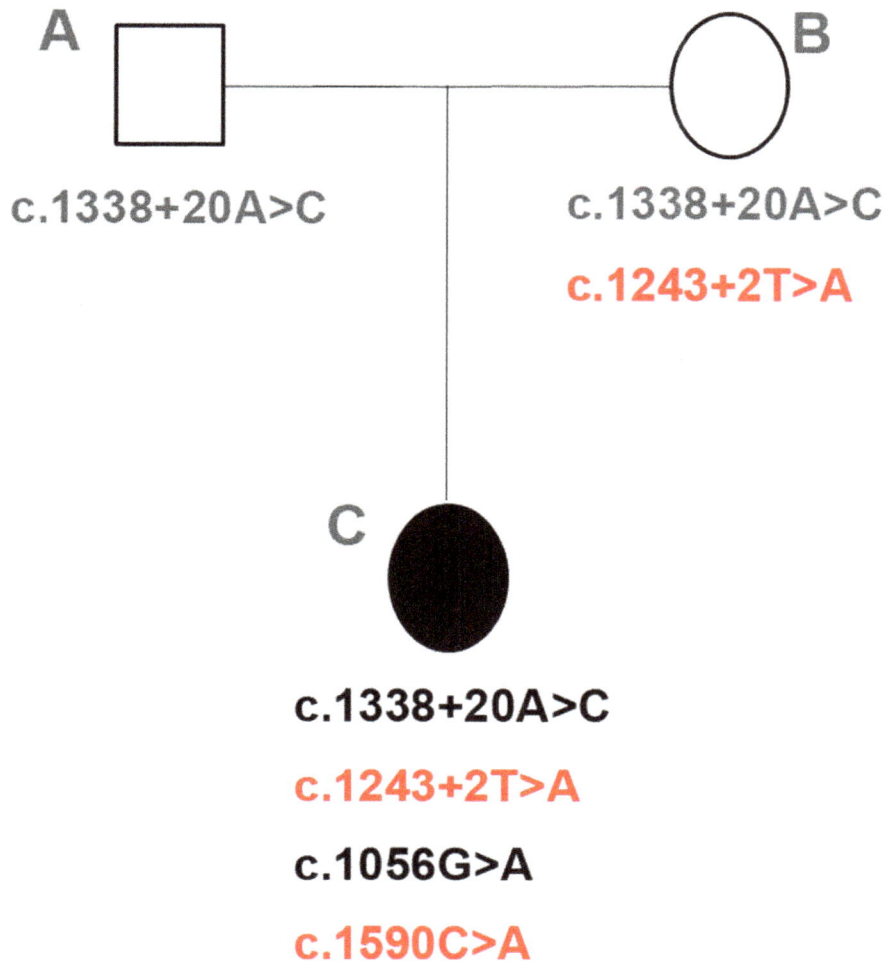

Figure 4. Pedigree of the Chinese family and mutations of *RPE65* gene. In the family structure, male and female are represented by squares and circles, respectively. The filled square symbol represents the ESORD-affected daughter (c). One mutation (c.1338+20A>C) is detected in *RPE65* gene of her father (a); two other mutations (c.1243+2T>A and c.1590C>A) are detected in her mother (b); four mutation are found in the daughter (a). The red color highlights the novel mutation.

These mutations were one insertion mutation (c.1059_1060insG) [51], four missense mutations (c.295G>A, c.997G>C, c.200 T>G, and c.1103A>G) [30,31], and four polymorphisms (c.643+22C>T, c.1338+20A>C, c.1056G>A, and c.*726_*727insAG) [31]. In this study, four mutations were found in the patient (Table 2), who carried two reported single nucleotide polymorphisms (SNPs) of c.1338+20A>C (rs12534647) and c.1056G>A (rs12145904) [32]. In the SNP database of GenBank, with benign allele was predicted for both c.1338+20A>C and c.1056G>A mutations.

Both c.1243+2T>A and c.1590C>A (F530L) are novel mutations and there are no previous reports. The c.1243+2T>A mutation is a point mutation at consensus sequences at the 5′ end of intron 11 of *RPE65* gene. It has been reported that mutations at consensus sequences uniformly result in aberrant splicing [50]. To confirm the effects of this mutation on splicing, we constructed *RPE65* minigene from three exons, containing either normal or mutant intron 11 sequences (Figure 5) and investigated their transcripts in 293T cell line by RT-PCR. A normal transcript consisting of three exons (264 bp) was obtained from the wild-type minigene (Figure 6a and b). For the mutant, the transcript is 358 bp in length that is longer than the normal transcript.

Sequence analysis showed that the mutant transcript is 94 bp longer than the normal transcript at the 3′ end of exon 11, whose sequence perfectly matches the sequences of intron 11 in *RPE65* gene containing the c.1243+2T>A mutation (Figure 6a and b). These results indicate that the c.1243+2T>A mutation results in aberrant splicing, which is consistent with the result of "splicing site abolised" by Automated Splice Site Analyses. Based on the result of *RPE65* minigene experiment *in vitro*, the c.1243+2T>A mutation may be pathogenic. Both the mother and the daughter had this mutation; however, the mother showed no symptoms of EOSRD. Since mutations of *RPE65* gene usually cause an autosomal recessive disease, either a single or a compound heterozygous or a homozygous mutation is expected to cause EOSRD. Therefore, the single heterozygous state of the c.1243+2T>A mutation in the mother does not rule out its pathogenicity.

The c.1590C>A change is the second novel mutation in this study. This mutation results in an amino acid transition from phenylalanine to leucine, but it is not detected in patient's parents. Based on an RPE65 topology diagram, the phenylalanine residue 530 in *RPE65* gene is conserved and located within blade VII of the seven-bladed β-propeller motif in the RPE65 protein [52]. Seven mutations found from LCA and RP patients are reported to

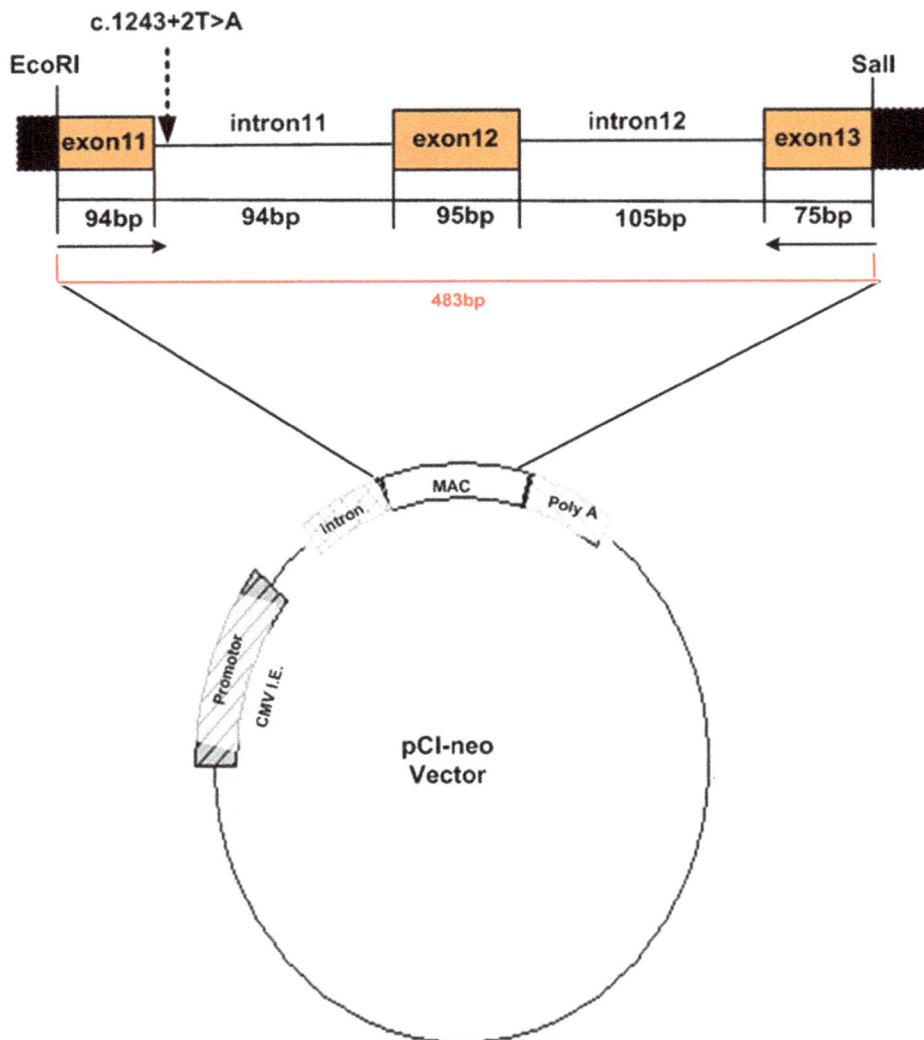

Figure 5. Structure of *RPE65* minigene. The pCIneo minigenes of *RPE65* gene were constructed to contain three exons (exon 11, 12, and 13) and flanking intronic sequences (intron 11 and 12) from wild or mutant type (c.1243+2T>A) of *RPE65* gene. *Eco*RI and *Sal*I represent restriction enzyme sites. Horizontal arrows indicate the positions and the directions of the primers. The red 483 bp indicates the amplified product.

be located within blade VII. They are L22P, P25L, G40S, R44Q, H68Y, Y79H, and G528V [14,15,17,24]. In our study, F530L (c.1590C>A) is found to be the eighth mutation in blade VII. Moreover, F530L and G528V are in the same sheet of blade VII. Both biochemical and crystal structure studies on RPE65 show that residues in any sheet of each blade of the propeller structure are essential for RPE65 isomerase activity [5,52,53]. In addition, the c.1590C>A (F530L) mutation was also analyzed by the online tools (PolyPhen and SIFT). The potential functional consequence of this nucleotide change was predicted to be "possibly damaging" and "deleterious". Therefore, the c.1590C>A (F530L) mutation could be responsible for the daughter's phenotype. It has also been verified to cause the pathogenesis of blade VII in *RPE65* gene, based on its isomerase activity and crystal structure [52,53]. If there were no other mutant genes involved in ESORD in this family, it could be concluded that this mutation played an important role in the pathogenesis of blade VII in *RPE65* gene.

From the above, we could infer that the c.1590C>A (F530L) mutation together with the c.1243+2T>A mutation is disease-causing mutation. However, *RPE65* is not the only gene associated with EOSRD. Although reports about mutations of the *RPE65* gene are mainly found in EOSRD patients, it is still difficult to say whether the daughter's phenotype is definitely caused by the two novel mutations, because the mother has one of these novel mutations and shows no symptoms of EOSRD. Either the c.1590C>A (F530L) mutation or other mutated genes in the daughter may be responsible for her phenotype. Thus, further studies should be performed to confirm if there is a definite genotype-phenotype correlation between *RPE65* gene and EOSRD.

Acknowledgments

We would like to thank the ophthalmologists at the Department of Ophthalmology in Wuhan General Hospital of Guangzhou Military Command for their help, and we also thank the patients for participation in this study. We deeply appreciate the time and critical comments of the editor and the two anonymous reviewers for improving the quality of this paper.

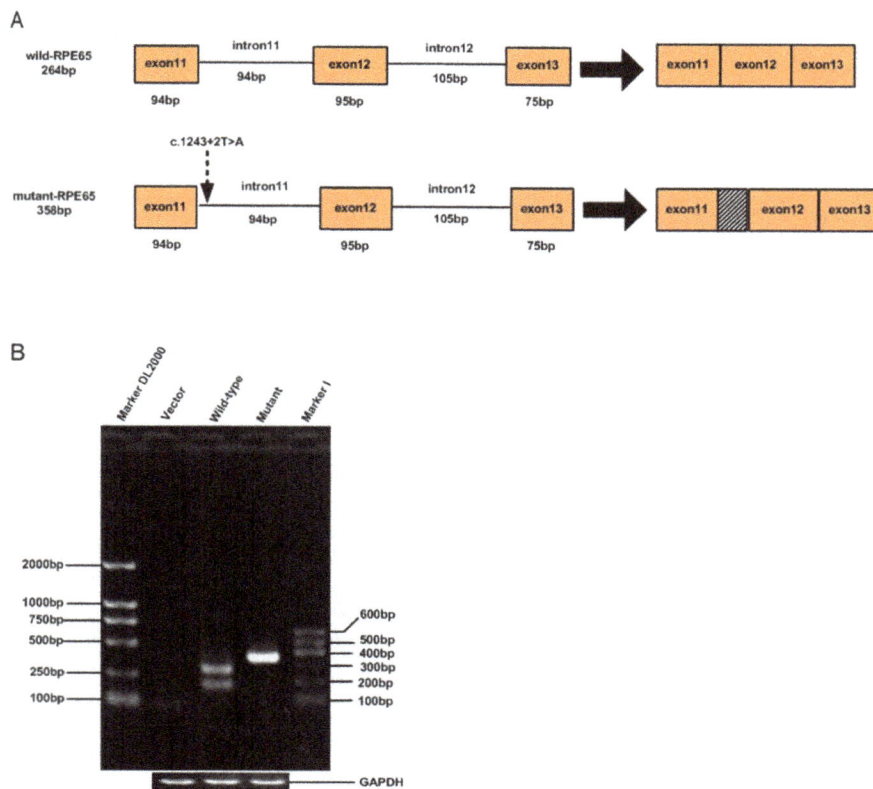

Figure 6. Analysis of pre-mRNA splicing of pClneo minigenes in the transfected 293T cell line. A. Graphic representation of pre-mRNA splicing of wild type and mutant (C.1243+2T>A) minigenes of *RPE65* gene. B. The isolated RNA of transfected cells was amplified by RT-PCR analysis. The different splicing products for wild type (264 bp) and mutant (358 bp) are shown on a 2% agarose gel. The mutant lane demonstrated that only a 358 bp band was obtained from the mutant-RPE65 minigene (a). The wild-type lane showed two different size DNA bands: one is a 264 bp band, and another is ~200 bp band. The 264 bp DNA band is the expected size (a). The 200 bp band is the amplification caused by mispriming.

Author Contributions

Conceived and designed the experiments: GYM YPS GHY. Performed the experiments: GYM. Analyzed the data: GYM GHY LJB QD. Contributed reagents/materials/analysis tools: GYM ZSC YBL MY. Wrote the paper: GYM YPS GHY.

References

1. Bavik CO, Busch C, Eriksson U (1992) Characterization of a plasma retinol-binding protein membrane receptor expressed in the retinal pigment epithelium. J Biol Chem 267: 23035–23042.
2. Hamel CP, Tsilou E, Harris E, Pfeffer BA, Hooks JJ, et al. (1993) A developmentally regulated microsomal protein specific for the pigment epithelium of the vertebrate retina. J Neurosci Res 34: 414–425.
3. Jin M, Li S, Moghrabi WN, Sun H, Travis GH (2005) Rpe65 is the retinoid isomerase in bovine retinal pigment epithelium. Cell 122: 449–459.
4. Moiseyev G, Chen Y, Takahashi Y, Wu BX, Ma JX (2005) RPE65 is the isomerohydrolase in the retinoid visual cycle. Proc Natl Acad Sci U S A 102: 12413–12418.
5. Redmond TM, Poliakov E, Yu S, Tsai JY, Lu Z, et al. (2005) Mutation of key residues of RPE65 abolishes its enzymatic role as isomerohydrolase in the visual cycle. Proc Natl Acad Sci U S A 102: 13658–13663.
6. Redmond TM, Yu S, Lee E, Bok D, Hamasaki D, et al. (1998) Rpe65 is necessary for production of 11-cis-vitamin A in the retinal visual cycle. Nat Genet 20: 344–351.
7. Woodruff ML, Olshevskaya EV, Savchenko AB, Peshenko IV, Barrett R, et al. (2007) Constitutive excitation by Gly90Asp rhodopsin rescues rods from degeneration caused by elevated production of cGMP in the dark. J Neurosci 27: 8805–8815.
8. Hamel CP, Jenkins NA, Gilbert DJ, Copeland NG, Redmond TM (1994) The gene for the retinal pigment epithelium-specific protein RPE65 is localized to human 1p31 and mouse 3. Genomics 20: 509–512.
9. Marlhens F, Bareil C, Griffoin JM, Zrenner E, Amalric P, et al. (1997) Mutations in RPE65 cause Leber's congenital amaurosis. Nat Genet 17: 139–141.
10. Morimura H, Fishman GA, Grover SA, Fulton AB, Berson EL, et al. (1998) Mutations in the RPE65 gene in patients with autosomal recessive retinitis pigmentosa or leber congenital amaurosis. Proc Natl Acad Sci U S A 95: 3088–3093.
11. Perrault I, Rozet JM, Ghazi I, Leowski C, Bonnemaison M, et al. (1999) Different functional outcome of RetGC1 and RPE65 gene mutations in Leber congenital amaurosis. Am J Hum Genet 64: 1225–1228.
12. Dharmaraj SR, Silva ER, Pina AL, Li YY, Yang JM, et al. (2000) Mutational analysis and clinical correlation in Leber congenital amaurosis. Ophthalmic Genet 21: 135–150.
13. Lotery AJ, Namperumalsamy P, Jacobson SG, Weleber RG, Fishman GA, et al. (2000) Mutation analysis of 3 genes in patients with Leber congenital amaurosis. Arch Ophthalmol 118: 538–543.
14. Thompson DA, Gyurus P, Fleischer LL, Bingham EL, McHenry CL, et al. (2000) Genetics and phenotypes of RPE65 mutations in inherited retinal degeneration. Invest Ophthalmol Vis Sci 41: 4293–4299.
15. Simovich MJ, Miller B, Ezzeldin H, Kirkland BT, McLeod G, et al. (2001) Four novel mutations in the RPE65 gene in patients with Leber congenital amaurosis. Hum Mutat 18: 164.
16. Sitorus RS, Lorenz B, Preising MN (2003) Analysis of three genes in Leber congenital amaurosis in Indonesian patients. Vision Res 43: 3087–3093.
17. Hanein S, Perrault I, Gerber S, Tanguy G, Barbet F, et al. (2004) Leber congenital amaurosis: comprehensive survey of the genetic heterogeneity, refinement of the clinical definition, and genotype-phenotype correlations as a strategy for molecular diagnosis. Hum Mutat 23: 306–317.
18. Al-Khayer K, Hagstrom S, Pauer G, Zegarra H, Sears J, et al. (2004) Thirty-year follow-up of a patient with leber congenital amaurosis and novel RPE65 mutations. Am J Ophthalmol 137: 375–377.

19. Zernant J, Kulm M, Dharmaraj S, den Hollander AI, Perrault I, et al. (2005) Genotyping microarray (disease chip) for Leber congenital amaurosis: detection of modifier alleles. Invest Ophthalmol Vis Sci 46: 3052–3059.
20. Jacobson SG, Aleman TS, Cideciyan AV, Sumaroka A, Schwartz SB, et al. (2005) Identifying photoreceptors in blind eyes caused by RPE65 mutations: Prerequisite for human gene therapy success. Proc Natl Acad Sci U S A 102: 6177–6182.
21. Galvin JA, Fishman GA, Stone EM, Koenekoop RK (2005) Evaluation of genotype-phenotype associations in leber congenital amaurosis. Retina 25: 919–929.
22. Yzer S, Leroy BP, De Baere E, de Ravel TJ, Zonneveld MN, et al. (2006) Microarray-based mutation detection and phenotypic characterization of patients with Leber congenital amaurosis. Invest Ophthalmol Vis Sci 47: 1167–1176.
23. Henderson RH, Waseem N, Searle R, van der Spuy J, Russell-Eggitt I, et al. (2007) An assessment of the apex microarray technology in genotyping patients with Leber congenital amaurosis and early-onset severe retinal dystrophy. Invest Ophthalmol Vis Sci 48: 5684–5689.
24. Simonelli F, Ziviello C, Testa F, Rossi S, Fazzi E, et al. (2007) Clinical and molecular genetics of Leber's congenital amaurosis: a multicenter study of Italian patients. Invest Ophthalmol Vis Sci 48: 4284–4290.
25. Stone EM (2007) Leber congenital amaurosis - a model for efficient genetic testing of heterogeneous disorders: LXIV Edward Jackson Memorial Lecture. Am J Ophthalmol 144: 791–811.
26. Jacobson SG, Cideciyan AV, Aleman TS, Sumaroka A, Schwartz SB, et al. (2007) RDH12 and RPE65, visual cycle genes causing leber congenital amaurosis, differ in disease expression. Invest Ophthalmol Vis Sci 48: 332–338.
27. den Hollander AI, Lopez I, Yzer S, Zonneveld MN, Janssen IM, et al. (2007) Identification of novel mutations in patients with Leber congenital amaurosis and juvenile RP by genome-wide homozygosity mapping with SNP microarrays. Invest Ophthalmol Vis Sci 48: 5690–5698.
28. Jacobson SG, Cideciyan AV, Aleman TS, Sumaroka A, Windsor EA, et al. (2008) Photoreceptor layer topography in children with leber congenital amaurosis caused by RPE65 mutations. Invest Ophthalmol Vis Sci 49: 4573–4577.
29. Jacobson SG, Aleman TS, Cideciyan AV, Roman AJ, Sumaroka A, et al. (2009) Defining the residual vision in leber congenital amaurosis caused by RPE65 mutations. Invest Ophthalmol Vis Sci 50: 2368–2375.
30. McKibbin M, Ali M, Mohamed MD, Booth AP, Bishop F, et al. (2010) Genotype-phenotype correlation for leber congenital amaurosis in Northern Pakistan. Arch Ophthalmol 128: 107–113.
31. Li L, Xiao X, Li S, Jia X, Wang P, et al. (2011) Detection of variants in 15 genes in 87 unrelated Chinese patients with Leber congenital amaurosis. PLoS One 6: e19458.
32. Xu F, Dong Q, Liu L, Li H, Liang X, et al. (2012) Novel RPE65 mutations associated with Leber congenital amaurosis in Chinese patients. Mol Vis 18: 744–750.
33. Verma A, Perumalsamy V, Shetty S, Kulm M, Sundaresan P (2013) Mutational screening of LCA genes emphasizing RPE65 in South Indian cohort of patients. PLoS One 8: e73172.
34. Leber T (1869) Ueber Retinitis pigmentosa und angeborene Amaurose. Archiv für Ophthalmologie 15: 1–25.
35. Leber T (1871) Ueber hereditäre und congenital-angelegte Sehnervenleiden. Albrecht von Graefes Archiv für Ophthalmologie 17: 249–291.
36. Hufnagel RB, Ahmed ZM, Correa ZM, Sisk RA (2012) Gene therapy for Leber congenital amaurosis: advances and future directions. Graefes Arch Clin Exp Ophthalmol 250: 1117–1128.
37. Gu SM, Thompson DA, Srikumari CR, Lorenz B, Finckh U, et al. (1997) Mutations in RPE65 cause autosomal recessive childhood-onset severe retinal dystrophy. Nat Genet 17: 194–197.
38. Foxman SG, Heckenlively JR, Bateman JB, Wirtschafter JD (1985) Classification of congenital and early onset retinitis pigmentosa. Arch Ophthalmol 103: 1502–1506.
39. Lorenz B, Gyurus P, Preising M, Bremser D, Gu S, et al. (2000) Early-onset severe rod-cone dystrophy in young children with RPE65 mutations. Invest Ophthalmol Vis Sci 41: 2735–2742.
40. Lorenz B, Poliakov E, Schambeck M, Friedburg C, Preising MN, et al. (2008) A comprehensive clinical and biochemical functional study of a novel RPE65 hypomorphic mutation. Invest Ophthalmol Vis Sci 49: 5235–5242.
41. Li Y, Wang H, Peng J, Gibbs RA, Lewis RA, et al. (2009) Mutation survey of known LCA genes and loci in the Saudi Arabian population. Invest Ophthalmol Vis Sci 50: 1336–1343.
42. Mamatha G, Srilekha S, Meenakshi S, Kumaramanickavel G (2008) Screening of the RPE65 gene in the Asian Indian patients with leber congenital amaurosis. Ophthalmic Genet 29: 73–78.
43. Klein D, Mendes-Madeira A, Schlegel P, Rolling F, Lorenz B, et al. (2014) Immuno-histochemical analysis of rod and cone reaction to RPE65 deficiency in the inferior and superior canine retina. PLoS One 9: e86304.
44. Song Y, Mo G, Yin G (2013) A novel mutation in the CYP4V2 gene in a Chinese patient with Bietti's crystalline dystrophy. Int Ophthalmol 33: 269–276.
45. Adzhubei IA, Schmidt S, Peshkin L, Ramensky VE, Gerasimova A, et al. (2010) A method and server for predicting damaging missense mutations. Nat Methods 7: 248–249.
46. Ng PC, Henikoff S (2001) Predicting deleterious amino acid substitutions. Genome Res 11: 863–874.
47. Hood DC, Lin CE, Lazow MA, Locke KG, Zhang X, et al. (2009) Thickness of receptor and post-receptor retinal layers in patients with retinitis pigmentosa measured with frequency-domain optical coherence tomography. Invest Ophthalmol Vis Sci 50: 2328–2336.
48. Hood DC, Lazow MA, Locke KG, Greenstein VC, Birch DG (2011) The transition zone between healthy and diseased retina in patients with retinitis pigmentosa. Invest Ophthalmol Vis Sci 52: 101–108.
49. Ehnes A, Wenner Y, Friedburg C, Preising MN, Bowl W, et al. (2014) Optical Coherence Tomography (OCT) Device Independent Intraretinal Layer Segmentation. Transl Vis Sci Technol 3: 1.
50. Nakai K, Sakamoto H (1994) Construction of a novel database containing aberrant splicing mutations of mammalian genes. Gene 141: 171–177.
51. Bereta G, Kiser PD, Golczak M, Sun W, Heon E, et al. (2008) Impact of retinal disease-associated RPE65 mutations on retinoid isomerization. Biochemistry 47: 9856–9865.
52. Kiser PD, Golczak M, Lodowski DT, Chance MR, Palczewski K (2009) Crystal structure of native RPE65, the retinoid isomerase of the visual cycle. Proc Natl Acad Sci U S A 106: 17325–17330.
53. Takahashi Y, Moiseyev G, Chen Y, Ma JX (2005) Identification of conserved histidines and glutamic acid as key residues for isomerohydrolase activity of RPE65, an enzyme of the visual cycle in the retinal pigment epithelium. FEBS Lett 579: 5414–5418.

6

Myocardial Metastases on 6-[^{18}F] fluoro-L-DOPA PET/CT: A Retrospective Analysis of 116 Serotonin Producing Neuroendocrine Tumour Patients

Walter Noordzij[1]*, **André P. van Beek**[2], **René A. Tio**[3], **Anouk N. van der Horst-Schrivers**[2], **Elisabeth G. de Vries**[4], **Bram van Ginkel**[5], **Annemiek M. Walenkamp**[4], **Andor W. Glaudemans**[1], **Riemer H. Slart**[1], **Rudi A. Dierckx**[1]

1 Department of Nuclear Medicine and Molecular Imaging, University of Groningen, University Medical Center Groningen, Groningen, The Netherlands, **2** Department of Endocrinology, University of Groningen, University Medical Center Groningen, Groningen, The Netherlands, **3** Department of Cardiology, University of Groningen, University Medical Center Groningen, Groningen, The Netherlands, **4** Department of Medical Oncology, University of Groningen, University Medical Center Groningen, Groningen, The Netherlands, **5** Faculty of Medicine, University of Groningen, University Medical Center Groningen, Groningen, The Netherlands

Abstract

Purpose: This study evaluates the prevalence of cardiac metastases in patients with serotonin producing neuroendocrine tumours (NET), examined with ^{18}F-FDOPA PET/CT, and the relationship of these metastases to the presence of carcinoid heart disease (CHD) based on echocardiography.

Background: CHD occurs in patients with serotonin producing NET. The diagnostic method of choice remains echocardiography. The precise prevalence of cardiac metastases is unknown given the limitations of standard technologies. Nuclear medicine modalities have the potential to visualize metastases of NET.

Methods: All patients who underwent ^{18}F-FDOPA PET/CT because of serotonin producing NET between November 2009 and May 2012 were retrospectively analyzed. The presence of cardiac metastasis was defined as myocardial tracer accumulation higher than the surrounding physiological myocardial uptake. Laboratory tests and transthoracic echocardiography (TTE) results were digitally collected.

Results: 116 patients (62 male) underwent ^{18}F-FDOPA PET/CT, mean age was 61±13 years. TTE was performed in 79 patients. Cardiac metastases were present in 15 patients, of which 10 patients also underwent TTE. One patient had both cardiac metastasis (only on ^{18}F-FDOPA PET/CT) and echocardiographic signs of CHD. There were no differences in echocardiographic parameters for CHD between patients with and without cardiac metastases. TTE in none of the 79 patients showed cardiac metastases.

Conclusion: The prevalence of cardiac metastases detected with ^{18}F-FDOPA PET/CT in this study is 13%. ^{18}F-FDOPA PET/CT can visualize cardiac metastases in serotonin producing NET patients. There appears to be no relationship between the presence of cardiac metastases and TTE parameters of CHD.

Editor: Carmine Pizzi, University of Bologna, Italy

Funding: The authors have no support or funding to report.

Competing Interests: The authors have declared that no competing interests exist.

* Email: w.noordzij@umcg.nl

Introduction

Neuroendocrine tumours (NET) are rare but well-defined neuroendocrine malignancies, with a low worldwide incidence; approximately 1–2 per 100,000 persons [1]. Nuclear medicine modalities and three-phase CT scans are the cornerstones in clinical staging of NET [1]. Indium-111 (^{111}In) labelled pentetreotide scintigraphy (SRS, planar whole body scan with or without additional single photon emission computed tomography and CT (SPECT/CT)) and gallium-68 (^{68}Ga) labelled (DOTA-Phe-Tyr)-octreotide (DOTATOC) positron emission tomography (PET) are both used to visualize somatostatin receptor density. 6-[^{18}F]fluoro-L-DOPA (^{18}F-FDOPA) uptake in NET is analogous to the uptake of amine precursors in these tumours. The overall sensitivity of ^{18}F-FDOPA PET/CT for the detection of (metastatic) NET lesions is higher than that of SRS [2]. All these nuclear medicine modalities have the potential to visualize tracer uptake in myocardial metastases in patient with NET [3,4].

NET of the small bowel frequently produces serotonin which, in case of metastatic disease, may lead to carcinoid syndrome, consisting of diarrhoea, flushing and carcinoid heart disease (CHD). CHD, present in up to 60% of patients with carcinoid syndrome, is characterized by plaque-like endocardial deposits of fibrous tissue on the ventricular aspect of the tricuspid valve leaflets, the arterial side of the pulmonary valve cusps, but also in the right atrium, and right ventricle [5,6]. This plaque formation and subsequent endocardial thickening eventually result in valve dysfunction [7]. Tricuspid valve involvement usually leads to regurgitation, whereas pulmonary valve involvement rather results into stenosis. Despite the indolent character of CHD, it is associated with a worse clinical outcome, especially when developing into heart failure [7].

Echocardiography is the modality of choice for diagnosing CHD [8,9]. Characteristic findings consist of thickening of leaflets/cusps that become retracted and eventually immobile, leading to the combination of valvular regurgitation and stenosis. Myocardial metastases are sometimes considered as a feature of CHD. However, these metastases are not always detected with echocardiography, and do not necessarily lead to typical valve dysfunction [10,11]. The prevalence of cardiac NET metastases is still not well established, partly due to lacking literature. Only few studies report on cardiac metastases, with a prevalence of 4% [12]. This is possibly an underestimation, partly due to low sensitivity of conventional imaging modalities.

The purpose of this retrospective study was to establish the prevalence of cardiac metastases in patients with serotonin producing NET, detected by ^{18}F-FDOPA PET/CT, and its relationship with the presence of echocardiography based CHD.

Patients and Methods

All patients who were referred to the Department of Nuclear Medicine and Molecular Imaging for an ^{18}F-FDOPA PET/CT between November 2009 and May 2012, were retrospectively analyzed. Selected were patients with serotonin producing NET based on elevated urinary 5-hydroxyindole acetic acid (5-HIAA, upper reference limit 3.8 mmol/mol creatinine) and elevated serotonin in platelets (upper reference limit 5.4 nmol/10^9 platelets). Serum creatinine level was used to determine the estimated glomerular filtration rate (eGFR). Presence of chronic kidney disease (CKD) was based on the Kidney Disease Outcomes Quality Initiative CKD classification [13].

Previous medical history was retrieved from the electronic patient chart, especially history of hypertension (defined as either systolic pressure higher than 140 mmHg, diastolic pressure higher than 90 mm Hg, or the use of anti-hypertensive medication), atrial fibrillation (AF) and myocardial infarction. Electrocardiograms (ECG) at the time point of the ^{18}F-FDOPA PET/CT scan (±3 months) were collected from the electronic patient chart, when available. ECGs were re-evaluated regarding rhythm, heart rate, QRS axis, PQ interval, QRS duration, presence of bundle branch block, QTc interval and STT segments. Transthoracic echocardiography (TTE) findings at the same time point were collected from the local digital archive of the Department of Cardiology of our hospital. Patients were followed until May 2013: one year after the ^{18}F-FDOPA PET/CT scan of the last included patient. Information on cardiac events (either myocardial infarction, or sudden cardiac death) or death during follow-up was retrieved from the electronic chart. This study was approved by the Institutional Ethics Review Board (name: 'medisch ethische toetsingscommissie' of the University Medical Center Groningen). According to the Dutch law, no additional informed consent was required. Patient information was anonymized and de-identified before data analysis.

^{18}F-FDOPA PET/CT scanning

All patients fasted for at least 6 hours and were allowed to continue all medication. Whole-body (from top of the skull through midthigh) three-dimensional PET images were acquired 60 minutes after intravenous administration of a standard dose of 200 MBq ^{18}F-FDOPA on a Biograph mCT (Siemens Medical Systems, Knoxville, TN, USA). ^{18}F-FDOPA PET/CT scans were performed with a mean amount of 140±15.5 mg carbidopa premedication, and mean administered activity of 186±39.8 MBq ^{18}F-FDOPA. Acquisition was performed in 7 bed positions of 2 minutes emission scan for patients 60–90 kg. Patient with body weight less than 60 kg and more than 90 kg body weight, were scanned with 1 minute and 3 minutes per bed position, respectively. Low dose transmission CT was used for attenuation correction. For the reduction of tracer decarboxylation and subsequent renal clearance, all patients received 2 mg/kg carbidopa (with a maximum of 150 mg) orally as pre-treatment, 1 hour before the ^{18}F-FDOPA injection, to decrease peripheral uptake and to increase tracer accumulation in tumor cells. Low dose CT and ^{18}F-FDOPA PET scans were automatically fused by use of three-dimensional fusion software (Siemens) with manual fine adjustments. All scans were interpreted by well trained nuclear medicine physicians as part of routine care. For this study, all scans were retrospectively analyzed for the presence of myocardial metastases.

Raw data were reconstructed through ultra high definition (Siemens) and guidelines based standardized algorithms [14,15], for visual assessment and standardized uptake value (SUV) calculations, respectively. Focal left and/or right ventricle ^{18}F-FDOPA uptake higher than the surrounding physiological myocardial uptake was considered abnormal, and thus suspicious for cardiac metastases.

Transthoracic echocardiography

The following variables were measured according to standard recommendations in the M-mode transthoracic echocardiographic examination: left ventricular internal end-diastolic and end-systolic dimensions, inter-ventricular wall thickness and left ventricular posterior wall thickness at end-diastole. An eyeballing left ventricular ejection fraction (LVEF) >55% was considered to be normal, between 55% and 40% mildly disturbed, between 30% and 40% moderately disturbed, and <30% was considered to represent a severely impaired systolic function.

Serotonin induced cardiac involvement was defined as tricuspid or pulmonary valvular dysfunction (i.e. valve leaflet thickening, shortening, retraction, hypomobility, or incomplete coaptation) associated with regurgitation or stenosis [16,17]. Pulmonary valve

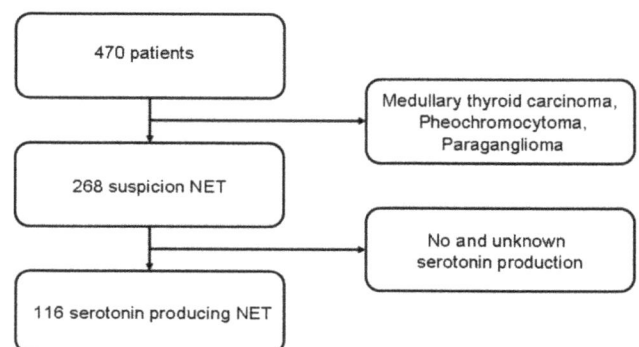

Figure 1. CONSORT diagram.

Table 1. Characteristics of all patients, and patients with and without abnormal cardiac ^{18}F-FDOPA uptake.

Parameter	All patients		No cardiac metastases		Cardiac metastases		p-value
	N (%)	Mean ± SD, or median (range)	N (%)	Mean ± SD, or median (range)	N (%)	Mean ± SD, or median (range)	
Age (y)	116 (100)	64±9.3	101 (87)	64±8.5	15 (13)	67±8.1	NS
Male patients	62 (53)		55 (54)		7 (47)		NS
History of							
- Hypertension	48 (41)		39 (39)		9 (60)		NS
- Atrial fibrillation	3 (3)		2 (1)		0		NS
- Myocardial infarction	7 (6)		6 (6)		1 (7)		NS
Cardiac medication							
- β blocker	34 (29)		28 (28)		6 (40)		NS
- Angiotensin converting enzyme inhibitor	18 (16)		16 (16)		2 (13)		NS
- Diuretic	21 (18)		15 (15)		6 (40)		0.021
- Angiotensin II antagonist	9 (8)		8 (8)		1 (7)		NS
- Statin	28 (24)		25 (25)		3 (20)		NS
- Calcium channel blocker	12 (10)		9 (9)		3 (20)		NS
Laboratory tests	116 (100)		101 (87)		15 (13)		
Serum							
- Creatinine (μmol/L)	114 (98)	84±29	99 (98)	84±30	15 (100)	80±6	NS
- Estimated glomerular filtration rate (mL/min/1.73 m²)	114 (98)	77±20	99 (98)	78±21	15 (100)	72±18	NS
- Chromogranin A (μg/L)	116 (100)	185 (29.0–44.6×10³)	101 (100)	168 (29.0–44.6×10³)	15 (100)	320 (48.0–19.1×10³)	NS
- Platelet serotonin (nmol/10⁹)	116 (100)	18 (3.8–58)	101 (100)	17 (3.8–48)	15 (100)	20 (8.2–58)	NS
Urine							
- Serotonin (μmol/mol creatinine)	98 (84)	69 (16–1.2×10³)	89 (88)	67 (16–1.2×10³)	9 (60)	96 (36–4.3×10²)	NS
- 5-Hydroxyindole acetic acid (mmol/mol creatinine)	110 (95)	8.5 (1.8–3.9×10²)	96 (95)	7.3 (1.8–2.3×10²)	14 (93)	11 (3.2–3.9×10²)	NS
Electrocardiography	60 (52)		51 (50)		9 (60)		
- Heart rate (bpm)	60 (100)	68±17	51 (100)	68±17	9 (100)	67±24	NS
- Sinus rhythm	58 (97)		50 (98)		8 (89)		NS
- Atrial fibrillation (n)	2 (3)		1 (1)		1 (11)		NS
- PQ duration (ms)	58 (97)	158±23	50 (98)	157±22.6	8 (89)	162±23.2	NS
- QRS duration (ms)	60 (100)	90±15	51 (100)	90±15	9 (100)	93±10	NS
- QTc duration (ms)	60 (100)	416±28	51 (100)	416±29.0	9 (100)	420±25.0	NS

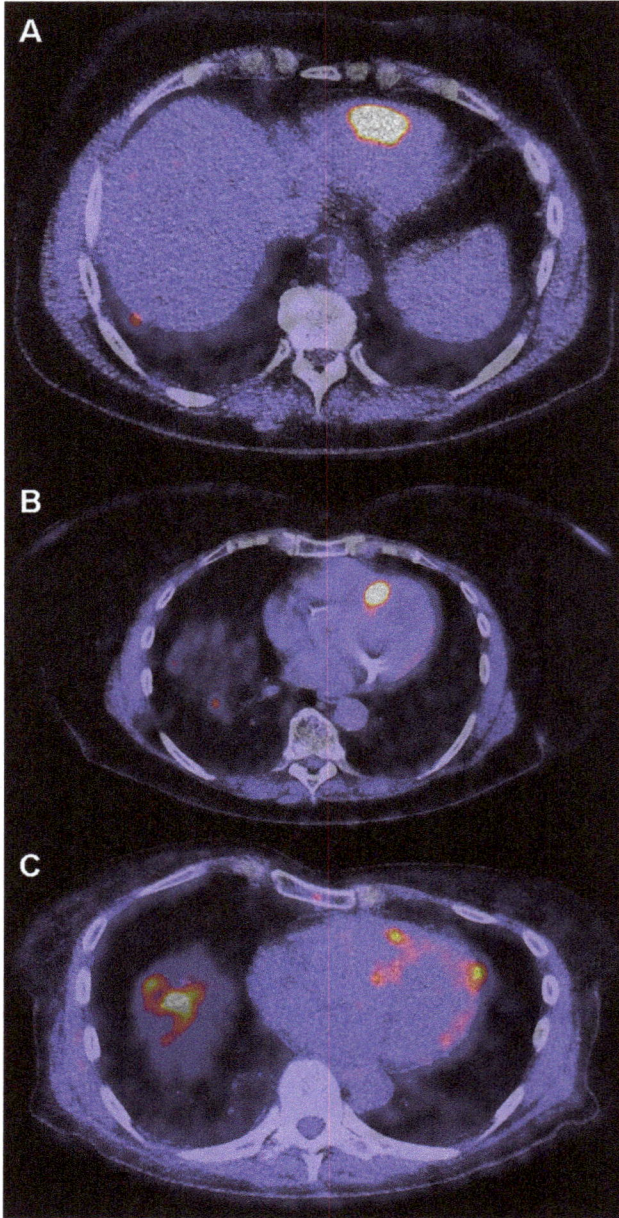

Figure 2. Three fusion images of ^{18}**F-FDOPA PET/CT scan in three different patients, indicating cardiac metastases.** A: Intense tracer accumulation in the apex of the right ventricle wall. B: Intense uptake in the inter-ventricular septum. C: One lesion in the apex of both the left and right ventricle, with physiological uptake in the rest of the myocardium. The more diffuse and intense uptake projected in the basal part of the right lung is actually located in large liver metastases.

(PV) stenosis (peak gradient across the valve) was graded as mild (<25 mmHg), moderate (25 to 50 mmHg), or severe (>50 mmHg). Tricuspid valve (TV) stenosis (mean gradient across the valve) was graded as mild (0 to 5 mmHg), moderate (5 to 8 mmHg), or severe (>8 mmHg) [18]. Tricuspid annular plane systolic excursion (TAPSE) was measured by M-mode echocardiography at the RV free wall in the apical four-chamber view [19].

Table 2. 6-[fluoride-18]fluoro-L-DOPA (^{18}F-FDOPA PET/CT) results.

Parameter	All patients		No cardiac metastases		Cardiac metastases		p-value
	N (%)	Mean ± SD	N (%)	Mean ± SD	N (%)	Mean ± SD	
^{18}F-FDOPA PET/CT scan	116 (100)		101 (87)		15 (13)		
SUV$_{max}$ right ventricle	116 (100)	2.1±1.6	101 (87)	1.9±0.41	15 (13)	3.9±4.4	<0.001
SUV$_{mean}$ right ventricle	116 (100)	1.4±0.37	101 (87)	1.3±0.32	15 (13)	1.6±0.65	0.015
SUV$_{max}$ left ventricle	116 (100)	2.9±1.6	101 (87)	2.8±1.3	15 (13)	3.7±2.8	0.029
SUV$_{mean}$ left ventricle	116 (100)	1.7±0.36	101 (87)	1.7±0.35	15 (13)	1.7±0.47	NS

SUV denotes Standardized Uptake Value.

Table 3. Echocardiography results of all patients, and patients with and without abnormal cardiac tracer uptake.

Parameter	All patients		No cardiac metastases		Cardiac metastases		p-value
	N (%)	Mean ± SD, or median (range)	N (%)	Mean ± SD, or median (range)	N (%)	Mean ± SD, or median (range)	
Heart rate (bpm)	72 (91)	71±18	64 (91)	72±17	8 (89)	68±27	NS
Inter-ventricular septal thickness (mm)	63 (88)	9.4±1.8	54 (77)	9.2±1.7	9 (100)	11±2.1	0.037
Left ventricle posterior wall thickness (mm)	63 (88)	8.5±1.7	54 (77)	8.4±1.6	9 (100)	9.3±2.0	NS
Left ventricle end diastolic volume (mL)	38 (48)	96.8 (41.3–214)	34 (49)	95.2 (41.3–214)	4 (44)	116 (87.2–160)	NS
Left ventricle end systolic volume (mL)	40 (51)	30 (18–95)	36 (51)	30 (18–95)	4 (44)	58 (20–90)	NS
Left ventricle diastolic internal diameter (mm)	63 (88)	46 (34–76)	54 (77)	46 (34–76)	9 (100)	50 (36–58)	NS
Left ventricle systolic internal diameter (mm)	64 (91)	28 (22–46)	55 (79)	28 (22–46)	9 (100)	34 (23–44)	NS
Left ventricle ejection fraction (%)	62 (78)	60±9.8	54 (77)	61±8.6	8 (89)	52±14	0.010
Left atrium diameter (mm)	57 (72)	35±5.6	50 (71)	35±5.6	7 (78)	35±6.3	NS
Right atrium length (mm)	55 (70)	52±5.3	49 (70)	52±5.3	6 (67)	55±5.0	NS
Right atrium wide (mm)	50 (63)	39±6.6	45 (64)	40±6.5	5 (56)	39±8.7	NS
Left atrium length (mm)	53 (67)	54±8.1	47 (67)	54±8.4	6 (67)	55±4.6	NS
Left atrium wide (mm)	53 (67)	40±6.0	47 (67)	39±5.9	6 (67)	45±4.8	0.019
Pulmonary valve peak flow (mmHg)	45 (57)	7.7±6.2	37 (53)	7.9±5.9	8 (89)	6.9±7.7	NS
- Mild pulmonary valve stenosis (<25 mmHg)	45 (100)		37 (100)		8 (100)		NS
Tricuspid valve peak gradient (mmHg)	11 (14)	3.3±3.1	10 (14)	3.4±3.3	1 (11)	2.2	NS
- Mild tricuspid valve stenosis (<5 mmHg)	7 (64)		6 (60)		1 (100)		NS
- Moderate tricuspid valve stenosis (5–8 mmHg)	4 (36)		4 (40)		0		NS
Tricuspid valve regurgitation peak flow (mmHg)	37 (47)	24±7.2	29 (41)	23±7.1	8 (89)	28±6.7	NS
TAPSE (mm)	63 (80)	24±4.4	56 (80)	24±4.3	7 (78)	26±4.7	NS

TAPSE denotes tricuspid annular plane systolic excursion.

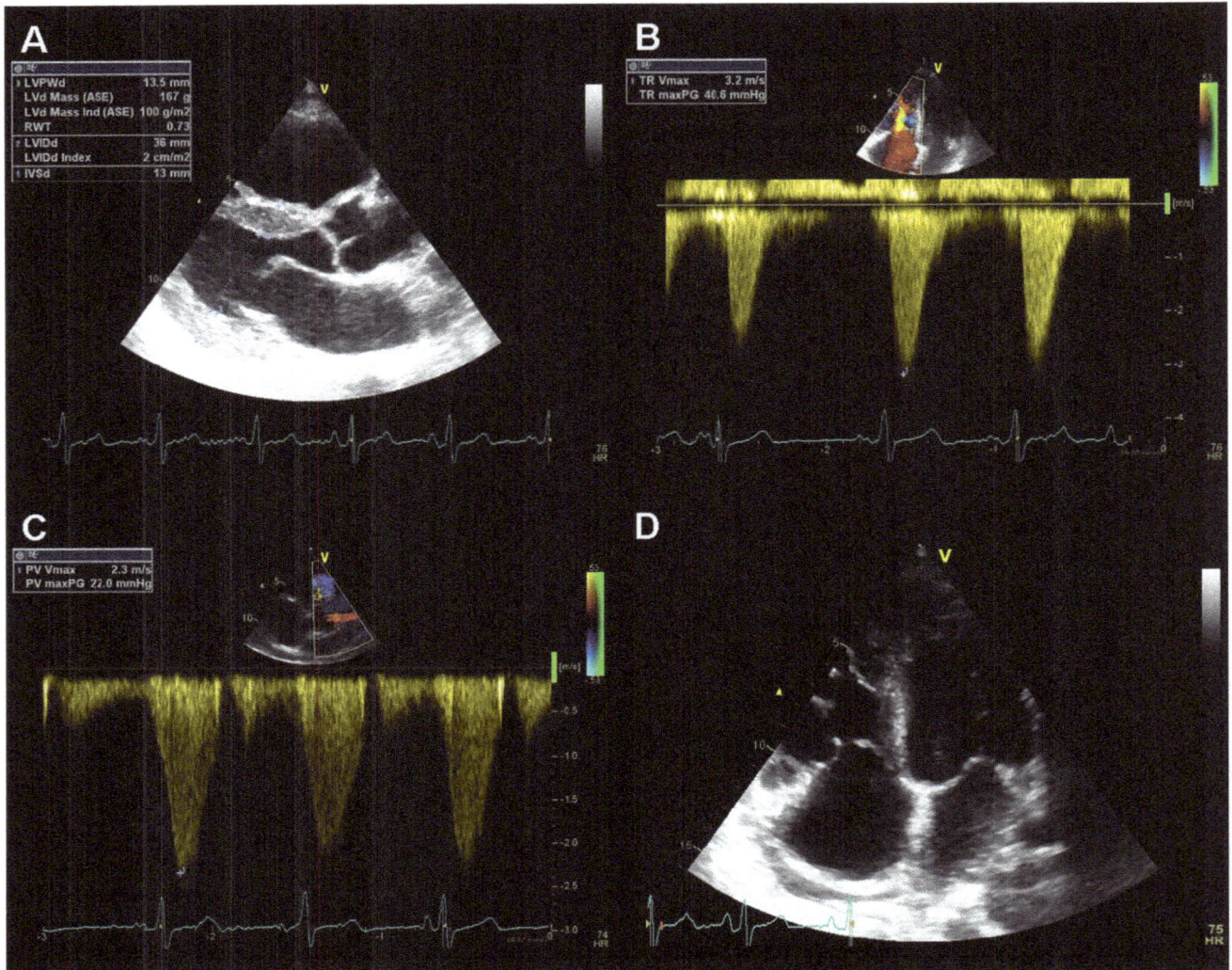

Figure 3. Example of echocardiographic characteristics of a patient with carcinoid heart disease. A: Parasternal long axis view showing thickened LV walls (inter-ventricular septum 13 mm, posterior wall 13 mm). B: Continuous wave Doppler of the tricuspid valve jet. The peak velocity (41 mm Hg) indicates severe tricuspid insufficiency. C: Continuous wave Doppler of the pulmonary valve. The peak gradient (22 mmHg) indicates mild pulmonary valve stenosis. D: 2D four chamber image. On the right in the image normal function of the mitral valve. On the left in the image retraction and immobilisation of the tricuspid valve. The leaflets of the tricuspid valves are also hyperechogenic than normal.

Statistical analysis

Results are expressed as mean value ± standard deviation, or median (range) in the case of an abnormal distribution. The differences between patient categories were evaluated using unpaired Student's t-tests (in case of normal distribution), independent sample test (Mann-Whitney U, in case of abnormal distribution), or Chi-square in case of categories. A p value <0.05 was considered significant. Survival was analyzed using log rank test. Statistical analysis was performed using the SPSS package version 20 (IBM Corp., Armonk, NY, USA).

Results

Patient characteristics

Patient selection is shown in Fig. 1. Of the 470 patients who underwent ^{18}F-FDOPA PET/CT, those with medullary thyroid carcinoma, pheochromocytoma and paraganglioma (n = 202) were excluded. Of the remaining 268 patients with any form of

NET, 116 patients had a serotonin producing NET. Of these patients 103 had a primary location in the small bowel, three a primary in lung, and in 10 patients the exact location of the primary tumour was unknown.

Characteristics of the 116 patients are presented in Table 1. There was a slight male predominance: 62 (53%) vs 54 female. None of the patients had recordings or complaints of ventricular dysrhythmia. During follow up (median 24, range 1–42 months), no cardiac event (either myocardial infarction, or sudden cardiac death) was reported. Eventually 30 patients (26%) died during follow-up. Metastatic disease was the main cause of death. Two patients died from non-disease related causes (one because of a cerebro-vascular accident, the other patient died due to pneumonia during the treatment of her co-existing non-Hodgkin's lymphoma).

In 114 patients (98%), eGFR as a marker for kidney function was determined. Mean eGFR was within normal ranges. In 22 patients, eGFR was moderately decreased (values 30–60 mL/

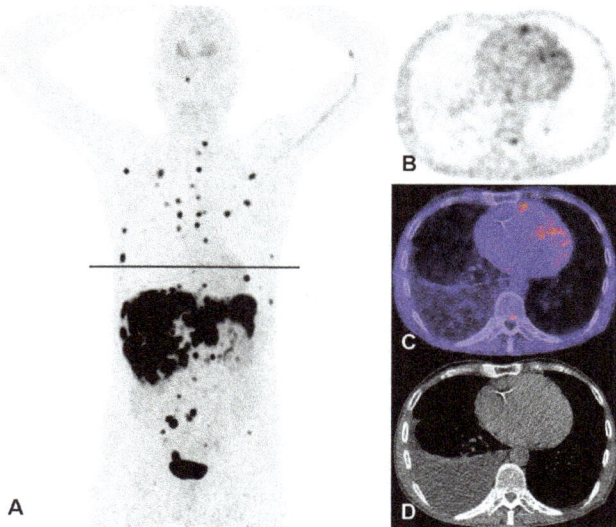

Figure 4. ^{18}F-FDOPA PET/CT scan of the patient illustrated in **Fig 2.** A: Maximum intensity projection showing multiple metastases of the carcinoid tumour in the mediastinum, thoracic wall, liver, mesentery and skeleton. Physiological uptake in the striatum. Administration artefact in the left elbow and vein in the left upper arm. The black line is the slice position of panels B, C, and D. PET alone (B), fused PET/CT (C) and CT alone (D) images on the slice position indicated in panel A. Physiological uptake in the myocardium with a focus of increased uptake in the right ventricle wall. Also small focal uptake in the posterior part of a thoracic vertebral body, right sided pleural effusion and atherosclerosis of the right coronary artery.

min*1.73 m^2), however, none of the patients had severe impaired kidney function, defined as eGFR <30 mL/min*1.73 m^2.

An ECG in the period of the ^{18}F-FDOPA PET/CT was available in 60 patients (52%). The majority of patients had sinus rhythm at the time of the ECG. In two patients (2%) AF was recorded. One of these patients was newly diagnosed with AF, whereas also one patient with previous reported AF was in sinus rhythm at the time of ECG registration.

^{18}F-FDOPA PET/CT findings

Table 2 shows the results of the ^{18}F-FDOPA PET/CT scans. Fifteen patients (13%) showed abnormal tracer uptake (focal myocardial uptake higher than the surrounding physiological myocardial uptake), suspected of being a result of myocardial metastases of the NET. Of these 15 patients, one patient had a serotonin producing NET originating from the lung. All others had serotonin producing NET originating from the small bowel. Three patients had manifestation of one cardiac metastasis in the left ventricle only, six patients only one metastasis in the right ventricle free wall, and six patients showed lesions in both left and right ventricle walls (Fig. 2).

Of these 15 patients, 4 (27%) died during follow-up after the diagnosis of cardiac metastasis (median 5, range 0–22 months). This was not significantly different from 26 (26%) patients who died with normal cardiac tracer distribution (median 17, range 2–37 months).

Echocardiography

Echocardiography was performed in 79 patients (68%, Table 3). The median time between the ^{18}F-FDOPA PET/CT and echocardiography was 0.80 (range 0.20–1.4) months. Mean LV wall thickness and atrial diameter measurements were within normal ranges. In 10 patients inter-ventricular septum thickness was more than 11 mm, whereas posterior wall was thicker than 11 mm in three patients.

Of these 79 patients, nine patients had abnormal cardiac ^{18}F-FDOPA uptake (Table 3). In six patients with abnormal cardiac uptake, no echocardiography was performed. All of these 15 patients had metastatic disease, based upon the ^{18}F-FDOPA PET/CT. Of the echocardiographic parameters, septum thickness, LVEF, left atrium (wide) measurement and mean peak flow across the aortic valve appeared to be significantly different in the patients with abnormal cardiac tracer distribution. Only one of the nine patients with abnormal ^{18}F-FDOPA uptake had echocardiographic signs of carcinoid heart disease: hypertrophic left ventricle (both septum and posterior wall thickness 13 mm), estimated ejection fraction of 30%, severe tricuspid valve (peak gradient 41 mmHg) and pulmonary valve insufficiency, and a mild pulmonary stenosis (peak gradient 22 mmHg, Figs. 3 and 4). In none of the patients with abnormal ^{18}F-FDOPA uptake in the LV wall who underwent echocardiography a patent foramen ovale could be retrieved on the saved images.

Seven patients with echocardiographic parameters of CHD showed no signs of myocardial metastases on the ^{18}F-FDOPA PET/CT. However, the right ventricle diameter in these patients appeared to be relatively wide (Fig. 5). In two of these patients CHD was based on relatively high maximum peak gradient of TV regurgitation (31 and 37 mm Hg) and peak gradient across the PV (22 and 16 mmHg). In this small group of CHD patients urine level of 5-HIAA was higher than those without echo-based CHD: median 153 (range 4.30–385) vs 5.70 (range 1.70–160) mmol/mol creatinine, $p = 0.001$.

Discussion

This study showed cardiac metastases in 15 out of 116 patients (13%). The presence of cardiac metastases was not related to the occurrence of CHD.

There is slowly growing awareness that cardiac metastases occur rather frequently. However, the early detection of these metastases, especially with echocardiography, remains a challenge. The main limitation is that lesions smaller than 10 mm are non-detectable [20]. The conventional nuclear medicine modality ^{111}In-SRS has the same limitation, especially in whole body imaging. The addition of SPECT/CT of the thorax contributes to a better spatial resolution, with more precise anatomic localization of abnormal tracer accumulation. The introduction of newer imaging modalities with PET tracers ^{68}Ga-DOTATOC and ^{18}F-FDOPA provide an even better spatial resolution (up to 4 mm) and overall more sensitive detection of metastases of NET [4]. This is the largest cohort of patients referred for ^{18}F-FDOPA PET/CT scans, showing that cardiac metastases of NET are more prevalent than previously assumed.

In a review of the reported literature thus far in 2010, a total of 45 patients with cardiac metastases based on imaging, surgery and autopsy findings were retrospectively analyzed [4]. In 21 cases, the presence of cardiac metastasis was based on echocardiographic findings, whereas nuclear medicine modalities were positive in 10 patients. PET scans visualized cardiac metastases in three out of those 10 cases. In all of these cases, the presence of cardiac metastases could be verified with other imaging modalities: echocardiography and MRI. This indicates that both PET tracers are accurately able to visualize cardiac metastases. A recent report on rare metastases of NET further confirms this statement [21]. In this study a total of 4,210 ^{68}Ga-somatostatin-receptor PET/CT

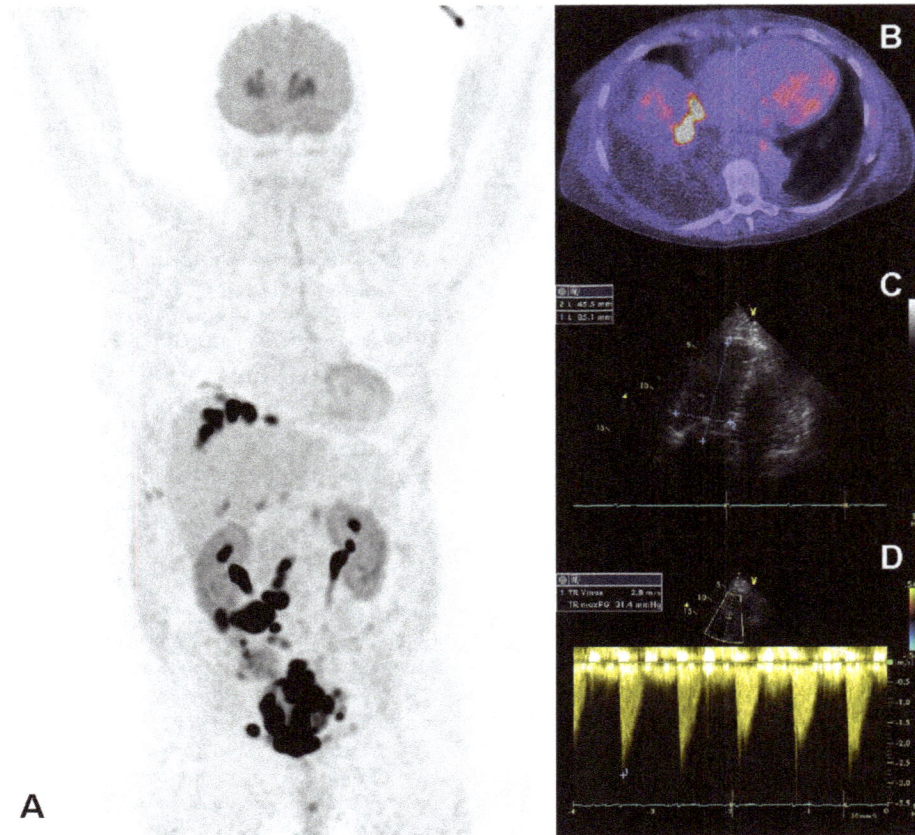

Figure 5. Maximum intensity projection (A) of an [18]**F-FDOPA PET/CT scan in a patient with echocardiographic signs of carcinoid heart disease, but without myocardial metastases on the** [18]**F-FDOPA PET/CT scan.** B: Fused PET/CT image showing only physiological tracer distribution in the myocardium. The intense uptake in liver is due to liver metastases. Ascites surrounding the right liver half. C: Measurements of the right ventricle (85 mm long, 46 mm wide). D: Continuous wave Doppler of the tricuspid valve (peak gradient 31 mmHg), indicating tricuspid insufficiency.

scans performed in a 5-year period were retrospectively analyzed. Cardiac metastases appeared to be rare: in merely 29 of all cases. Both these reports also included non-serotonin producing and non-metastatic NET. Therefore, the prevalence of cardiac metastases in these cohorts is less than 1%. However, this is even less than the low prevalence of 4%, as mentioned previously, and probably a result of selection bias [12]. On the other hand, the most recent study on the presence of cardiac metastases in patients with NET of the small bowel reported that cardiac metastases detected by ^{68}Ga-DOTATOC PET/CT were present in four out of 92 patients with ileal NET [22]. These four patients showed in total seven cardiac metastases, supporting the previously acclaimed prevalence of approximately 4%. As in our study, all patients with myocardial metastases had high tumour burden. Although cardiac metastases are usually detected in patients with widespread metastatic disease, the myocardium can occasionally be the only location of NET metastases [4]. Our study consists of the largest cohort of patients referred for ^{18}F-FDOPA PET/CT scans. We clearly add the novel information that cardiac metastases of NET occur more frequently than previously assumed, and that ^{18}F-FDOPA PET/CT appears to be more sensitive in detecting these metastases than other imaging modalities reported so far.

We showed no relationship between the presence of cardiac metastases and echocardiographic parameters for CHD. This suggests that myocardial metastases and typical CHD are two different entities, which do not seem to affect each other. We could not identify a patent foramen ovale in patients with cardiac metastases, which may support the idea that the presence of cardiac metastases is independent of flow. Lower eyeballing LVEF and wider left atrium measurements were considered to be coincidental findings due to the small group of patients. Urinary excretion of 5-HIAA was higher in patients with echocardiographic signs of CHD, but not in patients with cardiac metastases. Although the duration of the disease was not investigated in this retrospective study, this finding implies that CHD patients probably had long standing disease. Other laboratory tests, as well as ECG findings did not differ. This finding is concordant with the progression of CHD [23].

Conclusions

The prevalence of cardiac metastases found on ^{18}F-FDOPA PET/CT is higher that previously assumed. Cardiac metastases were not related with typical echocardiographic features of CHD, suggesting that these findings are two different entities within the same disease. Of importance, the clinical consequences of this higher incidence of cardiac metastases found on ^{18}F-FDOPA PET/CT may not be of high importance, due to the indolent character of the disease, leading to a comparable survival in patients without cardiac metastases. A large prospective study of serotonin producing NET patients with cardiac metastases should be performed to further establish the clinical role of ^{18}F-FDOPA PET/CT for this indication.

Acknowledgments

We would like to thank Adrienne H. Brouwers, MD PhD, for her expertise in the fields of nuclear medicine and neuroendocrine tumours, and Paul van Snick for reconstructing the raw PET data.

References

1. Pape UF, Perren A, Niederle B, Gross D, Gress T, et al (2012) ENETS Consensus Guidelines for the management of patients with neuroendocrine neoplasms from the jejuno-ileum and the appendix including goblet cell carcinomas. Neuroendocrinology 95: 135–56.
2. Koopmans KP, Neels OC, Kema IP, Elsinga PH, Sluiter WJ, et al (2008) Improved staging of patients with carcinoid and islet cell tumors with ^{18}F-dihydroxy-phenyl-alanine and ^{11}C-5-hydroxy-tryptophan positron emission tomography. J Clin Oncol 26: 1489–1495.
3. Fiebrich HB, Brouwers AH, Links TP, de Vries EGE (2008) Myocardial metastases of carcinoid visualized by F-18-dihydroxy-phenyl-alanine positron emission tomography. Circulation 118: 1602–1604.
4. Jann H, Wertenbruch T, Pape U, Ozcelik C, Denecke T, et al (2010) A matter of the heart: myocardial metastases in neuroendocrine tumors. Horm Metab Res 42: 967–976.
5. Anderson AS, Krauss D, Lang R (1997) Cardiovascular complications of malignant carcinoid disease. Am Heart J 134: 693–702.
6. Roberts WC, Sjoerdsma A (1964) The cardiac disease associated with the carcinoid syndrome (carcinoid heart disease). Am J Med 36: 5–34.
7. Palaniswamy C, Frishman WH, Aronow WS (2012) Carcinoid heart disease. Cardiol Rev 20: 167–176.
8. Bernheim AM, Connolly HM, Hobday TJ, Abel MD, Pellikka PA (2007) Carcinoid heart disease. Prog Cardiovasc Dis 49: 439–451.
9. Rudski LG, Lai WW, Afilalo J, Hua L, Handschumacher MD, et al (2010) Guidelines for the echocardiographic assessment of the right heart in adults: a report from the American Society of Echocardiography endorsed by the European Association of Echocardiography, a registered branch of the European Society of Cardiology, and the Canadian Society of Echocardiography. J Am Soc Echocardiogr 23: 685–713.
10. Møller JE, Pellikka PA, Bernheum AM, Schaff HV, Rubin J, et al (2005) Prognosis of carcinoid heart disease: analysis of 200 cases over two decades. Circulation 112: 3320–3327.
11. Bhattacharyya S, Toumpanakis C, Burke M, Taylor AM, Caplin ME, et al (2010) Features of carcinoid heart disease identified by 2- and 3-dimensional echocardiography and cardiac MRI. Circ Cardiovasc Imaging 3: 103–11.
12. Pellikka PA, Tajik AJ, Khandheria BK, Seward JB, Callahan JA, et al (1993) Carcinoid heart disease. Clinical and echocardiographic spectrum in 74 patients. Circulation 87: 1188–1196.
13. National Kidney Foundation (2002) KDOQI clinical practice guidelines for chronic kidney disease: evaluation, classification, and stratification. Kidney Disease Outcome Quality Initiative. Am J Kidney Dis 39: S1–S266.
14. Boellaard R, Oyen WJ, Hoekstra CJ, Hoekstra OS, Visser EP, et al (2008) The Netherlands protocol for standardisation and quantification of FDG whole body PET studies in multi-centre trials. Eur J Nucl Med Mol Imaging 35: 2320–2333.
15. Boellaard R, O'Doherty MJ, Weber WA, Mottaghy FM, Lonsdale MN, et al (2010) FDG PET and PET/CT: EANM procedure guidelines for tumour PET imaging: version 1.0. Eur J Nucl Med Mol Imaging 37: 181–200.
16. Castillo JG, Silvay G, Solis J (2013) Current concepts in diagnosis and perioperative management of carcinoid heart disease. Semin Cardiothorac Vasc Anesth 2013 17: 212–223.
17. Zoghbi WA, Enriquez-Sarano M, Foster E, Grayburn PA, Kraft CD, et al (2003) Recommendations for evaluation of the severity of native valvular regurgitation with two-dimensional and Doppler echocardiography. J Am Soc Echocardiogr 16: 777–802.
18. Bonow RO, Carabello BA, Chatterjee K, de Leon AC Jr, Faxon DP, et al (2006) ACC/AHA 2006 guidelines for the management of patients with valvular heart disease: a report of the American College of Cardiology/American Heart Association Task Force on Practice Guidelines. J Am Coll Cardiol 48: e1–148.
19. Koestenberger M, Ravekes W, Everett AD, Stueger HP, Heinzl B, et al (2009) Right ventricular function in infants, children and adolescents: reference values of the tricuspid annular plane systolic excursion (TAPSE) in 640 healthy patients and calculation of z score values. J Am Soc Echocardiogr 22: 715–719.
20. Pandya UH, Pellikka PA, Enriquez-Sarano M, Edwards WD, Schaff HV, et al (2002) Metastatic carcinoid tumor to the heart: Echocardiographic-pathologic study of 11 patients. J Am Coll Cardiol 40: 1328–1332.
21. Carreras C, Kulkarni HR, Baum RP (2013) Rare metastases detected by (68)Ga-somatostatin receptor PET/CT in patients with neuroendocrine tumors. Recent Results Cancer Res 194: 379–84.
22. Calissendorff J, Sundin A, Falhammar H (2014). 68Ga-DOTA-TOC-PET/CT detects heart metastases from ileal neuroendocrine tumors. Endocrine 47: 169–76.
23. Denney WD, Kemp WE Jr, Anthony LB, Oates JA, Byrd BF 3rd (1998). Echocardiographic and biochemical evaluation of the development and progression of carcinoid heart disease. J Am Coll Cardiol 32: 1017–22.

Author Contributions

Conceived and designed the experiments: APB AWG RAD. Performed the experiments: WN BG. Analyzed the data: WN. Contributed reagents/materials/analysis tools: AWG RHS RAD. Wrote the paper: WN APB RAT ANH EGV AMW AWG RHS RAD.

7

Percutaneous Resolution of Lumbar Facet Joint Cysts as an Alternative Treatment to Surgery

Feng Shuang[1,2], Shu-Xun Hou[1]*, Jia-Liang Zhu[1], Dong-Feng Ren[1], Zheng Cao[1], Jia-Guang Tang[1]*

1 Department of Orthopaedics, The First Affiliated Hospital of General Hospital of Chinese PLA, Beijing, China, 2 Department of Orthopedics, The 94th Hospital of Chinese PLA, Nanchang, China

Abstract

Purpose: A comprehensive review of the literature in order to analyze data about the success rate of percutaneous resolution of the lumbar facet joint cysts as a conservative management strategy.

Methods: A systematic search for relevant articles published during 1980 to May 2014 was performed in several electronic databases by using the specific MeSH terms and keywords. Most relevant data was captured and pooled for the meta-analysis to achieve overall effect size of treatment along with 95% confidence intervals.

Results: 29 studies were included in the meta-analysis. Follow-up duration as mean $\pm$ sd (range) was 16 ± 10.2 (5 days to 5.7 years). Overall the satisfactory results (after short- or long-term follow-up) were achieved in 55.8 [49.5, 62.08] % (pooled mean and 95% CI) of the 544 patients subjected to percutaneous lumbar facet joint cyst resolution procedures. 38.67 [33.3, 43.95] % of this population underwent surgery subsequently to achieve durable relief. There existed no linear relationship between the increasing average duration of follow-up period of individual studies and percent satisfaction from the percutaneous resolutions procedure.

Conclusion: Results shows that the percutaneous cyst resolution procedures have potential to be an alternative to surgical interventions but identification of suitable subjects requires further research.

Editor: Sam Eldabe, The James Cook University Hospital, United Kingdom

Funding: This work was supported by the National Natural Science Foundation of China (No. 81071514). The funders had no role in study design, data collection and analysis, decision to publish, or preparation of the manuscript.

Competing Interests: The authors have declared that no competing interests exist.

* Email: jiaguangtang@yahoo.com.cn (JGT); houshuxun_2000@163.com (SXH)

Introduction

Facet joint cysts of lumbar spine (LFJCs) are benign degenerative outgrowths which are most usually associated with low back pain and radiculopathy. Two types of cysts recognized under this category are the synovial cysts and ganglion cysts [1]. The synovial cysts have vascularized lining filled with xanthochromic fluid and have communication with facet joint while the ganglion cysts are covered by fibrocartilagenous capsule filled with proteinaceous and gelatinous material and do not communicate with joint [2].

These cysts can arise because of the chronic hypermobility of the spinal segments leading to increased and more frequent loading of the zygapophyseal joint (Z-joint; a synovial joint). This causes the accumulation of fibrocartilaginous substances which provide raw material for cyst formation [3,4]. The Z-joint is thought to be involved in the genesis of cysts owing to a degenerative process, not fully understood, though herniation of synovial tissue is frequently perceived [5–7]. The LFJCs are associated with spinal stenosis, nerve root compression, neurogenic claudication and many other neurological disturbances by encroaching the local foramen [8,9].

Although, small scale studies indicate that the prevalence of LFJCs in symptomatic patients is 0.7 to 2.5% (Ayberg et al., 2008) [10], but it may be higher and even increase with increasing longevity. This neuropathological agent is strongly associated with late decades of life and females harbor more than males [1].

Diagnosis of the LFJCs utilize magnetic resonance imaging (MRI) or computed tomography (CT) and to some extent CT myelography. Seldom these cysts resolve spontaneously; mostly require treatment. Various management strategies include bed rest, non-steroidal anti-inflammatory drugs, analgesics, physical therapies, transcutaneous electrical nerve stimulation (TENS), intra-articular steroid injections/epidural steroid instillation with or without cyst rupture and CT or flouroscopy guided aspiration of the cyst materials and surgical interventions such as laminectomy, facetectomy, flavectomy, cyst excision and microsurgery.

Long term relief from the symptoms associated with the LFJCs can be achieved with surgery or percutaneous resolution procedures, however. Surgery is the most effective treatment noted so far but studies indicate that percutaneous cyst resolution procedures can be an alternative to surgery in a well-sized subgroup of patients. Moreover, older and high risk patients who are abstained from surgical interventions due to many reasons can

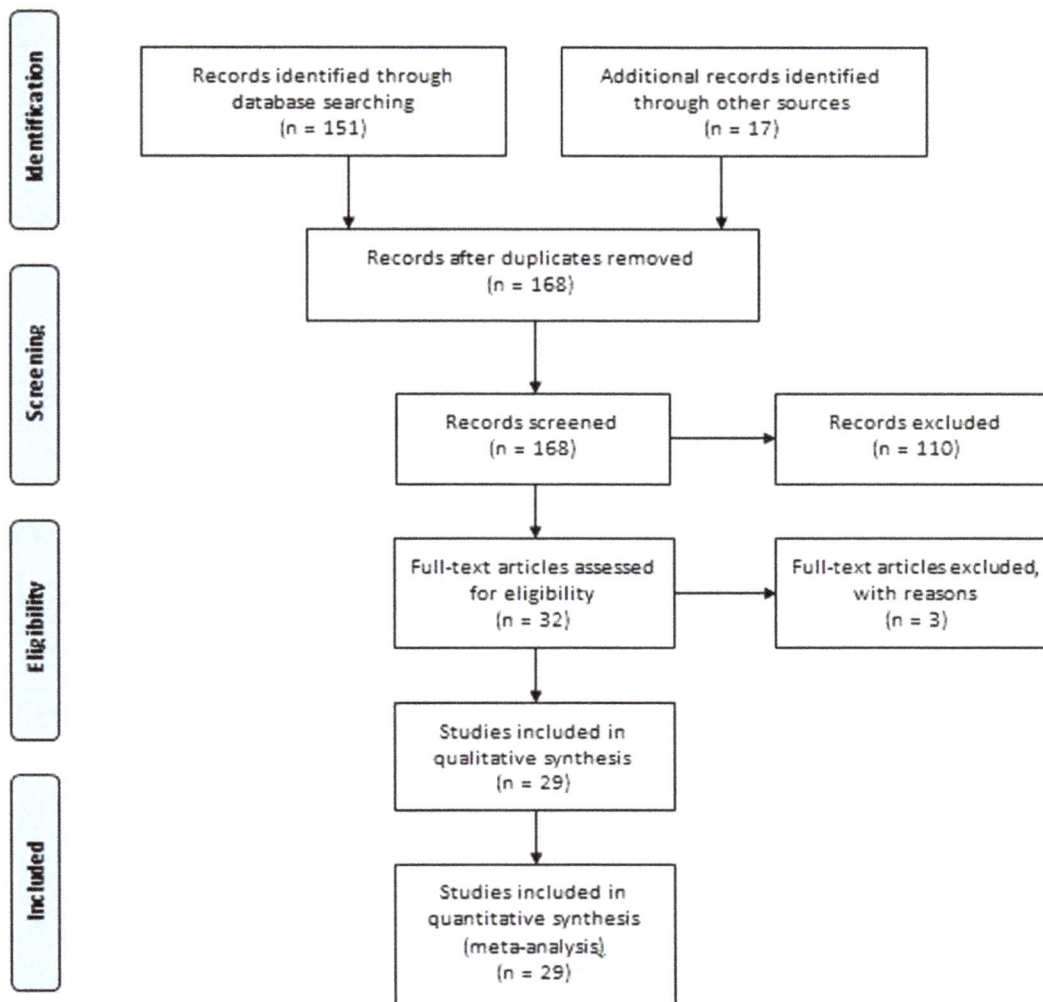

Figure 1. Flowchart of study screening and selection process.

also be benefited from later treatment regimen. In order to explore this avenue, this systematic review and meta-analysis is conducted to evaluate the success rate of percutaneous cyst resolution procedures in terms of durable relief and to attempt the identification of subgroup of patients in which chances success with this technique can be better than surgical intervention.

Materials and Methods

Study Identification

Detailed systematic search was made in several electronic databases including PubMed/Medline, Embase, EBSCO, CINAHL, Ovid SP, SCI Web of Science and Google Scholar under most relevant keywords. MeSH terms and keywords used in various logical combinations included: spinal, lumbar, cyst, synovial, ganglion, juxtafacet, facet, zygapophyseal, magnetic resonance imaging (MRI), computed tomography (CT), conservative management, percutaneous, puncture, rupture, steroid, injection, intra-articular, epidural, facet, joint, effusion. Literature search was restricted to a period from 1980 to May 2014. All retrospective analyses, prospective studies, and individual case reports were taken into consideration.

Selection criteria

The PRISMA guidelines were followed for this study. Because of the scarcity of well-designed clinical trials, selection of studies was made under a broader scope and all studies with prospective or retrospective designs and case reports were included. Inclusion criteria were: a) Studies mentioning percutaneous resolution procedures of LFJCs (synovial/ganglion) such as steroid injections, cyst rupture and cyst material aspiration by utilizing CT/fluoroscopically guided instrumentation; b) studies mentioning a short-term or long-term follow-up of the outcomes and related details, including the provision of data of the subjects who underwent surgical procedures in case of failure of the interventions. Exclusion criteria were: a) studies/case reports intervening other types of similar spinal cyst pathologies such as discal cysts, vertebroplasty etc; b) studies involving percutaneous procedures for the purpose of diagnosis only; and c) studies/case reports utilizing percutaneous procedures for the alleviation of back pain without a diagnosis of LFJC/s; d) studies/case reports which did not contain sufficient details of the outcomes of interventions of interest.

Table 1. Quality Assessment Tool for Observational Cohort and Cross-Sectional Studies.

Criteria	12	13	14	15	16	17	18	19	20	21	22	23	24	25
1. Was the research question or objective in this paper clearly stated?	Y	Y	Y	Y	Y	Y	Y	Y	Y	Y	Y	Y	Y	Y
2. Was the study population clearly specified and defined?	Y	Y	Y	Y	Y	Y	Y	Y	Y	Y	Y	Y	Y	Y
3. Was the participation rate of eligible persons at least 50%?	Y	Y	Y	Y	Y	Y	Y	Y	Y	Y	Y	Y	Y	Y
4. Were all the subjects selected or recruited from the same or similar populations (including the same time period)? Were inclusion and exclusion criteria for being in the study prespecified and applied uniformly to all participants?	Y	Y	Y	Y	Y	Y	Y	Y	Y	Y	Y	Y	Y	Y
5. Was a sample size justification, power description, or variance and effect estimates provided?	N	N	N	N	N	N	Y	N	N	N	N	Y	N	N
6. For the analyses in this paper, were the exposure(s) of interest measured prior to the outcome(s) being measured?	NA	NA	NA	NA	NA	NA	NA	NA	NA	NA	NA	NA	NA	NA
7. Was the timeframe sufficient so that one could reasonably expect to see an association between exposure and outcome if it existed?	N	N	N	Y	Y	N	Y	N	Y	N	N	N	N	N
8. For exposures that can vary in amount or level, did the study examine different levels of the exposure as related to the outcome (e.g., categories of exposure, or exposure measured as continuous variable)?	Y	Y	NA	Y	Y	NA	Y	Y	Y	Y	Y	Y	Y	Y
9. Were the exposure measures (independent variables) clearly defined, valid, reliable, and implemented consistently across all study participants?	Y	Y	Y	Y	Y	Y	Y	Y	Y	Y	Y	Y	Y	Y
10. Was the exposure(s) assessed more than once over time?	Y	Y	Y	Y	Y	NR	Y	Y	Y	Y	Y	NR	Y	NR
11. Were the outcome measures (dependent variables) clearly defined, valid, reliable, and implemented consistently across all study participants?	N	N	N	Y	Y	N	Y	N	Y	N	N	N	N	N
12. Were the outcome assessors blinded to the exposure status of participants?	N	N	N	N	N	N	N	N	N	N	N	N	N	N
13. Was loss to follow-up after baseline 20% or less?	CD	CD	CD	CD	CD	CD	CD	CD	CD	CD	CD	CD	CD	CD
14. Were key potential confounding variables measured and adjusted statistically for their impact on the relationship between exposure(s) and outcome(s)?	N	N	N	N	Y	N	Y	N	N	N	N	N	N	N

Legends: CD: Cannot be determined, NA: not applicable, NR: not reported, N: no, Y: yes.

Data extraction, synthesis and analysis

Data were extracted from each research article/case report regarding the demographics of patients, clinical and pathological characteristics, diagnostic tools, procedural features, follow-up period, and outcomes. Outcome measures were the percent satisfactory response of the patient after a reasonable follow-up and the percentage of patients who subsequently underwent surgery. Pooling of dichotomous data (satisfactory outcomes vs surgery requirement) was made by calculating standard errors and 95% confidence intervals (CI) of the data from individual studies and then overall effect size of the meta-analysis was calculated. Forest graphs were plotted manually on the spreadsheets from pooled data and the overall effect size. Descriptive data are presented as mean along with either standard deviation (sd) or range. Quality of the included studies was assessed by using Quality Assessment Tool for Observational Cohort and Cross-Sectional Studies [11].

Results

Search identified 29 articles [12–40] reporting 12 retrospective studies, 2 prospective studies and 15 case reports which are included in this analytical review. Study screening and selection process has been depicted in Figure 1. Quality assessment outcomes are presented in Table 1.

Major characteristics relevant to the manifesto of the present study are present in Table 2. Overall of the 544 subjects included in this meta-analysis, age of the participants as mean ± sd (range) was 62 ± 4.2 (28–87) years and proportion of females in this population was 64%. Spinal level of the cysts was L_{2-3} in 10, L_{3-4} in 69, L_{4-5} in 384 and L_5-S_1 in 96 cases (Figure 2). Size of the cyst ranged from 6×13 to 12×18 mm. Duration of symptoms before percutaneous resolution interventions ranged from 2 weeks to 60 months. Major conditions associated with the presence of LFJCs in these patients were lower back pain and radiculopathy, especially lower extremity radiculopathy. Symptomatic features at clinical presentation are presented in Table 3.

The procedures involved cyst puncture, rupture, aspiration, intra-articular steroid injection, epidural steroid injection, and local anesthetics injections. These procedures were performed under CT/fluoroscopic guidance, though, not all studies utilized each of these interventions. Arthrography was also performed in majority of cases. Majority of the subjects were diagnosed with MRI (about 85% vs CT about 15%) for harboring one or more

Table 2. Characteristics of the included studies which utilized percutaneous resolution of lumbar facet joint cyst procedures.

Study/Design	Patients' characteristics	Pathology	Diagnosis	Intervention	Follow up	Outcome
Allen et al., 2009 [12]/ Retrospective cohort	n: 32; age: 66 (46–86) y; females: 18; Location ($L_{3-4}/L_{4-5}/L_5$–S_1): 2/22/8 (left 18, right 13, bilateral 1)	LBP/LER since 5 mo	MRI	FCR/ESI	12 (6–24) mo	Satisfactory: 19 (60%), Repeats: 11 (34%), Required Surgery: 6 (19%)
Amoretti et al., 2012 [13]/ prospective	n: 120; age: 68.2 (52–84) y; Location ($L_{3-4}/L_{4-5}/L_5$–S_1): 16/84/20; VAS change; mean ± sd: 7.2±1.2 to 2.9±1.2	Disabling LBP/radiculopathy	MRI	CTISI	12 mo	Satisfactory: 90 (75%), Repeats: 43 (36%), Required Surgery: 30 (25%)
Bjorkengren et al., 1987 [14]/ prospective	n: 3; age: 59 (44, 56 & 77) y; females: 2; Location: L_{4-5} in all	LBP/LER	CT	CTISI	11 (6–14) mo	Satisfactory: 2 partially, Repeats: 1, Required surgery: 1/refused
Bureau et al., 2001 [17]/ retrospective	n: 12; age: 60 (45–79) y; females: 8; Location ($L_{3-4}/L_{4-5}/L_5$–S_1): 1/10/1; Cyst size: 11×13.6 (6–13×8–19)mm	LBP/radiculopathy	MRI	FCR/SI	23 (12–36) mo	Satisfactory: 9 (75%), Repeats: 7 (58%), Required Surgery: 3 (25%)
Cambron et al., 2013 [18]/ retrospective	n: 110; age: 63 (28–87) y; females: 71; Location ($L_{2-3}/L_{3-4}/L_{4-5}/L_5$–$S_1$): 6/17/89/22; Cyst size: 10.6 mm/intensity: H 48/L 65	LER	MRI	CT-guided FCR/SI	34 (7–93) mo	Satisfactory: 63 (57%), Repeats: 40 (36%), Required Surgery: 47 (43%)
Carrera, 1980 [19]/retrospective	n: 20; age (mean): 54 y; females: 12; Location ($L_{2-3}/L_{3-4}/L_{4-5}/L_5$–$S_1$): NA	LBP/symptomatic facet arthropathy	CT	IAFB	6–12 mo	Satisfactory: 6 (30%), Repeats: NA, Required Surgery: NA
Martha et al., 2009 [30]/ retrospective	n: 101; age: 59.8±1.3 y; females: 69; Location ($L_{2-3}/L_{3-4}/L_{4-5}/L_5$–$S_1$): 2/9/69/21	LBP/LER	MRI	FCR/SI	3.2±1.3 y (mean ± sd)	Satisfactory: 46 (46%), Repeats: 51 (51%), Required Surgery: 55 (55%)
Ortiz & Tekchandani, 2013 [32]/ retrospective	n: 20; age: 65.5 y average; females: 9; Location ($L_{2-3}/L_{3-4}/L_{4-5}/L_5$–$S_1$): 1/5/11/4; Cyst size: 7.3 (3–14) mm	LBP/LER	NA	CTISI/aspiration	18 (4–24)	Satisfactory: 18 (90%), Repeats: 4 (20%), Required Surgery: 2 (10%)
Parlier-Cuau et al., 1999 [33]/ retrospective	n: 30; age: 67 (44–82) y; females: 21; Location ($L_{2-3}/L_{3-4}/L_{4-5}/L_5$–$S_1$): 1/3/25/1; Symptom duration: at least 6 mo	Sciatic/femoral pain	CT: 27/MRI: 3/ arthrography	FISI	26 (8–50) mo	Satisfactory: 14 (47%), Repeats: 7 (23%), Required Surgery: 14 (47%)
Sabers et al., 2005 [35]/ retrospective	n: 23; age: 64 (28–81) y; females: 12; Location ($L_{3-4}/L_{4-5}/L_5$–S_1): 1/15/7; Symptom duration: 10.5 (2 wk–48 mo)	LBP/LER	MRI	FISI/aspiration	9.1 (1.5–21) mo	Satisfactory: 9 (50%), Repeats: 2 (1–4) per subject, Required Surgery: 9 (50%)
Sauvage et al., 2000 [36]/ retrospective	n: 13; age: 63 (42–87) y; females: 9; Location ($L_{3-4}/L_{4-5}/L_5$–S_1): 1/8/4; Cyst size: 9 (5–11) mm; largest 12×18 mm	radiculopathy	MRI	CTISI	9 (2–25) mo	Satisfactory: 6 (46%), Repeats: 6 (46%), Required Surgery: 3 (23%)
Schulz et al 2011 [37]/ prospective	n: 20; age: median 54.5 y; females: 17; Location ($L_{3-4}/L_{4-5}/L_5$–S_1): 1/19/0; Symptom duration: median 10.5 mo	radiculopathy	CT	CTISI	24 mo	Satisfactory: 8 (40%), Repeats: NA, Required Surgery: 12 (60%)
Shah and Lutz, 2003 [38]/ retrospective	n: 10; age: 60 (53–70) y; females: 8; Location ($L_{3-4}/L_{4-5}/L_5$–S_1): 0/8/2; Symptom duration: 7.9 (1–30) mo	LBP/LER	CT/MRI	FISI/aspiration/ESI	11.5 (3–30) mo	Satisfactory: 1 (10%), Repeats: 1 (10%), Required Surgery: 8 (80%)
Slipman et al, 2000 [40]/ retrospective	n: 14; age: 60.2 (39–87) y; females: 7; Location ($L_{3-4}/L_{4-5}/L_5$–S_1): 2/10/2; Symptom duration: 18.8 (3–60) mo	radiculopathy	CT/MRI	FISI/aspiration	1.4 (1–3) y	Satisfactory: 4 (40%), Repeats: NA, Required Surgery: 8(58%)
Case Reports						
Boissiere et al, 2013 [15]	57 y old male with cyst at L_{4-5}	Sciatica since 24 mo	CT	CTISI	6 mo	surgery (decompression + fusion)
Braza et al., 2005 [16]	48 y old man with cyst at L_{4-5} (7 mm)	Thigh and calf pain (7 mo)	MRI	FISI/aspiration	2 mo	80% improvement in pain relief
Casselman et al 1985 [20]	65 y old woman with cyst at L_{4-5}	LBP/LER	CT	Intra-articular SI	3 mo	Underwent surgery

Table 2. Cont.

Study/Design	Patients' characteristics	Pathology	Diagnosis	Intervention	Follow up	Outcome
Chang et al 2009 [21]	63 y old woman with cyst at L_5–S_1 (7 mm)	Left-sided radiculopathy	MRI	CT-guided FISI	1 mo	Satisfactory relief
Foley, 2009 [22]	44 y old man with cyst at L_{4-5}	LBP	MRI	FISI/rupture	1 mo	Satisfactory relief (0/10 VAS)
Gishen & Mill., 2001 [23]	65 y old woman with cyst at L_5–S_1	Hip osteoarthris/left sciatica	MRI	CTISI/ESI	12 mo	Satisfactory (asymptomatic)
Hong et al., 1995 [24]	51 y old woman with cyst at L_{4-5}	LBP/right knee pain (6 mo)	MRI	FCA, no SI	6 mo	Satisfactory (asymptomatic)
Imai et al., 1998 [25]	77/55 y old women with cysts at L_{4-5}/L_{3-4}	LBP/LER (15 mo/10 mo)	MRI	FISI/aspiration	5 d/2 mo	surgery for durable relief (both)
Kozar & Jer. 2014 [26]	77 y old man with cyst at L_{4-5} (3×5 mm)	LBP/LER (3 y)	MRI	CTISI/rupture	1 mo	Partial relief/surgery not feasible
Lim et al., 2001 [27]	67 y old woman with cyst at L_{4-5}	LBP/right LER	MRI	CTISI	9 mo	Satisfactory (asymptomatic)
Lin et al., 2014 [28]	52 y old man with cyst at L_{4-5}	LBP/right LER since 10 mo	MRI	UISI	18 mo	Satisfactory (asymptomatic)
Lutz and Shen, 2002 [29]	48 y old woman; cyst at L_{4-5} (7×15 mm)	LBP/right LER (4 mo)	MRI	FCA, no SI	1 mo	Satisfactory (asymptomatic)
Melfi & Aprill, 2005 [31]	72 y old woman with cyst at L_{4-5}/L_5–S_1	Chronic LBP/LER (7 mo)	MRI	FISI	30 mo	Satisfactory (asymptomatic)
Rauchwerger 2011 [34]	70 y old woman with cyst at L_5–S_1	LBP/radiculopathy (1 y)	MRI	FISI	1 day	Partial relief
Shin et al., 2012 [39]	51 y old man with cyst at L_{4-5}	LBP/LER (1mo)	MRI	FISI/aspiration	6 mo	Satisfactory (asymptomatic)

Values are presented as mean (range) unless otherwise stated. Abbreviations: CTISI (CT-guided Intra-cystic/Intra-articular SI), ESI (epidural SI), FCA (fluoroscopically-guided cyst aspiration), FCR (fluoroscopically guided cyst rupture), FISI (fluoroscopic intra-articular SI), IAFB (intra-articular facet block), LBP (lower back pain), LER (lower extremity radiculopathy), mo (month/s), NA (not available), SI (steroid injection), wk (week/s), y (year/s).

LFJCs. Cyst rupture outcomes were assessed by the loss of resistance method or by the extravasation of dye.

Follow-up duration as mean ± sd (range) was 16±10.2 (5 days to 5.7 years). Overall the satisfactory results (after short- or long-term follow-up) were achieved in 55.8 [49.5, 62.08] % (pooled mean and 95% CI) of the 544 patients subjected to percutaneous lumbar cyst resolution procedures (Figure 3). Repeat procedures were performed in 115 of 323 subjects at an average duration of 4.7 (range 0.06–26.3) months after first procedure (data from 7 studies only). On the other hand, 38.67 [33.3, 43.95] % of this population underwent surgery subsequently to achieve durable relief (Figure 4). Average time from percutaneous resolution procedure to surgery was 6.7 (range 0.13–34.4) months (data from six studies only).

There was no purposeful linear relationship between the increasing average duration of follow-up period of individual studies and percent satisfaction from the percutaneous resolutions procedure (correlation coefficient: 0.13; slope: 0.057; Figure 5). However, number of studies with around 1-year follow up was highest (10), with 2-year follow-up 4 and with 3-year follow-up 2 only. For this analysis individual case reports were lumped in to three groups according to follow-up period (1, 6 and 12 months). Only one case report had a follow-up of over 2-years duration (30 months).

Discussion

Usually, the LFJCs are found as rare incidental MRI findings of elderly patients (usually in their 6th or 7th decade) presenting with low back pain and lower extremity radiculopathy. However, discovery of LFJCs remains difficult because low back pain is one of the most common presentations in a visit to physician [41]. Frequently, small cohorts of patients often develop additional bony abnormalities, including instability and spondylolisthesis.

Previously, it was difficult to pinpoint a precise existence of a cyst. Rather, the physician relied on his/her clinical acumen. For example, bilateral examinations of L_4, L_5 and S_1, supplying the knee, foot dorsiflexion and plantar flexion, respectively, could give quick insight into the functioning of these spinal nerve roots. Added to these were lumbosacral flexion-extension plain film radiographs that could provide basic information about vertebral anatomy. However, with the advent of modern imaging modalities like CT scans and MRI, primary care physicians as well as specialists started utilizing these techniques in order to obtain more reliable anatomical features leading to pathology. This has resulted in better insights of pathoanatomical diagnoses that can provide sustained and earlier relief.

The present study utilizes almost all relevant data to appraise the success rate of the percutaneous resolution of the LFJCs and finds perhaps the highest rate (56%) reviewed so far [2 e.g.]. This appears to be because of inclusion of 15 case reports which provide considerable power to analysis. Overall success rate noted in the case reports was 70%, whereas, in the pooled analysis of 14 studies the success rate was noted to about 50%. Although, follow-up period of the case reports was much less than the pooled analysis of 14 studies, yet, in the subset of 4 case reports with 9, 12, 18, and 30 months follow-up, the success rate was 100%. Overall association between the follow-up and satisfactory results was also not providing indication of declined success rate with increments in follow up period. Such a difference of success rate of percutaneous procedures in the retrospective analyses and case reports can be attributed to publication bias or scarcity of prospective studies will be clarified in future research. Nevertheless, this point is

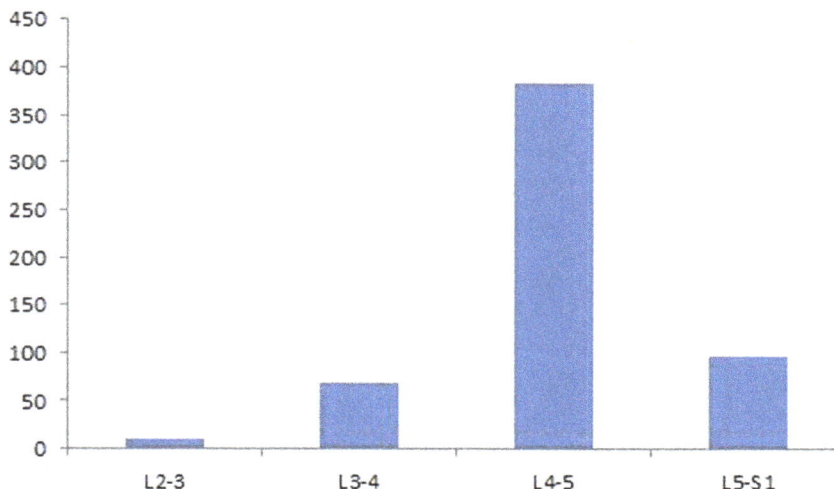

Figure 2. Spinal level of cysts diagnosed in the patients included in the meta-analysis.

encouraging enough to provide impetus for larger and longer trial/s to assess the potentials of this treatment strategy.

Natural history of the disease progression of LJFCs is not known. Frequently, patients with radicular pain may be advised for obtaining MRI scans and if there is incidental detection of LJC, detailed neurological examination is meritorious in order to seek insights into the associated pathophysiology. Patients presenting with any kind of radicular pain or associated claudication syndromes, cauda equina syndrome, or any lower extremity motor or sensory symptoms must be evaluated with advanced imaging like MRI. However, in order to avoid extra un-forecasted healthcare costs, there is sheer need of a good clinical examination at the presentation. Due to methodological issues, scarcity of categorical data and statistical power limitations, the present study could not arrive at an initiative of establishing criteria for the selection of suitable patients for percutaneous resolution procedures. Narrowing and ideally eliminating the gray areas of when to take the decision for percutaneous rupture versus the definitive strategy of cyst excision remains the hallmark of clinical research in this area. Surgical excision is precise, but is time consuming, expensive and still not risk-free. On the other hand complications may also develop following procedures such as paraplegia [42].

Because of a number of factors, the present study encounters significant limitations. Firstly, as the diagnosis of LJC remains incidental, there is only one considerable sized prospective study and all others are either retrospective analyses or case reports. Schulz et al. [37] utilized a prospective design to compare the efficacy of percutaneous resolution of LFJCs with microsurgery and noticed a clear-cut supremacy of microsurgery over percutaneous resolution attempts. Their study was not randomized but acts as a required initiative which noted satisfactory benefit of percutaneous treatment for 8 of 20 patients. Indeed, because of minimally invasiveness of this treatment, it remains a treatment of choice.

Secondly, follow-up period in the majority of studies was less than two years which makes it difficult to speculate long-term benefits of the intervention. Thirdly, data availability remained a major issue as it could be useful to apply meta-regression analyses for predicting factor by utilizing data such as age, gender cyst size, cyst type, cyst orientation/location, radiological intensity, preprocedure duration of symptoms and previous history of treatment/s. Although, case reports were considerably detailed yet in many all relevant data was not available. Cambron et al. [18] studied the effect of low or high signal intensity of MRI on the success rate of percutaneous resolution of LFJCs and noted that patients with T2-hyperintene LFJCs can be more reliably benefited from percutaneous resolution procedures.

Table 3. Common presenting conditions of lumbar facet joint cysts.

Low back pain	Disc herniation
Unilateral or bilateral radiculopathy	Spinal stenosis
Myelopathy	Neural foraminal stenosis
Neurogenic claudication	Herniated nucleus pulposus
Caudaequina syndrome	Osteoarthritis
Intracystic or epidural hemorrhage	Arachnoiditis
Spondylolisthesis	Cauda equina compression from cyst
Trochanteric bursitis	High-intensity zone in disk
Peripheral neuropathy	

Study / Case reports	Benefitted subjects	Total	Percent benefitted subjects and 95% CI		
			Percentage	Upper limit	Lower limit
Allen et al., 2009	19	32	59.37	32.68	86.07
Amoretti et al., 2012	90	120	75.0	59.5	90.5
Bjorkengren et 1987	1	3	33.33	-32.0	98.67
Bureau et al., 2001	9	12	75.0	26.0	124.0
Cambron et al 2013	63	110	57.27	43.13	71.42
Carrera, 1980	6	20	30.0	5.995	54.0
Martha et al., 2009	46	101	45.54	32.38	58.71
Ortiz & Tekch., 2013	18	20	90.0	48.42	131.6
Parlier-Cuau et 1999	14	30	46.66	22.22	71.11
Sabers et al., 2005	9	23	39.13	13.57	64.7
Sauvage et al., 2000	6	13	46.15	9.223	83.08
Schulz et al., 2011	8	20	40.0	12.28	67.72
Shah & Lutz, 2003	1	10	10.0	-9.6	29.6
Slipman et al., 2000	4	14	28.57	0.571	56.57
CR 1	4	8	50.0	1.0	99.0
CR 2	2	3	66.66	-25.7	159.1
CR 3	3	3	100	-13.2	213.2
Summary	303	543	55.80	49.52	62.08

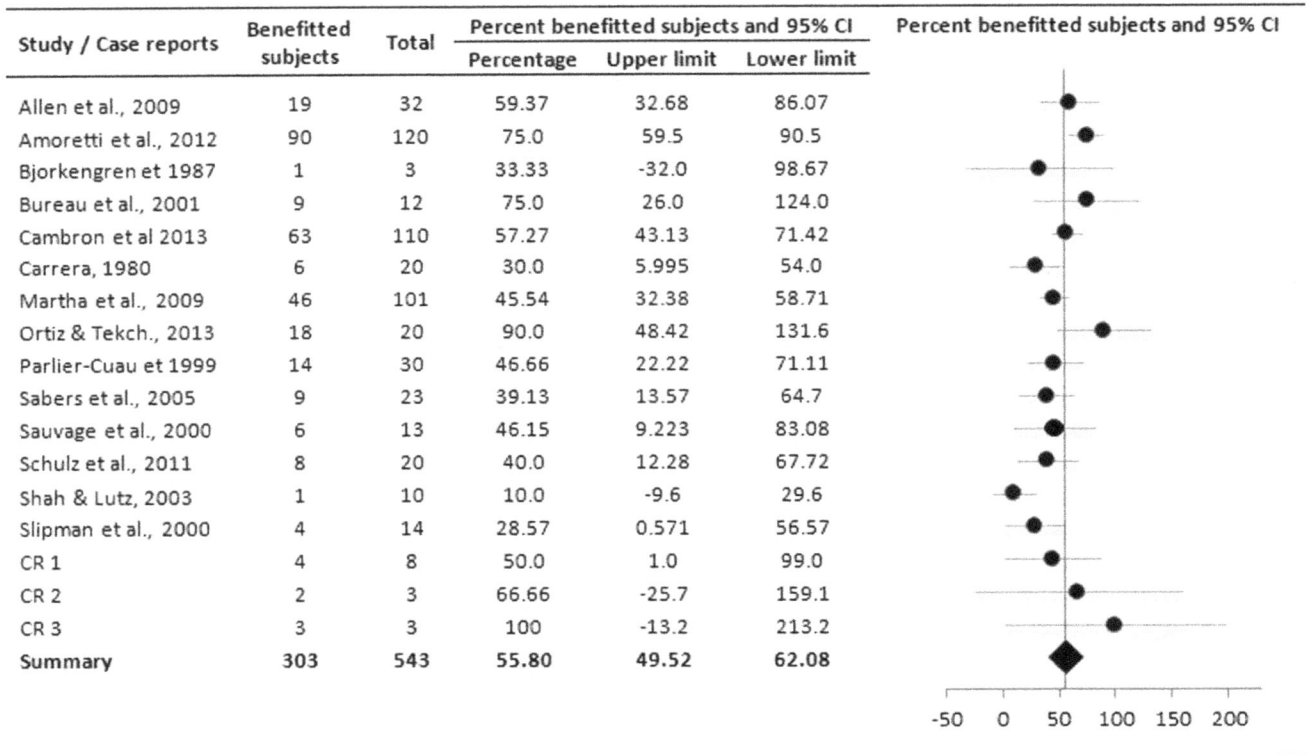

Figure 3. Forest plot showing effect sizes of satisfactory results of percutaneous treatments of the LFJCs after short- or long-term follow-up in individual studies (closed circles) and the overall effect size achieved in meta-analysis (diamond). CR 1 (follow-up 1 mo): Braza et al., 2005; Casselman et al., 1985; Chang, 2009; Foley, 2009; Imai et al., 1998; Kozar & Jeromal, 2014; Lutz and Shen, 2002; Rauchwerger et al., 2011/CR 2 (follow-up 6 month): Boissier et al., 2013; Hong et al., 1995; Shin et al., 2012/CR 3 (follow-up 1 year or more): Gishen et al., 2001; Lim et al., 2001; Lin et al., 2014; Melfi and Aprill, 2005.

Study / Case reports	Subsequent surgery	Total	Percent surgery subjects and 95% CI		
			Percentage	Upper limit	Lower limit
Allen et al., 2009	6	32	18.75	3.747	33.75
Amoretti et al., 2012	30	120	25.0	16.05	33.95
Bjorkengren et 1987	1	3	33.33	-32.0	98.67
Bureau et al., 2001	3	12	25.0	-3.29	53.29
Cambron et al 2013	47	110	42.72	30.51	54.94
Martha et al., 2009	55	101	54.45	40.06	68.85
Ortiz & Tekch., 2013	2	20	10.0	-3.86	23.86
Parlier-Cuau et 1999	14	30	46.66	22.22	71.11
Sabers et al., 2005	9	23	39.13	13.57	64.7
Sauvage et al., 2000	3	13	23.07	-3.04	49.19
Schulz et al., 2011	12	20	60.0	26.05	93.95
Shah & Lutz, 2003	8	10	80.0	24.56	135.4
Slipman et al., 2000	8	14	57.14	17.54	96.74
CR 1	2	8	25.0	-9.65	59.65
CR 2	1	3	33.33	-32.0	98.67
CR 3	0	3	0	-	-
Summary	201	523	38.62	33.30	43.95

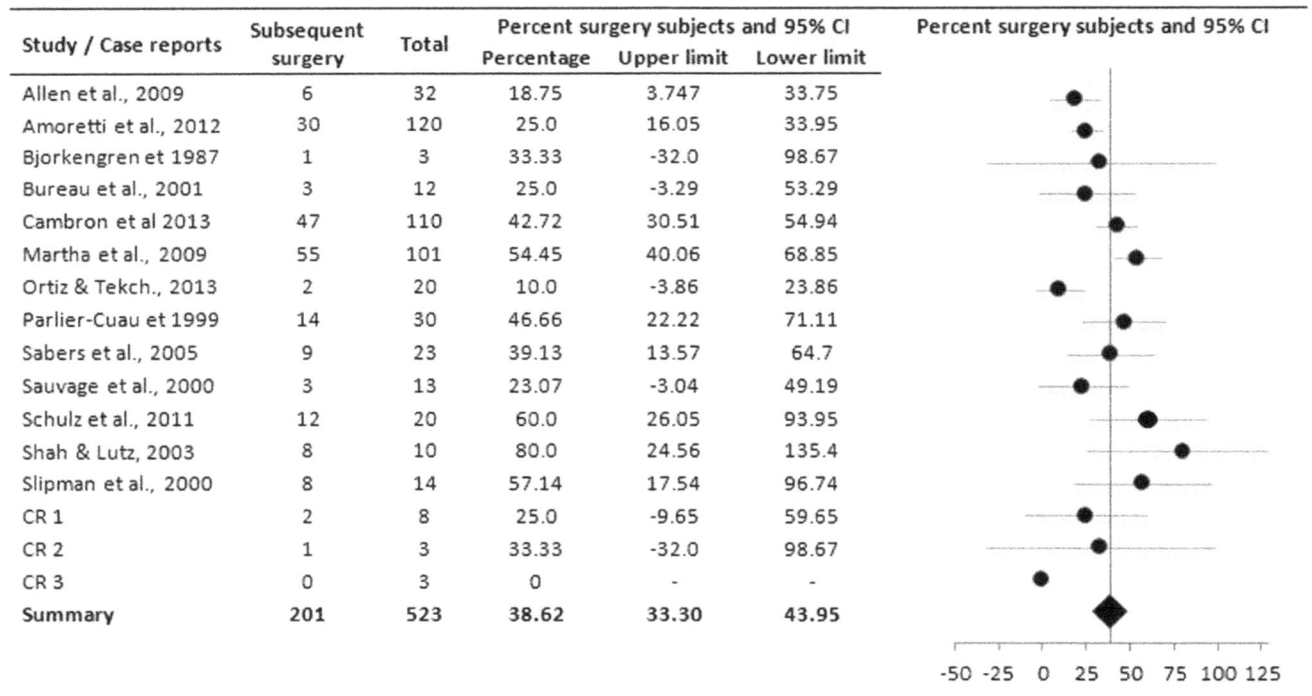

Figure 4. Forest plot showing effect sizes of subjects underwent surgical treatments subsequent to failure of percutaneous treatments of the LFJCs in individual studies (closed circles) and the overall effect size achieved in meta-analysis (diamond). CR 1/CR 2/CR 3 as given in Figure 2.

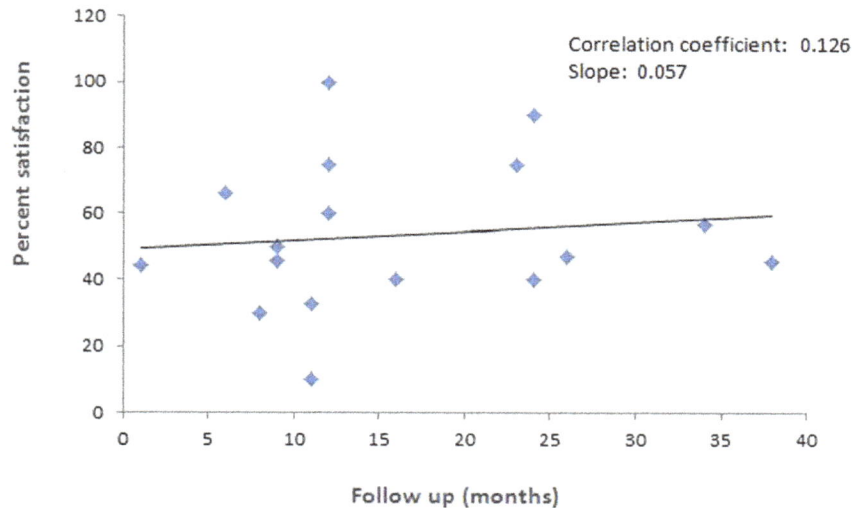

Figure 5. Scatter plot showing relationship between percent satisfaction of the subjects of percutaneous resolution procedures and follow-up duration in months.

It seems that the success rate of percutaneous resolution procedures will increase with the improvement in decision-making information and advancement in technology and skill training and exposure. However, of much importance is the availability of results of a few or a bigger, multi-center randomized controlled trial/s with adequate power to assess the success rate as well as the predicting factors for percutaneous resolution procedure selection. Without which as pointed out by Arnold et al. [43], patient is presented with the coin flip odds for percutaneous vs surgery choice.

Conclusion

By analyzing all available evidence pertaining to the efficacy of percutaneous cyst resolution procedures the present study finds this therapeutic regimen as an alternative to surgical interventions but is unable to identify subgroup/s of patients that can be benefited more reliably with this technique and therefore urges to conduct comparative studies with longer follow-up periods.

Author Contributions

Conceived and designed the experiments: JGT SXH. Performed the experiments: SXH FS JLZ DFR ZC. Analyzed the data: FS SXH JLZ DFR ZC JGT. Wrote the paper: FS SXH.

References

1. Epstein NE, Baisden J (2012) The diagnosis and management of synovial cysts: Efficacy of surgery vs cyst aspiration. Surg Neurol Int 3: 157–66.
2. DePalma MJ (2009) Driving the lane: a clearer view of facet joint cyst intervention. Spine J 9: 921–3.
3. Shipley JA, Beukes CA (1998) The nature of spondylolytic defect. Demonstration of a communicating synovial pseudoarthrosis in the pars interarticularis. J Bone Joint Surg Br 80: 662–4.
4. Alicioglu B, Sut N (2009) Synovial cysts of the lumbar facet joints: a retrospective magnetic resonance imaging study investigating their relation with degenerative spondylolisthesis. Prague Medical Report 110: 301–9.
5. Budris DM (1991) Radiologic case study, intraspinal lumbar synovial cyst. Orthopedics 14: 618–20.
6. Gheyi GY, Uppot RN, Flores C, Koyfman YU (1999) Unusual case of lumbar synovial cyst. Clin Imaging 23: 394–6.
7. Boviatsis EJ, Staurinou LC, Kouyialis AT, Gavra MM, Stavrinou PC, et al. (2008) Spinal synovial cysts: pathogenesis, diagnosis and surgical treatment in a series of seven cases and literature review. Eur Spine J 17: 831–7.
8. Abdullah AF, Chambers RW, Daut DP (1984) Lumbar nerve root compression by synovial cysts of the ligamentum flavum. Report of four cases. J Neurosurg 60: 617–20.
9. Kurz LT, Garfin SR, Unger AS, Thorne RP, Rothman RH (1985) Intraspinal synovial cyst causing sciatica. J Bone Joint Surg Am 67: 865–71.
10. Ayberg G, Ozveren F, Gok Yazgan A, Tosun H, Seçkin Z, et al. (2008) Lumbar synovial cysts: experience with nine cases. Neurol Med Chir 48: 298–303.
11. U.S. Department of Health & Human Services.Quality Assessment Tool for Observational Cohort and Cross-Sectional Studies. Available: http://www.nhlbi.nih.gov/health-pro/guidelines/in-develop/cardiovascular-risk-reduction/tools/cohort.htm. Accessed 2014 March.
12. Allen TL, Tatli Y, Lutz GE (2009) Fluoroscopic percutaneous lumbar zygapophyseal joint cyst rupture: a clinical outcome study. Spine J 9: 387–95.
13. Amoretti N, Huwart L, Foti P, Boileau P, Amoretti ME, et al. (2012) Symptomatic lumbar facet joint cysts treated by CT-guided intracystic and intra-articular steroid injections. Eur Radiol 22: 2836–40.
14. Bjorkengren AG, Kurz LT, Resnick D, Sartoris DJ, Garfin SR (1987) Symptomatic intraspinal synovial cysts: opacification and treatment by percutaneous injection. AJR Am J Roentgenol 149: 105–7.
15. Boissière L, Valour F, Rigal J, Soderlund C (2013) Lumbar synovial cyst calcification after facet joint steroid injection. BMJ Case Rep 2013. pii: bcr2012008029.
16. Braza DW, Dedianous D, Peterson B (2005) Lumbar synovial cyst. Am J Phys Med Rehabil 84: 911–2.
17. Bureau NJ, Kaplan PA, Dussault RG (2001) Lumbar facet joint synovial cyst: percutaneous treatment with steroid injections and distention—clinical and imaging follow-up in 12 patients. Radiol 221: 179–85.
18. Cambron SC, McIntyre JJ, Guerin SJ, Li Z, Pastel DA (2013) Lumbar facet joint synovial cysts: does T2 signal intensity predict outcomes after percutaneous rupture? AJNR Am J Neuroradiol 34: 1661–4.
19. Carrera GF (1980) Lumbar facet joint injection in low back pain and sciatica: preliminary results. Radiol 137: 665–7.
20. Casselman ES (1985) Radiologic recognition of symptomatic spinal synovial cysts. AJNR Am J Neuroradiol 6: 971–3.
21. Chang A (2009) Percutaneous CT-guided treatment of lumbar facet joint synovial cysts. HSS J 5: 165–8.
22. Foley BS (2009) Percutaneous rupture of a lumbar synovial facet cyst. Am J Phys Med Rehabil 88: 1046.
23. Gishen P, Miller FN (2001) Percutaneous excision of a facet joint cyst under CT guidance. Cardiovasc Intervent Radiol 24: 351–53.
24. Hong Y, O'Grady T, Carlsson C, Casey J, Clements D (1995) Percutaneous aspiration of lumbar facet synovial cyst. Anesthesiol 82: 1061–2.

25. Imai K, Nakamura K, Inokuchi K, Oda H (1998) Aspiration of intraspinal synovial cyst: recurrence after temporal improvement. Arch Orthop Trauma Surg 118: 103–5.

26. Kozar S, Jeromel M (2014) Minimally invasive CT guided treatment of intraspinal synovial cyst. Radiol Oncol 48: 35–9.

27. Lim AK, Higgins SJ, Saifuddin A, Lehovsky J (2001) Symptomatic lumbar synovial cyst: management with direct CT-guided puncture and steroid injection. Clin Radiol 56: 990–3.

28. Lin TL, Chung CT, Lan HH, Sheen HM (2014) Ultrasound-guided facet joint injection to treat a spinal cyst. J Chin Med Assoc 77: 213–6.

29. Lutz GE, Shen TC (2002) Fluoroscopically guided aspiration of a symptomatic lumbar zygapophyseal joint cyst: A case report. Arch Phys Med Rehabil 83: 1789–91.

30. Martha JF, Swaim B, Wang DA, Kim DH, Hill J, et al. (2009) Outcome of percutaneous rupture of lumbar synovial cysts: a case series of 101 patients. Spine J 9: 899–904.

31. Melfi RS, Aprill CN (2005) Percutaneous puncture of zygapophysial joint synovial cyst with fluoroscopic guidance. Pain Med 6: 122–8.

32. Ortiz AO, Tekchandani L (2013) Improved outcomes with direct percutaneous CT guided lumbar synovial cyst treatment: advanced approaches and techniques. J Neurointerv Surg doi: 10.1136/neurintsurg-2013-010891.

33. Parlier-Cuau C, Wybier M, Nizard R, Champsaur P, Le Hir P, et al. (1999) Symptomatic lumbar facet joint synovial cysts: clinical assessment of facet joint steroid injection after 1 and 6 months and long-term follow-up in 30 patients. Radiol 210: 509–13.

34. Rauchwerger JJ, Candido KD, Zoarski GH (2011) Technical and imaging report: fluoroscopic guidance for diagnosis and treatment of lumbar synovial cyst. Pain Pract 11: 180–4.

35. Sabers SR, Ross SR, Grogg BE, Lauder TD (2005) Procedure-based nonsurgical management of lumbar zygapophyseal joint cyst-induced radicular pain. Arch Phys Med Rehabil 86: 1767–71.

36. Sauvage P, Grimault L, Ben Salem D, Roussin I, Huguenin M, et al. (2000) Lumbar intraspinal synovial cysts: imaging and treatment by percutaneous injection. Report of thirteen cases. J Radiol 81: 33–8.

37. Schulz C, Danz B, Waldeck S, Kunz U, Mauer UM (2011) Percutaneous CT-guided destruction versus microsurgical resection of lumbar juxtafacet cysts. Orthopade 40: 600–6.

38. Shah RV, Lutz GE (2003) Lumbar intraspinal synovial cysts: conservative management and review of the world's literature. Spine J 3: 479–88.

39. Shin KM, Kim MS, Ko KM, Jang JS, Kang SS, et al. (2012) Percutaneous aspiration of lumbar zygapophyseal joint synovial cyst under fluoroscopic guidance - A case report. Korean J Anesthesiol 62: 375–8.

40. Slipman CW, Lipetz JS, Wakeshima Y, Jackson HB (2000) Nonsurgical treatment of zygapophyseal joint cyst-induced radicular pain. Arch Phys Med Rehabil 81: 973–7.

41. Deyo RA, Weinstein JN (2001) Low back pain. N Engl J Med 344: 363–70.

42. Kennedy DJ, Dreyfuss P, Aprill CN, Bogduk N (2009) Paraplegia following image-guided transforaminal lumbar spine epidural steroid injection: two case reports. Pain Med 10: 1389–94.

43. Arnold PM (2009) Efficacy of injection therapy for symptomatic lumbar synovial cysts. Spine J 9: 919–20.

8

Frequency of and Predictive Factors for Vascular Invasion after Radiofrequency Ablation for Hepatocellular Carcinoma

Yoshinari Asaoka[1], Ryosuke Tateishi[1]*, Ryo Nakagomi[1], Mayuko Kondo[1], Naoto Fujiwara[1], Tatsuya Minami[1], Masaya Sato[1], Koji Uchino[1], Kenichiro Enooku[1], Hayato Nakagawa[1], Yuji Kondo[1], Shuichiro Shiina[2], Haruhiko Yoshida[1], Kazuhiko Koike[1]

1 Department of Gastroenterology, Graduate School of Medicine, The University of Tokyo, Tokyo, Japan, 2 Department of Gastroenterology, Graduate School of Medicine, Juntendo University, Tokyo, Japan

Abstract

Background: Vascular invasion in patients with hepatocellular carcinoma (HCC) is representative of advanced disease with an extremely poor prognosis. The detailed course of its development has not been fully elucidated.

Methods: We enrolled 1057 consecutive patients with HCC who had been treated with curative intent by radiofrequency ablation (RFA) as an initial therapy from 1999 to 2008 at our department. We analyzed the incidence rate of and predictive factors for vascular invasion. The survival rate after detection of vascular invasion was also analyzed.

Results: During a mean follow-up period of 4.5 years, 6075 nodules including primary and recurrent lesions were treated by RFA. Vascular invasion was observed in 97 patients. The rate of vascular invasion associated with site of original RFA procedure was 0.66% on a nodule basis. The incidence rates of vascular invasion on a patient basis at 1, 3, and 5 years were 1.1%, 5.9%, and 10.4%, respectively. Univariate analysis revealed that tumor size, tumor number, alpha-fetoprotein (AFP), des-gamma-carboxy prothrombin (DCP), and Lens culinaris agglutinin-reactive fraction of alpha-fetoprotein were significant risk predictors of vascular invasion. In multivariate analysis, DCP was the most significant predictor for vascular invasion (compared with a DCP of ≤100 mAu/mL, the hazard ratio was 1.95 when DCP was 101–200 mAu/mL and 3.22 when DCP was >200 mAu/mL). The median survival time after development of vascular invasion was only 6 months.

Conclusion: Vascular invasion occurs during the clinical course of patients initially treated with curative intent. High-risk patients may be identified using tumor markers.

Editor: Yujin Hoshida, Icahn School of Medicine at Mount Sinai, United States of America

Funding: This work was supported by Health Sciences Research Grants of The Ministry of Health, Labour and Welfare of Japan (Research on Hepatitis). No additional external funding received for this study. The funders had no role in study design, data collection and analysis, decision to publish, or preparation of the manuscript.

Competing Interests: The authors have declared that no competing interests exist.

* Email: tateishi-tky@umin.ac.jp

Introduction

Hepatocellular carcinoma (HCC) is a leading cause of cancer death. It has a particularly high incidence in Asian countries, including Japan [1,2]. To control this disease, close surveillance using advanced diagnostic modalities including ultrasonography (US), computed tomography (CT), and gadolinium-ethoxybenzyl-diethylenetriamine pentaacetic acid-enhanced magnetic resonance imaging (EOB-MRI) in designated high-risk patients has facilitated HCC detection at a very early stage at which surgical resection, liver transplantation, and percutaneous ablative therapies are feasible [3]. Although surgical resection is usually the first-choice treatment option for early stage disease, it is not frequently indicated in patients with underlying liver function impaired by

chronic infection of hepatitis B or C virus [4]. Liver transplantation can treat both cancer and liver dysfunction; it has shown excellent survival rates in patients with early stage HCC [5]. However, in countries where cadaveric donor organs are scarce, as in Japan, the application of liver transplantation is limited.

Radiofrequency ablation (RFA) is currently considered to be the most effective first-line percutaneous ablative therapy because it has greater efficacy in terms of local cure than does ethanol injection [6]. The survival outcomes for patients who achieve a complete response by RFA are comparable with those for patients treated by hepatic resection [7,8]. However, even after locally curative resection or ablation, patients encounter frequent recurrence in the remnant liver because of intrahepatic spread of tumor cells and metachronous multicentric carcinogenesis; the rate of recurrence at 5 years is as high as 70–80% [9,10]. Although repeated resection or ablation can be performed in patients with recurrent HCC [11,12], the tumor tends to be out of control during the clinical course of frequent recurrence and retreatment. This is a major reason for the poor long-term survival after curative resection or ablation [13].

The development of vascular invasion and extrahepatic metastasis are representative events of an advanced stage of HCC [14,15]. Once tumor cells have invaded the portal vein, they progressively spread and increase the portal venous pressure, resulting in ascites and the rupture of esophageal varices. The spread also decreases portal flow into the hepatic parenchyma,

causing fatal liver failure [16–18]. Hepatic venous invasion causes tumor thrombi to form in the pulmonary arteries and lung tissue [19], and biliary invasion may cause jaundice, hemobilia, or cholangitis [20]. Previous studies have reported that patients with HCC with vascular invasion survive for only three months [15].

The detailed course of development of vascular invasion could not be fully elucidated by analyzing the cases who unfortunately encountered the advanced disease with vascular invasion at the time of the initial diagnosis. Because patients who undergo RFA are rigorously followed up for recurrence, the use of imaging modalities might allow for the identification of the early form of vascular invasion.

In this paper, we analyzed the incidence and predictive factors of vascular invasion as well as its detailed characteristics in patients with HCC treated with RFA with curative intent as the initial therapy.

Patients and Methods

Ethics statement

This retrospective study was conducted according to the ethical guidelines for epidemiological research of the Japanese Ministry of Education, Culture, Sports, Science and Technology and Ministry of Health, Labour and Welfare. The study design was included in a comprehensive protocol at the Department of Gastroenterology, The University of Tokyo Hospital and approved by the University of Tokyo Medical Research Center Ethics Committee (approval number 2058). Informed consent was waived because of the retrospective design. The following statements were posted at a website (http://gastro.m.u-tokyo.ac.jp/med/0602A.htm) and participants who do not agree to the use of their clinical data can claim deletion of them.

Department of Gastroenterology at The University of Tokyo Hospital contains data from our daily practice for the assessment of short-term (treatment success, immediate adverse events etc.) and long-term (late complications, recurrence etc.) outcomes. Obtained data were stored in an encrypted hard disk separated from outside of the hospital. When reporting analyzed data, we protect the anonymity of participants for the sake of privacy

Table 1. Patients' characteristics at initial RFA (n = 1057).

Variable	
Age in years	
Median	68.8
IQR	63.4–74.4
Male sex, n (%)	685 (64.8)
Etiology	
HBsAg-positive only, n (%)	119 (11.3)
Anti-HCVAb-positive only, n (%)	789 (74.6)
Both positive, n (%)	11 (1.0)
Both negative, n (%)	138 (13.0)
Alcohol consumption>80 g/day	154 (14.6)
Platelet count (×10^9/L)	
Median	108
IQR	78–146
Child-Pugh classification, n (%)	
Class A	781 (73.9)
Class B	265 (25.1)
Class C	11 (1.0)
Tumor number, n (%)	
1	622 (58.8)
2–3	350 (33.1)
>3	85 (8.0)
Maximal tumor size (mm)	
Median	24
IQR	18–31
AFP, n (%)	
≤100 ng/mL	832 (78.7)
>100 and ≤200 ng/mL	72 (6.8)
>200 ng/mL	153 (14.5)
DCP, n (%)*	
≤100 mAU/mL	878 (83.6)
>100 and ≤200 mAU/mL	72 (6.9)
>200 mAU/mL	100 (9.5)
AFP-L3, n (%)	
≤10%	878 (83.1)
>10%	179 (16.9)

* Not determined in seven patients due to warfarin use.
Abbreviations: HBsAg, hepatitis B surface antigen; HCVAb, hepatitis C virus antibody; AFP, alpha-fetoprotein; AFP-L3, *Lens culinaris* agglutinin-reactive fraction of AFP; DCP, des-gamma-carboxyprothrombin; IQR, interquartile range.

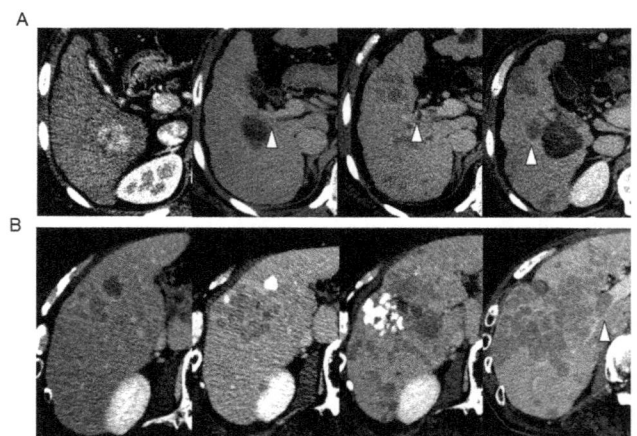

Figure 1. Images of vascular invasion developing adjacent (A) and apart (B) from the ablated area. (Case A: left panel: primary lesion before RFA, middle left panel: development of VI, middle right and right panel: evident development of VI after 4 months, Case B: left panel: multiple recurrence after RFA, middle left panel: after TACE, middle right and right panel: VI development after repeated TACE). Arrowheads denote portal venous invasion.

Table 2. Patients' characteristics at diagnosis of vascular invasion (n = 97).

Variable	
Extension of vascular invasion, n (%)	
Portal invasion within subsegmental branch	20 (20.6)
Portal invasion within segmental branch	22 (22.6)
Portal invasion within first branch	30 (30.9)
Portal invasion to main trunk	12 (12.3)
Bile duct invasion	17 (17.5)
Hepatic venous invasion	4 (4.1)
Tumor location	
Adjacent to previously ablated area, n (%)	40 (41.2)
Apart from previously ablated area, n (%)	57 (58.8)
Tumor number, n (%)	
1	10 (10.3)
2–3	8 (8.3)
4–10	14 (14.4)
>10	44 (45.4)
Undetectable*	21 (21.6)
Maximal tumor size	
Median (mm)	27.5
IQR	15.5–41.0
Diffuse/infiltrative, n (%)	36 (37.1)
Extrahepatic metastasis, n (%)	28 (28.9)
AFP, n (%)	
≤100 ng/mL	34 (35.1)
>100 and ≤200 ng/mL	9 (9.3)
>200 ng/mL	54 (55.7)
DCP, n (%)†	
≤100 mAU/mL	31 (32.3)
>100 and ≤200 mAU/mL	10 (10.4)
>200 mAU/mL	55 (57.3)
AFP-L3, n (%)	
≤10%	42 (43.3)
>10%	55 (56.7)

*Intrahepatic tumor was not clearly identified. †DCP was not measured in one patient due to warfarin use.
Abbreviations: HR, hazard ratio; HBsAg, hepatitis B surface antigen; HCVAb, hepatitis C virus antibody; AFP, alpha-fetoprotein; AFP-L3, Lens culinaris agglutinin-reactive fraction of AFP; DCP, des-gamma-carboxyprothrombin.

protection. If you do not wish the utilization of your data for the clinical study or have any question on the research content, please do not hesitate to make contact with us.

Patients

From 1999 to 2008, a total of 1057 patients with HCC underwent RFA as the initial treatment for naïve HCC. All the patients were included in this study and followed. The inclusion criteria for RFA were: 1) no prior HCC treatment other than TACE as part of sequential TACE-RFA treatment protocol; 2) three or fewer lesions of ≤3 cm in diameter; 3) a total bilirubin level of <3 mg/dL; 4) a platelet count of $\geq 50 \times 10^3/mm^3$; and 5) a prothrombin activity level of ≥50%. Exclusion criteria were: 1) portal vein tumor thrombosis; 2) refractory ascites; or 3) extrahepatic metastasis However, we also performed RFA on

patients outside these criteria if treatment was predicted to be clinically effective [21].

Diagnosis and treatment of primary HCC

HCC was diagnosed using dynamic computed tomography (CT); hyperattenuation in the arterial phase with washout in the late phase was considered to be a definitive sign of this disease [22]. Most nodules were also confirmed histopathologically via ultrasound (US)-guided biopsy. All patients underwent dynamic CT with a slice thickness of 5 mm within 1 month prior to RFA for comparison. The detailed protocol for RFA is described elsewhere [21]. Briefly, a 17-gauge, cooled tip electrode was inserted into the lesion under real-time ultrasound guidance. We started ablation at 60 W for the 3-cm exposed tip and 40 W for the 2-cm exposed tip. The power was increased to 140 W at a rate of 20 W/min. When a rapid increase in impedance was observed

A

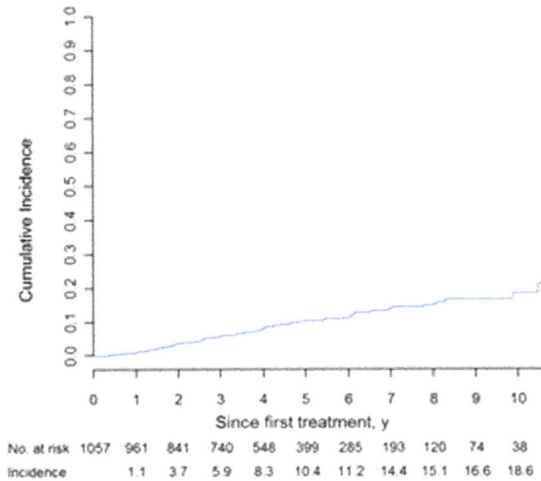

B

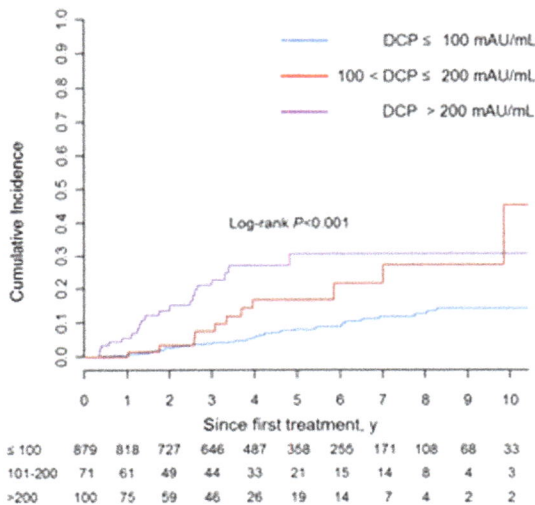

C

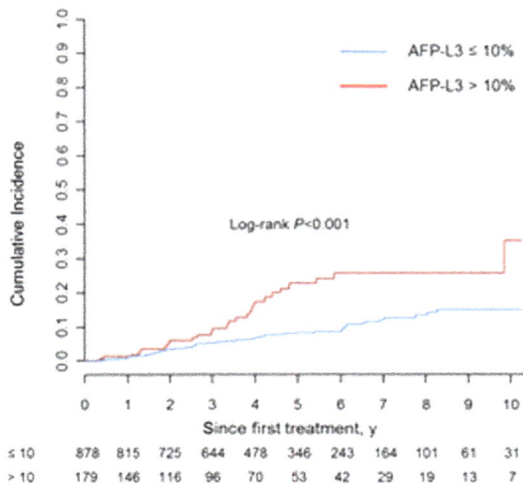

Figure 2. Cumulative incidence of vascular invasion after the initial treatment (A) and incidence stratified based on the DCP (B) and AFP-L3 (C) levels at the initial treatment.

during thermal ablation, we minimized the output for 15 seconds and restarted the emission at a lower output. The duration of a single ablation was 12 minutes for the 3-cm electrode and 6 minutes for the 2-cm electrode. During the treatment evaluation, a lesion was judged to be completely ablated when the nonenhanced area shown in the late phase of post-ablation CT covered the entire lesion shown in both the early and late phases of pre-ablation CT with a safety margin in the surrounding liver parenchyma. We confirmed complete ablation in all slices in which the target nodule was visualized. Patients underwent additional sessions until complete ablation was confirmed in each nodule.

Follow-up and assessment of vascular invasion

The follow-up regimen comprised blood tests to monitor tumor markers in an outpatient setting. Dynamic CT was also performed every 4 months. When HCC recurrence was identified, patients who met the same criteria used for primary HCC underwent RFA. When RFA was not indicated for the recurrent nodules due to their multiplicity, the patient underwent TACE if liver function was categorized as Child-Pugh class B or better. Those with extrahepatic tumor metastasis received systemic chemotherapy if they had well-preserved liver function and a good performance status. Vascular invasion was defined as invasion of an HCC tumor into the first and/or second branch or the main trunk of the vasculature. Vascular invasion was confirmed by demonstrating the following imaging characteristics: 1) a low-attenuation intraluminal mass that expanded the vasculature on CT, MRI, or conventional US[23,24] or 2) attenuation of portal blood flow and detection of vascularity in the thrombi by contrast-enhanced CT, MRI, or US [25,26]. The follow-up period was defined as the interval from the date of the initial RFA until the date of diagnosis of vascular invasion development, the date of death, or the end of December 2011.

Statistical analysis

Cumulative incidence of vascular invasion was calculated using the Kaplan–Meier method. Predictive factors for the development of vascular invasion were analyzed using univariate and multivariate Cox proportional hazard regression. The following factors at the initial therapy were used for the analyses: age, sex, hepatitis B surface antigen positivity, hepatitis C antibody positivity, Child-Pugh class, platelet count, alanine aminotransferase level, maximum tumor size, number of lesions, alpha-fetoprotein (AFP) level, des-gamma-carboxyprothrombin (DCP) level, and *Lens culinaris* agglutinin-reactive fraction of AFP (AFP-L3). In the multivariate analysis, stepwise variable selection based on the Akaike information criterion was used to build the final model. Scatter plots were used to assess the relationship between tumor marker values immediately before the initial treatment and at the time of diagnosis of vascular invasion. We also estimated survival rates after the development of vascular invasion using the Kaplan–Meier method. Survival curves were stratified according to the mode of vascular invasion, which was classified by the level of portal vein invasion. For the survival analysis, the follow-up was censored on 31 December 2012. Differences with a P value of < 0.05 were considered to be statistically significant. All statistical analyses were performed with R 2.13.0 (http://www.R-project.org).

Table 3. Predictors of vascular invasion after RFA (n = 1057).

Variable	Univariate Analysis		Multivariate Analysis	
	HR (95% CI)	P	HR (95% CI)	P
Age (per 1 year)	1.01 (0.98–1.03)	0.69		
Male sex	0.85 (0.55–1.30)	0.45		
HCVAb-positive	1.10 (0.69–1.75)	0.70		
HBsAg-positive	1.54 (0.93–2.55)	0.11		
Platelet count (per 10^9/L)	1.00 (0.97–1.04)	0.97		
ALT>80 U/L	0.88 (0.53–1.46)	0.62		
Child Pugh (per 1 point)	1.05 (0.87–1.26)	0.65		
Tumor size (mm)				
≤20	1		1	
21–30	1.54 (0.92–2.57)	0.098	1.30 (0.77–2.19)	0.320
>30	2.51 (1.49–4.22)	<0.001	1.74 (1.01–3.01)	0.048
Tumor number				
1	1		1	
2–3	1.59 (1.04–2.43)	0.033	1.61 (1.05–2.47)	0.029
>3	2.18 (1.13–4.20)	0.002	2.02 (1.05–3.92)	0.037
AFP (ng/mL)				
≤100	1			
101–200	1.41 (0.68–2.94)	0.36		
>200	1.93 (1.18–3.15)	0.008		
DCP (mAU/mL)				
≤100	1		1	
101–200	2.34 (1.23–4.43)	0.008	1.99 (1.03–3.84)	0.041
>200	4.33 (2.62–7.16)	<0.001	3.24 (1.90–5.51)	<0.001
AFP-L3 (%)				
≤10	1		1	
>10	2.22 (1.42–3.48)	<0.001	1.75 (1.10–2.78)	0.018

Abbreviations: HR, hazard ratio; HBsAg, hepatitis B surface antigen; HCVAb, hepatitis C virus antibody; AFP, alpha-fetoprotein; AFP-L3, *Lens culinaris* agglutinin-reactive fraction of AFP; DCP, des-gamma-carboxyprothrombin.

Results

Patient profiles and development of vascular invasion

The enrolled HCC patient cohort in this study comprised 685 males and 372 females with a median age of 68.8 years (Table 1). Approximately 75% of cases were hepatitis C-related. The median [interquartile range (IQR)] maximal tumor size was 2.4 [1.8–3.1] cm. The mean (± standard deviation) number of nodules was 1.7±1.2.

During the mean follow-up period of 4.5 years, 735 of the 1057 enrolled patients underwent 2288 RFA treatments for tumor recurrence in addition to the initial RFA. Thus, the total number of RFA treatments and target nodules were 3345 and 6075, respectively. Vascular invasion was observed in 97 patients, developing adjacent and apart from the ablated area in 40 and 57 patients, respectively (Fig. 1). Therefore, the rate of vascular invasion development associated with site of original RFA was 0.66% on a nodule basis. The detailed tumor characteristics of the patients at the time of diagnosis of vascular invasion are shown in Table 2. The sites of vascular invasion were the portal vein in 85, biliary tract in 17, and hepatic vein in 4. The cumulative incidence

rates of vascular invasion on a patient basis at 1, 3, 5, and 10 years were 1.1%, 5.9%, 10.4%, and 18.6%, respectively (Fig. 2A).

Predictive factors related to vascular invasion

Univariate Cox proportional regression revealed that the following factors were significantly associated with vascular invasion: tumor size, tumor number, AFP, DCP, and AFP-L3. Multivariate analysis with step-wise variable selection showed that the final model included tumor size, tumor number, DCP, and AFP-L3 (Table 3, Fig. 2B and C). We assessed the relationship of tumor marker values prior to ablation and at the time of diagnosis of vascular invasion. As shown in Figure 3, the sensitivities of tumor markers were higher at the time of diagnosis of vascular invasion than at the time of initial treatment: 64.9% for AFP, 67.7% for DCP, and 47.4% for AFP-L3 at the diagnosis of vascular invasion when cut-off values of 100 ng/mL, 100 mAU/mL, and 15% were adopted, respectively. Although DCP at the time of the initial treatment showed a high ability to predict vascular invasion, DCP at the initial treatment was also positive in only 23 (41.8%) of the 55 patients with a DCP of >100 mAU/mL

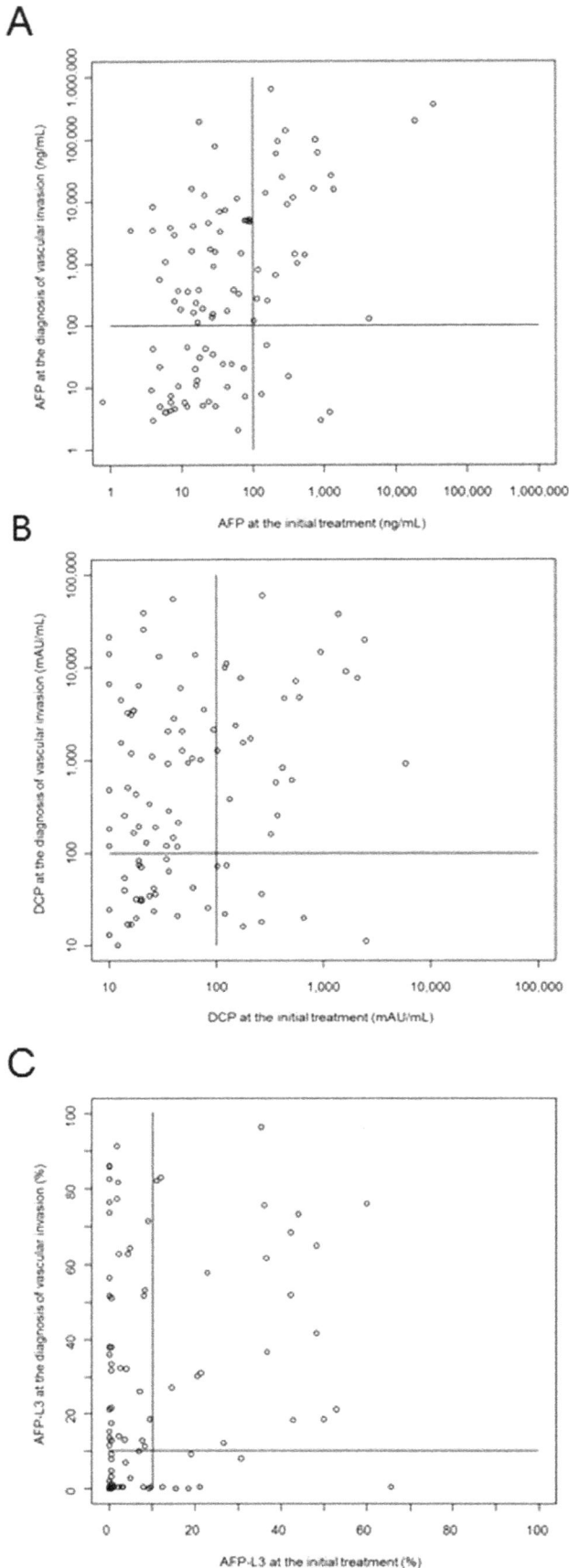

Figure 3. Scatter plots of AFP (A), DCP (B), and AFP-L3 (C) at initial treatment and at diagnosis of vascular invasion.

at the time of vascular invasion development. This result indicates that the tumor characteristics changed during the clinical course.

Treatment of vascular invasion and associated survival outcomes

Among the 97 patients diagnosed with vascular invasion, 53 (55%) underwent hepatic arterial infusion chemotherapy. Four patients underwent hepatic resection because of a localized tumor in three and tumor shrinkage due to hepatic arterial chemotherapy in one. Six patients received systemic chemotherapy including sorafenib. The remaining patients were treated with combination therapies including TACE, irradiation, and chemotherapy. Twenty-four patients (25%) received supportive therapy due to liver dysfunction or a poor performance status. The 1-, 3-, and 5-year survival rates after development of vascular invasion were 33.1%, 10.6%, and 6.4%, respectively (Fig. 4A). Survival rates differed with the severity of vascular invasion (Fig. 4B), but even in the mildest disease group with Vp1 (invasion within the second branch of the portal vein), survival was still poor (1-, 2-, and 3-year survival rates were 58.9%, 12.0%, and 6.0%, respectively). The survival rate did not change whether the vascular invasion developed adjacent to or apart from the ablated area (Fig. 4C).

Discussion

Vascular invasion is one of the most important predictors of poor survival of HCC patients [15–18]. This study showed that vascular invasion occurred in 10% of patients within 5 years when HCC was initially diagnosed at an early stage. The fact that tumor-related factors at the initial diagnosis could predict the appearance of vascular invasion as a late event may suggest that intrahepatic metastasis of primary tumors can determine overall survival. However, more than half of patients in whom a tumor marker was elevated at the diagnosis of vascular invasion were negative for the tumor marker at the initial diagnosis, which suggests that the appearance of a more aggressive tumor during the clinical course was the direct cause of vascular invasion.

Compatible with our previous report on patients with HCC treated with ethanol injection and microwave ablation, DCP was strongly related to the development of vascular invasion [27]. Some cross-sectional studies reported that DCP was correlated with microvascular invasion [28,29]. As high DCP tumors were suggested to possess invasive capacity, a high DCP level is proposed to be regarded as a contraindication for liver transplantation in several institutions in Japan [30,31]. One suggested mechanism behind the relationship between vascular invasion and DCP was that hypoxia in the tumor, which is a key trigger of epithelial-mesenchymal transition, correlates with DCP elevations [32]. It is quite reasonable that tumors with such an invasive phenotype finally develop macrovascular invasion. One concern is that patients with high DCP level may not be suitable for RFA. However, considering the fact that a high DCP level is regarded as a contraindication for liver transplantation and there is no evidence that TACE is superior to RFA in terms of local cure, it would be reasonable to consider resection in patients with good liver function[33] or to perform RFA with a wider margin in unresectable cases with deteriorated liver function when patients show a high DCP level [34].

Several reports have suggested that incomplete thermal ablation might increase tumor aggressiveness. In this study, only 0.66% of

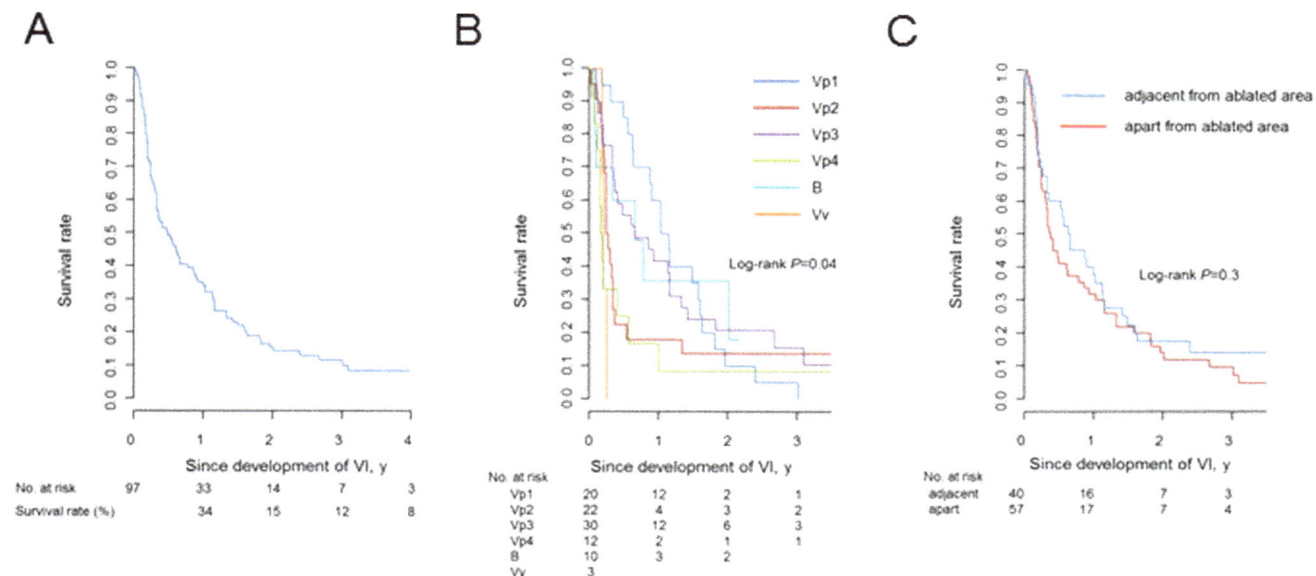

Figure 4. Overall survival rate after development of vascular invasion (A) and survival rate stratified based on severity of invasion (B). Survival rates of patients with vascular invasion developing adjacent to (blue) and apart from (red) the ablated area (C).

ablated nodules developed vascular invasion as local tumor progression [35]. This rate is acceptable considering the low mortality rate related to RFA compared with resection [36], although there is room for technical improvement. In addition, the survival rates of patients with vascular invasion adjacent to and apart from the ablated area were similar. This suggests that vascular invasion might not be a consequence of malignant transformation caused by RFA.

Vascular invasion was diagnosed in an advanced form in 52 of 97 patients, although most of them were followed closely by imaging modalities. One possible reason is that once a tumor invades the vasculature, it extends quite rapidly, probably because there is no obstacle within the lumen. Another reason would be that tumors located in the hilar region of the liver directly invaded the main trunk in some cases. This suggests that early diagnosis of vascular invasion is quite difficult. In addition, it should be noted that even when a minimal extent of portal invasion is diagnosed, the outcome is disappointing with a median survival of 1 year.

After the development of vascular invasion in this study, the therapeutic options were limited and the prognosis was poor. Surgical resection may be preferable in patients with limited tumor extension, but only four patients were indicated for resection; 25% of patients were ineligible for aggressive treatment and received best supportive care because of liver dysfunction caused by the vascular invasion itself or because of repeated recurrence and

treatment. Sorafenib is now the treatment of choice for patients with vascular invasion. However, the survival outcome is still unsatisfactory, even in patients with Child-Pugh class A [37], probably because tumors in the portal vein rarely decrease in size with the use of sorafenib and liver function may deteriorate with reduced portal blood flow.

In conclusion, vascular invasion occurs during the clinical course of patients with HCC initially treated with curative intent. The serum DCP level is the most useful predisposing parameter for the development of vascular invasion after RFA. Once vascular invasion has developed, the prognosis is poor. We must develop another strategy by which to improve the survival of these patients.

Author Contributions

Conceived and designed the experiments: YA RT KK. Analyzed the data: RT. Contributed reagents/materials/analysis tools: YA RN MK NF TM MS KU KE HN YK SS. Wrote the paper: YA RT. Critical revision of manuscript: SS HY KK.

References

1. Parkin DM, Bray F, Ferlay J, Pisani P (2005) Global cancer statistics, 2002. CA Cancer J Clin 55: 74–108.
2. Matsuda T, Marugame T, Kamo K, Katanoda K, Ajiki W, et al. (2009) Cancer incidence and incidence rates in Japan in 2003: based on data from 13 population-based cancer registries in the Monitoring of Cancer Incidence in Japan (MCIJ) Project. Jpn J Clin Oncol 39: 850–858.
3. Sato T, Tateishi R, Yoshida H, Ohki T, Masuzaki R, et al. (2009) Ultrasound surveillance for early detection of hepatocellular carcinoma among patients with chronic hepatitis C. Hepatol Int 3: 544–550.
4. Shiratori Y, Shiina S, Imamura M, Kato N, Kanai F, et al. (1995) Characteristic difference of hepatocellular carcinoma between hepatitis B- and C- viral infection in Japan. Hepatology 22: 1027–1033.

5. Mazzaferro V, Regalia E, Doci R, Andreola S, Pulvirenti A, et al. (1996) Liver transplantation for the treatment of small hepatocellular carcinomas in patients with cirrhosis. N Engl J Med 334: 693–699.
6. Lin SM, Lin CJ, Lin CC, Hsu CW, Chen YC (2004) Radiofrequency ablation improves prognosis compared with ethanol injection for hepatocellular carcinoma < or = 4 cm. Gastroenterology 127: 1714–1723.
7. Livraghi T, Meloni F, Di Stasi M, Rolle E, Solbiati L, et al. (2008) Sustained complete response and complications rates after radiofrequency ablation of very early hepatocellular carcinoma in cirrhosis: Is resection still the treatment of choice? Hepatology 47: 82–89.
8. Shiina S, Tateishi R, Arano T, Uchino K, Enooku K, et al. (2012) Radiofrequency ablation for hepatocellular carcinoma: 10-year outcome and prognostic factors. Am J Gastroenterol 107: 569–577; quiz 578.

9. Tateishi R, Shiina S, Yoshida H, Teratani T, Obi S, et al. (2006) Prediction of recurrence of hepatocellular carcinoma after curative ablation using three tumor markers. Hepatology 44: 1518–1527.

10. Okada S, Shimada K, Yamamoto J, Takayama T, Kosuge T, et al. (1994) Predictive factors for postoperative recurrence of hepatocellular carcinoma. Gastroenterology 106: 1618–1624.

11. Nagasue N, Kohno H, Hayashi T, Uchida M, Ono T, et al. (1996) Repeat hepatectomy for recurrent hepatocellular carcinoma. Br J Surg 83: 127–131.

12. Liang HH, Chen MS, Peng ZW, Zhang YJ, Zhang YQ, et al. (2008) Percutaneous radiofrequency ablation versus repeat hepatectomy for recurrent hepatocellular carcinoma: a retrospective study. Ann Surg Oncol 15: 3484–3493.

13. Ikai I, Arii S, Okazaki M, Okita K, Omata M, et al. (2007) Report of the 17th Nationwide Follow-up Survey of Primary Liver Cancer in Japan. Hepatol Res 37: 676–691.

14. Llovet JM, Bru C, Bruix J (1999) Prognosis of hepatocellular carcinoma: the BCLC staging classification. Semin Liver Dis. pp. 329–338.

15. Giannelli G, Pierri F, Trerotoli P, Marinosci F, Serio G, et al. (2002) Occurrence of portal vein tumor thrombus in hepatocellular carcinoma affects prognosis and survival. A retrospective clinical study of 150 cases. Hepatol Res 24: 50.

16. Albacete RA, Matthews MJ, Saini N (1967) Portal vein thromboses in malignant hepatoma. Ann Intern Med 67: 337–348.

17. Adachi E, Maeda T, Kajiyama K, Kinukawa N, Matsumata T, et al. (1996) Factors correlated with portal venous invasion by hepatocellular carcinoma: univariate and multivariate analyses of 232 resected cases without preoperative treatments. Cancer 77: 2022–2031.

18. Fujii T, Takayasu K, Muramatsu Y, Moriyama N, Wakao F, et al. (1993) Hepatocellular carcinoma with portal tumor thrombus: analysis of factors determining prognosis. Jpn J Clin Oncol 23: 105–109.

19. Sawabe M, Nakamura T, Kanno J, Kasuga T (1987) Analysis of morphological factors of hepatocellular carcinoma in 98 autopsy cases with respect to pulmonary metastasis. Acta Pathol Jpn 37: 1389–1404.

20. Qin LX, Tang ZY (2003) Hepatocellular carcinoma with obstructive jaundice: diagnosis, treatment and prognosis. World J Gastroenterol 9: 385–391.

21. Tateishi R, Shiina S, Teratani T, Obi S, Sato S, et al. (2005) Percutaneous radiofrequency ablation for hepatocellular carcinoma. An analysis of 1000 cases. Cancer 103: 1201–1209.

22. Torzilli G, Minagawa M, Takayama T, Inoue K, Hui AM, et al. (1999) Accurate preoperative evaluation of liver mass lesions without fine-needle biopsy. Hepatology 30: 889–893.

23. Inamoto K, Sugiki K, Yamasaki H, Miura T (1981) CT of hepatoma: effects of portal vein obstruction. AJR Am J Roentgenol 136: 349–353.

24. Van Gansbeke D, Avni EF, Delcour C, Engelholm L, Struyven J (1985) Sonographic features of portal vein thrombosis. AJR Am J Roentgenol 144: 749–752.

25. Mathieu D, Grenier P, Larde D, Vasile N (1984) Portal vein involvement in hepatocellular carcinoma: dynamic CT features. Radiology 152: 127–132.

26. Mitani T, Nakamura H, Murakami T, Nishikawa M, Maeshima S, et al. (1992) Dynamic MR studies of hepatocellular carcinoma with portal vein tumor thrombosis. Radiat Med 10: 232–234.

27. Koike Y, Shiratori Y, Sato S, Obi S, Teratani T, et al. (2001) Des-gamma-carboxy prothrombin as a useful predisposing factor for the development of portal venous invasion in patients with hepatocellular carcinoma: a prospective analysis of 227 patients. Cancer 91: 561–569.

28. Shimada M, Yonemura Y, Ijichi H, Harada N, Shiotani S, et al. (2005) Living donor liver transplantation for hepatocellular carcinoma: a special reference to a preoperative des-gamma-carboxy prothrombin value. Transplant Proc 37: 1177–1179.

29. Shirabe K, Itoh S, Yoshizumi T, Soejima Y, Taketomi A, et al. (2007) The predictors of microvascular invasion in candidates for liver transplantation with hepatocellular carcinoma-with special reference to the serum levels of des-gamma-carboxy prothrombin. J Surg Oncol 95: 235–240.

30. Ito T, Takada Y, Ueda M, Haga H, Maetani Y, et al. (2007) Expansion of selection criteria for patients with hepatocellular carcinoma in living donor liver transplantation. Liver Transpl 13: 1637–1644.

31. Hasegawa K, Imamura H, Ijichi M, Matsuyama Y, Sano K, et al. (2008) Inclusion of tumor markers improves the correlation of the Milan criteria with vascular invasion and tumor cell differentiation in patients with hepatocellular carcinoma undergoing liver resection (#JGSU-D-07-00462). J Gastrointest Surg 12: 858–866.

32. Murata K, Suzuki H, Okano H, Oyamada T, Yasuda Y, et al. (2009) Cytoskeletal changes during epithelial-to-fibroblastoid conversion as a crucial mechanism of des-gamma-carboxy prothrombin production in hepatocellular carcinoma. Int J Oncol 35: 1005–1014.

33. Kobayashi M, Ikeda K, Kawamura Y, Yatsuji H, Hosaka T, et al. (2009) High serum des-gamma-carboxy prothrombin level predicts poor prognosis after radiofrequency ablation of hepatocellular carcinoma. Cancer 115: 571–580.

34. Takahashi S, Kudo M, Chung H, Inoue T, Ishikawa E, et al. (2008) PIVKA-II is the best prognostic predictor in patients with hepatocellular carcinoma after radiofrequency ablation therapy. Oncology 75 Suppl 1: 91–98.

35. Baldan A, Marino D, M DEG, Angonese C, Cillo U, et al. (2006) Percutaneous radiofrequency thermal ablation for hepatocellular carcinoma. Aliment Pharmacol Ther 24: 1495–1501.

36. Sato M, Tateishi R, Yasunaga H, Horiguchi H, Yoshida H, et al. (2012) Mortality and morbidity of hepatectomy, radiofrequency ablation, and embolization for hepatocellular carcinoma: a national survey of 54,145 patients. J Gastroenterol 47: 1125–1133.

37. Jeong SW, Jang JY, Shim KY, Lee SH, Kim SG, et al. (2013) Practical effect of sorafenib monotherapy on advanced hepatocellular carcinoma and portal vein tumor thrombosis. Gut Liver 7: 696–703.

9

Comparison of Optic Disc Morphology of Optic Nerve Atrophy between Compressive Optic Neuropathy and Glaucomatous Optic Neuropathy

Masayuki Hata*, Kazuaki Miyamoto, Akio Oishi, Yukiko Makiyama, Norimoto Gotoh, Yugo Kimura, Tadamichi Akagi, Nagahisa Yoshimura

Department of Ophthalmology and Visual Sciences, Kyoto University Graduate School of Medicine, Kyoto, Japan

Abstract

Objectives: To compare the optic nerve head (ONH) structure between compressive optic neuropathy (CON) and glaucomatous optic neuropathy (GON), and to determine whether selected ONH quantitative parameters effectively discriminate between GON and CON, especially CON cases presenting with a glaucoma-like disc.

Methods: We prospectively assessed 34 patients with CON, 34 age-matched patients with moderate or severe GON, and 34 age-matched healthy control subjects. The quantitative parameters of ONH structure were compared using the Heidelberg Retina Tomograph 2 (HRT2) and Spectralis optical coherence tomography with an enhanced depth imaging method.

Results: The mean and maximum cup depths of CON were significantly smaller than those with GON ($P<0.001$ and $P<0.001$, respectively). The distance between Bruch's membrane opening and anterior surface of the lamina cribrosa (BMO-anterior LC) of CON was also significantly smaller than that of glaucoma but was similar to that of the healthy group ($P<0.001$ and $P=0.47$, respectively). Based on Moorfields regression analysis of the glaucoma classification of HRT2, 15 eyes with CON were classified with a glaucoma-like disc. The cup/disc area ratio did not differ between cases of CON with a glaucoma-like disc and cases of GON ($P=0.16$), but the BMO-anterior LC and mean and maximum cup depths of CON cases with a glaucoma-like disc were smaller than those in GON ($P=0.005$, $P=0.003$, and $P=0.001$, respectively).

Conclusions: Measurements of the cup depths and the LC depth had good ability to differentiate between CON with a glaucoma-like disc and glaucoma. There was no laminar remodeling detected by laminar surface position in the patients with CON compared to those with GON.

Editor: Louis R. Pasquale, Harvard Medical School, United States of America

Funding: The authors have no support or funding to report.

Competing Interests: The authors have declared that no competing interests exist.

* Email: trj74h6@kuhp.kyoto-u.ac.jp

Introduction

Enlargement of optic disc cupping is a classical sign of glaucoma, but it also can result from nonglaucomatous neurological lesions, such as ischemic optic neuropathy, hereditary optic neuropathy, traumatic optic neuropathy, and compressive optic neuropathy (CON) [1–6]. Many reports indicate that intracranial lesions often mimic the clinical presentation of glaucoma and result in misdiagnosis [2,3,7–9]. Detecting CON among eyes with glaucoma and a glaucoma-like disc is critically important because intracranial lesions, including a brain tumor and intracranial aneurysm, are life-threatening and require treatments that are entirely different from that of glaucoma, and the delay in diagnosis or misdiagnosis can be fatal.

Differentiating glaucomatous from nonglaucomatous disc cupping is often difficult. Trobe and associates showed that pallor of the neuroretinal rim is useful in predicting nonglaucomatous

cupping in a review of optic nerve head (ONH) photographs, but such funduscopic characteristics are subjective; the degree of pallor is influenced by disturbances of the ocular media and variations in photographic technique, and even experienced observers often misdiagnose the etiology of the cupping [2]. Other clinical findings such as dyscromatopsia or certain visual field characteristics can help differentiate between the two diseases; however, their usefulness is limited. The depth of optic disc cupping is considered one of the most important objective findings of the ONH, which helps to differentiate nonglaucomatous optic neuropathy from glaucoma. Mashima and associates compared the ONH between eyes with glaucoma and those with hereditary optic neuropathy using the Heidelberg Retina Tomograph (HRT) parameters [10]. They reported that 73% of eyes with hereditary optic neuropathy were misdiagnosed with glaucoma, but the mean cup depth and maximum cup depth of eyes with hereditary optic neuropathy were significantly smaller than those of eyes with glaucoma.

However, characteristics of cupping depth for eyes with CON remained unknown. The quantitative analysis of optic disc cupping may provide useful data to distinguish CON from glaucoma. Additionally, other ONH structures characteristic of glaucoma, such as lamina cribrosa (LC) degeneration [11–13], are candidates for objective parameters for differentiating sight-threatening and life-threatening optic atrophy from glaucoma. However, in vivo evaluation of the LC was not easy.

Recently, a new approach to optical coherence tomography (OCT), known as enhanced depth imaging (EDI) OCT, allows visualization of deeper layers of the ONH, including the LC [14–18]. These studies showed that the LC was located posteriorly and significantly thinner in patients with glaucoma than in healthy controls. However, the morphology of these ONH structures in eyes with an enlarged optic cup caused by nonglaucomatous optic neuropathy has not been elucidated. In this prospective study, we compare, for the first time, the ONH quantitative parameters, including cup/disc (C/D) area ratio, cup depth, disc size, LC depth and prelamina tissue thickness (PLT), between CON and glaucomatous optic neuropathy and determine whether these ONH parameters effectively discriminate between eyes with glaucoma and eyes with CON, especially in eyes with CON presenting with a glaucoma-like disc.

Methods

This prospective, cross-sectional, comparative study was carried out with approval by the Institutional Review Board (IRB) at Kyoto University Graduate School of Medicine, and all studies conducted adhered to the tenets of the Declaration of Helsinki. Written informed consent was obtained from each participant after a detailed explanation of the nature and possible consequences of the study procedures and the IRB approve this consent procedure. Compressive optic neuropathy patients who visited the Neuro-ophthalmology Clinic of Kyoto University Hospital between August 2012 and September 2013 were recruited for this study. Age-matched open-angle glaucoma and healthy control subjects were also recruited during the same study period from the Glaucoma Clinic of the same hospital. Subjects were included only

if they fulfilled the eligibility requirements detailed below and signed an informed consent form at the screening visit. When both eyes were eligible, 1 eye was randomly selected for inclusion in the study.

All subjects underwent comprehensive ophthalmic assessment, including visual acuity measurements with a Landort chart, intraocular pressure (IOP) measurement using a Goldmann applanation tonometry, slit-lamp examinations, stereo disc photography with a 3-Dx simultaneous stereo disc camera (Nidek Co., Ltd, Gamagori, Japan), axial length measurement with an IOLMaster biometer (Carl Zeiss Meditec, Inc., Dublin, California, USA), and standard automated perimetry with the Humphrey Visual Field Analyzer using the 24–2 Swedish Interactive Threshold Algorithm (SITA) standard strategy (Carl Zeiss Meditec, Inc., Dublin, CA, USA) within 3 months from the date of OCT. Experienced ophthalmologists performed spectral domain (SD)-OCT (Spectralis; Heidelberg Engineering GmbH, Dossenheim, Germany) and the Heidelberg Retina Tomograph 2 (HRT2; Heidelberg Engineering GmbH, Heidelberg, Germany).

Inclusion criteria

Inclusion criteria for compressive optic neuropathy subjects included the following: (1) optic nerve atrophy caused by compression of the anterior visual pathway by a brain tumor or aneurysm confirmed by cranial neuroimaging with magnetic resonance imaging, (2) history of surgical treatment for the causative disease more than 1 year before this study, (3) mean deviation (MD) measured with the Humphrey visual field analyzer of −6 dB or less, and (4) IOP of 20 mm Hg or less. Inclusion criteria for open-angle glaucoma subjects were as follows: (1) a clinical diagnosis of open-angle glaucoma with documented progressive optic disc change, such as a vertical cup-to-disc ratio of 0.7 or greater, intraindividual asymmetry of 0.2 or more, or the presence of focal thinning, notching, and disc hemorrhage, and associated glaucomatous loss of visual field; (2) repeatable glaucomatous visual field loss as measured with the Humphrey field analyzer with the standard 24–2 SITA program on at least 2 subsequent tests; (3) treated IOP of 20 mm Hg or less; and (4) MD

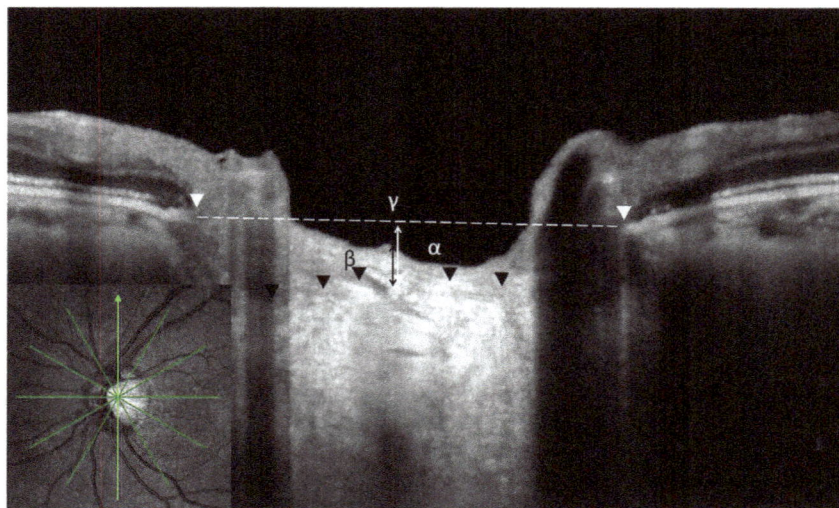

Figure 1. Optic nerve head quantitative parameters measured with enhanced depth imaging optical coherence tomography (OCT). A radial OCT scans at the optic disc were obtained. White arrowheads show Bruch's membrane opening (BMO). Dotted line shows BMO reference plane. Black arrowhead shows the anterior surface of the lamina cribrosa (LC). The distance between BMO reference plane and anterior LC (α), prelamina tissue thickness (β) at the center of BMO reference plane, and the diameters of the BMOs (γ) are also indicated.

Table 1. Baseline Patient Characteristics.

	CON	Glaucoma	P value*	normal subjects	P value[†]
Number of eyes	34	34	-	34	-
Age (years)	59.2±13.2	59.5±13.5	0.94	59.4±14.6	0.95
Sex (male/female)	12/22	19/15	0.14	14/20	0.80
Spherical equivalent (Diopter)	−1.7±2.5	−2.0±2.3	0.63	−1.1±2.6	0.31
Axial length (mm)	24.0±1.3	24.3±1.2	0.31	24.1±1.2	0.56
Intraocular pressure (mm Hg)	15.8±3.7	16.3±3.7	0.58	16.3±3.5	0.51
Mean deviation (dB)	−18.9±8.1	−17.3±6.4	0.38	−0.6±1.7	<0.001

CON = compressive optic neuropathy
*comparison between CON and glaucoma
[†]comparison between CON and normal subjects

measured with Humphrey visual field analyzer of -6 dB or less. Inclusion criteria for healthy normal eyes included (1) an IOP of 20 mm Hg or less with no history of increased IOP, (2) normal visual field testing results, and (3) an absence of glaucomatous optic disc appearance on stereo disc photography.

The appearance of the optic disc on stereoscopic photographs was evaluated by glaucoma specialist (YK and TA) who was masked to all other information about the eyes. Determination of the appearance of the optic disc (glaucomatous or normal) was performed in accordance with the assessments of the two examiners. For all subjects in the three groups, a vertical cup-to-disc ratio was measured on stereo disc photography.

Exclusion criteria

Exclusion criteria were as follows: (1) high myopia defined as less than −6.0 diopters (D); (2) astigmatism more than 3 D; (3) any other ophthalmic disease, including media opacity, diabetic retinopathy, or other diseases affecting the visual fields, such as ischemic optic neuropathy, optic neuritis, uveitis, retinal or choroidal diseases, and trauma; (4) a tilted optic disc, which was defined as an index of tilt (ratio of minimum to maximum optic

disc diameter) less than 0.75 on stereo disc photography [19]; and (5) a history of intraocular surgery or laser treatment except for uncomplicated cataract surgery.

Age matching in the glaucoma patients and healthy subjects was performed by randomly selecting one subject within 2 years of the same age for CON.

Confocal scanning laser tomography

Confocal scanning laser tomography of the optic disc was performed on all participants in this study with HRT2 (Heidelberg Engineering GmbH, Heidelberg, Germany) to evaluate the optic disc size, cup/disc area ratio, and mean and maximum cup depths. Three images were acquired automatically after initial positioning by an experienced operator. Qualified HRT scans were well-centered and well-focused. The ONH contour line was then drawn by the same operator with the ONH margin defined as the inner border of Elschnig's ring, and global stereometric parameters for HRT2 were acquired. Moorfields regression analysis (MRA) categorical classification (within normal limits, borderline, or outside normal limits) was also recorded. We defined CON with a glaucoma-like disc as those classified as

Table 2. Comparison of OCT and HRT parameters among CON, glaucoma, and normal subjects.

	CON (N = 34)	glaucoma (N = 34)	P value*	normal subjects (N = 34)	P value[†]
cpRNFL (μm)	51.3±14.5	58.6±12.5	0.03	97.2±8.8	<0.001
PLT (μm)	116.3±59.6	111.7±59.8	0.75	183.5±97.7	0.001
Width of BMO (μm)	1659.2±155.7	1655.2±168.1	0.92	1617.5±217.6	0.37
cpCT (μm)	169.8±52.6	157.2±48.9	0.32	171.1±44.3	0.92
Disc size (mm)	2.03±0.53	2.21±0.46	0.16	2.04±0.57	0.96
BMO-anterior LC (μm)	324.0±114.2	508.4±157.8	<0.001	348.2±156.8	0.47
C/D area ratio	0.35±0.15	0.52±0.17	<0.001	0.25±0.14	0.006
Mean cupping depth (mm)	0.19±0.07	0.33±0.11	<0.001	0.22±0.08	0.16
Max cupping depth (mm)	0.46±0.14	0.74±0.21	<0.001	0.58±0.16	0.002

CON = compressive optic neuropathy; OCT = optical coherence tomography; HRT = Heidelberg Retina Tomograph; cpRNFL = circumpapillary retinal nerve fiber layer; PLT = prelamina tissue thickness; BMO = Bruch's membrane opening; cpCT = circumpapillary choroidal thickness; BMO-anterior LC = distance between BMO and anterior surface of lamina cribrosa.
*comparison between CON and glaucoma.
[†]comparison between CON and normal subjects.

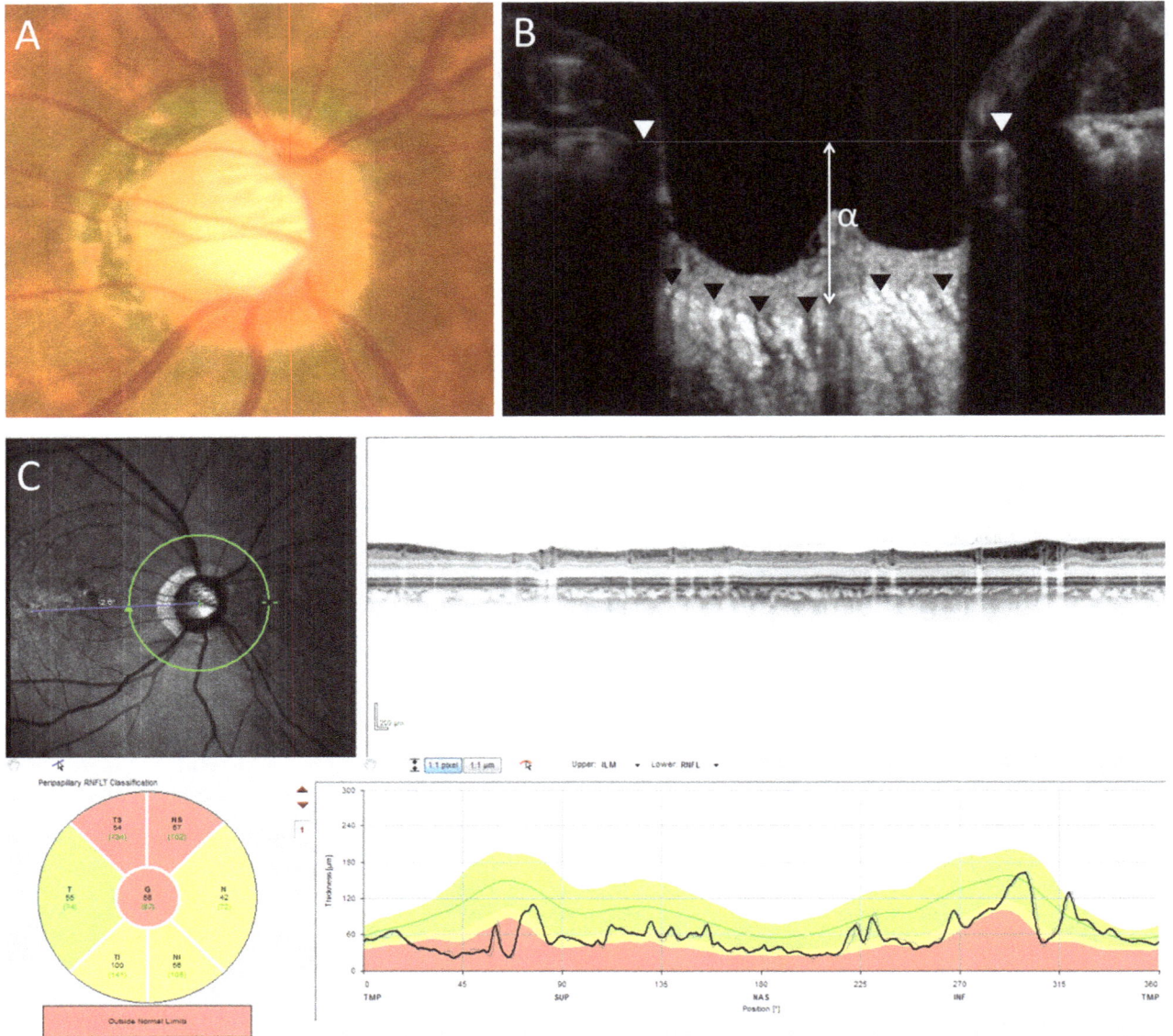

Figure 2. Representative case of eye with glaucoma. A fundus photograph (A) shows a glaucomatous disc with enlarged optic disc cupping and upper rim loss. A vertical OCT scan (B) shows a distance of 406 μm between Bruch's membrane opening reference line and the anterior lamina cribrosa (α). A circular OCT (C) scan shows thinning of the circumpapillary retinal nerve fiber layer (58 μm).

abnormal or borderline by the glaucoma classification of HRT2 MRA.

Spectral-domain optical coherence tomography

After pupillary dilation, the optic nerve was imaged using Spectralis OCT (Heidelberg Engineering GmbH, Dossenheim, Germany). For peripapillary retinal nerve fiber layer measurement and peripapillary choroidal thickness, a 3.46-mm-diameter circular scan, centered around the optic disc center, was used. The mean circumpapillary retinal nerve fiber layer (cpRNFL) thickness and circumpapillary choroidal thickness (cpCT) on the OCT image obtained by averaging 50 circular B-scans was used for analysis.

The EDI technique was also used for measuring the PLT, diameter of Bruch's membrane opening (BMO), and distance

between BMO and the anterior surface of the LC (BMO-anterior LC; Figure 1). The details and advantages of this technology for evaluating the LC have been described previously [14,20]. A radial scanning pattern centered on the optic disc (24 high-resolution 15° radial scans, each averaged from 50 B-scans with 768 A-scans per B-scan acquired with a scanning speed of 40,000 A-scans per second). The LC appeared as a highly reflective plate-like structure in B-scan images. The start of the highly reflective region within the ONH was considered the anterior border of the LC [21]. We adjusted the brightness and contrast of the images to identify LC border as precisely as possible. The PLT was defined as the distance between the optic cup surface and the anterior border of the highly reflective region that corresponded to the LC. The BMO was defined as the termination of the Bruch's membrane, and we measured the diameter of BMO [22]. The

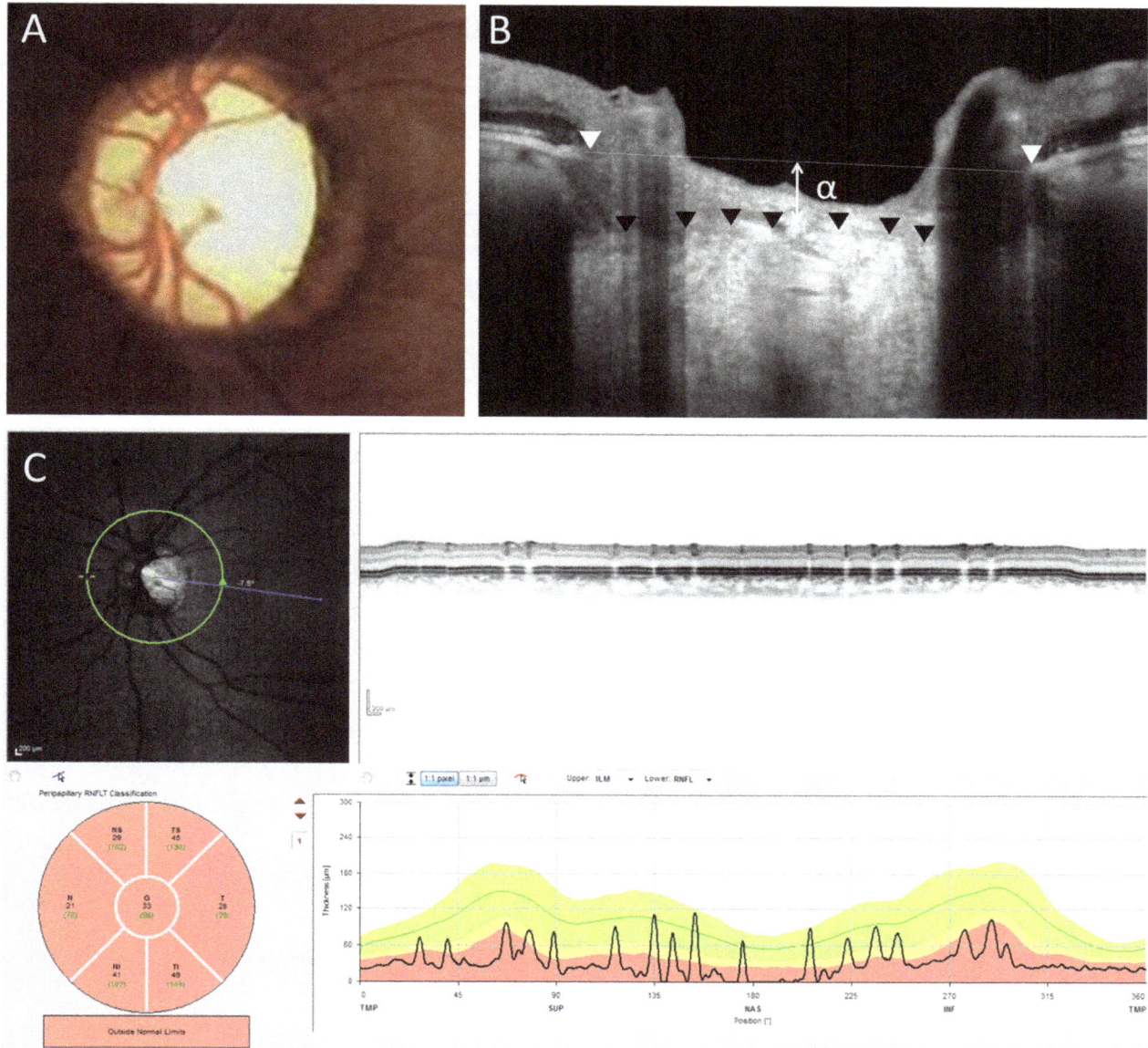

Figure 3. Representative case of eye with compressive optic neuropathy caused by a meningioma. A fundus photograph (A) shows optic nerve atrophy with pallor and enlarged optic disc cupping. A vertical OCT (B) scan shows a distance of 165 µm between Bruch's membrane opening reference line and the anterior lamina cribrosa (α). A circular OCT (C) scan shows severe thinning of the circumpapillary retinal nerve fiber layer (33 µm).

BMO-anterior LC was defined as the vertical distance between the reference line connecting BMO and the anterior laminar surface. In principle, we measured the PLT, diameter of BMO, and BMO-anterior LC at the midpoints between the BMOs on both vertical and horizontal images. An average value was obtained from two images.

Statistical analyses

All values are presented as mean ± standard deviation. Differences in parameters between two groups were compared by using the unpaired t-test or the Mann-Whitney U test, and differences among the 3 groups were compared by analysis of variance (ANOVA) followed by the Tukey post hoc test. Differences in categorical variables were evaluated by χ^2 tests.

To evaluate the interobserver reproducibility of our measuring method for cpCT, PLT, diameter of BMO, and BMO-anterior LC, all SD-OCT datasets from each group were evaluated by 2 examiners (MH and KM), and the interclass correlation coefficient (ICC) was calculated. The diagnostic accuracy was determined by computing the area under the receiver operating characteristic curve (AUROC), and the sensitivity at the fixed specificity was determined to differentiate between CON eyes with a glaucoma-like disc and eyes with glaucoma [23]. The unpaired t-test scores, Mann-Whitney U test, ANOVA, and ICC were calculated using SPSS version 19.0.0 statistical software (IBM Japan, Tokyo, Japan), and the AUROCs were compared using MedCalc version 12 (MedCalc Software, Ostend, Belgium). The cutoff points were calculated with MedCalc version 12 as the points with the best

Table 3. Comparison of OCT and HRT parameters between eyes with CON with a glaucoma-like disc and eyes with glaucoma.

	CON (N = 15)	glaucoma (N = 34)	P value
cpRNFL (μm)	49.0±15.0	58.6±12.5	0.02
PLT (μm)	124.5±70.0	111.7±59.8	0.52
Width of BMO (μm)	1699.0±128.2	1655.1±168.1	0.37
Disc size (mm)	2.17±0.46	2.21±0.46	0.80
BMO-anterior LC (μm)	376.2±102.6	508.4±157.8	0.005
C/D area ratio	0.46±0.11	0.52±0.17	0.16
Mean cupping depth (mm)	0.23±0.07	0.33±0.11	0.003
Max cupping depth (mm)	0.52±0.14	0.74±0.21	0.001

CON = compressive optic neuropathy; OCT = optical coherence tomography; HRT = Heidelberg Retina Tomograph; BMO-anterior LC = distance between Bruch's membrane opening and anterior surface of lamina cribrosa.

sensitivity-specificity balance. Sensitivity at fixed specificities of 90% and 95% (10% and 5% false positive rate, respectively) and positive and negative likelihood ratios were also calculated. A P value <0.05 was considered statistically significant.

Results

During the enrollment period, 34 subjects with compressive optic neuropathy were included. Furthermore, 63 glaucoma and 60 healthy control subjects were initially included. After age matching, this study included 68 eyes of 68 subjects (34 eyes of 34 age-matched glaucoma subjects and 34 eyes of 34 age-matched normal control subjects).

Of the 34 subjects with CON, 13 had pituitary adenomas, 9 had intracranial meningiomas, 9 had craniopharyngiomas, 2 had intracranial aneurysms, and 1 had a sinus mucocele. The descriptive data of the participants are summarized in Table 1. No significant differences were found with regard to age, refraction, sex, axial length, and intraocular pressure when the CON group was compared to either the glaucoma or healthy group. The MD of the visual field was −18.9±8.1, −17.3±6.4, and −0.6±1.7 in the CON, glaucoma, and healthy groups, respectively. There was no significant difference in the MD between the CON and glaucoma groups (P = 0.38), but both groups had a significantly poorer MD than the healthy group (P< 0.001).

Table 2 shows the comparison of the OCT and HRT parameters of the CON group to the glaucoma and healthy groups. The ICC for cpCT, PLT, the diameter of BMO, and the BMO-anterior LC were 0.92, 0.92, 0.96, and 0.96, respectively; these findings indicate good reliability in the measurement of these parameters. There were no significant differences in the diameter of the BMO and disc size in HRT measurements among the 3 groups. The mean cpRNFL of the CON group was significantly thinner than that of the healthy group and that of the glaucoma group (P<0.001 and P = 0.03, respectively). The C/D area ratio of the glaucoma group was significantly greater than that of the CON group, and the ratio of the CON group was significantly greater compared to that of the healthy group (P<0.001 and P = 0.006, respectively). The mean PLT of the CON group was thinner than that of normal subjects but was almost the same as that of the glaucoma group (P = 0.001 and P = 0.75, respectively). Among HRT parameters, the mean and maximum cup depths of glaucoma were significantly greater than those in the CON group (P<0.001 and P<0.001, respectively). In EDI-OCT, the BMO-anterior LC of the glaucoma group was also significantly greater

than that of the CON group, and the BMO-anterior LC of the CON group was similar to that of the healthy group (P<0.001 and P = 0.47, respectively) (Figures 2 and 3). In the CON group, the mean cpCT was 169.8±52.6 μm, which was similar to that of the healthy group (171.1±44.3 μm, P = 0.92). The mean cpCT in the glaucoma group was 157.2±48.9 μm, and there was no significant difference between the glaucoma group and the CON group (P = 0.32).

Of 34 eyes with CON, 17 eyes (50%) presented with a cup-to-disc ratio of 0.8 or greater on stereoscopic photographs. Based on the glaucoma classification of HRT2 MRA, 15 (44.1%) of 34 eyes with CON were classified as abnormal or borderline (defined as CON with a glaucoma-like disc). Table 3 shows the comparison of OCT and HRT parameters between CON with a glaucoma-like disc by HRT classification and glaucoma. The BMO-anterior LC and the mean and maximum cup depths of CON subjects with a glaucoma-like disc were smaller than those of the glaucoma group (P = 0.005, P = 0.003, and P = 0.001, respectively).

To differentiate between eyes with CON with a glaucoma-like disc and eyes with glaucoma, the AUROCs, best sensitivity-specificity balance, and sensitivity at 90% and 95% specificities were calculated for BMO-anterior LC, mean cup depth, and maximum cup depth (Table 4). Overall, the AUROCs of the mean cup depth and maximum cup depth were above 0.800.

Discussion

The purpose of the current study was to determine whether there are any differences in quantitative parameters of the ONH between eyes with CON and eyes with glaucoma and to identify parameters useful in detecting intracranial lesions among eyes with enlarged optic disc cupping. Compared to eyes with glaucoma, eyes with CON had a shallower cup depth. Additionally, 50% of eyes with CON presented with enlargement of the optic cup on fundus photographs, and 44.1% were judged to have a glaucoma-like disc by HRT classification. For distinguishing CON with a glaucoma-like disc from glaucoma, ONH parameters, specifically a shallow maximum cup depth, increase the likelihood of identifying an intracranial mass lesion.

This study elucidated the difference in ONH deeper structures between glaucoma and CON. Our results indicate that different mechanisms may result in disc cup enlargement. Glaucomatous cupping has been histologically shown to result from the loss of both axons and astroglia in the optic disc [24,25] and posterior LC displacement and thinning of the LC [11,26–28]. Compression of the afferent visual pathway also causes enlargement of the optic

Table 4. Diagnostic accuracy determined by computing the AUROCs, best sensitivity-specificity balance, likelihood ratios, and sensitivity at the fixed specificities for the optic nerve head parameters of OCT and HRT to discriminate between CON eyes with a glaucoma-like disc and glaucoma eyes.

OCT and HRT parameters	AUROC	95% CI	AUROCs P Value	Cutoff Point	Sensitivity (%)	Specificity (%)	+LR	–LR	Sensitivity Specificity 90%	Specificity 95%
BMO-anterior LC	0.754	0.610–0.866	0.0009	395 μm	73.33	79.41	3.56	0.34	33.33	13.33
Mean cupping depth	0.803	0.662–0.903	<0.0001	0.27 mm	85.71	67.65	2.65	0.21	41.43	14.29
Maximum cupping depth	0.829	0.692–0.922	<0.0001	0.6 mm	85.71	73.53	3.24	0.19	57.14	28.57

AUROC = area under the receiver operating characteristic curve; OCT = optical coherence tomography; HRT = Heidelberg Retina Tomography; CI = confidence interval; +LR = positive likelihood ratio; –LR = negative likelihood ratio; BMO-anterior LC = distance between Bruch's membrane opening and anterior surface of lamina cribrosa.
Note: The cutoff points were calculated using the MedCalc software as the points with the best sensitivity-specificity balance. Sensitivities at fixed specificities of 90% and 95% are shown.

nerve cup. Portney and associates conducted a pathological study in a case of disc cupping associated with compression of the optic nerve and showed loss of axons and reported that glial tissue within the optic nerve head would account for the cupping [7]. However, whether axonal loss alone is a sufficient explanation for cupping in CON has been unknown.

This study used a new EDI-OCT technique, which has been shown to reliably capture the LC and the deep structures of the ONH in normal eyes and eyes with glaucoma. Our study showed that eyes with CON had a smaller LC depth than eyes with glaucoma and that LC depth of the CON group was similar to that of the healthy group. Previous studies have reported that eyes with glaucoma presented with posterior LC displacement and a thinner LC than normal eyes [14,15,17,29]. Our results indicated that retrograde axonal degeneration caused by optic nerve compression does not accompany laminar remodeling, which is unlike that observed in glaucomatous optic neuropathy. This result was consistent with the hypothesis that the pathogenesis of optic nerve degeneration in glaucomatous optic neuropathy is located at the LC, while the pathogenesis of other optic neuropathies is not [11,30–32].

Our study revealed that disc cupping depth and LC depth are useful diagnostic parameters in detecting CON with a glaucoma-like disc. Compressive anterior visual pathway lesions can mimic both glaucomatous disc cupping [3] and field defects [33], and distinguishing them from glaucoma is often difficult. Ahmed and associates state that it would be difficult for a normal clinician rather than a neuro-ophthalmologist to diagnose most forms of optic neuropathy and, thus, advocates routine neuroimaging [34]. However, routine neuroimaging for subjects suspected to have glaucoma has a low sensitivity for detecting intracranial lesions [35,36]. To improve the cost-to-benefit ratio of neuroimaging, a more selective approach is needed. Among quantitative parameters investigated in this study, maximum cupping depth has good specificity and sensitivity. A detailed assessment of the ONH provides the information necessary to distinguish cupping caused by glaucoma versus compression.

The LC depth in the patients with CON was smaller than that in the glaucoma group, but this is not a useful diagnostic parameter in detecting CON with glaucoma-like discs. In our study, we measured the LC depth as the distance between the BMO and the anterior surface of the LC, as has been previously reported [18]. However, the use of the BMO as a reference plane for deep optic nerve structures may be influenced by the choroidal thickness [37]. In fact, the peripapillary choroidal thickness has been reported to be thinner in patients with normal tension glaucoma compared to normal subjects [38]. Although there was no significant difference in the cpCT between the CON and glaucoma groups in the present study, the difference of choroidal thickness could underestimate the differences between CON and glaucoma.

This study has several limitations. In addition to the relatively small sample size, poor fixation of patients could impair the reliability of visual field testing because some CON and glaucoma patients had poor visual acuity. Additionally, the results of visual field testing do not represent all visual fields. In the present study, all patients with glaucoma and CON were Japanese and of Asian ancestry, and high prevalence of glaucoma is reported among Japanese individuals. Differences in glaucoma prevalence according to race might be a factor in differentiating between the two diseases [39]. Diagnostic tests are indicated for use in patients with suspected disease and not in patients with confirmed CON or glaucoma; however, we compared only patients who had already been diagnosed with CON or glaucoma. A further prospective study should be performed in a larger population. As for the HRT measurement, the cup size and rim can be artifactually smaller using the HRT because the reference plane is selected to be temporal, in which the papillo-maculo bundle is the first to be affected in eyes with CON [40]. In fact, the incidence of a glaucoma-like disc in eyes with CON was smaller with evaluation by HRT than that by stereo disc photography in our study. In addition, although as many as one-half of patients with CON presented with a glaucoma-like disc, we could not exclude the possibility that some of them may have had an underlying glaucomatous process. Despite these limitations, quantitative analysis of ONH morphology provides the necessary evidence to distinguish cupping caused by intracranial lesions from that caused by glaucoma.

Supporting Information

File S1 Specific data of each group. Detail data of group1 (glaucoma), group2 (normal), group3 (compressive optic neuropathy), and group4 (compressive optic neuropathy accompanying with glaucomatous disc).

Author Contributions

Conceived and designed the experiments: MH KM AO YM NG YK TA NY. Performed the experiments: MH KM AO YM NG YK TA NY. Analyzed the data: MH KM AO YM NG. Contributed reagents/materials/analysis tools: MH KM AO YM NG YK TA NY. Wrote the paper: MH KM AO YM NG YK TA NY.

References

1. Quigley H, Anderson DR (1977) Cupping of the optic disc in ischemic optic neuropathy. Trans Sect Ophthalmol Am Acad Ophthalmol Otolaryngol 83: 755–762.
2. Trobe JD, Glaser JS, Cassady J, Herschler J, Anderson DR (1980) Nonglaucomatous excavation of the optic disc. Arch Ophthalmol 98: 1046–1050.
3. Kupersmith MJ, Krohn D (1984) Cupping of the optic disc with compressive lesions of the anterior visual pathway. Ann Ophthalmol 16: 948–953.
4. Rebolleda G, Noval S, Contreras I, Arnalich-Montiel F, Garcia-Perez JL, et al. (2009) Optic disc cupping after optic neuritis evaluated with optic coherence tomography. Eye (Lond) 23: 890–894.
5. Fournier AV, Damji KF, Epstein DL, Pollock SC (2001) Disc excavation in dominant optic atrophy: differentiation from normal tension glaucoma. Ophthalmology 108: 1595–1602.
6. Ortiz RG, Newman NJ, Manoukian SV, Diesenhouse MC, Lott MT, et al. (1992) Optic disk cupping and electrocardiographic abnormalities in an American pedigree with Leber's hereditary optic neuropathy. Am J Ophthalmol 113: 561–566.
7. Portney GL, Roth AM (1977) Optic cupping caused by an intracranial aneurysm. Am J Ophthalmol 84: 98–103.
8. Bianchi-Marzoli S, Rizzo JF 3rd, Brancato R, Lessell S (1995) Quantitative analysis of optic disc cupping in compressive optic neuropathy. Ophthalmology 102: 436–440.
9. Pruett RC, Wepsic JG (1973) Delayed diagnosis of chiasmal compression. Am J Ophthalmol 76: 229–236.
10. Mashima Y, Kimura I, Yamamoto Y, Ohde H, Ohtake Y, et al. (2003) Optic disc excavation in the atrophic stage of Leber's hereditary optic neuropathy: comparison with normal tension glaucoma. Graefes Arch Clin Exp Ophthalmol 241: 75–80.
11. Quigley HA, Hohman RM, Addicks EM, Massof RW, Green WR (1983) Morphologic changes in the lamina cribrosa correlated with neural loss in open-angle glaucoma. Am J Ophthalmol 95: 673–691.
12. Tezel G, Trinkaus K, Wax MB (2004) Alterations in the morphology of lamina cribrosa pores in glaucomatous eyes. Br J Ophthalmol 88: 251–256.
13. Fontana L, Bhandari A, Fitzke FW, Hitchings RA (1998) In vivo morphometry of the lamina cribrosa and its relation to visual field loss in glaucoma. Curr Eye Res 17: 363–369.
14. Lee EJ, Kim TW, Weinreb RN, Park KH, Kim SH, et al. (2011) Visualization of the lamina cribrosa using enhanced depth imaging spectral-domain optical coherence tomography. Am J Ophthalmol 152: 87–95 e81.
15. Park SC, De Moraes CG, Teng CC, Tello C, Liebmann JM, et al. (2012) Enhanced depth imaging optical coherence tomography of deep optic nerve complex structures in glaucoma. Ophthalmology 119: 3–9.
16. Park HY, Park CK (2013) Diagnostic capability of lamina cribrosa thickness by enhanced depth imaging and factors affecting thickness in patients with glaucoma. Ophthalmology 120: 745–752.
17. Furlanetto RL, Park SC, Damle UJ, Sieminski SF, Kung Y, et al. (2013) Posterior displacement of the lamina cribrosa in glaucoma: in vivo interindividual and intereye comparisons. Invest Ophthalmol Vis Sci 54: 4836–4842.
18. Seo JH, Kim TW, Weinreb RN (2014) Lamina cribrosa depth in healthy eyes. Invest Ophthalmol Vis Sci 55: 1241–1251.
19. Jonas JB, Kling F, Grundler AE (1997) Optic disc shape, corneal astigmatism, and amblyopia. Ophthalmology 104: 1934–1937.
20. Spaide RF, Koizumi H, Pozzoni MC (2008) Enhanced depth imaging spectral-domain optical coherence tomography. Am J Ophthalmol 146: 496–500.
21. Inoue R, Hangai M, Kotera Y, Nakanishi H, Mori S, et al. (2009) Three-dimensional high-speed optical coherence tomography imaging of lamina cribrosa in glaucoma. Ophthalmology 116: 214–222.
22. Fatehee N, Yu PK, Morgan WH, Cringle SJ, Yu DY (2011) Correlating morphometric parameters of the porcine optic nerve head in spectral domain optical coherence tomography with histological sections. Br J Ophthalmol 95: 585–589.
23. DeLong ER, DeLong DM, Clarke-Pearson DL (1988) Comparing the areas under two or more correlated receiver operating characteristic curves: a nonparametric approach. Biometrics 44: 837–845.
24. Anderson DR, Cynader MS (1997) Glaucomatous optic nerve cupping as an optic neuropathy. Clin Neurosci 4: 274–278.
25. Hernandez MR, Pena JD (1997) The optic nerve head in glaucomatous optic neuropathy. Arch Ophthalmol 115: 389–395.
26. Hayreh SS (1974) Pathogenesis of cupping of the optic disc. Br J Ophthalmol 58: 863–876.
27. Quigley HA, Green WR (1979) The histology of human glaucoma cupping and optic nerve damage: clinicopathologic correlation in 21 eyes. Ophthalmology 86: 1803–1830.
28. Quigley HA, Addicks EM (1981) Regional differences in the structure of the lamina cribrosa and their relation to glaucomatous optic nerve damage. Arch Ophthalmol 99: 137–143.
29. Park HY, Jeon SH, Park CK (2012) Enhanced depth imaging detects lamina cribrosa thickness differences in normal tension glaucoma and primary open-angle glaucoma. Ophthalmology 119: 10–20.
30. Quigley H, Anderson DR (1976) The dynamics and location of axonal transport blockade by acute intraocular pressure elevation in primate optic nerve. Invest Ophthalmol 15: 606–616.
31. Crawford Downs J, Roberts MD, Sigal IA (2011) Glaucomatous cupping of the lamina cribrosa: a review of the evidence for active progressive remodeling as a mechanism. Exp Eye Res 93: 133–140.
32. Bellezza AJ, Rintalan CJ, Thompson HW, Downs JC, Hart RT, et al. (2003) Deformation of the lamina cribrosa and anterior scleral canal wall in early experimental glaucoma. Invest Ophthalmol Vis Sci 44: 623–637.
33. Blazar HA, Scheie HG (1950) Pseudoglaucoma. AMA Arch Ophthalmol 44: 499–513.
34. Ahmed, II, Feldman F, Kucharczyk W, Trope GE (2002) Neuroradiologic screening in normal-pressure glaucoma: study results and literature review. J Glaucoma 11: 279–286.
35. Shiose Y, Kitazawa Y, Tsukahara S, Akamatsu T, Mizokami K, et al. (1991) Epidemiology of glaucoma in Japan—a nationwide glaucoma survey. Jpn J Ophthalmol 35: 133–155.
36. Greenfield DS, Siatkowski RM, Glaser JS, Schatz NJ, Parrish RK 2nd (1998) The cupped disc. Who needs neuroimaging? Ophthalmology 105: 1866–1874.
37. Johnstone J, Fazio M, Rojananuangnit K, Smith B, Clark M, et al. (2014) Variation of the axial location of Bruch's membrane opening with age, choroidal thickness, and race. Invest Ophthalmol Vis Sci 55: 2004–2009.
38. Hirooka K, Tenkumo K, Fujiwara A, Baba T, Sato S, et al. (2012) Evaluation of peripapillary choroidal thickness in patients with normal-tension glaucoma. BMC Ophthalmol 12: 29.
39. Iwase A, Suzuki Y, Araie M, Yamamoto T, Abe H, et al. (2004) The prevalence of primary open-angle glaucoma in Japanese: the Tajimi Study. Ophthalmology 111: 1641–1648.
40. Nagai-Kusuhara A, Nakamura M, Kanamori A, Nakanishi Y, Kusuhara S, et al. (2008) Evaluation of optic nerve head configuration in various types of optic neuropathy with Heidelberg Retina Tomograph. Eye (Lond) 22: 1154–1160.

10

Multimodal Retinal Vessel Analysis in CADASIL Patients

Florian Alten[1][*][⑨], **Jeremias Motte**[2][⑨], **Carina Ewering**[2], **Nani Osada**[3], **Christoph R. Clemens**[1], **Ella M. Kadas**[4], **Nicole Eter**[1], **Friedemann Paul**[4,5], **Martin Marziniak**[2]

1 Department of Ophthalmology, University of Muenster Medical Center, Muenster, Germany, **2** Department of Neurology, University of Muenster Medical Center, Muenster, Germany, **3** Department of Medical Informatics and Biomathematics, University of Muenster, Muenster, Germany, **4** Department of Neurology, Charite University Medicine Berlin, Berlin, German, **5** NeuroCure Clinical Research Center, Berlin, Germany

Abstract

Purpose: To further elucidate retinal findings and retinal vessel changes in Cerebral autosomal dominant arteriopathy with subcortical infarcts and leukoencephalopathy (CADASIL) patients by means of high resolution retinal imaging.

Methods: 28 eyes of fourteen CADASIL patients and an equal number of control subjects underwent confocal scanning laser ophthalmoscopy (cSLO), spectral-domain optical coherence tomography (SD-OCT), retinal nerve fibre layer (RNFL) measurements, fluorescein and indocyanine angiography. Three vessel measurement techniques were applied: RNFL thickness, a semiautomatic software tool based on cSLO images and manual vessel outlining based on SD-OCT.

Results: Mean age of patients was 56.2 ± 11.6 years. Arteriovenous nicking was present in 22 (78.6%) eyes and venous dilation in 24 (85.7%) eyes. Retinal volume and choroidal volume were 8.77 ± 0.46 mm^3 and 8.83 ± 2.24 mm^3. RNFL measurements showed a global increase of 105.2 µm (Control group: 98.4 µm; p = 0.015). Based on semi-automatic cSLO measurements, maximum diameters of arteries and veins were 102.5 µm (106.0 µm; p = 0.21) and 128.6 µm (124.4 µm; p = 0.27) respectively. Manual SD-OCT measurements revealed significantly increased mean arterial 138.7 µm (125.4 µm; p < 0.001) and venous 160.0 µm (146.9; p = 0.003) outer diameters as well as mean arterial 27.4 µm (19.2 µm; p < 0.001) and venous 18.3 µm (15.7 µm; p < 0.001) wall thicknesses in CADASIL patients.

Conclusions: The findings reflect current knowledge on pathophysiologic changes in vessel morphology in CADASIL patients. SD-OCT may serve as a complementary tool to diagnose and follow-up patients suffering from cerebral small-vessel diseases.

Editor: Knut Stieger, Justus-Liebig-University Giessen, Germany

Funding: The authors have no support or funding to report.

Competing Interests: Alten F, Heidelberg Engineering, Novartis, Bayer, Allergan; Motte J, none; Ewering C, none; Osada N, none; Clemens CR, Heidelberg Engineering, Novartis, Bayer, Allergan; Kadas EM, none; Eter N, Heidelberg Engineering, Bayer, Novartis, Allergan, Pfizer, Bausch and Lomb; Paul F, BiogenIdec, Teva, SanofiGenzyme, Merck, Novartis, Heidelberg Engineering; supported by German Research Foundation (DFG Exc 257), German Ministry for Education and Research (BMBF Competence Network Multiple Sclerosis); Marziniak M, none.

* Email: florian.alten@ukmuenster.de

⑨ These authors contributed equally to this work.

Introduction

Cerebral autosomal dominant arteriopathy with subcortical infarcts and leukoencephalopathy (CADASIL) is a hereditary vascular small-vessel disease caused by Notch3 mutations [1]. It is distinguished from similar vascular disorders by the unique accumulation of granular osmiophilic material in systemic and particularly brain vasculature [2]. CADASIL represents a genetic model for small vessel diseases without the confounding factors of advanced age and other vascular diseases such as diabetes mellitus or arteriosclerosis. Besides migraine, transient ischemic attacks and strokes leading to severe disability and dementia in adult midlife in the absence of common vascular risk factors, CADASIL is clinically also characterized by various ophthalmologic findings [3–11]. Knowledge on the pathophysiology of CADASIL mainly derives from post mortem data due to the challenge of inspecting brain microvessels in vivo. Immunohistochemistry and electron microscopy have been proposed as useful diagnostic tools for CADASIL patients, yet, diagnostic sensitivity is still discussed controversially [12–14].

Architecture and properties of retinal blood vessels can provide essential clinical information not only in ocular disease but also in systemic disorders. Given the strong need for improved biomarkers in systemic vascular diseases, in-vivo imaging of retinal vessels appears to be a promising diagnostic approach. Recent technologic advances in imaging resolution and acquisition speed of commercial spectral-domain optical coherence tomography (SD-OCT) and confocal scanning laser ophthalmoscopy (cSLO) allow analysis of retinal morphology and retinal vessel morphology in greater detail and have contributed to our understanding of various retinal diseases. SD-OCT scans provide an 'in-vivo histologic' view and allow the differentiation of the various retinal layers as well as morphologic changes within these layers. Recently, high resolution SD-OCT proved to be capable of reliably measuring retinal vessel diameters and vessel wall thickness in vivo [15–17]. As CADASIL represents a model for small vessel diseases, this pathology is particularly suitable for research on vessel imaging. This study aims to evaluate three methods of retinal vessel analysis as well as to re-evaluate and to further elucidate retinal findings and retinal vessel changes in CADASIL patients using high resolution retinal imaging technology.

Methods

Demographics

Fourteen participants were recruited from the Department of Neurology at University of Muenster Medical Center. Diagnosis of CADASIL was confirmed in 12 patients by detection of Notch3 gene mutations and in two patients by vessel biopsy. Personal medical history was collected for each patient. Clinical investigations have been conducted according to the principles expressed in the Declaration of Helsinki. Informed consent, written and oral, have been obtained from the participants. The institutional review board of the ethics committee of the University of Berlin, Charité, approved the study.

All patients went through a test battery containing the Montreal Cognitive Assessment (MoCA), a questionnaire for migraine and vascular risk factors. The cut-off for a cognitive impairment was < 26 points in the MoCA. The MoCA offers a high sensitivity for mild cognitive impairment (MCI) and therefore, it is well suited to detect early stages of dementia in CADASIL patients [18]. Common risk factors and co-morbidities for vascular diseases (smoking, hypertension, diabetes mellitus, overweight, coronary heart disease, arterial obstructive disease and stroke) were recorded. Furthermore, a detailed medical history for migraine was taken. A staging regarding the course of disease based on the classification by Verin et al. was performed [19]. Every patient was assigned to stage I through IV. Stage I includes common migraine episodes, abnormal MRI as well as a reliable diagnosis of

CADASIL. Stage II includes psychiatric abnormality, transient ischemic attack while stage III requires history of stroke and dementia. Patients of stage IV show a progressed disease with severe dementia and frequent strokes.

All patients underwent a complete ophthalmic evaluation, including assessment of best-corrected visual acuity (BCVA), tonometry, slit-lamp biomicroscopy and fundus ophthalmoscopy. The visual field (VF) was defined by standard automated perimetry using a 30-2 central threshold test (Humphrey 740i, Zeiss Meditec, Germany). Heidelberg retina tomography (HRT, Heidelberg Engineering, Germany) was performed to rule out any glaucomatous damage. Age-matched healthy control subjects were attributed to CADASIL patients and underwent a complete ophthalmic evaluation as well.

Imaging protocol

Color fundus photography (CFP) was performed according to standard 7-field-method (Visucam, Carl Zeiss Meditech, Germany). cSLO near infrared (IR) imaging ($\lambda = 820$ nm; Spectralis; Heidelberg Engineering, Germany) was performed with a minimum resolution of 768×768 pixels. The field of view was set at $30° \times 30°$ and centered on the macula as well as on the optic disc. Scans were saved for evaluation after 100 frames had been averaged using the automatic averaging and eye-tracking feature of the Spectralis device.

Imaging of the choroid was performed using enhanced depth imaging (EDI) OCT and indocyanine green angiography (ICG). EDI-OCT is a new approach to improve depth imaging and proved to be able to reliably image the full thickness of the choroid [20]. EDI-OCT volume scans were obtained consisting of 49 scans centered on the fovea. As previously described by Tanabe and colleagues, in each EDI-OCT scan, the cursor line marking the internal limiting membrane was moved manually to the outer border of the retinal pigment epithelium (RPE) [21]. Choroidal volume (CV) values in the posterior pole were obtained using the circular grid of the Early Treatment Diabetic Retinopathy Study (ETDRS) which is an integrated feature of the Heidelberg Eye Explorer software. This technique of manual CV measurements

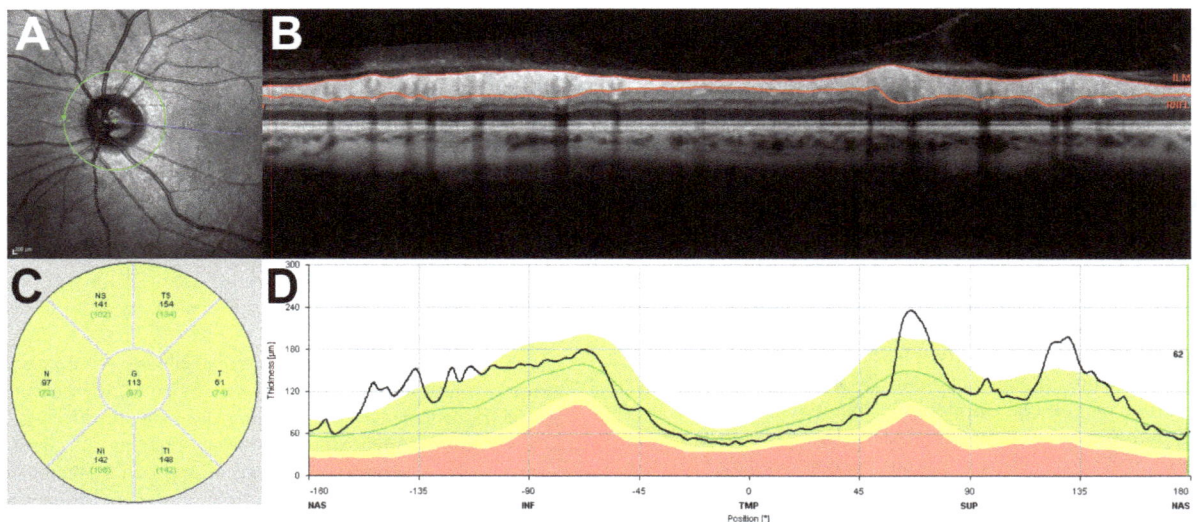

Figure 1. A–D Measurement of retinal nerve fiber layer (RNFL) thickness, using a circular B-scan placed around the optic disc. A Confocal scanning laser ophthalmoscopy infrared image shows optic disc with circular scan (diameter: 3.5 mm). **B** Corresponding spectral domain optical coherence tomography scan. Red marks delineate automatically borders of RNFL layer. **C** Presentation of RNFL thickness values for individual sectors and global measurement. **D** Individual measurement graphically compared to a healthy population.

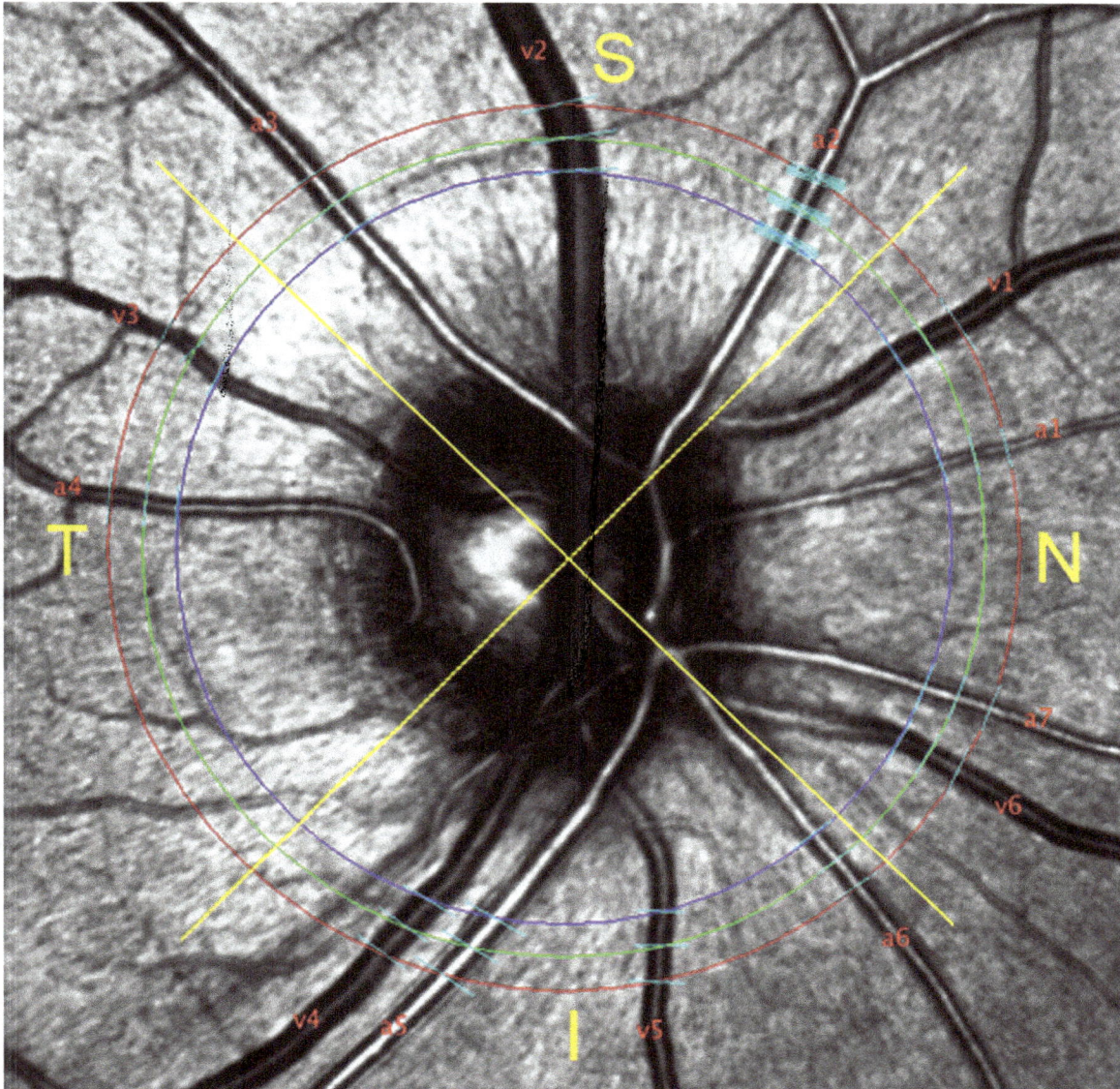

Figure 2. Confocal scanning laser (cSLO) infrared image illustrating semi-automatic measurement tool. Three concentric circles (blue 3.2 mm, green 3.5 mm, red 3.8 mm) are placed around the optic disc. Vessel labelling marks arteries (a) and veins (v). Measurement lines (cyan) are defined by the software user. Additional measurement lines automatically produced by the software are shown exemplary in artery two (a2; set of five lines). Yellow lines separate superior (S), inferior (I), nasal (N) and temporal (T) quadrant.

proved to be highly reproducible and repeatable and has a very small range of variability [22]. According to recorded EDI-OCT scans, additional SD-OCT volume scans were obtained to assess macular retinal volume (RV) within the ETDRS grid.

ICG allows for clearly displaying choroidal circulation and for identifying and delineating of choroidal watershed zones (CWZ) [23]. ICG was performed using 5 mg ICG dye (ICG-Pulsion, Pulsion Medical Systems, Germany) diluted in 5 ml aqueous solvent, injected into a peripheral vein in the arm. The field of view was set at 30° and centered on fovea. Recordings were performed according to the 7-field method. Excitation wavelength was at 787 nm and the range of transmitted light through the barrier filter was above 800 nm (Spectralis; Heidelberg Engineering, Germany). ICG of CADASIL patients were evaluated for the presence of CWZ as well as any other angiographic findings.

Fluorescence angiography (FA) was performed in the same manner using an injection of 3 ml fluorescein (Fluorescein, Alcon, Germany). Excitation wavelength was at 488 nm and the range of transmitted light through the barrier filter was 500–700 nm (Spectralis; Heidelberg Engineering, Germany).

Retinal nerve fiber layer measurements in SD-OCT

Measurement of retinal nerve fiber layer (RNFL) thickness was performed using a circular B-scan placed around the optic disc (diameter: 3.5 mm) [24]. The exactly located placement around the center of the optic disc was carefully reviewed. Sectorial analysis of mean RNFL thickness is illustrated in Figure 1.

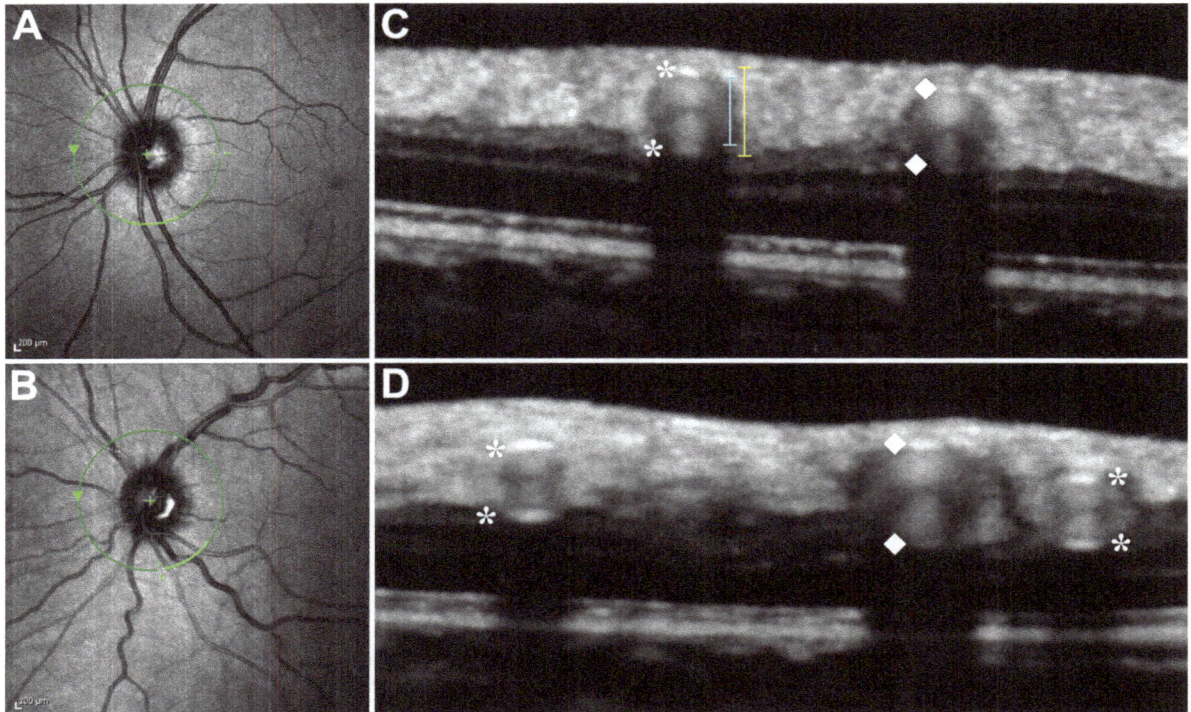

Figure 3. A–D Combined simultaneous confocal scanning laser ophthalmoscopy (cSLO) and spectral-domain optical coherence tomography (SD-OCT). A–B Infrared cSLO image centered on the optic disc of a healthy control subject (A) and a CADASIL patient (B). Green circle indicates the position of corresponding SD-OCT scan. Light green section inferiorly on the circle marks the localization of corresponding SD-OCT scan shown aside. **C–D** Magnified SD-OCT scans of healthy control subject (C) and CADASIL patient (D) show sections of major retinal vessels appearing as a group of heterogeneous reflectivities in a round-shaped configuration. Asterisks mark the inner and outer reflections of arterial vessel walls and diamonds indicate inner and outer reflections of venous vessel walls. Hyperreflectivities representing the vessel walls seem thicker and more accentuated in the CADASIL patient. Particularly in veins, demarcation of the inferior vessel wall (towards the retinal pigment epithelium) often remains challenging due to absorption effects also seen as acoustical shadow underneath the vessel (towards the retinal pigment epithelium). Note the typical hour-glass shaped configuration within the vessel lumen in both subjects. Lateral vessel walls cannot be visualized as OCT laser beam is not projected perpendicularly to them.

Retinal vessel diameter measurements in cSLO

Vessel identification in cSLO IR images was performed according to previously reported criteria [25]. Vessel measurements in native cSLO IR images were performed by a semi-automatic "Image-J"-Plugin. The Plugin creates three concentric rings (diameter: small - 3.2 mm, medium - 3.5 mm, large - 3.8 mm) in the cSLO IR images (Figure 2). The medium ring lies exactly at the level of the circular SD-OCT scan used in RNFL measurement (diameter 3.5 mm). The other two rings of the semi-automated software lie slightly peripherally and centrally to the medium ring. The user labels each vessel as artery or vein and defines vessel measurement lines on all three rings. The software algorithm produces four additional measurements, two above and two below, based on the localization and orientation of each defined measurement point. In total, every vessel is measured at 15 different points. The rings are divided into four quadrants according to RNFL and SD-OCT measurements. A particular strength of the semi-automated technique based on cSLO is that vessel diameters are measured perpendicularly, while the applied SD-OCT scan crosses vessels tangentially according to the peripapillary circle.

cSLO IR images of retinal vessels show a central light reflex (CLR) and a dark vessel edge [25]. The software recognizes strong contrasts in reflectivity between outer vessel borders and surrounding retinal tissue, and between the CLR and inner vessel

borders respectively (Figure 2). Changes in the vessel wall may alter the reflectivity in cSLO IR images. The reflex diameter may be interpreted as an indicator for the vessel architecture. Measurements were performed for the maximum measurable vessel diameter as well as for the reflex diameter. In both groups, artery-to-vein ratios (AVR) were calculated.

Retinal vessel diameter and vessel wall thickness measurements in SD-OCT

SD-OCT measurements of vessel diameter and vessel wall thickness around the optic disc proved to be highly reproducible and results correlate well with previous histologic studies [17,18,26]. Cross-sectional SD-OCT images reveal major retinal vessels as oval configurations with heterogeneous reflectivities, mainly in the RNFL and occasionally in the inner plexiform layer. Physiologic vessels show four distinctive hyperreflectivities. The top and bottom of the vessel walls correlate to the innermost and outermost hyperreflectivities. The arterial walls generally have higher reflectivity compared with the venous walls. Muraoka and colleagues previously reported that retinal vessels with physiologic blood flow show paired hyperreflectivities inside, which are frequently hourglass-shaped (Figure 3) [17]. According to this study, inner and outer vessel diameters of the four largest retinal arteries and veins were measured vertically by two blinded, independent readers (FA, JM) using the built-in manufacturer's software (Heidelberg Eye Explorer) [17]. A mean value of the two readers as well as AVR values of outer and inner diameter were calculated in CADASIL patients and healthy controls.

Notably, the same circular SD-OCT scan centered on the optic disc that was used for RNFL analysis was used for manual SD-OCT vessel measurements. Moreover, this scan position is analogous to the medium size ring in cSLO IR vessel measurements. Thus, vessel diameter measurements in cSLO IR and SD-OCT as well as RNFL thickness measurements were performed exactly at the same anatomical localization warranting a thorough comparability of all three methods. As vessel diameters decrease as they run peripherally from the optic disk margin measurement localization is an important criterion [18].

Statistical methods

HRT, ICG, FA and EDI-OCT volume scan was performed in the CADASIL group only while cSLO IR, SD-OCT volume scan and RNFL imaging was conducted in both groups. Both groups were homogeneous in age and gender. Statistical analysis was performed using IBM SPSS Statistics Ver. 22.0.0.0. Vessel diameter values were presented as mean ± standard deviation (SD). In cSLO IR images, all labelable and measureable vessels were used for analysis. Vessel diameters based on manual SD-OCT measurements were calculated using the four largest arteries and four largest veins. U-test and t-test were used to identify differences between control group and study group. A probability value of $p < 0.05$ was considered indicative of statistical significance.

Results

Demographics

Mean age was 56.2 ± 11.6 (control group: 54.5 ± 10.1) years. Disease severity was as following: Stage I: 5 patients; St. II: 4 patients, St. III: 3 patients, St. IV: 2 patients. Two patients (14%) were clinically asymptomatic. Four (29%) had strokes in the medical history. The MoCA indicated dementia or MCI in 10 patients (71%). Four patients (29%) showed strong signs of dementia. A history of migraine was reported in 7 patients (50%), of whom one suffered from migraine with aura. Two (14%) of them reported a decrease of symptoms with increasing age.

BCVA was 0.75 ± 0.25 given as decimal visual acuity values. Spherical equivalent was $+0.27 \pm 1.39$ diopters. One eye suffered from refractive amblyopia. Intraocular pressures were within normal limits. Slit lamp examination revealed no signs of iris atrophy as well as no signs of intraocular inflammation. One patient had a history of unilateral central retinal artery occlusion and showed panretinal laser coagulation spots with ghost vessels as well as an atrophy of the optic nerve head and was consequently excluded from RNFL and vessel analysis. One eye showed a drusen papilla that was excluded from RNFL evaluation. Two patients presented with macro papilla. No functional or morphological signs of glaucoma were present in any patient. Neuroretinal rim volume measured by HRT was 0.33 ± 0.15 mm^3. VF testing was performed in all patients except for one patient who was not capable of performing the examination due to his state of health. One patient showed scattered reduction of central and peripheral sensitivity secondary to his history of stroke. One examination was not evaluable due to fixation mistakes. The remaining VF tests were normal (-1.85 ± 1.10 dB MD).

Imaging

CFP and FA revealed neither cotton wool spots nor signs of ischemia in any eye. Sheathed arteries were detected in three eyes of two patients while no patient presented with tortuous arteries. No capillary leakage from blood vessels was seen during FA. Vessels with vascular sheathing also appeared normal during angiography. CFP further revealed arteriovenous nicking in 22 (78.6%) eyes and venous dilation in 24 (85.7%) eyes. RV in OCT volume measurements did not differ significantly between both groups (study group: 8.77 ± 0.46 mm^3; control group: 8.85 ± 0.35 mm^3; p = 0.341). CV in EDI-OCT volume scans was 8.83 ± 2.24 mm^3 in CADASIL patients. ICG revealed a CWZ in 6 (42.9%) CADASIL patients. Otherwise, there was no evidence for choroidal vascular occlusion or hypoperfusion.

Table 1. Retinal nerve fiber layer thickness (RNFL) measured by spectral-domain optical coherence tomography: healthy controls compared to CADASIL patients.

Peripapillary sector	Mean RNFL thickness [μm ± SD]				p-value
	healthy controls		CADASIL		
	n = 28		n = 23		
nasal sup.	115.3	±26.4	121.7	±25.2	0.368
nasal	75.9	±13.1	85.3	±13.8	0.027
nasal inf.	105.1	±28.3	116.2	±24.1	0.173
temporal inf.	138.1	±19.9	143.2	±18.3	0.289
temporal	69.9	±9.4	73.0	±8.2	0.254
temporal sup.	136.5	±20.8	143.3	±21.6	0.244
superior*	125.9	±18.5	132.5	±19.6	0.349
inferior*	121.6	±20.4	129.7	±16.4	0.08
global	98.4	±10.5	105.2	±9.5	0.015

(n) number of eyes.

*superior and inferior measurements were calculated based on data from nasal superior and temporal superior quadrants and from nasal inferior and temporal inferior quadrants respectively.

Table 2. Semi-automated vessel measurements based on confocal scanning laser ophthalmoscopy (cSLO): healthy controls compared to CADASIL patients.

Vessel	Peripapillary sector	Mean [μm ± SD]					p-value
		healthy controls			CADASIL		
		n = 28		v	n = 25		v	
Arteries								
Max diameter	nasal	94.16	±20.33	53	88.95	±20.96	51	0.201
	superior	109.98	±29.32	66	110.43	±24.94	63	0.926
	temporal	89.03	±21.39	11	85.03	±21.56	16	0.639
	inferior	112.55	±27.99	60	109.48	±27.39	60	0.545
	global	*105.99*	*±27.92*	*190*	*102.49*	*±26.74*	*190*	*0.213*
Inner reflex diameter	nasal	25.68	±10.54	40	27.93	±8.23	43	0.280
	superior	32.10	±8.00	64	34.47	±8.26	61	0.106
	temporal	26.25	±10.03	11	27.01	±8.15	14	0.836
	inferior	33.22	±8.44	55	34.53	±9.25	54	0.441
	global	*30.68*	*±9.42*	*170*	*32.19*	*±9.17*	*172*	*0.134*
Veins								
Max diameter	nasal	111.33	±19.07	30	103.93	±20.32	35	0.137
	superior	123.02	±27.26	66	133.61	±36.28	58	0.067
	temporal	81.34	±4.96	1	54.42	±1.93	2	n/a
	inferior	132.62	±31.02	51	139.98	±36.44	50	0.277
	global	*124.38*	*±28.74*	*148*	*128.61*	*±36.60*	*145*	*0.272*
Inner reflex diameter	nasal	32.66	±7.07	21	31.26	±8.80	26	0.558
	superior	34.80	±8.29	63	37.88	±10.47	51	0.082
	temporal	25.21	±2.83	1	2.83	±5.11	1	n/a
	inferior	38.45	±7.77	47	40.80	±11.64	48	0.251
	global	*35.74*	*±8.22*	*132*	*37.22*	*±11.53*	*126*	*0.235*

(n) number of total eyes; (v) number of total vessels; (n/a) too few vessels in the respective sector to calculate p-value.

Table 3. Manual vessel measurements using spectral-domain optical coherence tomography (SD-OCT): healthy controls compared to CADASIL patients.

Vessel	Mean [μm±SD]					
		healthy controls		CADASIL		p-value
		n = 28		n = 25		
Arteries	Outer diameter	125.38	±19.42	138.71	±20.25	<0.001
	Inner diameter	87.02	±17.06	83.99	±18.76	0.238
	Vessel wall	19.18	±3.03	27.36	±4.47	<0.001
Veins	Outer diameter	146.92	±25.72	159.95	±32.97	0.003
	Inner diameter	115.47	±24.38	123.35	±30.63	0.05
	Vessel wall	15.73	±2.99	18.30	±4.91	<0.001

(n) number of eyes.

Retinal nerve fiber layer measurements in SD-OCT

Mean number of averaging frames was 91.2 ± 17.4. Both groups showed a regular retinal layer configuration. Global RNFL measurements revealed significant differences between both groups (Study group: 105.2 μm; control group: 98.4 μm; $p = 0.015$). Consequently, a clear significance towards a thicker RNFL in CADASIL patients is evident. (Table 1).

Retinal vessel diameter measurements in cSLO

In the study group, maximum diameters of arteries and veins were 102.5 μm (Control group: 106.0 μm; $p = 0.21$) and 128.6 μm (124.4 μm; $p = 0.27$) respectively. Inner reflex diameters of arteries and veins were 32.2 μm (Control group: 30.7 μm; $p = 0.13$) and 37.2 μm (35.7 μm; $p = 0.23$) (Table 2). AVR of all vessels based on the maximum diameter was 0.80 for CADASIL patients and 0.85 for healthy controls.

Retinal vessel diameter and vessel wall thickness measurements in SD-OCT

High quality SD-OCT images are crucial to perform accurate vessel diameter and vessel wall thickness measurements. A clear demarcation was required between inner vessel wall and vessel lumen as well as outer vessel wall and retinal tissue. Due to questionable border discrimination of vessel walls, two arteries and three veins were excluded in the healthy control group as well as three veins in the study group. At vessel crossing points and in case of close vicinity of vessels, SD-OCT offers better vessel border discrimination compared to cSLO. Modification of contrast in SD-OCT scans slightly improved border discrimination particularly in arteries.

Mean arterial and venous outer diameters were 138.7 μm (Control group: 125.38 μm; $p < 0.001$) and 160.0 μm (146.9 μm; $p = 0.003$). Mean inner arterial and venous diameters were 84.0 μm (87.0 μm; $p = 0.238$) and 123.4 μm (115.5 μm; $p = 0.05$). Vessel wall thickness was calculated as difference between outer and inner vessel diameter measurements. Mean wall thickness was 27.4 μm (19.2 μm; $p < 0.001$) in arteries and 18.3 μm (15.7 μm; $p < 0.001$) in veins (Table 3). AVR values of inner and outer diameters of CADASIL patients were AVR_{out} 0.87, AVR_{in} 0.68 and for healthy controls AVR_{out} 0.85, AVR_{in} 0.75.

Discussion

CADASIL has gained increasing interest as a model for the more common forms of ischemic cerebral small-artery diseases and subcortical ischemic vascular dementia [27]. CADASIL is characterized by a thickening of the arterial wall leading to lumen stenosis, the presence of a non-amyloid granular osmiophilic material within the media extending into the adventitia, as well as morphological alterations of smooth-muscle cells [28,29]. Cerebral and retinal arterioles share a similar anatomy, physiology, and embryology and there is evidence for an association between retinal vessel changes and cerebral small vessel disease [30,31]. The aim of our study was to benefit from recent advances in in-vivo retinal imaging and to analyze and re-evaluate previously reported retinal findings and retinal vessel changes in CADASIL patients. To our knowledge, this is the first study to apply these refined in-vivo imaging tools to CADASIL patients and to report detected changes in vessel architecture due to this pathology.

Functional data as well as funduscopic findings like vascular sheathing, arteriovenous nicking and venous dilation are in line with previous reports [3–12]. The prevalence of single findings may vary as different study groups are certainly heterogeneous regarding the clinical stage of included patients and usually contain only a limited number of patients.

Previous histologic data revealed that ocular vessel pathologies in CADASIL patients are limited to retinal vessels only, while choroidal vessels are unaffected [5]. For the first time, we report in-vivo imaging data on the choroid of CADASIL patients that clinically confirm former histologic findings. Neither ICG nor EDI-OCT imaging revealed pathologic findings in the study group. The CV as well as the number of CWZ are in line with previously reported data of healthy probands [23,32,33].

RNFL measurements in CADASIL patients based on previous generation time-domain OCT instruments consistently showed a significant reduction in peripapillary RNFL thickness [6–8]. SD-OCT allows a refined RNFL analysis around the optic disc with a differentiated eight sector analysis grid. Interestingly, our measurements revealed an increased global RNFL thickness in CADASIL patients. As retinal vessels run within the RNFL for the most part, this finding suggests that a pathologic thickening of peripapillary retinal vessels in CADASIL patients, as seen histopathologically, may result in an increase of global RNFL thickness [2]. Considering the anatomic distribution of peripapillary vessel trunks one may consequently hypothesize that this finding must be particularly found in the vessel rich superior and

Table 4. Data overview regarding manual retinal vessel measurements based on spectral-domain optical coherence tomography.

Vessel	Mean [μm ± SD]	Goldberg et al* n = 29		Muraoka et al# n = 238		healthy controls# n = 14		CADASIL# n = 14	
Arteries	Outer diameter	127.8	±13.4	122.5	±13.1	125.38	±19.42	138.71	±20.25
	Inner diameter			87.8	±9.4	87.02	±17.06	83.99	±18.76
	Vessel wall			17.4	±2.4	19.18	±3.03	27.36	±4.47
Veins	Outer diameter	145.3	±15	141	±13.1	146.92	±25.72	159.95	±32.97
	Inner diameter			113.7	±12.5	115.47	±24.38	123.35	±30.63
	Vessel wall			13.7	±2.1	15.73	±2.99	18.30	±4.91

(n) number of patients.
*measurements performed at 960 μm from the optic disc edge.
#circular SD-OCT scan 3.5 mm in diameter.

inferior sectors potentially serving as an additional marker of vessel alteration in CADASIL patients. Yet, a significant increase in those vessel rich sectors was not found for supporting this thesis. An increase in RNFL thickness in CADASIL patients certainly is an interesting finding, and it might be interpreted as a result of vessel thickening. However, previous studies on RNFL measurements in CADASIL patients report a decrease in RNFL thickness [6–8]. These contradictory results suggest that RNFL measurements currently do not appear suitable as screening or follow-up tool in this patient group and require further research.

Fischer et al. previously described the challenge of visualizing and measuring outer vessel diameters in native cSLO IR images as borders between retinal vessels and surrounding tissue often become indistinct. Similarly to funduscopy, the authors postulate that native cSLO IR only captures inner vessel diameter, while vessel outer diameters as well as vessel walls remain undetectable [34].

We found no significant changes in the arterial and venous maximum diameter in CADASIL patients using native cSLO IR imaging. Based on the hypothesis by Fischer and colleagues, these measurements can be interpreted as inner vessel diameter. Previous studies controversially discussed the value of retinal vessel characteristics such as AVR representing factors for assessing vascular status or even risk assessment. Ikram and co-workers reported that increased retinal venous calibers are associated with stroke and progression of cerebral small vessel disease [35,36].

As CADASIL patients represent a high risk group for stroke, a venous dilatation in retinal vessels could be expected in these patients. Contrary, Chui et al. recently postulated that vessel walls are detectable using adaptive optics cSLO [37]. Additionally, our data shows AVR values higher than 0.8 in cSLO IR imaging in both groups, which gives rise to doubts whether cSLO IR in fact measures inner vessel diameters considering that AVR values of about 2/3 for the inner vessel diameter were reported previously [34,38]. We use the term 'maximum vessel diameter' for the diameter measured in cSLO IR images. Regardless of the question whether cSLO records the inner or outer diameter, we did not find significant changes in the maximum diameters between healthy controls and CADASIL patients suggesting that pathologic structural vessel changes in CADASIL are not accessible to native cSLO IR imaging.

Goldenberg et al recently proposed a non-invasive, in-vivo method for measuring retinal vessel caliber based on SD-OCT [18]. Furthermore, Muraoka and colleagues proved that measuring retinal vessel walls in healthy subjects and in patients is reliable using a manual measurement tool in SD-OCT [16,17]. A paired, frequently hourglass-shaped hyperreflectivity inside the vessels was observed in healthy subjects and interpreted as result of physiologic blood flow. As previously described, this pattern is substantially altered in patients suffering from retinal vein occlusion [16]. In our study group as well as in our control group, the hourglass-shaped hyperreflectivity was consistently seen suggesting that blood flow is not severely disturbed in major retinal vessels of CADASIL patients (Figure 3).

Manual vessel measurements using SD-OCT revealed that the outer diameter in arteries and veins in CADASIL patients was highly significantly thicker than in healthy subjects. Moreover, the vessel wall was highly significantly thicker in both venous and arterial vessels. An important difference between arteries and veins is the inner diameter. In veins, the inner diameter i.e. the lumen showed significantly higher values in CADASIL subjects. The inner diameter of arteries in CADASIL patients did not reveal a significant difference, yet, the arterial lumina tended to narrow. If thickening of arteries in CADASIL patients affects lumen diameters is still subject of debate. Dong et al recently confirmed a substantial thickening of leptomeningeal arteries of CADASIL patients, which is primarily a result of distinct intimal hyperplasia that does not affect lumen diameter [39]. AVR values of healthy controls revealed a considerable difference between outer and inner diameters suggesting that unlike cSLO IR, SD-OCT allows for differentiating between outer and inner diameters. In 2006, Roine et al reported significantly lower AVR values (0.53) in 33 CADASIL patients compared to healthy controls (0.61) based on fundus photography, which approximately corresponds to our inner diameter AVR values based on manual SD-OCT [10]. This additionally supports the notion that fundus photography shows inner diameters, while cSLO IR does not.

Measurements of our healthy control group are in accordance with recently reported data [16,17]. In summary, using manual SD-OCT measurements CADASIL patients revealed a distinct difference in inner and outer diameter as well as in vessel wall thickness in both arteries and veins not only compared to our control group but also to measurements of larger healthy populations from the literature (Table 4).

Manual vessel measurements in peripapillary SD-OCT scans allow for in-vivo identification of vessel walls, outer and inner diameter of retinal arteries and veins in CADASIL patients. This technique visualizes morphologic changes in vessel architecture reflecting histologic and pathophysiologic knowledge on this disease.

Obviously, the small number of subjects included in the study precludes any definitive interpretation. Yet, CADASIL is a rare disease and in those patients included diagnosis was confirmed by genetic testing and vessel biopsy. Furthermore, the clinical stage of the disease was heterogeneous within the study group. As automated software is not commercially available, retinal vessel diameters had to be measured manually on SD-OCT sections. Study results must be interpreted cautiously bearing in mind that SD-OCT does allow for highlighting differences of reflectivity within the human retina in-vivo, however, no strict correlations with histology have been demonstrated yet. So far it remains unclear, for instance, which vessel wall layer or which property of the vessel wall results in hyper- or hyporeflectivities seen in SD-OCT. Therefore, one cannot assume for sure that the identified and measured reflectivities in this study in fact represent the entire vessel wall. Furthermore, all depicted vessels within an SD-OCT scan are captured by the laser beam in various angles, which may lead to altered reflection properties of each individual vessel wall. Finally, absorption effects of the inner vessel tissue (towards the vitreous) may cause a challenging demarcation of outer vessel walls (towards the RPE) particularly in venous vessels since veins exhibit a weaker reflectivity signal compared to arteries due to their different wall architecture. These facts certainly limit the validity of morphologic changes in vessel wall thickness observed in SD-OCT.

Regarding continuous improvements in retinal imaging, retinal vessel analysis may become more relevant not only in ophthalmologic but also in systemic and neurologic diseases [40]. In the near future, adaptive optics SLO appears to be the next step in in-vivo retinal imaging as it is increasingly capable of non-invasively detecting and monitoring morphological changes within retinal vascular wall morphology [37]. Image acquisition using adaptive optics systems and the subsequent image processing is extremely time consuming, which currently limits widespread clinical application.

This is the first study to report retinal findings and retinal vessel measurements in CADASIL patients based on high resolution imaging. CADASIL patients revealed a thicker RNFL caused by enlarged vessel diameters. Increased retinal venous lumina, a known risk factor for stroke, were found in manual SD-OCT measurements. Thickened vessel walls as found in manual SD-OCT measurements correspond to previous histologic reports. Finally, reduced arterial vessel lumina as shown in SD-OCT represent the ischemic component of this disease.

In the future, retinal imaging will certainly not replace MRI in CADASIL patients as it is indispensable for detection of cerebral damage as well as for differential diagnosis. Nevertheless, besides MRI, genetic diagnostic and immunohistology, high resolution retinal vessel imaging may be accounted as a complementary tool to diagnose and follow-up CADASIL patients and other cerebral small-vessel diseases in the future.

Author Contributions

Conceived and designed the experiments: FA JM NE FP MM. Performed the experiments: FA JM CE MM. Analyzed the data: FA JM EMK NO FP MM. Contributed reagents/materials/analysis tools: NO EMK NE FP MM. Contributed to the writing of the manuscript: FA JM CC NE FP MM.

References

1. Joutel A, Corpechot C, Ducros A, Vahedi K, Chabriat H, et al. (1996) NOTCH3 mutations in CADASIL, a hereditary adult-onset condition causing stroke and dementia. Nature 383: 707–10.

2. Tikka S, Mykkänen K, Ruchoux M-M, Bergholm R, Junna M, et al. (2009) Congruence between NOTCH3 mutations and GOM in 131 CADASIL patients. Brain 132: 933–939.

3. Dichgans M, Mayer M, Uttner I, Brüning R, Müller-Höcker J, et al. (1998) The phenotypic spectrum of CADASIL: clinical findings in 102 cases. Ann Neurol. 44: 731–739.

4. Haritoglou C, Rudolph G, Hoops JP, Opherk C, Kampik A, et al (2004) Retinal vascular abnormalities in CADASIL. Neurology 62: 202–1205.

5. Haritoglou C, Hoops JP, Stefani FH, Mehraein P, Kampik A, et al. (2004) Histopathological abnormalities in ocular blood vessels of CADASIL patients. Am J Ophthalmol. 138: 302–5.

6. Pretegiani E, Rosini F, Dotti MT, Bianchi S, Federico A, et al. (2013) Visual System Involvement in CADASIL. J Stroke Cerebrovasc Dis. 22: 1377–84.

7. Parisi V, Pierelli F, Coppola G, Restuccia R, Ferrazzoli D, et al. (2007) Reduction of optic nerve fiber layer thickness in CADASIL. Eur J Neurol 14: 627–631.

8. Rufa A, Pretegiani E, Frezzotti P, De Stefano N, Cevenini G, et al. (2011) Retinal nerve fiber layer thinning in CADASIL: an optical coherence tomography and MRI study. Cerebrovasc Dis. 31: 77–82.

9. Robinson W, Galetta SL, McCluskey L, Forman MS, Balcer LJ (2001) Retinal findings in cerebral autosomal dominant arteriopathy with subcortical infarcts and leukoencephalopathy (CADASIL). Surv Ophthalmol 45: 445–448.

10. Roine S, Harju M, Kivelä TT, Pöyhönen M, Nikoskelainen E, et al. (2006) Ophthalmologic findings in cerebral autosomal dominant arteriopathy with subcortical infarcts and leukoencephalopathy: a cross-sectional study. Ophthalmology 13: 1411–7.

11. Liu Y, Wu Y, Xie S, Luan XH, Yuan Y (2008) Retinal arterial abnormalities correlate with brain white matter lesions in cerebral autosomal dominant arteriopathy with subcortical infarcts and leucoencephalopathy. Clin Experiment Ophthalmol. 36: 532–6.

12. Joutel A, Favrole P, Labauge P, Chabriat H, Lescoat C, et al. (2001) Skin biopsy immunostaining with a Notch3 monoclonal antibody for CADASIL diagnosis. Lancet 358: 2049–2051.

13. Lesnik Oberstein SA, van Duinen SG, van den Boom R, Maat-Schieman ML, van Buchem MA, et al. (2003) Evaluation of diagnostic NOTCH3 immunostaining in CADASIL. Acta Neuropathol 106: 107–111.

14. Malandrini A, Gaudiano C, Gambelli S, Berti G, Serni G, et al. (2007) Diagnostic value of ultrastructural skin biopsy studies in CADASIL. Neurology 68: 1430–1432.

15. Muraoka Y, Tsujikawa A, Murakami T, Ogino K, Kumagai K, et al. (2013) Morphologic and functional changes in retinal vessels associated with branch retinal vein occlusion. Ophthalmology. 120: 91–9.

16. Muraoka Y, Tsujikawa A, Kumagai K, Akiba M, Ogino K, et al. (2013) Age- and hypertension-dependent changes in retinal vessel diameter and wall thickness: an optical coherence tomography study. Am J Ophthalmol. 156: 706–714.

17. Goldenberg D, Shahar J, Loewenstein A, Goldstein M (2013) Diameters of retinal blood vessels in a helathy cohort as measured by spectral domain optical coherence tomography. Retina 33: 1888–94.

18. Lonie JA, Tierney KM, Ebmeier KP (2009) Screening for mild cognitive impairment: a systematic review. Int J Geriatr Psychiatry. 24: 902–15.

19. Vérin M, Rolland Y, Landgraf F, Chabriat H, Bompais B, et al. (1995) New phenotype of the cerebral autosomal dominant arteriopathy mapped to chromosome 19: migraine as the prominent clinical feature. J Neurol Neurosurg Psychiatry. 59: 579–85.

20. Spaide RF, Koizumi H, Pozzoni MC (2008) Enhanced depth imaging spectral-domain optical coherence tomography. Am J Ophthalmol. 146: 496–500.

21. Tanabe H, Ito Y, Terasaki H (2012) Choroid is thinner in inferior region of the optic disk of normal eyes. Retina 32: 134–139.

22. Chhablani J, Barteselli G, Wang H, El-Emam S, Kozak I, et al. (2012) Repeatability and reproducibility of manual choroidal volume measurements using enhanced depth imaging optical coherence tomography. Invest Ophthalmol Vis Sci. 53: 2274–80.

23. Yannuzzi LA, Slakter JS, Sorenson JA, Guyer DR, Orlock DA (1992) Digital indocyanine green videoangiography and choroidal neovascularization. Retina. 12: 191–223.

24. Oberwahrenbrock T, Ringelstein M, Jentschke S, Deuschle K, Klumbies K, et al. (2013) Retinal ganglion cell and inner plexiform layer thinning in clinically isolated syndrome. Mult Scler. 19: 1887–95.

25. Motte J, Alten F, Ewering C, Osada N, Kadas EM, et al. (2014) Vessel labeling in combined confocal scanning laser ophthalmoscopy and optical coherence tomography images: Criteria for blood vessel discrimination. PLoS One. 9(9): e102034.

26. Hogan MJ, Alvarado JA, Weddell JE (eds) (1971) Histology of the Human Eye: An Atlas and Textbook. Saunders: Philadelphia, PA, 393–522.

27. Roman GC, Erkinjuntti T, Wallin A, Pantoni L, Chui HC (2002) Subcortical ischaemic vascular dementia. Lancet Neurol 1: 426–36.

28. Baudrimont M, Dubas F, Joutel A, Tournier-Lasserve E, Bousser MG (1993) Autosomal dominant leukoencephalopathy and subcortical ischemic stroke. A clinicopathological study. Stroke 24: 122–25.

29. Viswanathan A, Gray F, Bousser MG, Baudrimont M, Chabriat H (2006) Cortical neuronal apoptosis in CADASIL. Stroke 37: 2690–95.

30. Kwa VI, van der Sande JJ, Stam J, Tijmes N, Vrooland JL (2002) Retinal arterial changes correlate with cerebral small-vessel disease. Neurology 59: 1536–1540.

31. Wong TY, Klein R, Couper DJ, Cooper LS, Shahar E, et al. (2001) Retinal microvascular abnormalities and incident stroke: the atherosclerosis risk in communities study. Lancet 358: 1134–1140.

32. Barteselli G, Chhablani J, El-Emam S, Wang H, Chuang J, et al. (2012) Choroidal volume variations with age, axial length, and sex in healthy subjects: a three-dimensional analysis. Ophthalmology. 119: 2572–8.

33. Giuffrè G (1989) Main posterior watershed zone of the choroid. Variations of its position in normal subjects. Doc Ophthalmol. 72: 175–80.

34. Fischer MD, Huber G, Feng Y, Tanimoto N, Mühlfriedel R, et al. (2010) In Vivo Assessment of Retinal Vascular Wall Dimensions. Invest Ophthalmol Vis Sci. 51: 5254–9.

35. Ikram MK, de Jong FJ, Bos MJ, Vingerling JR, Hofman A, et al. (2006) Retinal vessel diameters and risk of stroke: the Rotterdam Study. Neurology 66: 1339–1343.

36. Ikram MK, De Jong FJ, Van Dijk EJ, Prins ND, Hofman A, et al. (2006) Retinal vessel diameters and cerebral small vessel disease: the Rotterdam Scan Study. Brain. 129: 182–8.

37. Chui TY, Gast TJ, Burns SA (2013) Imaging of vascular wall fine structure in human retina using adaptive optics scanning laser ophthalmoscopy. Invest Ophthalmol Vis Sci. 54: 7115–24.

38. Brinchmann-Hansen O, Sandvik L (1986) The width of the light reflex on retinal arteries and veins. Acta Ophthalmol (Copenh). 64: 433–438.

39. Dong H, Ding H, Young K, Blaivas M, Christensen PJ, et al. (2013) Advanced intimal hyperplasia without luminal narrowing of leptomeningeal arteries in CADASIL. Stroke. 44: 1456–8.

40. Ouyang Y, Shao Q, Scharf D, Joussen AM, Heussen FM (2014) Retinal Vessel Diameter Measurements by Spectral Domain Optical Coherence Tomography. Graefes Arch Clin Exp Ophthalmol. Aug 17. [Epub ahead of print].

11

High Fidelity System Modeling for High Quality Image Reconstruction in Clinical CT

Synho Do[1]*, William Clem Karl[2], Sarabjeet Singh[1], Mannudeep Kalra[1], Tom Brady[1], Ellie Shin[1], Homer Pien[1]

1 Department of Radiology, Massachusetts General Hospital and Harvard Medical School, Boston, Massachusetts, United States of America, **2** Department of Electrical and Computer Engineering, Boston University, Boston, Massachusetts, United States of America

Abstract

Today, while many researchers focus on the improvement of the regularization term in IR algorithms, they pay less concern to the improvement of the fidelity term. In this paper, we hypothesize that improving the fidelity term will further improve IR image quality in low-dose scanning, which typically causes more noise. The purpose of this paper is to systematically test and examine the role of high-fidelity system models using raw data in the performance of iterative image reconstruction approach minimizing energy functional. We first isolated the fidelity term and analyzed the importance of using focal spot area modeling, flying focal spot location modeling, and active detector area modeling as opposed to just flying focal spot motion. We then compared images using different permutations of all three factors. Next, we tested the ability of the fidelity terms to retain signals upon application of the regularization term with all three factors. We then compared the differences between images generated by the proposed method and Filtered-Back-Projection. Lastly, we compared images of low-dose in vivo data using Filtered-Back-Projection, Iterative Reconstruction in Image Space, and the proposed method using raw data. The initial comparison of difference maps of images constructed showed that the focal spot area model and the active detector area model also have significant impacts on the quality of images produced. Upon application of the regularization term, images generated using all three factors were able to substantially decrease model mismatch error, artifacts, and noise. When the images generated by the proposed method were tested, conspicuity greatly increased, noise standard deviation decreased by 90% in homogeneous regions, and resolution also greatly improved. In conclusion, the improvement of the fidelity term to model clinical scanners is essential to generating higher quality images in low-dose imaging.

Editor: Arrate Muñoz-Barrutia, University of Navarra, Spain

Funding: The authors have no funding or support to report.

Competing Interests: The authors have declared that no competing interests exist.

* Email: sdo@mgh.harvard.edu

Introduction

Computed tomography (CT) is one of the most commonly used diagnostic imaging modalities in modern medicine. CT enables rapid, non-invasive image acquisition at high resolutions. However, CT also exposes the patient to radiation [1,2]. CT dosage can be decreased by lowering either the voltage or the flux. Lowering the voltage implies that the emitted photons are less energetic, reducing their ability to penetrate through the body. Lowering the flux reduces the number of photons emitted, further degrading the signal-to-noise ratio of the acquired data. Therefore, the consequence of low-dose CT imaging is that the resulting images are considerably noisier than images acquired with todays clinical doses [3].

The drive towards lower dose CT imaging (while maintaining the diagnostic quality of CT) has been an area of focus for the entire CT community [4–9]. Numerous approaches to dose reduction have been implemented in commercial systems including the use of filters [10–12], collimators [13], dose modulation [14,15], prospective triggering [6], patient-specific protocols

[16,17], and more [12,18]. One additional component to the current repertoire of low-dose CT scanning techniques is the use of new image reconstruction techniques.

Through recent studies, iterative reconstruction (IR) algorithms have been shown to be more robust than FBP algorithms in regards to the presence of noise and artifacts [8,19–25]. Numerous researchers have discussed different aspects of formulations [26–31] and optimization approaches [32–36]. However, we have found that having a high fidelity model of the imaging system is also a critical factor in the reconstruction of high quality images; this is an aspect of iterative reconstruction algorithms which has often been either neglected or substantially simplified [37,38].

A critical component of tomographic IR algorithms is the accuracy of the forward system model. In positron emission tomography (PET), the forward system model consists of a geometric projection matrix and a sinogram blurring matrix, which can be either measured or simulated [39,40]. It is shown that the combined model improves resolution and contrast-to-noise ratio in PET imaging [41]. It is also possible to reuse the

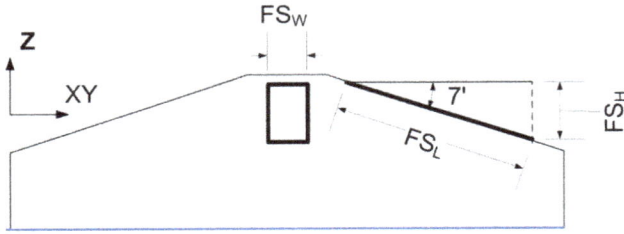

Figure 1. Focal spot area diagram: The length (FSL), width (FSW), and height ($FSH = FSL \times sin(7)$) of the focal spot area (rectangular shape) are denoted in the diagram.

stored system matrix to improve computation time because the PET scanner is stationary, making it relatively easy to factorize the system model based on symmetric geometry. A similar method is applied to single photon emission computed tomography (SPECT) for the estimation of the depth-dependent component of the point spread function (PSF) [42]. However, it is a challenging task to derive an explicit system matrix in clinical CT for the following reasons: i) each scan has a different scan length and pitch based on the scanning protocol, and ii) it is very hard to find symmetries in cone beam helical CT scans because the source-detector set has a functional misalignment (i.e., a quarter of a detector offset [43]) and view-by-view deflections of the X-ray source spot (i.e., flying focal spot (FFS) [44]).

In this paper, we show the systematic implementation of accurate system modeling for an IRT in clinical CT. A similar approach for PET [45] was derived from an analytical formula for calculating error propagation in a reconstructed image from the system matrix. In addition, in the cone-beam CT, the beam divergence and the rotation of the X-ray source and detector unit give space-variant effect on image. Since we do not use a system matrix as in PET, we integrate all the functional misalignment and fabrication limitations with on-the-fly calculation method so that the space-invariant nature is embedded in the forward model. Therefore, when we run image reconstruction algorithm, we set up on/off parameters for each modular model. That is one of

major differences of our results compared to the previous 2D or phantom simulation works.

Also, there are algorithms (ASIR, IRIS, iDose, VEO, etc.) implemented in clinical scanners by vendors, but the technical description and detailed methods are not available to the research community. In this paper, we systematically demonstrate the necessity of implementing focal spot area, flying focal spot, and detector area in the forward system model to generate higher quality images. We also compare our raw-data-domain IRT with a mathematical formulation of image domain iteration called Iterative Reconstruction in Image Space (IRIS). The purpose of this paper is to examine the role of high-fidelity system models in the performance of the iterative image reconstruction approach minimizing energy functional. This paper is organized as follows. In section 2, we mathematically describe iterative image reconstruction and the components of proposed system models. In section 3, we present some initial results on phantom and in vivo data. In section 4, we summarize our findings and conclusions.

Methods

In this section, we describe the mathematical formulation of IRT and a detailed forward system modeling method. The forward system modeling method can be decomposed into a series of components to increase modeling accuracy. We structure a three-component model that incorporates the most important elements of the system model. Each component can be replaced by a specific scanner parameter or vendor-specific model. The accuracy of this system model is critical in the improvement of image quality of a reconstructed image.

On-the-fly System Modeling and Reconstruction Formulation for Clinical Scanner

We assume a transmission CT system with a field of x-ray attenuation coefficients x and projection operator H as modeled by:

$$y = Hx + \eta \qquad (1)$$

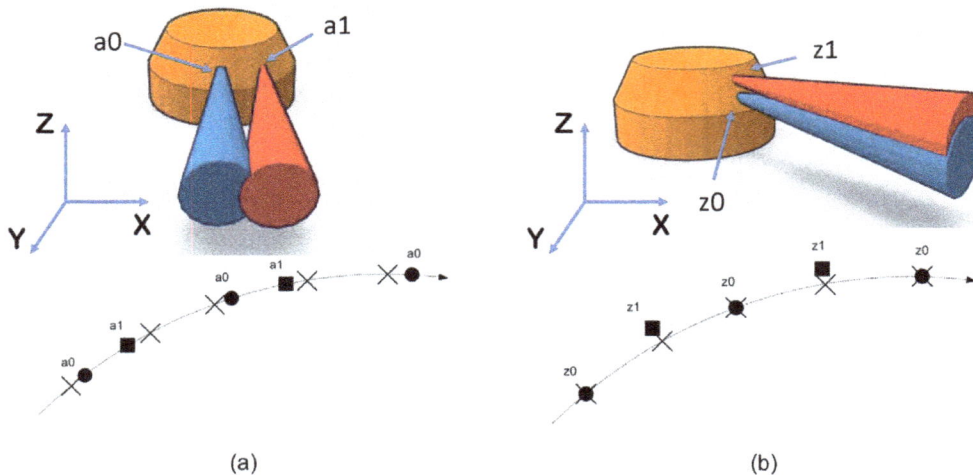

(a)   (b)

Figure 2. Flying Focal Spot (FFS) modeling: (a) $\alpha - FFS$ model shows deflected FFSs to the angular direction and (b) $z - FFS$ model shows z-directional deflections.

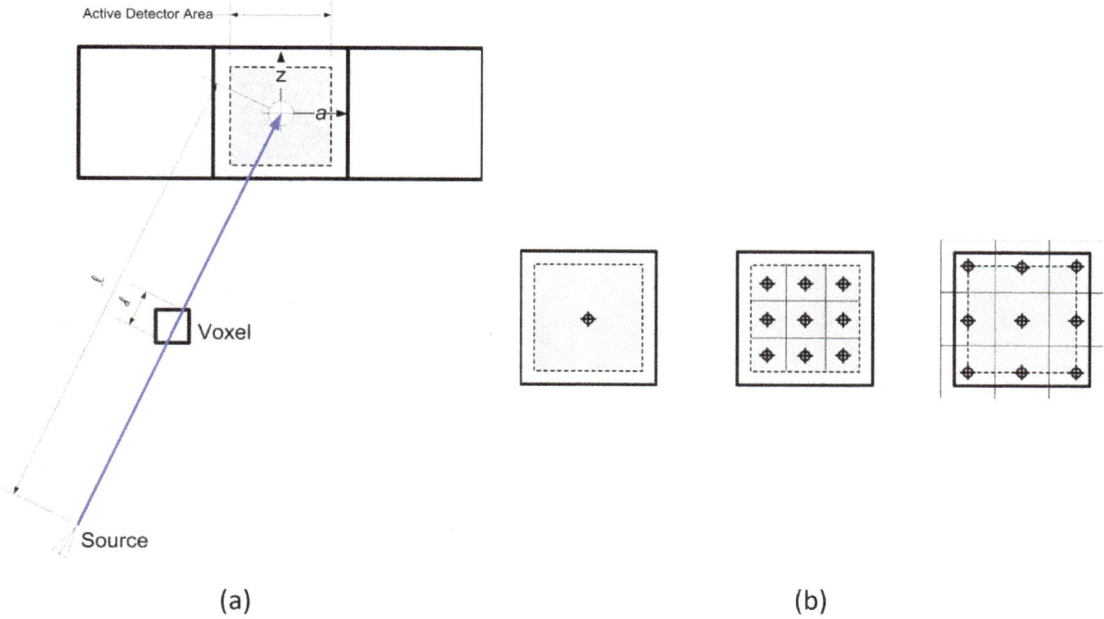

Figure 3. Diagram of active area of detector element: (a) Siddon-type ray-based projector calculates the ratio of intersections of the ray (i.e., d/l), (b) Gray area is the active region of single detector element, Left: single element model, middle: multiple elements by limiting active area of detector, right: multiple elements by assigning rays to the boundary of active area of detector element.

where y denotes the projection sinogram, and η denotes noise. We formulate our reconstruction problem by the following equation:

$$\hat{x} = \operatorname*{argmin}_{x} E_d(y,x) + \alpha E(x) \qquad (2)$$

where $E_d(y,x)$ is the data fidelity term between image x and sinogram y via the projection process. The second term $E(x)$ is the prior, or regularization term, and α is the weighting term. We formulate the fidelity term as:

$$E_d(y,x) = \|y - Hx\|_2^2 \qquad (3)$$

where H is the system matrix, or projection process. One example of the regularization term $E(x)$ is the L_p norm:

$$E(x) = \|Lx\|_p^p = (\|Lx\|_p)^p = ((|Lx_1|^p + |Lx_2|^p + \cdots + |Lx_n|^p)^{\frac{1}{p}})^p \quad (4)$$

When $L = \nabla$ and $p = 1$, $E(x)$ becomes a Total Variation (TV) regularizer, which is commonly used to suppress noise and preserve edges in the image [46,47]. From a modeling perspective, we make the assumption that H, the system matrix, can be decomposed into a series of component models:

$$H = A_{det} A_{fs} P_{geom} \qquad (5)$$

The models include a geometric projector (P_{geom}), a focal spot model (A_{fs}), and an active detector response function (A_{det}). By decomposing a system matrix H into sub-components, the implementation of complex clinical scanner modeling becomes more feasible. This approach also increases the usability of a single

developed code across multiple CT systems, as opposed to requiring entirely different projectors for each system.

In this paper, we used the least-squares (LS) solution without the regularization term and TV solution in Equation (2) and (4) for comparison. The lagged diffusivity fixed-point method [46,48], where we iteratively approximated the cost by a weighted quadratic cost and then solved the resulting linear normal equations using pre-conditioned conjugated gradient (CG) iterations, is used to minimize the energy functional in Equation (2) [49].

Focal Spot Area Modeling

A focal spot is the region where electrons transfer their energy to target atoms in order to generate X-rays. In many cases, the focal spot is approximated as a point model, but in reality, the focal spot consists of a finite area (i.e., 0.3 mm to 0.8 mm) [50]. Furthermore, the size of this area changes with scanner settings (kVp or mA), an important consideration in regards to image reconstruction of low dose scans. Figure 1 illustrates the focal spot area with the length (FS_L), width (FS_W), and height ($FS_H = FS_L \times sin(7)$) of the area in the diagram. This sub-module should be included for accurate forward system modeling.

Flying Focal Spot (FFS) Modeling

The detector elements form an equiangular concentric cylindrical structure with 32 rows and 672 channels (i.e., 1st generation Dual Source CT, Siemens, Definition) with FFS models as shown in Figure 2. We assume the active area of all detector elements (i.e., $32 \times 672 = 21504$) is identical for all elements according to manufacturer specifications. In Siddon-type ray-based projectors, a single ray sum is calculated for a single detector element by using the ratio of intersections of the ray with equally spaced parallel lines [51]. For our IR technique, we calculate a bundle of rays to simulate the virtual ray, which shapes the volume from the focal spot area to the active detector area. The ratio of the active

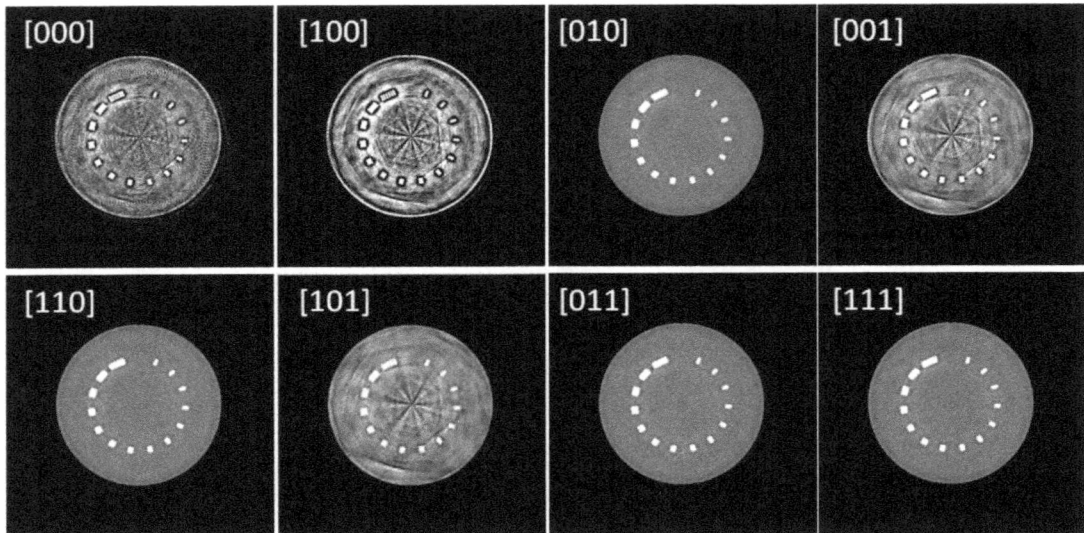

(a)

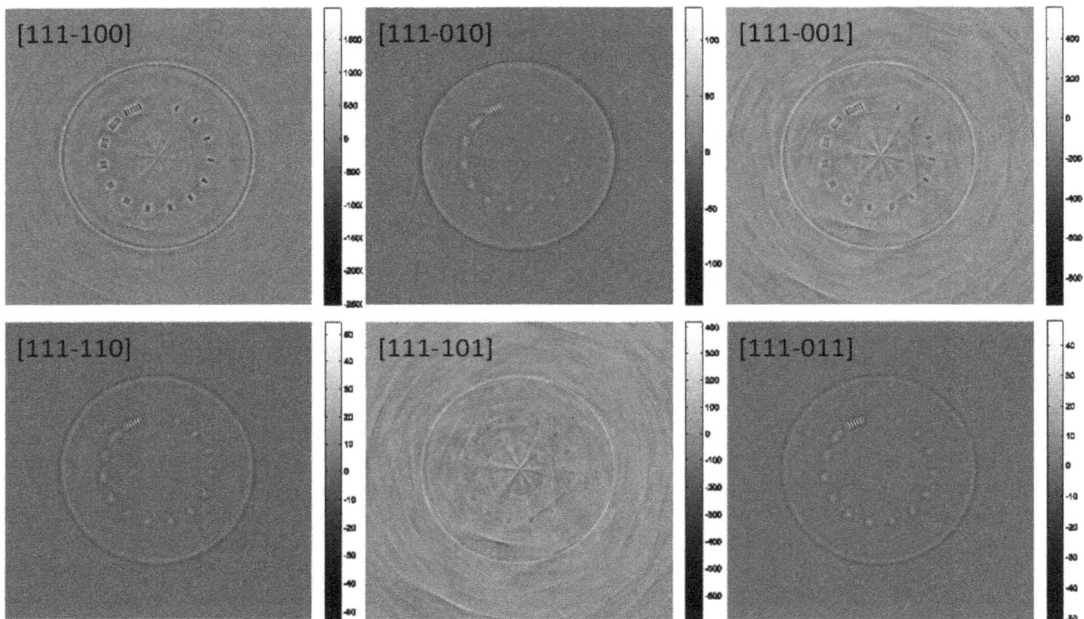

(b)

Figure 4. Modular system model effects: (a) Images are displayed in $[-1000,500]$ **HU and (b) difference maps are displayed in dynamic contrast range.** $[FS,FFS,DM]$: *FS*: Focal Spot model, *FFS*: Flying Focal Spot model, and *DM*: Detector model.

detector area to physical spacing between detector elements was provided to us by the scanner manufacturer as 85% in the angular direction and 80% in the z-direction as shown in Figure 3. These ratios can be changed for different systems.

The Siddon projector calculates only the weighted sums of the portion of the ray that intersects through each voxel without considering and compensating for the neighboring voxels, generating aliasing artifacts [52]. Multiple rays in the volume beam can be used to compensate for this aliasing effect at the expense of over-sampling the image grid [53]. We have additionally implemented a version of the Siddon projector which does not require recursion [54], thus making it amendable to parallel implementations [55].

Figure 3-(b) shows how we divide active sub-elements to compute ray-sums. In Figure 3-(b), a single element model, as well as a multiple element model that strictly limits the active area of the detector (i.e., middle sub-figure), is depicted. We have noticed, however, that applications with reconstructions on voxel

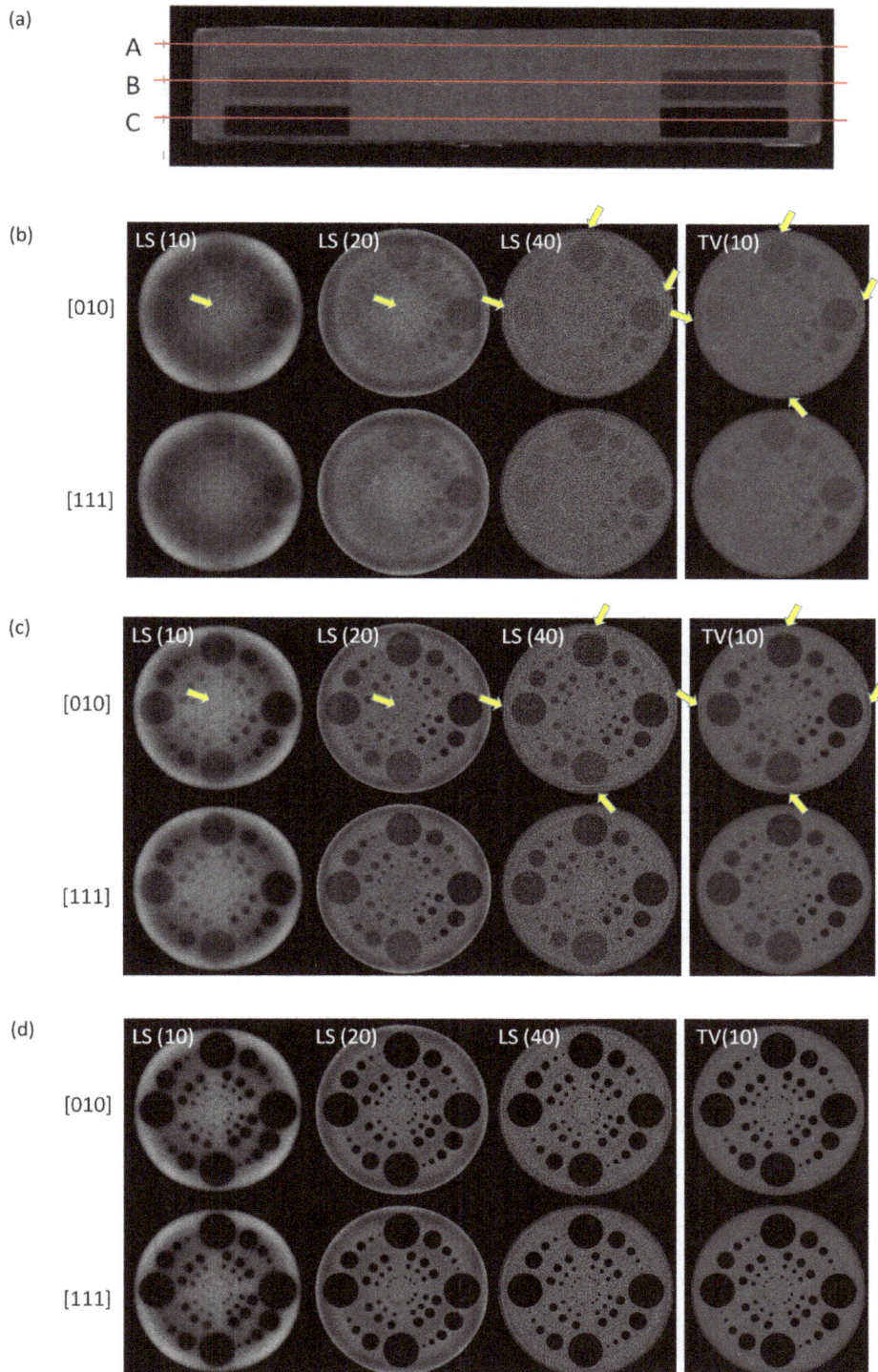

Figure 5. A modeling effect comparison on LS and TV images: (a) Coronal view of soft contrast section of phantom, (b), (c), and (d) show axial views of line A, B, and C respectively. The FFS only model (so called Siddon Model, (0,1,0)) shows circular line artifacts in LS and TV as well. In contrast, the proposed model ((1,1,1)) shows high quality image even in LS without regularization term and significant noise suppression effect on TV.

sizes that are finer than the detector size itself requires a greater over-sampling of the detector. In this case, not only does the computational demand increase, but the gap between the active areas of two adjacent detectors begin to introduce artifacts. As such, we have implemented the active area model depicted in the right sub-figure of Figure 3-(b), where the rays intersect the major boundary points, leading to a higher quality reconstruction.

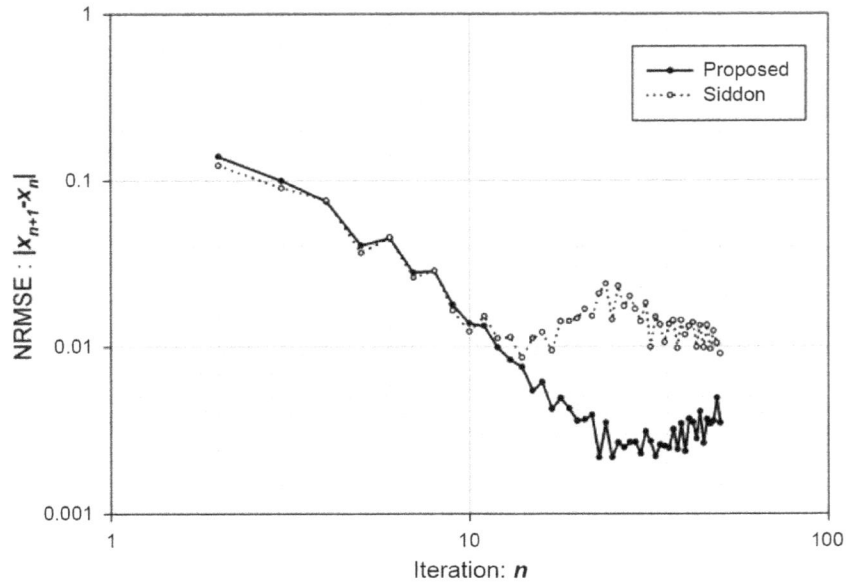

Figure 6. Consecutive error plot of Siddon (0,1,0) **and the proposed method** (1,1,1)**.** The NRMSEs of two consecutive images are calculated and displayed in log-log plot. The proposed method exhibits smaller consecutive errors after 15 iterations compared to Siddon method and reaches smaller modeling error.

Results

We show two experimental results in this section. For the phantom study, we focus on the comparison between the effects of each model on the LS images with a cone beam phantom (QRM, Moehrendorf, Germany) with respect to conspicuity improvement, noise statistics, and resolution. In an in vivo study, we show clinical evidence that supports the proposed approach with subjective assessment. The proposed method is compared with conventional FBP and image domain IR (IRIS) algorithms in a low dose scan. In this case, we used the same raw data for image reconstructions.

Phantom Study

A cone beam phantom with a spatial resolution section with 14 circularly aligned line-patterns varying from 4 to 30 lp/cm was scanned on a dual source 64-slice multi-detector row CT (Definition, Siemens Healthcare, Forchheim, Germany) using the following parameters: detector collimation $= 0.6mm$, table speed $= 3.8mm$ per gantry rotation, gantry rotation $= 330msec$, tube current $= 515mA$, and tube voltage $= 120kV$.

In the following sections we demonstrate the impact of our various system modules. We will use the following notation: the triplet (FS, FFS, DM) to denote with a 1 or 0, whether the focal spot model, flying focal spot model, and detector model, respectively, are turned on $(= 1)$ or off $(= 0)$. Thus, for example, $(FS, FFS, DM) = (0,1,0)$ indicates that the flying focal spot model is turned on, while the other two system models are turned off.

Figure 4 shows the LS solutions reconstructed using all permutations of (FS, FFS, DM). Additionally, the differences between these permutations and the case in which all models are turned on $((FS, FFS, DM) = (1,1,1))$ are shown. All reconstructed images are shown with a windowing level of $[-1000, 500]$, and difference images are shown with the full dynamic range of each difference so that patterns of artifacts are visible. The model without FFS generates the stellar shape artifact from the center of the rotation and it causes major deterioration of image quality. Therefore, FFS modeling is one of the most important compo-

nents of clinical system modeling. The image quality evaluations in analytic reconstruction methods are shown in papers [44,56]. In analytic reconstruction methods, the locations of X-ray source and detector elements are the only models that can be implemented in the algorithm, so it is easy to overlook the importance of FS and DM.

In Figure 4, we can visually compare image qualities of Siddon-type model with FFS (0,1,0) and the proposed method (1,1,1) including focal spot and detector models to acquire a more accurate system model and to remove Moire patterns. There are only small differences between the two models, especially around the edges of the image, but eventually these will cause a significant change in the final image (i.e., TV regularization), especially in low dose scans. To suppress noise in low dose imaging, we frequently use regularization terms in Equation (2) with which we suppress noise by keeping the structure components of the image. When there are small model discrepancies related to the fidelity term in Equation (3), the mismatches can be concealed by noise and may cause resolution degradation and eventually poor contrast.

To compare artifact propagation, we compare the LS and TV images with a soft contrast section of the phantom. The three cross-sections of the soft contrast region are displayed in Figure 5-(a). Figure 5-(b), (c), and (d) show the axial views of line A, B, and C respectively. The top images are from Siddon-type model with $FFS(0,1,0)$ and the bottom images are from the proposed method (1,1,1). By the number of iteration (i.e., LS: 10,20, and 40 iteration, TV: 10 iteration), we can observe circular line artifacts on LS and TV, as well as on the Siddon-type model. It is especially more obvious in a very low contrast case (Figure 5-(b)). However, the images reconstructed by the proposed method show high quality images without any artifacts in both LS and TV. As expected, the TV images show significant noise suppression.

To observe the effects of iterations, we simulated a Siddon-type projector with proper FFS model (0,1,0) without FS and DM, and a complete model (1,1,1) including all modular models in Section 2. Both methods used the same optimization algorithm

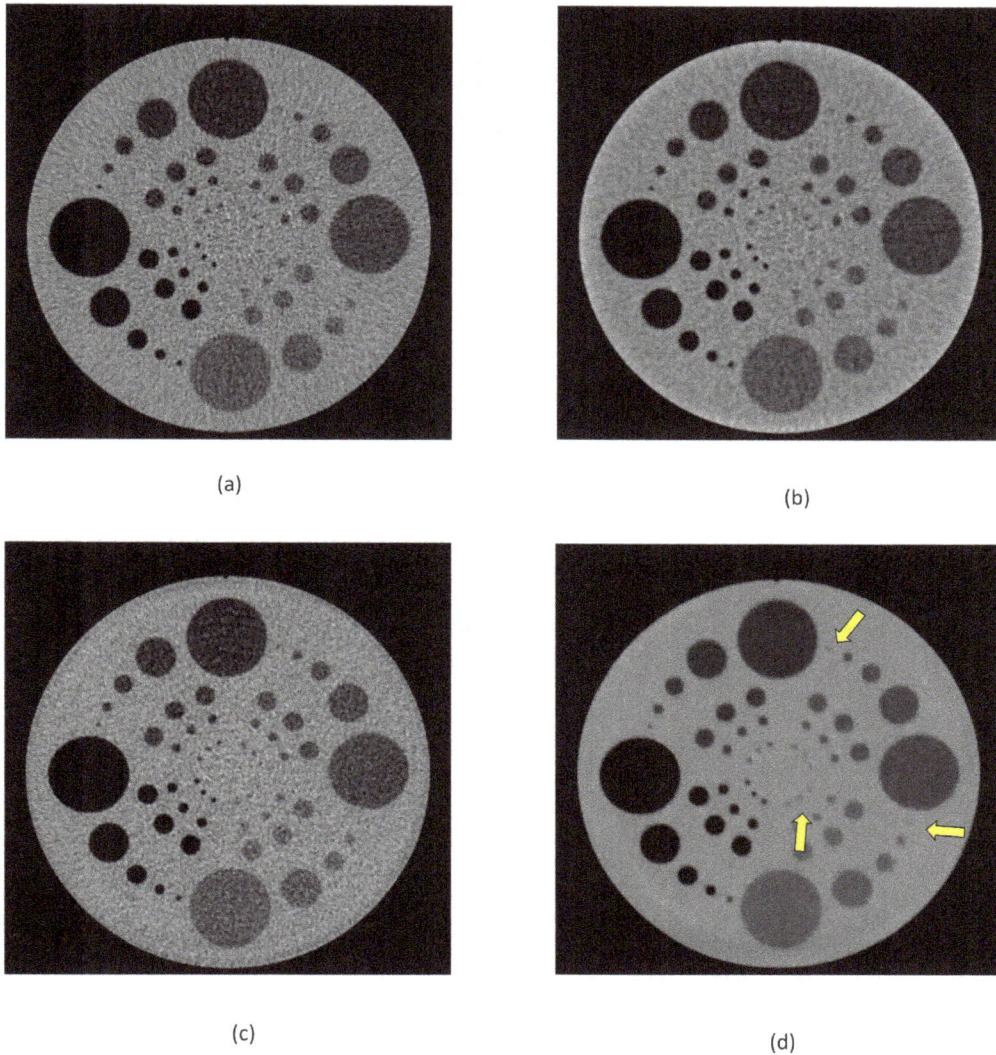

Figure 7. Soft contrast and conspicuity comparison for (a) FBP with sharp kernel filtering, (b) FBP with soft kernel filtering, (c) Least-Squares solution after 30-iteration, and (d) Total Variation (TV) image after 10-iteration with (c) initialization [−200,300].

and code (C++ and Open MPI) to reconstruct images and consecutively calculate the NRMSE (Normalized Root Mean Square Error):

$$\varepsilon = \sqrt{\frac{\sum(\|X_n - X_{n+1}\|^2)}{\sum(\|X_{n+1}\|^2)}} \qquad (6)$$

where X_n is the $n-th$ iteration result of LS-solution with L elements.

Figure 6 compares the consecutive errors with iteration for Siddon $(0,1,0)$ and the proposed method $(1,1,1)$ in the log-log scale. The Siddon-type projector shows similar updates to the proposed method until iteration-15, where it plateaus and then fluctuates. The resulting image from the Siddon projector does not provide the best image even though it reaches the solution of Equation (3). In contrast, the NRMSEs for our proposed method become smaller even after 15-iterations because the modeling error decreases with increasing iterations. However, the high

frequency and noise components of the 30 iterations become dominant in the system modeling.

Note that the proposed method exhibits significant modeling error reduction in terms of visual evaluation and NRMSE taking into account the nonlinear scaling of log-log plot.

Conspicuity Improvements. In Figure 7, we display a contrast resolution section of QRM phantoms scanned in the clinical system. We show four groups of circles with different attenuation coefficients in Hounsfield Units (HU) $(-60, -90, -120,$ and -200 HU) in tissue equivalent background (35 HU) at $120kVp$. Each group consists of 14 circular inserts with different diameters $(2,4,8,16,$ and $32mm)$. We used the same raw data for the comparison of four different reconstruction methods: Figure 7-(a) FBP with sharp kernel filtering, (b) FBP with soft kernel filtering, (c) Least-Squares (LS) solution after 30-iterations, and (d) Total Variation (TV) image after 10-iterations with (c) initialization.

We found that it is difficult to detect low contrast circles (for example, $2mm$ circles in -60 and -90 HU groups) visually as shown in Figure 7-(a), (b), and (c). Notice that there is no improvement of conspicuity in small circles with low contrast even

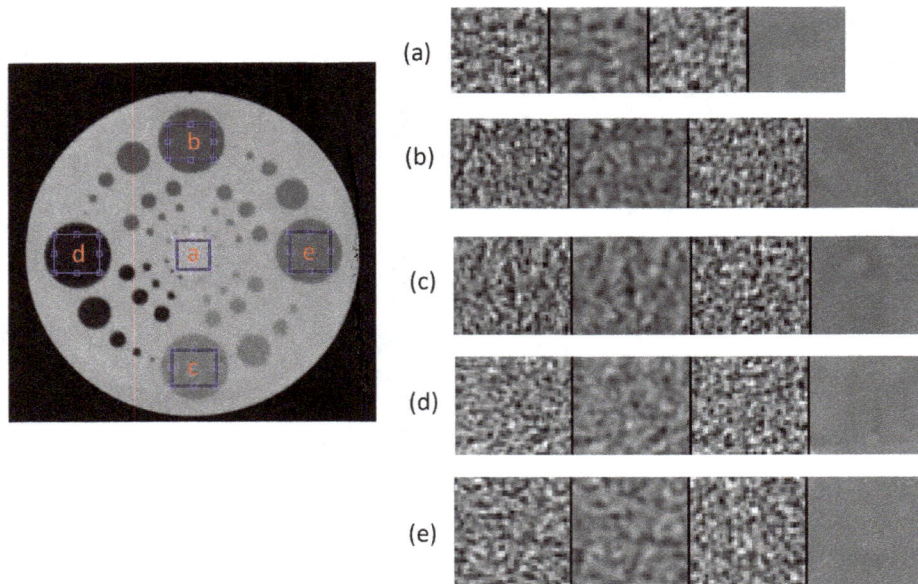

Figure 8. Noise patches comparison for the four images in Figure 8. Each sampled region is concatenated with dividing columns (zeros) and displayed in dynamic contrast window to show noticeable differences. From left to right, FBP with sharp kernel filtering, FBP with soft kernel filtering, IRT (LS), and IRT (TV).

with the smoothing kernel, Figure 7-(b). Basically, it suppresses high frequency noise components on the image without keeping small and low contrast information, which is key to the evaluation of low contrast tissues and lesions in most soft tissues such as the brain, liver, spleen, and lymph nodes, given subtle or low differences in HU values between organs and several of these legions (i.e., neoplasms and infarcts).

However, we can easily identify $2mm$ circles in -60 and -90 HU groups from Figure 7-(d). The TV image can be initialized on FBP image and can replace the LS solution.

Noise Statistics. Figure 8 compares noise patches from five noise regions for each image in Figure 7: one from each tissue equivalent region at the center of the Phantom and four $32mm$ circles from different HU groups ($-60, -90, -120,$ and -200 HU). Each sampled region is concatenated with dividing columns

(zeros) and displayed in a dynamic contrast window to show noticeable differences. The FBP with sharp kernel filtering and LS solutions show similar noise patterns. As shown in Table 1, a smoother and lower spatial frequency kernel FBP with soft kernel filtering has lower noise compared to that of a sharper and higher spatial frequency kernel FBP (sharp kernel). However, TV shows a strong noise suppression capability and retains visibility of small and low-contrast circular objects that are, in our opinion, from accurate system modeling.

The image reconstruction formulation in Equation (2) emphasizes that the energy functional aggregates a fidelity term and a regularization term. When the system model is not accurate enough to model details of the system, the TV-regularization (Equation (4)) of the energy functional (Equation (2)) smears or even loses the signal components associated with lower HU rather

Table 1. Shows the measurements of noise mean (m) and standard deviation (σ) for each patch from four difference reconstruction images.

		FBP(sharp kernel)	FBP(soft kernel)	IRT(LS)	IRT (TV)
Patch a	m	35.41	35.67	43.09	40.82
	σ	28.39	17.78	26.60	2.31
Patch b	m	-83.25	-84.19	-78.41	-78.92
	σ	21.81	13.14	22.35	2.04
Patch c	m	-26.99	-27.02	-24.23	-24.58
	σ	20.25	12.09	23.11	2.05
Patch d	m	-163.35	-164.98	-163.40	-163.64
	σ	19.07	11.66	21.90	2.29
Patch e	m	-54.57	-54.60	-51.37	-52.48
	σ	21.04	12.40	21.60	1.28

FBP (soft kernel) has smaller standard deviation than FBP (sharp kernel) and IRT (LS) but the IRT (TV) shows the smallest noise standard deviation.

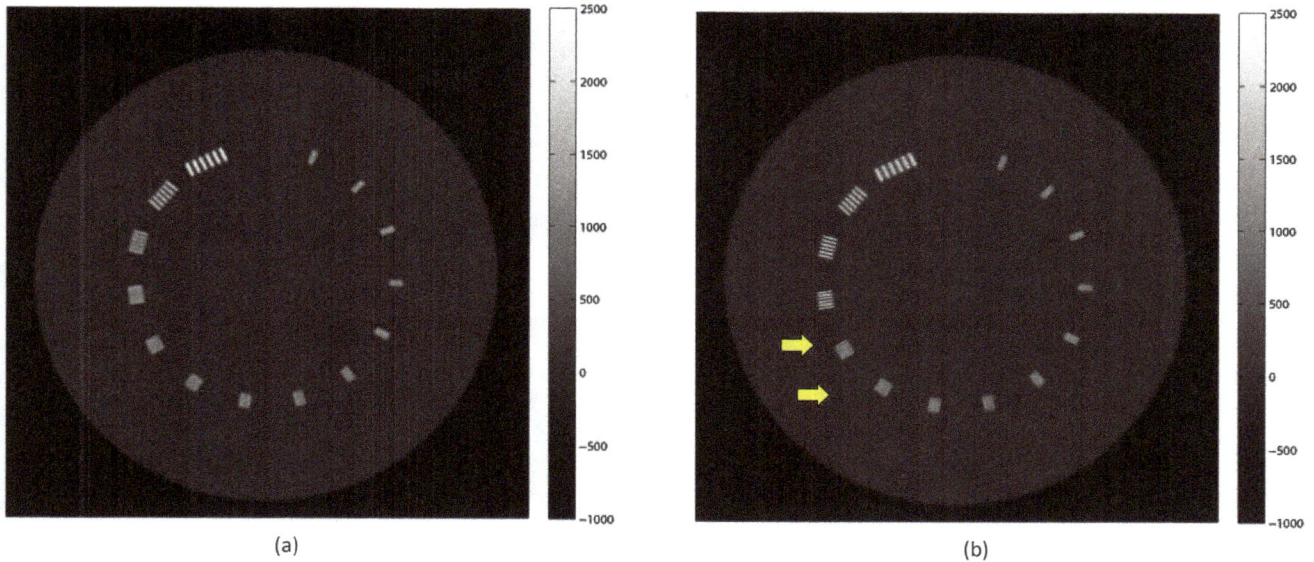

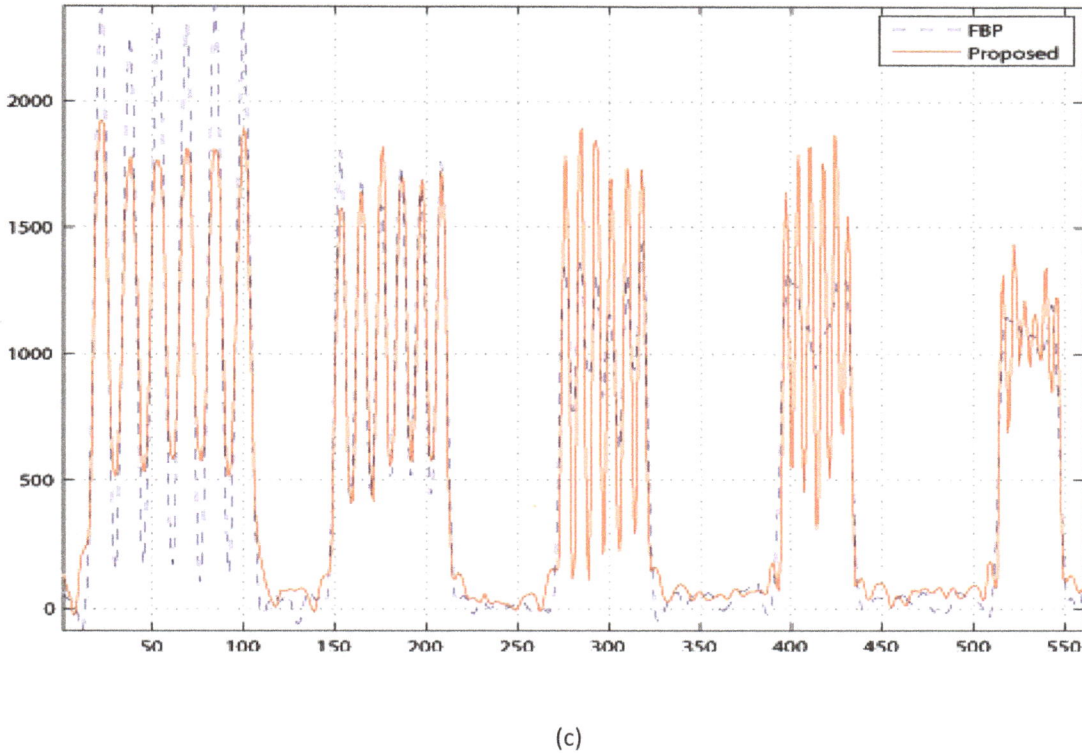

Figure 9. Spatial resolution bar pattern comparison: (a) FBP (sharp kernel) and (b) TV with high fidelity term image with proposed model (111) are displayed in $[800, 2300]$ **HU.** (a) shows clear separations of 4, 6, and 8 lp/cm and (b) presents improved resolution showing 10 and 12 lp/cm bar patterns. (c) compares profiles of spatial resolution inserts.

than noise when enforcing the smoothness constraint (i.e., L_1-norm) as in Equation (4). This can even occur to greater signal components in low dose CT data, when the system model is inaccurate and iteration proceeds to suppress amplified noise.

On the other hand, the accurate system model sustains small signal components in the fidelity term so that it eventually reveals hidden signal components under the noise components.

Resolution. The reconstruction parameters of FBP and the proposed IRT method $(1,1,1)$ are set to be the same as slice-thickness $(0.6mm)$.

The spatial resolution bar patterns are displayed in Figure 9 with a $[800,2300]$ contrast window. FBP (sharp kernel) and FBP (soft kernel) had similar resolutions, so only the better FBP (sharp kernel) is displayed in Figure 9-(a) and compared to the TV with

(a)

(b)

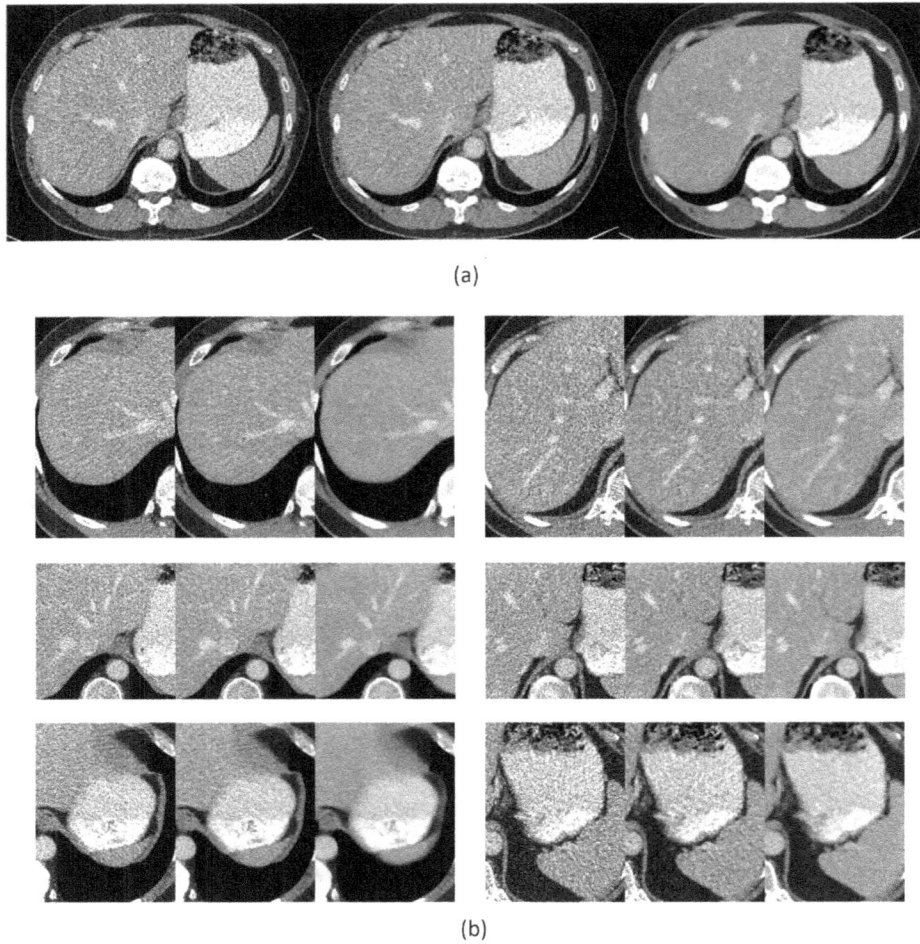

Figure 10. Comparison of reconstruction methods on half-dose images: (a) Reconstructed images, with (L) FBP, (M) IRIS, and (R) TV with advanced system modeling, (b) Zoomed images from different slices; each sub-figure shows (L) FBP, (M) IRIS, and (R) TV with advanced system modeling. Display in [5,155] **HU.**

advanced model in Figure 9-(b). Note that the arrows in Figure 9-(b) indicate 10 and 12 lp/cm inserts, which points to clear improvement of spatial resolution on the TV with advanced modeling image.

In vivo study

In the in vivo study, we only show clinical evidences of the proposed approach with subjective assessment. The proposed method is compared with conventional FBP and image domain IR algorithm (IRIS) in a low dose scan. In this case, we used the same raw data for image reconstructions. This study was conducted in

compliance with the Health Insurance Portability and Accountability Act (HIPAA) and used a scan protocol approved by the Massachusetts General Hospital Institutional Review Board (IRB). We obtained written informed consent as per Federal U.S. guidelines. All procedures in this study were performed in accordance with the approved protocol.

A patient was scanned on a dual source 64-slice MDCT (1st generation DSCT Definition, Siemens Medical Solutions) using routine abdominal CT protocols. The scan parameters were $120kV$, $177mA$, and 0.5 second gantry rotation. The reconstruct-

Table 2. SNR comparison of the three reconstruction methods for the half-dose dataset in Figure 10.

	FBP	IRIS	TV with high fidelity term
m	173.43	169.78	169.60
σ	43.66	20.99	13.17
SNR (dB)	27.59	41.81	51.11

Table 3. CNR comparison of the three reconstruction methods for the half-dose dataset in Figure 10.

	FBP	IRIS	TV with high fidelity term
$S_A - S_B$	192.24	192.40	198.52
σ	35.78	18.55	6.88
CNR	5.37	10.37	28.84

ed images show low dose image quality by reconstructing images with only half the data (i.e., detector A).

For this case, images with the volume $512 \times 512 \times 100$ were reconstructed. For FBP, the sharp kernel on the scanner was utilized. For Iterative Reconstruction in Image Space (IRIS) [57,58], the corresponding sharp kernel was chosen. IRIS is developed on a novel mathematical algorithm through iterative formation. The image domain iteration is initiated after it reconstructs a master volume, which is reconstructed based on how the scan projections provide image detail information, while reducing noise and enhancing object contrast step by step. IRIS utilizes well-established convolution kernels so that it is very fast compared to raw data domain iterative reconstruction.

In this experiment, we compare three different reconstruction approaches: the conventional FBP method, image domain iterative IRIS, and raw data domain IRT with the proposed methods. We have used 10-iterations with $\alpha = 2^5$ for IRT reconstruction with the proposed system modeling method.

To compare images, we defined a priori the regions of comparison. For SNR, the signal is defined over the region containing the hepatic artery, while the background standard deviation is chosen from patches (over 45 slices) of the liver without vasculature. We define CNR as:

$$CNR = \frac{|S_A - S_B|}{\sigma} \qquad (7)$$

where S_A and S_B are mean signal intensities of signal producing structures of the liver (S_A) and the mean signal of the camper's fascia (S_B), respectively. To obtain CNR background statistics, the standard deviation of the camper's fascia over 45 slices was computed, and is denoted by σ by in Equation (7).

A comparison of reconstruction algorithms for the half-dose scan is shown in Figure 10. Although the added noise associated with this low-dose scan is apparent, no undesired texturing appears in this set of images either. The proposed method shows better visual impression compared to FBP and IRIS.

We also tabulate the SNR and CNR of the low-dose scans, in Table 2 and 3, respectively. The proposed method preserves the signal/contrast at much reduced noise for the low-dose acquisition. In this paper, we choose the regularization parameter based on clinician's feedback so it can be improved by processing more cases with broad feedback from multiple radiologists.

In this study, we showed the efficacy and impact of the proposed method in the real clinical scanner.

Discussions and Conclusions

Modern CT systems are highly complex, and different reconstruction algorithms go to various lengths to model such complexities. In this paper, we show that the accurate modeling of system components such as focal spot area, flying focal spot, and active detector area can make a significant difference in the quality of reconstructed images.

Our phantom and patient studies show that the proposed technique can improve image quality (low contrast, noise statistics, spatial resolution, and visual impression). We have introduced a modular system modeling framework for a sophisticated clinical CT scanner. Even within the same system, some functions can be turned off or manipulated for clinical purposes. The advanced functions of state-of-art CT scanners need to be modeled accordingly for high quality image reconstruction. These parameter changes are meticulously recorded in the header files of raw data. None of these functions can be ignored for accurate system modeling to develop high-fidelity characteristics of an iterative algorithm.

As shown in Figure 4, there are sub-modules of the system that cause a small mismatch in system modeling, but these can be propagated through iterations, making them very hard to correct or compensate for by post-processing or utilization of regularization terms. Many studies claim that they can produce high quality SNR images with simple phantoms (having a few high density structures with homogeneous background) in low dose imaging; however, it is very hard to contain the small low-contrast structure in the final results without advanced system modeling. Without satisfying the fidelity term of the energy functional in Equation (3), we cannot guarantee that the reconstructed image is "the only stable solution" of this ill-posed image reconstruction problem.

At 50% dose, both IRIS and the proposed TV with advanced system modeling were found to be diagnostically acceptable. Although the proposed TV provided objectively superior images in terms of SNR and CNR, this image quality was achieved through a significant amount of processing. As a technique that achieves fast computations while maintaining good image quality, a hybrid method (such as IRIS) may potentially be a promising approach.

Future work will also address a variety of dose reductions on cadavers, and we anticipate being able to reduce computation time for the proposed advanced system modeling by implementing it on parallel computing architectures.

Acknowledgments

The authors gratefully acknowledge Dr. Herbert Bruder, Dr. Karl Stierstofer, Christianne Leidecker, and Dr. Thomas G. Flohr (Siemens Healthcare) for providing system geometry and data structure information of CT sinogram.

Author Contributions

Conceived and designed the experiments: SD WCK TB HP. Performed the experiments: SS MK TB HP. Analyzed the data: SD WCK HP. Contributed reagents/materials/analysis tools: SD. Wrote the paper: SD ES HP.

References

1. Brenner DJ, Elliston CD, Hall EJ, Berdon WE (2001) Estimated risks of radiation-induced fatal cancer from pediatric CT. American Journal of Roentgenology 176: 289–296.
2. Brenner DJ, Hricak H (2010) Radiation Exposure From Medical Imaging. JAMA: The Journal of the American Medical Association 304: 208.
3. Kalra MK, Maher MM, Sahani DV, Blake MA, Hahn PF, et al. (2003) Low-Dose CT of the Abdomen: Evaluation of Image Improvement with Use of Noise Reduction Filters-Pilot Study1. Radiology 228: 251–256.
4. Pontana F, Duhamel A, Pagniez J, Flohr T, Faivre J-B, et al. (2011) Chest computed tomography using iterative reconstruction vs filtered back projection (Part 2): image quality of low-dose CT examinations in 80 patients. European radiology 21: 636–643.
5. Scheffel H, Alkadhi H, Leschka S, Plass A, Desbiolles L, et al. (2008) Low-dose CT coronary angiography in the step-and-shoot mode: diagnostic performance. Heart 94: 1132–1137.
6. Husmann L, Valenta I, Gaemperli O, Adda O, Treyer V, et al. (2007) Feasibility of low-dose coronary CT angiography: first experience with prospective ECG-gating. European heart journal.
7. Marin D, Nelson RC, Schindera ST, Richard S, Youngblood RS, et al. (2009) Low-Tube-Voltage, High-Tube-Current Multidetector Abdominal CT: Improved Image Quality and Decreased Radiation Dose with Adaptive Statistical Iterative Reconstruction Algorithm-Initial Clinical Experience 1. Radiology 254: 145–153.

8. Prakash P, Kalra MK, Kambadakone AK, Pien H, Hsieh J, et al. (2010) Reducing abdominal CT radiation dose with adaptive statistical iterative reconstruction technique. Investigative radiology 45: 202–210.

9. Fazel R, Krumholz HM, Wang Y, Ross JS, Chen J, et al. (2009) Exposure to low-dose ionizing radiation from medical imaging procedures. New England Journal of Medicine 361: 849–857.

10. Kan MW, Leung LH, Wong W, Lam N (2008) Radiation dose from cone beam computed tomography for image-guided radiation therapy. International Journal of Radiation Oncology* Biology* Physics 70: 272–279.

11. Kwan AL, Boone JM, Shah N (2005) Evaluation of x-ray scatter properties in a dedicated cone-beam breast CT scanner. Medical physics 32: 2967–2975.

12. Kalra MK, Maher MM, Toth TL, Hamberg LM, Blake MA, et al. (2004) Strategies for CT Radiation Dose Optimization 1. Radiology 230: 619–628.

13. Hsieh J (2009) Computed tomography: principles, design, artifacts, and recent advances. SPIE Bellingham, WA.

14. Hentschel D, Popescu S, Strauss K-E, Wolf H (1999) Adaptive dose modulation during CT scanning. Google Patents.

15. Kalra MK, Maher MM, D'Souza RV, Rizzo S, Halpern EF, et al. (2005) Detection of Urinary Tract Stones at Low-Radiation-Dose CT with Z-Axis Automatic Tube Current Modulation: Phantom and Clinical Studies 1. Radiology 235: 523–529.

16. McCollough CH, Bruesewitz MR, Kofler Jr JM (2006) CT Dose Reduction and Dose Management Tools: Overview of Available Options 1. Radiographics 26: 503–512.

17. Singh S, Kalra MK, Moore MA, Shailam R, Liu B, et al. (2009) Dose Reduction and Compliance with Pediatric CT Protocols Adapted to Patient Size, Clinical Indication, and Number of Prior Studies 1. Radiology 252: 200–208.

18. Li J, Udayasankar UK, Toth TL, Seamans J, Small WC, et al. (2007) Automatic patient centering for MDCT: effect on radiation dose. American Journal of Roentgenology 188: 547–552.

19. Shepp LA, Vardi Y (1982) Maximum likelihood reconstruction for emission tomography. Medical Imaging, IEEE Transactions on 1: 113–122.

20. Wang G, Snyder DL, O'Sullivan J, Vannier M (1996) Iterative deblurring for CT metal artifact reduction. Medical Imaging, IEEE Transactions on 15: 657–664.

21. Thibault J-B, Sauer KD, Bouman CA, Hsieh J (2007) A three-dimensional statistical approach to improved image quality for multislice helical CT. Medical physics 34: 4526.

22. Bittencourt MS, Schmidt B, Seltmann M, Muschiol G, Ropers D, et al. (2011) Iterative reconstruction in image space (IRIS) in cardiac computed tomography: initial experience. The international journal of cardiovascular imaging 27: 1081–1087.

23. Tang J, Nett BE, Chen G-H (2009) Performance comparison between total variation (TV)-based compressed sensing and statistical iterative reconstruction algorithms. Physics in medicine and biology 54: 5781.

24. Sidky EY, Pan X, Reiser IS, Nishikawa RM, Moore RH, et al. (2009) Enhanced imaging of microcalcifications in digital breast tomosynthesis through improved image-reconstruction algorithms. Medical physics 36: 4920.

25. Park JC, Song B, Kim JS, Park SH, Kim HK, et al. (2012) Fast compressed sensing-based CBCT reconstruction using Barzilai-Borwein formulation for application to on-line IGRT. Medical Physics 39: 1207.

26. Andersen A, Kak A (1984) Simultaneous algebraic reconstruction technique (SART): a superior implementation of the ART algorithm. Ultrasonic imaging 6: 81–94.

27. Levitan E, Herman GT (1987) A maximum a posteriori probability expectation maximization algorithm for image reconstruction in emission tomography. Medical Imaging, IEEE Transactions on 6: 185–192.

28. Fessler JA (1994) Penalized weighted least-squares image reconstruction for positron emission tomography. Medical Imaging, IEEE Transactions on 13: 290–300.

29. Browne JA, Boone JM, Holmes TJ (1995) Maximum-likelihood x-ray computed-tomography finite-beamwidth considerations. Applied optics 34: 5199–5209.

30. Fu L, Wang J, Rui X, Thibault J-B, De Man B (2013) Modeling and estimation of detector response and focal spot profile for high-resolution iterative CT reconstruction. Nuclear Science Symposium and Medical Imaging Conference (NSS/MIC), 2013 IEEE. IEEE. pp. 1–5.

31. Little K, La Riviere P (2012) An algorithm for modeling non-linear system effects in iterative CT reconstruction. Nuclear Science Symposium and Medical Imaging Conference (NSS/MIC), 2012 IEEE. IEEE. pp. 2174–2177.

32. Sauer K, Bouman C (1993) A local update strategy for iterative reconstruction from projections. Signal Processing, IEEE Transactions on 41: 534–548.

33. De Man B, Nuyts J, Dupont P, Marchal G, Suetens P (2001) An iterative maximum-likelihood polychromatic algorithm for CT. Medical Imaging, IEEE Transactions on 20: 999–1008.

34. Hudson HM, Larkin RS (1994) Accelerated image reconstruction using ordered subsets of projection data. Medical Imaging, IEEE Transactions on 13: 601–609.

35. Wang G, Snyder DL, O'Sullivan JA, Vannier M (1996) Iterative deblurring for CT metal artifact reduction. Medical Imaging, IEEE Transactions on 15: 657–664.

36. Ramani S, Fessler J (2010) A splitting-based iterative algorithm for accelerated statistical X-ray CT reconstruction. Medical Imaging, IEEE Transactions on: 1–1.

37. Do S, Cho S, Karl WC, Kalra MK, Brady TJ, et al. (2009) Accurate model-based high resolution cardiac image reconstruction in dual source CT. IEEE. pp. 330–333.

38. Hofmann C, Knaup M, Kachelrie M (2014) Effects of ray profile modeling on resolution recovery in clinical CT. Medical physics 41: 021907.

39. Alessio AM, Kinahan PE, Lewellen TK (2006) Modeling and incorporation of system response functions in 3-D whole body PET. Medical Imaging, IEEE Transactions on 25: 828–837.

40. Panin VY, Kehren F, Michel C, Casey M (2006) Fully 3-D PET reconstruction with system matrix derived from point source measurements. Medical Imaging, IEEE Transactions on 25: 907–921.

41. Tohme MS, Qi J (2009) Iterative image reconstruction for positron emission tomography based on a detector response function estimated from point source measurements. Physics in Medicine and Biology 54: 3709.

42. Beekman FJ, Slijpen ETP, de Jong HWAM, Viergever MA (1999) Estimation of the depth-dependent component of the point spread function of SPECT. Medical physics 26: 2311.

43. La Riviere PJ, Pan X (2004) Sampling and aliasing consequences of quarter-detector offset use in helical CT. Medical Imaging, IEEE Transactions on 23: 738–749.

44. Kachelrie M, Knaup M, Penel C, Kalender WA (2006) Flying focal spot (FFS) in cone-beam CT. Nuclear Science, IEEE Transactions on 53: 1238–1247.

45. Qi J, Huesman RH (2005) Effect of errors in the system matrix on maximum a posteriori image reconstruction. Physics in Medicine and Biology 50: 3297.

46. Vogel CR, Oman ME (1996) Iterative methods for total variation denoising. SIAM Journal on Scientific Computing 17: 227–238.

47. Sidky EY, Pan X (2008) Image reconstruction in circular cone-beam computed tomography by constrained, total-variation minimization. Physics in Medicine and Biology 53: 4777.

48. Chan TF, Mulet P (1999) On the convergence of the lagged diffusivity fixed point method in total variation image restoration. SIAM Journal on Numerical Analysis: 354–367.

49. Do S, Karl WC, Liang Z, Kalra M, Brady TJ, et al. (2011) A decomposition-based CT reconstruction formulation for reducing blooming artifacts. Physics in Medicine and Biology 56: 7109.

50. Hsieh J (2003) Computed tomography: principles, design, artifacts, and recent advances. Society of Photo Optical.

51. Siddon RL (1985) Fast calculation of the exact radiological path for a three-dimensional CT array. Medical Physics 12: 252.

52. Siddon RL (1985) Fast calculation of the exact radiological path for a three?dimensional CT array. Medical physics 12: 252–255.

53. Sunnegardh J, Danielsson PE (2007) A new anti-aliased projection operator for iterative CT reconstruction. pp. 124–127.

54. Jacobs F, Sundermann E, De Sutter B, Christiaens M, Lemahieu I (1998) A fast algorithm to calculate the exact radiological path through a pixel or voxel space. Journal of computing and information technology 6: 89–94.

55. Jang B, Do S, Pien H, Kaeli D (2009) Architecture-aware optimization targeting multithreaded stream computing. ACM. pp. 62–70.

56. Flohr T, Stierstorfer K, Ulzheimer S, Bruder H, Primak A, et al. (2005) Image reconstruction and image quality evaluation for a 64-slice CT scanner with z-flying focal spot. Medical physics 32: 2536.

57. Tipnis S, Ramachandra A, Huda W, Hardie A, Schoepf J, et al. Iterative reconstruction in image space (IRIS) and lesion detection in abdominal CT. pp. 76222K.

58. Bittencourt MS, Schmidt B, Seltmann M, Muschiol G, Ropers D, et al. (2010) Iterative reconstruction in image space (IRIS) in cardiac computed tomography: initial experience. The International Journal of Cardiovascular Imaging (formerly Cardiac Imaging): 1–7.

12

Impact of Emphysema Heterogeneity on Pulmonary Function

Jieyang Ju[1]*, Ruosha Li[2]*, Suicheng Gu[1], Joseph K. Leader[1], Xiaohua Wang[3], Yahong Chen[3], Bin Zheng[4], Shandong Wu[1], David Gur[1], Frank Sciurba[5], Jiantao Pu[1,6]*

1 Department of Radiology, University of Pittsburgh, Pittsburgh, Pennsylvania, United States of America, 2 Department of Biostatistics, University of Pittsburgh, Pittsburgh, Pennsylvania, United States of America, 3 Peking University Third Affiliated Hospital, Beijing, People's Republic of China, 4 School of Electrical and Computer Engineering, University of Oklahoma, Norman, Oklahoma, United States of America, 5 Department of Medicine, University of Pittsburgh, Pittsburgh, Pennsylvania, United States of America, 6 Department of Bioengineering, University of Pittsburgh, Pittsburgh, Pennsylvania, United States of America

Abstract

Objectives: To investigate the association between emphysema heterogeneity in spatial distribution, pulmonary function and disease severity.

Methods and Materials: We ascertained a dataset of anonymized Computed Tomography (CT) examinations acquired on 565 participants in a COPD study. Subjects with chronic bronchitis (CB) and/or bronchodilator response were excluded resulting in 190 cases without COPD and 160 cases with COPD. Low attenuations areas (LAAs) ($\leq$950 Hounsfield Unit (HU)) were identified and quantified at the level of individual lobes. Emphysema heterogeneity was defined in a manner that ranged in value from -100% to 100%. The association between emphysema heterogeneity and pulmonary function measures (e.g., FEV1% predicted, RV/TLC, and DLco% predicted) adjusted for age, sex, and smoking history (pack-years) was assessed using multiple linear regression analysis.

Results: The majority (128/160) of the subjects with COPD had a heterogeneity greater than zero. After adjusting for age, gender, smoking history, and extent of emphysema, heterogeneity in depicted disease in upper lobe dominant cases was positively associated with pulmonary function measures, such as FEV1 Predicted ($p<.001$) and FEV1/FVC ($p<.001$), as well as disease severity ($p<0.05$). We found a negative association between HI% , RV/TLC ($p<0.001$), and DLco% (albeit not a statistically significant one, $p = 0.06$) in this group of patients.

Conclusion: Subjects with more homogeneous distribution of emphysema and/or lower lung dominant emphysema tend to have worse pulmonary function.

Editor: Harm Bogaard, VU University Medical Center, Netherlands

Funding: This work is supported in part by grants from the National Institutes of Health (RO1 HL096613), the Bonnie J. Addario Lung Cancer Foundation, and the National Health and Family Planning Commission of the R.R. China (No. 201402013). The funders had no role in study design, data collection and analysis, decision to publish, or preparation of the manuscript.

Competing Interests: The authors have declared that no competing interests exist.

* Email: puj@upmc.edu

⑨ These authors contributed equally to this work.

Introduction

As the most common phenotype of chronic obstructive pulmonary disease (COPD), emphysema is one of the leading cause of disability and death in the United States and worldwide [1]. This disease often goes undiagnosed for many years and irreversibly destroys lung parenchyma (alveoli), causes hyperinflation, and reduces lung elasticity [2]. In clinical practice, emphysema is typically diagnosed by pulmonary function tests (PFTs), medical history, and physical examination. However, traditional PFTs have a low sensitivity for diagnosing early stage COPD. It was reported that 30% of patients may have emphysema before exhibiting any detectable decline in pulmonary function [3]. In contrast, computed tomography (CT) is highly sensitive to depiction of the presence of emphysema. The extent of parenchyma destruction is often quantified as the fraction of lung voxels with Hounsfield Units (HU) value below a specific threshold (e.g., <-950 HU) [4]. Although pulmonary function and the amount of emphysema are significantly correlated, there is frequently a large variability in the computed fractional values of emphysema at a specific pulmonary function value and vice verse [5]. Hence, it is widely believed that spatial distribution and pattern of emphysema may be important for understanding the observed lack of concordance between pulmonary function and the amount of diseased lung.

Emphysema is widely classified into three pathological phenotypes: centrilobular, panlobular, and paraseptal [6–7]. It has been shown that panlobular emphysema was associated with *alpha 1-antitrypsin* deficiency, while centrilobuar emphysema was associated with tobacco exposure [8–9]. Recently, by classifying a population of 9,313 smokers into five subgroups in terms of emphysema patterns (i.e., mild centrilobular, moderate centrilobular, severe centrilobular, panlobular, and paraseptal emphysema), Castaldi et al. [10] showed that these phenotypes were strongly associated with a wide range of respiratory physiology and function measures. Other investigations assessed the spatial distribution of emphysema in different patient groups by dividing the lungs into: thirds [9], twelfths [8], and/or core and rind [11]. Different and at times conflicting findings have been reported [12–16]. However, all findings strongly and consistently suggest that the distribution patterns of emphysema have significant clinical implications and better understanding of the relationship between different patterns and lung function may aid in more precise patient stratification for optimal personalized management or treatment.

Anatomically the human lungs are comprised of five lobes that are serviced by their own of bronchovascular system and function somewhat independently from a mechanical, ventilation, and perfusion perspectives. Lobar independence may be what drives the different relations between pulmonary function and emphysema distribution and patterns. In particular, there are anatomical differences between the right and left lungs. For example, the right lung consists of three lobes, while the left lung is slightly smaller with only two lobes. Also, with respect to the trachea, the entering (branching) angle of the right bronchus is typically smaller than that of the left one because of the presence of the heart. Given the close relationship between structure and function, it is interesting to assess which lung tends to be more vulnerable to the disease. In this study, we quantified emphysema by lobes and investigated the possible impact of emphysema heterogeneity on pulmonary function in a well characterized cohort of participants in a chronic obstructive pulmonary disease (COPD) study.

Methods and Materials

A. Study population

We initially collected a dataset consisting of 565 CT exams from an NIH-sponsored Specialized Center for Clinically Oriented Research (SCCOR) in COPD at the University of Pittsburgh. The CT exams originate from the baseline data collection of the first 565 SCCOR participants who were recruited from those previously enrolled in the Pittsburgh Lung Screening Study (PLuSS) cohort [17]. The inclusion criteria for SCCOR were age >40 years and at least a 10 pack-year history of tobacco exposure. SCCOR participants underwent pre- and post-bronchodilator spirometry and plethysmography, measurement of lung diffusion capacity by single breath carbon monoxide (DLco), a chest CT examination and answered demographic as well as medical history questionnaires. The guidelines [18] published by American Thoracic Society were followed when performing these lung function tests. All data acquisition procedures and the CT scans were performed under a University of Pittsburgh Institutional Review Board-approved protocol (#0612016) with written informed consent obtained from all participants. The dataset included 346 subjects with COPD as defined by the Global Initiative for Obstructive Lung Disease (GOLD), and 219 subjects without COPD (Figure 1). Among the subjects with COPD, 137 had bronchodilator response (BR) and were excluded. An increase of 12% and 200 ml in the forced expiratory volume in one second (FEV1) was considered as a positive response to bronchodilator. We also excluded 49 patients who were either diagnosed with

chronic bronchitis (CB) or had no related information on CB (Figure 1). CB was assessed based on series of questionnaires completed by the subjects and determined by whether there is a cough productive of sputum over three months' duration during two consecutive years and airflow obstruction. The demographics of the 160 subjects with COPD and the 190 subjects without COPD included in analysis are summarized in Table 1.

B. Acquisition of thin-section CT examinations

CT examinations were acquired without the use of radiopaque contrast using a 64-detector CT scanner (LightSpeed VCT, GE Healthcare, Waukesha, WI, USA) while subjects held their breath at end inspiration. Scans were acquired using a helical technique at the following parameters: 32×0.625 mm detector configuration, 0.969 pitch, 120 kVp tube energy, 250 mA tube current, and 0.4-s gantry rotation (or 100 mAs). Images were reconstructed to encompass the entire lung field in a 512×512 pixel matrix using the GE "bone" kernel at 0.625-mm section thickness and 0.625-mm interval. Pixel dimensions ranged from 0.549 to 0.738 mm, depending on participant body size. The "bone" kernel was used because of its ability to visualize both parenchyma and airways [19]. The subjects were instructed in breathing to reach TLC prior to scanning; however, no real-time measures were employed to ensure breathing compliance such as spirometry-gated CT acquisition. The CT exams were reviewed to ensure compliance with the above mentioned chest CT protocol and were reviewed for artifacts that would contribute to poor image quality and/or quantification (e.g., subject motion and/or metal artifacts).

C. Heterogeneity of emphysema distribution in different lobes

In-house developed software was used to segment the lungs and the lobes [20–22]. Similar to other investigations [23–24], low attenuation area (LAA) was defined as the volume of image voxels with HU values lower than −950 HU [25]. The percentage of low attenuation areas (%LAA) was computed as the sum of LAAs divided by the lung volume, and values were computed for the entire lung and each lobe. Small LAA clusters were removed to limit possible over-estimation of emphysema due to image noise and/or artifacts. Considering that CT images are reconstructed in a slice-by-slice manner and in-plane image pixel size ranges typically from approximately 0.65 mm to 0.90 mm, low attenuation areas with

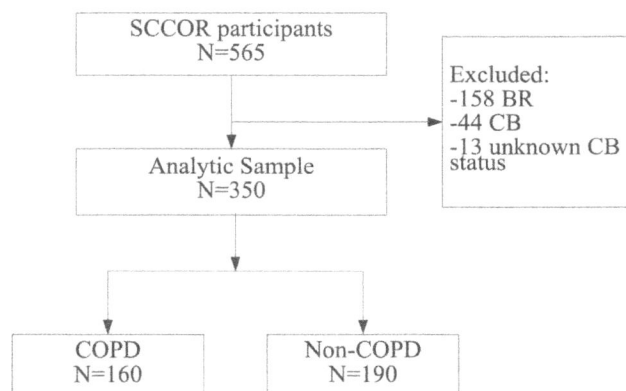

Figure 1. Flowchart illustrating how the final dataset analytic sample was obtained in which COPD by was defined by GOLD classification. (BR: subjects with bronchodilator response, and CB: subjects with chronic bronchitis).

Table 1. Patient characteristics.

characteristics	All	COPD	non-COPD
	N = 350	N = 160	N = 190
Sex: male [A]	201(57%)	104(65%)	97(51%)
Age (yrs) [B]	64(61,69)	67(61,70)	63(60,67)
Pack years, N = 287 [B]	50(35,70)	57(40,77)	45(32,63)
FEV1%Predicted (%)[B]	91(74,101)	71(48,85)	98(91,105)
FEV1/FVC% (%) [B]	72(62,77)	61(44,66)	77(75,81)
RV/TLC (%) [B]	38(34,43)	43(35,53)	36(33,40)
DLco Predicted (%) [B]	74(58,86)	61(42,75)	82(71,90)
LAA% [B]	1.2(0.5,4.4)	4.5(1.5,12.2)	0.5(0.2,1.3)
HI% [B]	17(4,36)	23(2,42)	14(4,27)
GOLD classification [A]			
None COPD	190(54%)	0(0%)	190(100%)
Gold I	55(16%)	55(34%)	0(0%)
Gold II	64(18%)	64(40%)	0(0%)
Gold III–IV	41(12%)	41(26%)	0(0%)

Categorical variables were summarized by frequency (%). Continuous variables were summarized by medians and interquartile ranges (IQR).
[A]Summarized by frequency (%);
[B]Summarized by median (IQR).
Abbreviations:
FVC – functional vital capacity.
FEV1% – forced expiratory volume in one second percent predicted.
RV –residual volume.
TLC –total lung capacity.
DLco% – diffusing lung capacity of carbon monoxide percent.

in-plane area less than 3 mm^2 (approximately 4~5 pixels in an image slice) were discarded and were not included in the %LAA computation. Considering that a median filter or other smoothing filters may alter pixel values, we chose not to use any smoothing filter. The clustering operation was performed after application of a threshold.

After the identification of regions associated with emphysema regions, an emphysema heterogeneity index (*HI*) between upper and lower lobes was computed (Eq. (1)), which results in values ranging from -100% to +100%. For the right lung, $\%LAA_{upper}$ was computed as the sum of emphysema volume in the right upper and middle lobes. For the entire lung, $\%LAA_{upper}$ was computed as the combination of the emphysema in the left upper, right upper, and right middle lobes, while $\%LAA_{lower}$ was the summed values for the left lower and right lower lobes. When emphysema is equally distributed among the lobes or its computed extent in the entire lung is less than 1%, *HI* has a zero value.

$$HI\% = \begin{cases} 0\%, & \text{if the total LAA\% is less than 1\%} \\ \frac{\%LAA_{upper} - \%LAA_{lower}}{\%LAA_{upper} + \%LAA_{lower}} \times 100\%, & \text{otherwise} \end{cases} \quad (1)$$

D. Statistical analyses

We summarized the patient characteristics using the frequencies and proportions for categorical variables (e.g., sex and GOLD classification score) and median values and quartiles for continuous variables (e.g., age and FEV1% predicted). Considering that a large portion of patients may have emphysema but do not

exhibit any detectable decline in pulmonary function [3], subgroups with COPD and without COPD were analyzed separately. We investigated the distribution of HI% and differences in HI% values between left lung and right lung using histograms. A one-sample chi-square test was used to examine whether the proportion of subjects with positive HI% was different from 50%. We used the sign test of location to examine whether the median difference in HI% values between the left and right lungs was different from zero.

The post-bronchodilator measurements used in the analyses include: (1) FEV1% predicted, (2) FEV1/FVC, (3) RV/TLC, and DLco%. We compared the distributions of these four pulmonary function measures between subjects with upper lung dominant emphysema (i.e., HI%>0%) and those with lower lung dominant emphysema (i.e., HI%≤0%) using the nonparametric Wilcoxon rank-sum test. In addition, we combined the GOLD classification score into two categories (I and II combined vs. III and IV combined) and compared the differences in distributions, if any, between the two groups.

To investigate the univariate association between HI% and lung function measures, we used piecewise linear regression method with a knot at 0, by defining $HI\%^+ = \max (0\%, HI\%)$ and $HI\%^- = \min(HI\%, 0\%)$. The piecewise linear regression is a generalization of the conventional linear regression method, which corresponds to situations where the slopes of $HI\%^+$ and $HI\%^-$ are equivalent. Note that a piecewise linear regression model provides more flexibility in characterizing the relationship between HI% and outcomes of interest when compared to the conventional linear regression model. Next, we performed multiple linear regression modeling between HI% and the four lung function measures respectively, adjusting for age, sex, smoking history, and overall emphysema (LAA%). A multiple logistic regression model was adopted to model the odds of having higher GOLD classification results for GOLD III and IV combined, and the results were summarized in terms of odds ratios (OR). Statistical significance was defined by $p<.05$ (two sided). Analyses were performed using SAS (SAS Institute Inc, NC), version 9.3.

Results

In the participants with COPD, median age was 67, 65% were male, median pack-years was 57, median FEV1% predicted was 71%, and median FEV1/FVC% was 61%. Forty-one (26%) of the COPD subjects had a GOLD classification scores greater than II (Table 1). In the participants without COPD, median age was 63, 51% were male, median pack-years was 45, median FEV1% predicted was 98%, and median FEV1/FVC% was 77%. Upper lobe dominant emphysema (positive HI%) was significantly more prevalent in both subjects with COPD (129/160 or 80.6%) and without COPD (161/190 or 84.7%) compared to lower lobe dominant emphysema ($p<0.05$ in both sets of subjects) (Figures 2A and 2C). The HI between the left and right lungs was not significantly different ($p>0.05$) in both sets of subjects (Figure 2B and 2D).

Lung function in COPD subjects was significantly correlated with upper lobe dominant emphysema. Subjects with COPD and upper lung dominant emphysema (i.e., HI%>0) had significantly higher FEV1% predicted ($p = 0.01$) and, consequently, lower GOLD scores ($p = 0.02$) than COPD subjects with lower lung dominant emphysema (Table 2). In subjects without COPD and upper lobe dominant emphysema DLco% predicted was signifi-

cantly lower than non-COPD subjects (Table 2). When HI was greater than zero (i.e., upper lobe dominant emphysema) it was significantly and directly correlated with FEV1 % predicted ($p<0.001$) and FEV1/FVC% ($p = 0.002$) and significantly and inversely correlated with RV/TLC% ($p<0.001$) among subjects with COPD (Figure 3). COPD subjects with lower lung dominant emphysema (i.e., HI%<0%) did not have a statistically significant correlation with lung function measures.

Emphysema heterogeneity in COPD subjects significantly contributed to linear regression models of lung function that included overall emphysema (LAA%), HI, age, gender, and smoking history. Heterogeneity index significantly and positively contributed to the linear model of FEV1% predicted ($p<.001$) and FEV1/FVC% ($p = 0.002$) and significantly and negatively to the linear model of RV/TLC% ($p<.001$) among COPD subjects with upper lung dominant emphysema (Table 3). A one percent increase in HI was associated with 0.28% (95% CI 0.14–0.42%) increase in FEV1% predicted. For GOLD classification score, in a multiple logistic regression model of GOLD COPD classification including overall emphysema (LAA%), HI, age, gender, and smoking history, HI significantly and negatively contributed to GOLD classification with the probability of having higher GOLD classification scores (i.e. III or IV) among COPD subjects with upper lung dominant emphysema (Table 4). A one percent increase in HI resulted in decreasing the odds of having high GOLD classification score by a multiplicative factor of 0.953 (95% CI 0.91–0.99, $p = 0.03$). In a multiple linear regression model of subjects without COPD that included overall emphysema, HI, age, gender, and smoking history, HI% significantly and

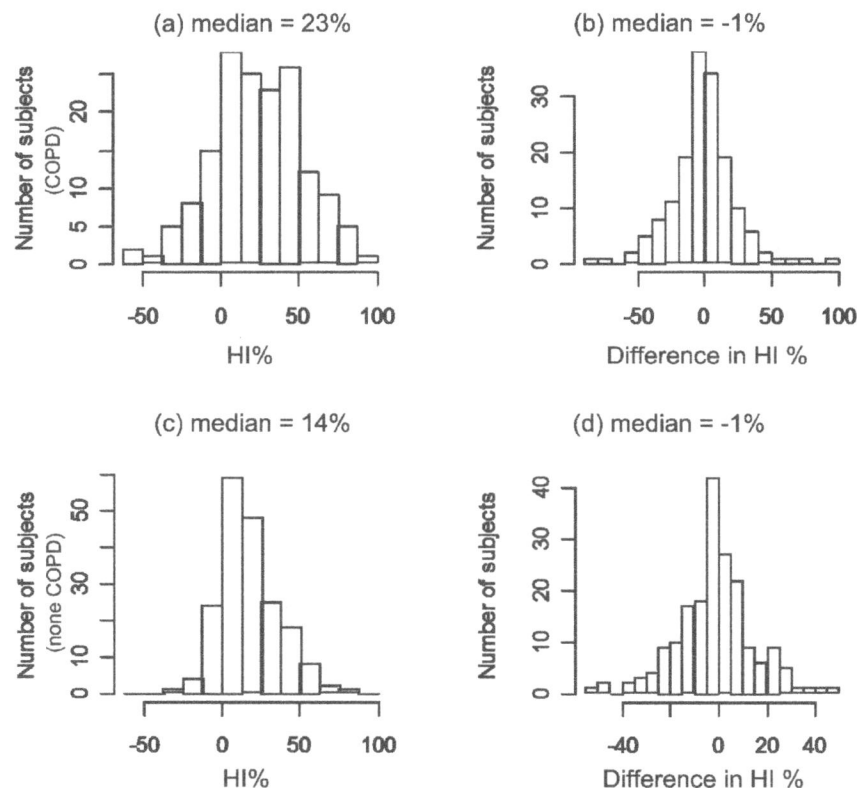

Figure 2. Distributions of computed HI% (left) and differences in computed HI% between the left and the right lungs (right). The top row represents the COPD patients (N = 160), and the bottom row represents the non-COPD patients (N = 190).

Table 2. Pulmonary function measures and COPD classification of subjects classified as having lower and upper lung dominant emphysema, stratified by emphysema heterogeneity and disease severity.

	COPD, N = 160			non-COPD, N = 190		
	HI< = 0%	HI>0%	p-value	HI< = 0%	HI>0%	p-value
	N = 31	N = 129		N = 29	N = 161	
FEV1% Predicted (%)[B]	55(32,80)	74(55,88)	0.01	99(91,108)	98(92,104)	0.8
FEV1/FVC (%)[B]	53(34,66)	62(51,66)	0.1	78(76,81)	77(75,81)	0.3
RV/TLC (%)[B]	45(39,57)	42(35,52)	0.1	35(34,40)	36(33,40)	0.9
DLco Predicted (%) [B]	56(42,76)	62(43,75)	0.7	89(83,92)	79(70,89)	0.01
GOLD classification [A]			0.02			
GOLD I–II	18(58%)	101(78%)				
GOLD III–IV	13(42%)	28(22%)				

[A]Summarized by frequency (%);
[B]Summarized by median (IQR).

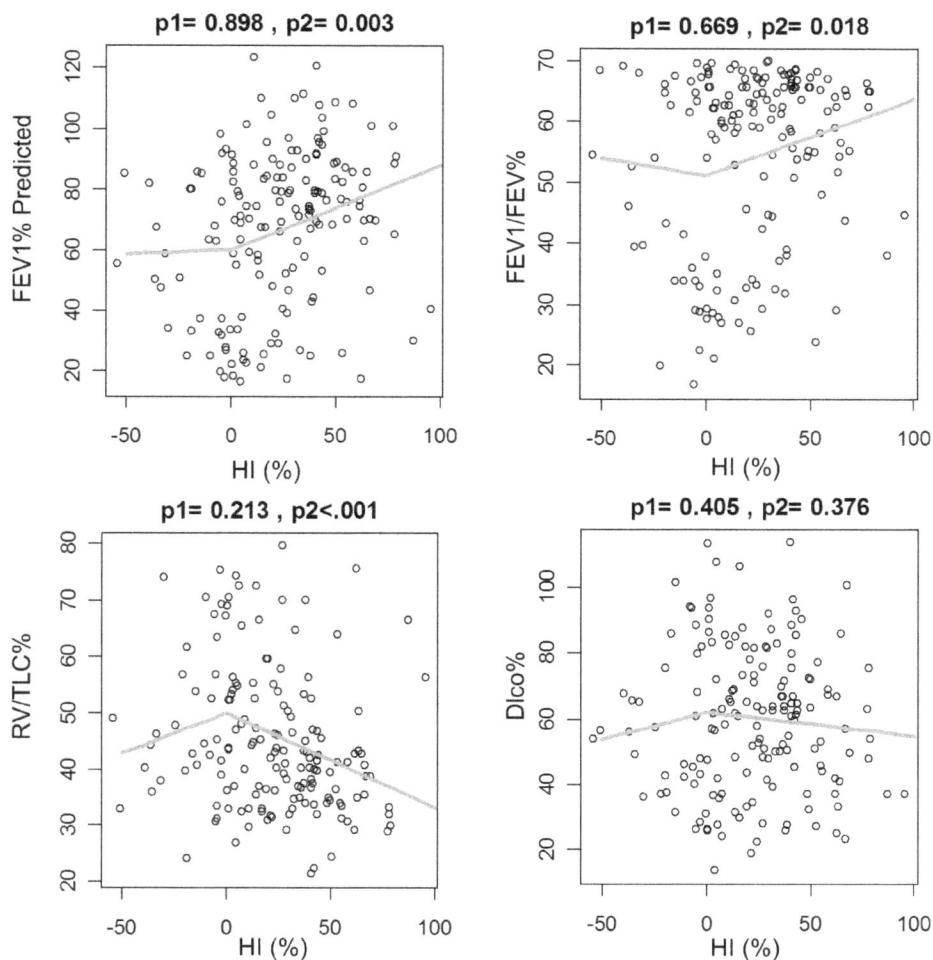

Figure 3. Scatter plots of pulmonary function measures and emphysema heterogeneity (HI%) for COPD patients. The grey line represents the estimated pulmonary function as a function of HI%. p1 denotes the p-value of $HI\%^- = \min(0\%, HI\%)$ in the piecewise linear regression, and p2 corresponds to the p-value of $HI\%^+ = \max(0\%, HI\%)$.

Table 3. Multiple linear regression results for different pulmonary function measures among subjects with COPD (n = 160).

	FEV1% Predicted Coef (CI)	FEV1/FVC% Coef (CI)	RV/TLC% Coef (CI)	DLCO% Coef (CI)
LAA%	−1.54 (−1.83,−1.26)	−1.09 (−1.22, −0.97)***	0.58 (0.43,0.74)***	−1.43 (−1.67, −1.18)***
HI%⁺	0.28 (0.14,0.42)***	0.09 (0.03,0.15)**	−0.15 (−0.23, −0.08)***	−0.11 (−0.23,0.01)
HI%⁻	0.02 (−0.29,0.33)	−0.03 (−0.17,0.11)	0.16 (−0.01,0.34)	0.19 (−0.08,0.46)
Age (yrs)	0.73 (0.17,1.29)*	0.06 (−0.18,0.31)	0.05 (−0.26,0.36)	0.18 (−0.3,0.66)
Male	9.53 (3.37,15.68)**	2.47 (−0.22,5.16)	−7.3 (−10.71, −3.88)***	6.46 (1.17,11.75)*
Packyear	−0.02 (−0.1,0.06)	0.00 (−0.04,0.03)	−0.02 (−0.07,0.02)	−0.01 (−0.08,0.06)

The cells represent the regression coefficients and estimated 95% confidence intervals (in parentheses).
*means $0.01 \leq p < 0.05$,
** means $0.001 \leq p < 0.01$, and *** means $p < 0.001$.

negatively contributed to RV/TLC%, but was not significantly associated with other lung function metrics (Table 5).

Discussion

The importance of emphysema distribution has been widely recognized. Accurate phenotypic description of emphysema may aid in predicting prognosis of emphysema and designing efficacy personalized therapy or management for preventing disease progression. In 1957, Leopold et al. [26] differentiated emphysema into two categories: centrilobular and panlobular. Presently, paraseptal emphysema is considered a third category of emphysema. This classification is based on the lobular locations of emphysema in the lungs. Castaldi et al. [10] found that emphysema phenotypes were strongly associated with respiratory physiology and function. Other investigators subdivided the lungs into varying number of zones and compared lung function across the zones [8–9,11]. In contrast, we quantified emphysema by lobes and assessed the association between inter-lobar heterogeneity, COPD severity, and lung function. Unlike the traditional "gravitational" division of the lungs, this strategy takes the unique lung anatomy into account when characterizing the emphysema distribution. Three-hundred and fifty subjects were included in our analysis after exclusion of subjects with CB and positive bronchodilator response, which consisted of 160 subjects with and 190 subjects without COPD by GOLD classification. As compared to previous investigation [6–7,27], this exclusion may enable more reliable assessment of the impact of emphysema on lung function. In our cohort, subjects with or without COPD and upper lobe dominant emphysema had significantly better pulmonary function compared with subjects with lower lobe dominant emphysema. However, smokers do not always have upper

predominant emphysema. Also, subjects with or without COPD had similar levels of emphysema in the right versus left lungs despite the relatively large differences in anatomical structure.

Our findings agreed with Tanabe et al. [6] who reported that a more homogeneous distribution of emphysema was associated with an accelerated decline in FEV1 independently of baseline pulmonary function and overall emphysema severity. In their study, 131 male patients were involved. Similarly, Haraguchi et al. [27] reported similarly that uniformity of emphysema distribution correlated with severity of airway obstruction in pulmonary embolism (PE) patients, which is consistent with our finding in that subjects with lower lung dominant emphysema had significantly worse pulmonary function. According to this observation, the chance of a rapid decline in lung function is relatively lower in subjects with upper dominant and heterogeneous emphysema. In contrast, Gietema et al. [7] observed that an apical distribution was associated with more severe air-flow impairment when the emphysema was quantified at a threshold of −910 HU, but they found no significant impact when emphysema was quantified at a threshold of −950 HU.

As Tanabe et al. [6] explained, it is not easy to identify the exact factors behind the variety of emphysema distribution among smokers and explain why homogeneous distribution and lower lung dominant emphysema is critical for lung function. However, on the basis of previous investigations [13–14], where specific genes (e.g., MMP-9) were found to associate with upper lung dominant emphysema, we believe that specific genes could be associated with susceptibility to homogeneous emphysema. Also, given the close relationship between structure and function in the biological system, the morphology of specific structures (e.g., airway tree) that affect airflow could contribute to emphysema distribution as well, because airway morphology, which could be

Table 4. Multiple logistic regression model for GOLD classification score among subjects with COPD (n = 160).

	OR (CI)
LAA%	1.28 (1.16, 1.41)***
HI%⁺	0.95 (0.91, 0.99)*
HI%⁻	1.03 (0.94, 1.13)
Age (yrs)	0.88 (0.76, 1.02)
Male	0.25 (0.05, 1.29)
packyear	1.00 (0.98, 1.03)

The cells represent the estimated odds ratio (OR) and the corresponding confidence intervals.

Table 5. Multiple linear regression model for pulmonary function measures among subjects without COPD (n = 190).

	FEV1% Predicted	FEV1/FVC%	RV/TLC%	DLCO%
	Coef (CI)	Coef (CI)	Coef (CI)	Coef (CI)
LAA%	−0.82 (−2.17,0.53)	−0.78 (−1.23, −0.32)***	0.54 (−0.05,1.13)	−1.37 (−2.96,0.23)
HI%+	0.08 (−0.04,0.19)	−0.04 (−0.08,0)	−0.06 (−0.11, −0.01)*	−0.11 (−0.24,0.03)
HI%−	−0.4 (−0.88,0.09)	−0.03 (−0.2,0.13)	−0.01 (−0.22,0.21)	−0.6 (−1.18, −0.02)*
Age (yrs)	0.47 (0.04,0.9)*	−0.16 (−0.3, −0.01)*	0.43 (0.24,0.62)***	−0.27 (−0.78,0.24)
Male	2.27 (−1.57,6.1)	−0.3 (−1.59,0.99)	−5.38 (−7.06, −3.7)***	5.21 (0.66,9.76)*
Packyear	−0.04 (−0.11,0.03)	0 (−0.02,0.03)	0 (−0.03,0.03)	−0.09 (−0.17, −0.01)*

The cells represent the regression coefficients and estimated 95% confidence intervals (in parentheses).

the result of specific genes, may alter the interaction between the harmful chemicals in the air and lung tissues. Therefore, in our opinion, a fully understanding of the variety of emphysema distribution may need multi-disciplinary investigative effort involving both imaging and genetics.

We note that there are limitations with this study. First, our study was performed at a single institution with a modest number of subjects and may or may not be generalizable to other cohorts or institutions. Although 350 subjects were included, the variety of emphysema extent and disease heterogeneity is still very limited. Non-smokers were not included. This data selection bias may somewhat affect the conclusion. To largely alleviate this issue, we proposed to exclude the asthmatic and CB patients to enable a relatively reliable analysis of the impact of emphysema heterogeneity on lung function. Second, the heterogeneity index may have oversimplified the complexity of heterogeneous distribution patterns of emphysema. Hence, more precise strategy for quantifying 3D distribution patterns of emphysema in the lung may be needed for improved phenotyping of emphysema. Third, we removed very small clusters of voxels below the threshold under the assumption they represent "image noises" or "artifacts." However, further effort may be needed to assess whether the approach taken is optimal for this purpose. Fourth, the number of subject with lower lobe dominant emphysema was relatively small in both the COPD (n = 31) and non-COPD (n = 29) subjects, which may have hinder this phenotype from reaching statistical significance in some of the analyses. Finally, this retrospective cross-sectional study did not consider the impact of longitudinal changes in emphysema distribution patterns on pulmonary function or disease progression, but was outside the scope of this preliminary study.

Conclusions

We investigated the association between inter-lobar heterogeneity of emphysema and pulmonary function measures. Our primary observation was that upper lone dominant emphysema was associated with significantly better lung function and significantly milder COPD compared to subjects with lower lobe dominant emphysema in both COPD and non-COPD subjects. We conclude that the chance of a rapid decline in lung function is relatively lower in subjects with upper dominant and heterogeneous emphysema.

Author Contributions

Conceived and designed the experiments: JP DG FS. Performed the experiments: SG JJ RL. Analyzed the data: RL JP SG JJ YC XW. Contributed reagents/materials/analysis tools: SW BZ JL YC XW. Wrote the paper: JJ RL JL BZ DG.

References

1. National Institute of Health (NIH) website. Available: http://www.nhlbi.nih.gov/health/health-topics/topics/copd/. Accessed 2014 Oct 30.
2. Minai OA, Benditt J, Martinez FJ (2008) Natural history of emphysema. Proc Am Thorac Soc 5(4): 468–474.
3. Gurney JW, Jones KK, Robbins RA, Gossman GL, Nelson KJ, et al. (1992) Regional distribution of emphysema: correlation of high-resolution CT with pulmonary function tests in unselected smokers. Radiology 183(2): 457–463.
4. Stolk J, Stoel BC (2011) Lung densitometry to assess progression of emphysema in chronic obstructive pulmonary disease: time to apply in the clinic? Am J Respir Crit Care Med 183(12): 1578–1580.
5. Boschetto P, Miniati M, Miotto D, Braccioni F, De Rosa E, et al. (2003) Predominant emphysema phenotype in chronic obstructive pulmonary. Eur Respir J 21(3): 450–454.
6. Tanabe N, Muro S, Tanaka S, Sato S, Oguma T, et al. (2012) Emphysema distribution and annual changes in pulmonary function in male patients with chronic obstructive pulmonary disease. Respir Res 13: 31.
7. Gietema HA, Zanen P, Schilham A, van Ginneken B, van Klaveren RJ, et al. (2010) Distribution of emphysema in heavy smokers: impact on pulmonary function. Respir Med 104(1): 76–82.
8. Parr DG, Stoel BC, Stolk J, Stockley RA (2004) Pattern of emphysema distribution in alpha1-antitrypsin deficiency influences pulmonary function impairment. Am J Respir Crit Care Med 170(11): 1172–1178.

9. Holme J, Stockley RA (2007) Radiologic and clinical features of COPD patients with discordant pulmonary physiology: lessons from alpha1-antitrypsin deficiency. Chest 132(3): 909–915.
10. Castaldi PJ, San José Estépar R, Mendoza CS, Hersh CP, Laird N, et al. (2013) Distinct quantitative computed tomography emphysema patterns are associated with physiology and function in smokers. Am J Respir Crit Care Med 188(9): 1083–1090.
11. Nakano Y, Coxson HO, Bosan S, Rogers RM, Sciurba FC, et al. (2001) Core to rind distribution of severe emphysema predicts outcome of lung volume reduction surgery. Am J Respir Crit Care Med 164(12): 2195–2199.
12. Fishman A, Martinez F, Naunheim K, Piantadosi S, Wise R, et al. (2003) National Emphysema Treatment Trial Research Group. A randomized trial comparing lung-volume-reduction surgery with medical therapy for severe emphysema. N Engl J Med 348(21): 2059–2073.
13. Ito I, Nagai S, Handa T, Muro S, Hirai T, et al. (2005) Matrix metalloproteinase-9 promoter polymorphism associated with upper lung dominant emphysema. Am J Respir Crit Care Med 172(11): 1378–1382.
14. DeMeo DL, Hersh CP, Hoffman EA, Litonjua AA, Lazarus R, et al. (2007) Genetic determinants of emphysema distribution in the national emphysema treatment trial. Am J Respir Crit Care Med 176(1): 42–48.
15. Haruna A, Muro S, Nakano Y, Ohara T, Hoshino Y, et al. (2010) CT scan findings of emphysema predict mortality in COPD. Chest 138(3): 635–640.

16. Zulueta JJ, Wisnivesky JP, Henschke CI, Yip R, Farooqi AO, et al. (2012) Emphysema scores predict death from COPD and lung cancer. Chest 141(5): 1216–1223.
17. Wilson DO, Weissfeld JL, Fuhrman CR, Fisher SN, Balogh P, et al. (2008) The Pittsburgh Lung Screening Study (PLuSS): outcomes within 3 years of a first computed tomography scan. Am J Respir Crit Care Med 178(9): 956–961.
18. American Thoracic Society (1991) Lung Function Testing: Selection of Reference Values and Interpretative Strategies. Am Rev Respir Dis 1991; 144: 1202–1218.
19. Pauls S, Gulkin D, Feuerlein S, Muche R, Krüger S, et al. (2010) Assessment of COPD severity by computed tomography: correlation with lung functional testing. Clin Imaging 34(3): 172–178.
20. Pu J, Roos JE., Rubin GD, Napel S, Paik DS (2008) Adaptive border marching algorithm: automatic lung segmentation on chest CT images. Comp Med Imaging Graph 32(6): 452–462.
21. Pu J, Zheng B, Leader JK, Fuhrman C, Knollmann F, et al. (2009) Pulmonary lobe segmentation in CT examinations using implicit surface fitting. IEEE Trans. Medical Imaging 28(12): 1986–1996.
22. Pu J, Leader JK, Zheng B, Knollmann F, Fuhrman C, et al. (2009) A computational geometry approach to automated pulmonary fissure segmentation in CT examinations. IEEE Trans Med Imaging 28(5): 710–719.
23. Yuan R, Hogg JC, Paré PD, Sin DD, Wong JC, et al. (2009) Prediction of the rate of decline in FEV(1) in smokers using quantitative Computed Tomography. Thorax; 64(11): 944–949.
24. Han MK, Kazerooni EA, Lynch DA, Liu LX, Murray S, et al. (2011) Chronic obstructive pulmonary disease exacerbations in the COPDGene study: associated radiologic phenotypes. Radiology 261(1): 274–282.
25. Wang Z, Gu S, Leader JK, Kundu S, Tedrow JR, et al. (2013) Optimal threshold in CT quantification of emphysema. Eur Radiol 23(4): 975–984.
26. Leopold JG, Gough J (1957) The centrilobular form of hypertrophic emphysema and its relation to chronic bronchitis. Thorax 12(3): 219–235.
27. Haraguchi M, Shimura S, Hida W, Shirato K (1998) Pulmonary function and regional distribution of emphysema as determined by high-resolution computed tomography. Respiration 65(2): 125–129.

13

The Kinetics of Glomerular Deposition of Nephritogenic IgA

Kenji Yamaji[1], Yusuke Suzuki[1], Hitoshi Suzuki[1], Kenji Satake[1], Satoshi Horikoshi[1], Jan Novak[2], Yasuhiko Tomino[1]*

1 Division of Nephrology, Department of Internal Medicine, Juntendo University School of Medicine, Tokyo, Japan, 2 Department of Microbiology, University of Alabama at Birmingham, Birmingham, Alabama, United States of America

Abstract

Whether IgA nephropathy is attributable to mesangial IgA is unclear as there is no correlation between intensity of deposits and extent of glomerular injury and no clear mechanism explaining how these mesangial deposits induce hematuria and subsequent proteinuria. This hinders the development of a specific therapy. Thus, precise events during deposition still remain clinical challenge to clarify. Since no study assessed induction of IgA nephropathy by nephritogenic IgA, we analyzed sequential events involving nephritogenic IgA from IgA nephropathy-prone mice by real-time imaging systems. Immunofluorescence and electron microscopy showed that serum IgA from susceptible mice had strong affinity to mesangial, subepithelial, and subendothelial lesions, with effacement/actin aggregation in podocytes and arcade formation in endothelial cells. The deposits disappeared 24-h after single IgA injection. The data were supported by a fluorescence molecular tomography system and real-time and 3D in vivo imaging. In vivo imaging showed that IgA from the susceptible mice began depositing along the glomerular capillary from 1 min and accumulated until 2-h on the first stick in a focal and segmental manner. The findings indicate that glomerular IgA depositions in IgAN may be expressed under the balance between deposition and clearance. Since nephritogenic IgA showed mesangial as well as focal and segmental deposition along the capillary with acute cellular activation, all glomerular cellular elements are a plausible target for injury such as hematuria.

Editor: Johan van der Vlag, Radboud university medical center, Netherlands

Funding: A part of this study was supported by research funds from Grant-in-Aids for Progressive Renal Disease Research, Research on intractable disease, from the Ministry of Health, Labor and Welfare of Japan, a grant from Strategic Japanese (JST)-Swiss (ETHZ) Cooperative Scientific Program and a grant from the Study Group on IgA Nephropathy in Japan. The funders had no role in study design, data collection and analysis, decision to publish, or preparation of the manuscript.

Competing Interests: The authors have declared that no competing interests exist.

* Email: yasu@juntendo.ac.jp

Introduction

Immunohistological analysis is the crux of the diagnosis of IgA nephropathy (IgAN) for which dominant or co-dominant mesangial deposition of IgA is essential. Significant number of patients is reported to have elevated levels of circulating IgA immune complexes (IC), presumably due to aberrantly glycosylated IgA and endogenous antiglycan antibodies [1–3]. Thus, primary IgAN is an IC-mediated glomerulonephritis that is immunohistologically defined by the presence of glomerular IgA deposits accompanied by various histopathologic lesions. However, whether IgAN is attributable to mesangial IgA or IgA IC deposition remains unclear. One mystery is the lack of correlation between the intensity of deposits and the extent of glomerular injury; in addition, a long-standing question remains whether these mesangial IgA deposits directly induce hematuria [3–6]. To the best of our knowledge, no definitive study provides a comprehensive answer to these questions.

In contrast, we also know patients who exhibit minor clinical symptoms, such as very low levels of hematuria and proteinuria but have massive glomerular IgA depositions, suggesting that not all IgA immune deposits possess equivalent pathogenic potential.

These conflicting clinical findings make it difficult to identify the true therapeutic target of this disease, thereby hindering the development of a specific therapy [7], [8]. Thus, despite almost half a century of clinical and basic research, the immunologic processes that induce and perpetuate glomerular IgA deposition and the detailed mechanism underlying deposition events remain unknown. IgAN may represent multiple diseases with abnormal urinary findings, sharing common pathogenic markers, such as mesangial IgA immune deposits, and having unknown mechanisms whereby damage is propagated in a discontinuous pattern [5]. The deposition of circulating IgA/IgA-containing IC may be the most likely mechanism; an understanding of the detailed sequential events in pathogenesis is the key to developing a successful therapy [2], [3], [9], [10].

We recently established a strain of spontaneous IgAN-prone gddY mice in which the disease phenotype and genetic regulation largely overlap with human IgAN [11–13]. Although abnormal glycosylation of O-linked glycans in the hinge region of human IgA1 is linked to human IgAN [2], [3], it has long been believed that O-glycans are absent in the hinge region of murine IgA. However, our recent paper [12] revealed that more severe disease in gddY mice occurs in those with an IgA allotype that has less sugar content in the hinge region. Thus, modification of carbohydrate structures may change the conformational or biochemical properties of murine IgA, thereby altering the nephritogenicity or formation of IgA-IC, as seen in human IgAN [2]. Moreover, aberrantly glycosylated IgA may induce macromolecular IgA complex formation, leading to the complement activation and subsequent progression to IgAN [14], as seen in human IgAN [2], [9]. Furthermore, serum levels of IgA-IgG IC correlate with the severity of renal damage in IgAN-prone mice [15]. Our recent reports demonstrate that cells responsible for producing nephritogenic IgA are disseminated in the mucosa-bone marrow axis [15–18] and are regulated by the innate immune system [19–21], as seen in human IgAN [13], [19], [22], [23]. Accordingly, experimental, immunological, and histopathological findings in this susceptible strain seem to recapitulate the clinical features of human IgAN [11–13]. Details of the sequence of events in glomerular deposition of nephritogenic IgA from IgAN have not been described in the literature. In the present study, we use nephritogenic IgA from this susceptible mouse strain to examine this sequence of events using a real-time imaging system. Sequential analysis of IgA-induced IgAN may provide clues to the pathogenesis of this disease and strategies for its treatment.

Materials and Methods

Mice

The gddY mice were established by the selective mating of early-onset ddY mice for more than 20 generations and have a 100 % incidence of severe disease, even at a young age [11–16]. The gddY mice were maintained on a regular chow (MF; Oriental Yeast, Tokyo, Japan) and water *ad libitum* in a specific pathogen-free (SPF) room at the animal facility of Juntendo University, Tokyo, Japan.

Same-age female Balb/c (Balb/c) mice were used as controls. Female Balb/c AJcl-nu/nu (nude) mice were used for the injection of serum or IgA from the gddY mice with early-stage disease and from the Balb/c mice. Balb/c and nude mice were purchased from CLEA Japan Inc., Tokyo, Japan. The experimental protocol of the present study was approved by the Ethics Review Committee for Animal Experimentation of Juntendo University Faculty of Medicine.

The serum single-injection model

Serum samples were obtained from gddY mice aged between 20 and 25 weeks who showed severe renal injury with glomerular IgA deposits. Serum from age-matched healthy Balb/c mice was also collected as the control serum. Serum levels of IgA were measured using a single radioimmunodiffusion assay (SRL, Tokyo, Japan). The obtained serum samples, including 2 mg IgA of gddY or Balb/c mice (300 μL, diluted with saline) were injected once into the tail vein of nude mice aged between 10 and 12 weeks. The nude mice were euthanized either 2 or 24 h after the injection of serum. Kidneys were collected from the nude mice after perfusion with normal saline solution. The serum samples and kidneys were stored at −80°C until use. Renal histological analysis was performed using electron and confocal microscopy.

Snap-frozen 3-μm-thick renal sections were used for immunofluorescence with a fluorescein isothiocyanate-conjugated goat antimouse IgA antibody (BD Biosciences, San Diego, CA, USA; Pharmingen, San Diego, CA, USA). For electron microscopy, the renal specimens were fixed in 2 % glutaraldehyde, washed in phosphate buffer, and postfixed in 1 % osmic acid. The specimens were washed, dehydrated, and embedded in Epon 812. The ultrathin sections were contrasted with uranyl acetate and lead citrate and then examined under an electron microscope (Hitachi 7100, Tokyo, Japan).

Purification of IgA

Serum samples were obtained from the gddY and Balb/c mice aged between 20 and 25 weeks. Each serum sample was incubated with a rat antimouse IgA antibody with CNBr Sepharose overnight at 4°C. After washing with phosphate-buffered saline (PBS), IgA was eluted with 0.1 M glycine (pH 2.5) using a fraction collector. Molecular size of purified IgA obtained from ddY and Balb/c mice were analyzed by Western blot analysis. The purified IgA samples were used for fluorescence molecular tomography and confocal laser microscopy analyses.

Kinetic studies using a fluorescence molecular tomography system

These studies were conducted on female nude mice (n = 3). The purified IgA samples obtained from gddY or Balb/c mice were labeled with Vivo Tag-S 750 (VisEn Medical Inc. Woburn, MA, USA). Purified IgA samples were dissolved at 2 mg/mL in PBS, and 0.5 mL of the solution was alkalized with 50 μL of 1 M sodium bicarbonate solution. The mixture was incubated with Vivo Tag-S 750 for 1 h at room temperature, with stirring. The labeled IgA was purified using resin column chromatography. Fluorescein-labeled IgA (0.5 mg/mL) was dissolved in 200 μL PBS and injected into nude mice aged between 10 and 12 weeks. After 2, 4, and 24 h, IgA signals were measured using a fluorescence molecular tomography system (VisEn Medical Inc. Woburn, MA, USA).

Kinetic studies by confocal laser microscopy

Kinetic studies by confocal laser microscopy were performed in female nude mice (n = 3). Purified IgA obtained from gddY or Balb/c mice was labeled using an Alexa Fluor 633 protein labeling kit (Molecular probes, Inc., Eugene, OR, USA). Purified IgA samples were dissolved at 2 mg/mL in PBS, and 0.5 mL of the solution was alkalized with 50 μL of a 1 M sodium bicarbonate solution. The mixture was incubated with Alexa Fluor 633 dye at room temperature for 1 h, with stirring. The labeled IgA was purified using resin column chromatography. Before analysis, the nude mice were anesthetized with sodium pentobarbital. An incision of approximately 10 mm was made on the lower back, and a kidney was removed using small forceps. The surface of the lower pole of the kidney was sliced and placed on a microscope stage. Dextran (500 kDa) is not filtered and is a good marker for blood vessel wall integrity. First, fluorescein-labeled 500-kDa dextran (Sigma–Aldrich Inc., St. Louis, MO, USA) was injected into nude mice to confirm the staining of glomeruli. Following this, fluorescein-labeled IgA (0.5 mg/mL) was dissolved in 200 μL PBS and injected into mice. After 1 and 120 min, the kinetics of labeled IgA in glomeruli were analyzed using confocal laser microscopy (ZEISS, LSM 510 META, Germany). Single or time-series images of glomeruli were recorded in fluorescence mode.

The procedure of BMT

The procedure for murine BMT was previously described in detail [15–18]. In brief, BMC were harvested from the tibia, femur, and humerus of control Balb/c mice at 8–10 weeks of age under sterile conditions. Red blood cells were removed from the collected BMC. Grouped ddY mice develop glomerular lesions with mesangial IgA deposits within 6–8 weeks of age [11], [12]. Young and old gddY mice aged 8 and 20 weeks who were at the early stage of the disease were used as recipients. Following this,

10^7 BMCs were injected into the tail vein of irradiated recipient mice (n = 3) at 700 rad. The recipient mice were housed under SPF conditions. Young and old gddY transplant recipients were euthanized 12 weeks after BMT. IgA deposits were assessed by immunofluorescence and electron microscopy, and urinary protein was measured by immunoassay (DCA 2000 system; Siemens Healthcare Diagnostics, Tokyo, Japan).

Results

A single injection of serum from gddY mice, but not from Balb/c mice, induced glomerular IgA deposition with an activation of glomerular podocytes and endothelial cells

We first tested whether a serum from gddY mice induced glomerular IgA deposition in nude mice. Serum from Balb/c mice was used as a control. Renal tissue was obtained from nude mice euthanized 2 and 24 h after a single injection of the serum. Serum from gddY mice, but not Balb/c mice, induced mesangial IgA deposition 2 h after the injection (Fig. 1a). The electron-dense deposits in the paramesangial areas were confirmed using electron microscopy (Fig. 1b). After 2 h, in some glomeruli of the mice injected with the gddY mouse serum, electron-dense deposits were detectable in subepithelial and subendothelial lesions, with effacement and actin aggregation in the podocytes and arcade formation in some endothelial cells. This data is indicative of the activation of those cells (Fig. 1c). Such morphological changes were not found with injections of Balb/c IgA (serum to be precise; data not shown). In this single-injection model, mesangial IgA deposition and electron-dense deposits almost disappeared after 24 h (Fig. 1a and b, right panels).

IgA from gddY mice showed high affinity for kidney tissue

We next labeled serum IgA from gddY mice and control Balb/c mice with Vivo Tag-S 750 and analyzed the *in vivo* kinetics of IgA using a fluorescence molecular tomography system after a single injection in nude mice. After the injection of IgA from gddY or Balb/c mice, fluorescence signals in the kidneys, liver, and bladder were evaluated after 10 min and 2, 4, and 24 h. There was no difference in the signals in the liver and bladder between the mouse groups that received labeled IgA from either gddY or Balb/c mice (Fig. 2, middle and lower panels). Two hours after injection, IgA signals were detected in the kidneys of both groups by molecular tomography (Fig. 2 upper panels). However, the renal signals in mice injected with IgA from gddY mice increased, with a peak at 4 h after the injection, whereas renal signals in controls were weak and gradually decreased.

IgA from gddY mice is deposited along the glomerular capillary wall in a focal and segmental manner

To further clarify the sequential manner of the deposition process, we injected Alexa Fluor 633 protein-labeled IgA (red) from gddY and Balb/c mice and fluorescein-labeled 500-kDa Dextran (green) to visualize the glomerular capillary in the nude mice. We then analyzed the glomerular capillaries using confocal laser microscopy from 1 min to 2 h after the single injection (Fig. 3). Yellow images indicate IgA deposition along the glomerular capillaries. This *in vivo* real-time/3D imaging (Fig. 3a and supporting information in video and 3D images) confirmed the data from previous immunofluorescent analysis, electron microscopy, and tomography, in that IgA from gddY has a higher affinity for the glomerulus than that from Balb/c mice. Nevertheless, this gddY-derived IgA was deposited along the glomerular

capillary in a focal and segmental manner. This *in vivo* imaging with a focus on the glomerular capillary showed initial deposition after only 1 min (Fig. 3b). IgA accumulated on top of these first aggregates or microdeposits (Fig. 3c); however, this accumulation was not diffuse. Two hours after the injection, the amount of labeled IgA in the glomerular capillary gradually decreased in both groups of mice. Nonetheless, a clear accumulation of IgA in glomerular mesangial areas was found in the *in vivo* imaging with a focus on mesangial areas after 2 h in the group injected with IgA from gddY mice, but not in that from Balb/c mice. Molecular forms of both IgA purified from ddY and Balb/c mice were analyzed by Western blotting under non-reducing condition. IgA purified from ddY mice serum was predominantly polymeric with a small peak of dimeric IgA. IgA purified from Balb/c mice was monomeric and dimeric dominant (data not shown).

Glomerular IgA deposits in old gddY mice remained after bone marrow transplantation (BMT) despite improved proteinuria

To clear IgAN in gddY mice [14], [15], we transplanted bone marrow cells (BMC) from Balb/c (healthy) mice into gddY mice. We confirmed the disappearance of proteinuria in both young and old recipients 12 weeks after BMT [albuminuria before vs. after BMT (μg/day): young recipients, 121.3±21.2 vs. 26.3±6.7; old recipients, 198.0±23.0 vs. 30.3±12.9]. However, fluorescence analysis still detected glomerular IgA deposition in old but not young gddY recipients (Fig. 4 left panels). Electron microscopy detected dense paramesangial deposits in the old recipients; however, these dense deposits showed fibrous and lattice structures.

Discussion

The primary abnormal clinical manifestation of IgAN in patients is recurring bouts of hematuria with or without associated proteinuria [3], [4]. In the complex web of potential mechanisms implicated in the pathogenesis of IgAN, mesangial IgA deposits remain a *sine qua non*. This notion may lead us to believe that mesangial IgA deposition directly induces hematuria. However, there are no studies proving a direct relationship between the amount mesangial IgA immune deposits and the extent of glomerular injury leading to hematuria. Our earlier comprehensive observations emphasized the variable characteristics of the IgA/IgA IC, particularly the nature of antigens and the molecular form of IgA, as major determinants of glomerular injury [10]. Several physical characteristics, including size, lattice composition, electric charge, and glycosylation, may also influence the probability of deposition in the glomerular mesangium [2], [3], [9], [10], [24–31]. Sequential events were analyzed in the experiments with artificially modified IgA or IgA IC. Even these observations failed to provide a sufficient explanation for the mechanisms leading to hematuria in IgAN. This may be partly due to the absence of experiments with IgA preparations that have been confirmed to induce a chronic progression of IgAN with mesangial cell proliferation and matrix expansion. Thus, this appears to be the first study to assess the kinetics of glomerular deposition of nephritogenic IgA in IgAN [11–16].

The present analysis using tomography showed a similar time course of liver signals peaking at 2 h in both the groups of mice, indicating that most of the injected IgA from the gddY and control mice was trapped in the liver in a similar fashion. The parts of injected IgA from both the groups of mice passed through into the bladder in a similar manner. Nevertheless, renal signals were conspicuously stronger in the group injected with IgA from gddY

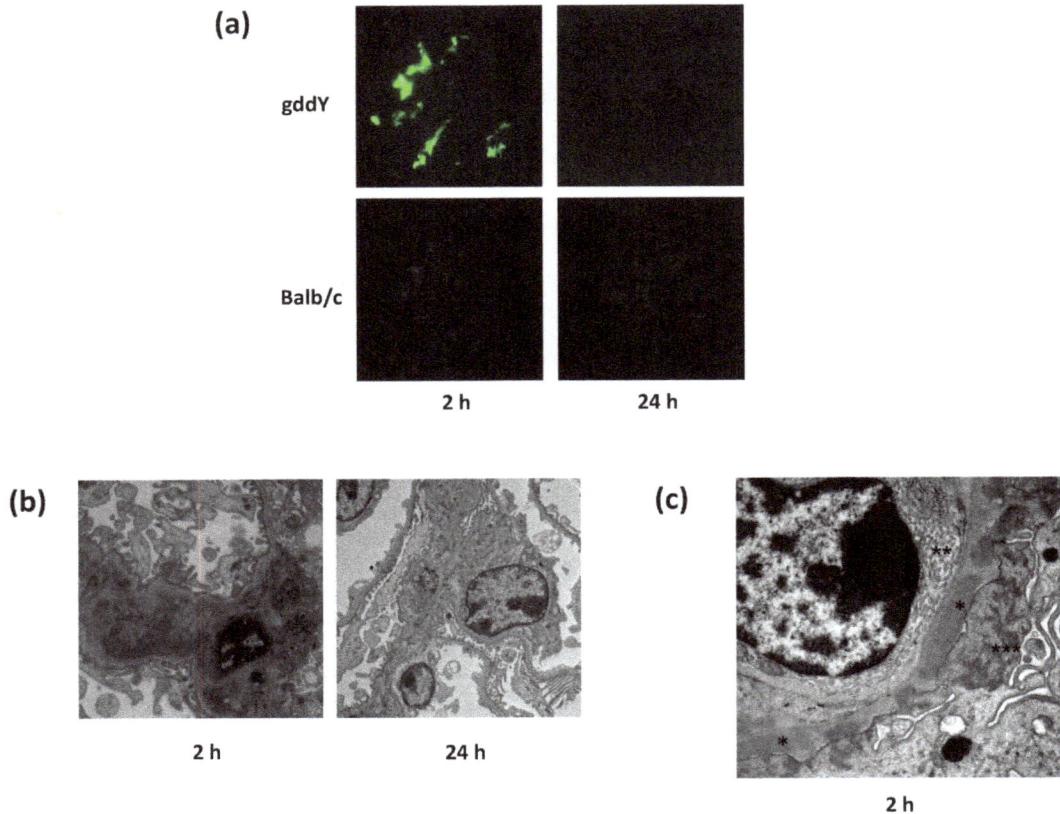

Figure 1. A single injection of serum from gddY mice induced glomerular IgA deposition with activation of glomerular podocytes and endothelial cells. (a) Glomerular IgA deposits were found at 2 h in mice injected with serum from gddY mice but not from Balb/c mice. These fluorescent signals disappeared after 24 h in this single-injection model. (b) These deposits and clearance were confirmed using electron microscopy. Electron-dense deposits were mainly detected in paramesangial lesions. (c) Some glomeruli showed subendothelial and subepithelial deposits (*) with arcade formation in glomerular endothelial cells (**) and effacement and actin aggregation in podocytes (***) 2 h after the injection.

mice than in those injected with IgA from healthy mice. This finding indicates that some clones of IgA in gddY mice have a strong affinity for kidney tissues and may be nephritogenic. Our recent studies have shown that IgA in gddY mice is polymeric and that it has a high capacity for activating complement cascades, including the lectin pathway [14]. The renal prognosis of this susceptible model is likely to be dependent on the content of carbohydrates in the hinge region of IgA [12]. Recent research has also suggested that aberrant N-glycan glycosylation may be involved in the pathogenesis of IgAN in mice [32], [33]. These findings suggest that aberrant modifications of serum IgA carbohydrate side chains are involved in the development of IgAN, not only in humans but also in mice, regardless of whether the carbohydrates are O-glycans or N-glycans [2], [3], [13]. Recent studies have revealed that aberrantly glycosylated IgA1 (GdIgA1) plays a nephritogenic role in this disease [1–3], [9], [34]. The serum level of GdIgA1 is associated with the disease activity of IgAN [35]. On the other hand, anomalous glycosylation of IgA is a key determinant of glomerular affinity [31]. Thus, the high glomerular affinity found in the present study may be partly due to the basic molecular nature of IgA, presumably with aberrant glycosylation.

The disappearance of the glomerular deposits in this single-injection model is one of most important findings of the present study. This finding indicates that a continuous clearance mechanism of IgA deposition may be at work in the glomerulus.

Thus, glomerular IgA deposits in IgAN may be explained as an imbalance between deposition and clearance. Although most IgAN patients have undoubtedly had glomerulonephritis for years before a renal biopsy, it seems that a certain percentage of IgAN patients may go through a clinical period just after the onset, when neither IgA nor C3 is detectable in the renal biopsy but when there are histological lesions and aberrant urinary test results [7], [8]. Thus, our results indicate that the intensity of staining for IgA in the kidney may wax or wane based on the balance in the glomeruli or mesangium.

Increasing evidences suggest that mucosal type polymeric IgA1 is produced in BM of IgAN patients [36]. Furthermore, BMT in patients with leukemia and IgAN resulted in the cure of not only leukemia but also IgAN [37]. Therefore, cross talk between the mucosa and BM is suspected in the pathogenesis of IgAN [13], [38], [39]. We previously showed that murine IgAN can be reconstituted via BMT from ddY mice to healthy mice [15–18], [40]. We also showed that early-stage IgAN in ddY mice can be cured by removing glomerular IgA via BMT from healthy mice [15], [16]. However, glomerular IgA deposits in the present BMT model from healthy mice to ddY mice disappeared in young but not old ddY recipients; proteinuria in both young and old recipients was alleviated by BMT. This finding suggests that incompletely cleared IgA deposition in the disease course of gddY mice may change in conformation or biochemical properties as a result of their organization or fibrosis with mesangial matrix

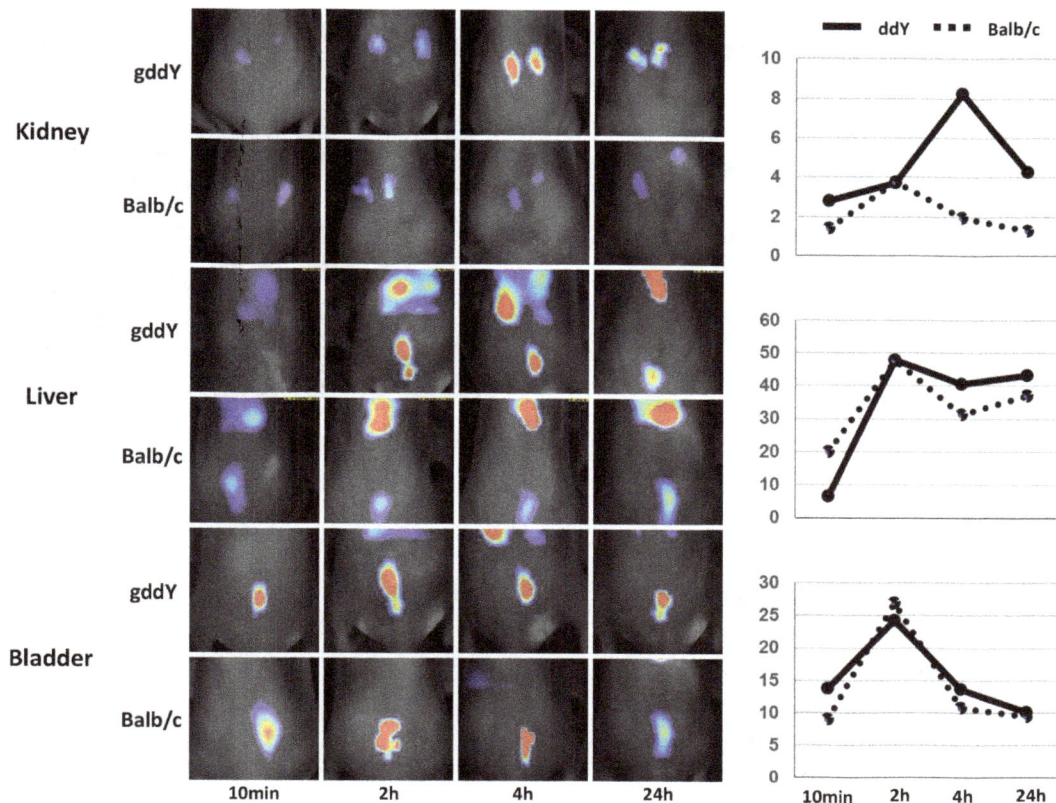

Figure 2. Kinetics of injected fluorescently labeled IgA in a fluorescence molecular tomography system. A fluorescence molecular tomography system (FMT) is capable of resolving size and concentration of fluorochromes in deep tissue *in vivo*. Fluorescein-labeled IgA samples from gddY and Balb/c mice were injected into nude mice and monitored from 10 min to 24 h postinjection by FMT. After 2 h, IgA signals in the liver and bladder were found in a similar manner in both the groups of nude mice. However, IgA signals in the kidneys clearly differed between them. Mice injected with gddY IgA showed strong signals in the kidneys, with a peak at 4 h.

components, losing nephritogenicity. However, because these deposits were present in old ddY recipients after BMT, such organized IgA may still have epitopes that the fluorescence-labeled anti-IgA antibody recognizes. Therefore, present BMT models indicate that glomerular IgA in IgAN patients may be mixed with freshly-delivered nephritogenic IgA and non-inflammatory organized IgA, particularly in those with a longer disease history. This finding may also partly explain the discrepancy between the amount of IgA deposition and severity of glomerular lesions in human IgAN.

Although most glomeruli in mice injected with gddY IgA showed mesangial IgA deposition, deposits along capillaries were detected in a focal and segmental manner. *In vivo* serial imaging showed that such subendothelial/subepithelial IgA deposits seemed to be formed as a result of an accumulation on the focal/segmental initial aggregates of IgA, suggesting that the initial aggregates (microdeposits) may change the local physiological conditions, thereby leading to the increased glomerular affinity of IgA. These physiological changes may include the local deceleration of the glomerular capillary flow or increased permeability of the glomerular basement membrane interposed between the endothelial and epithelial layers [41–43]. These deposits along glomerular capillaries were indeed found along with morphological changes in glomerular endothelial cells and podocytes, even after 2 h. This phenomenon is suggestive of a rapid activation of glomerular resident cells by IgA deposition. We can speculate that

such rapid activation (particularly in the endothelial cells, presumably in combination with slow blood flow) may facilitate leukocyte adhesion to the deposits and their subsequent clearance and/or inflammatory responses [44], [45], leading to hematuria in IgAN. This real-time imaging showed increased passage of IgA into glomerular mesangial lesions and the relevant glomerular pole after 2 h (data not shown), suggesting that subendothelial/subepithelial deposits may induce permeability factors, such as vascular endothelial growth factor (VEGF), and increase the flow of plasma into the mesangium and subsequent interstitium/lymph via the glomerular pole. Thus, nephritogenic IgA deposition may induce dynamic alterations in the glomerulus and subsequent glomerular and interstitial injury.

This study revealed the kinetics of glomerular deposition over the course of IgA-induced IgAN. These IgA molecules have a strong affinity for focal and segmental subendothelial, subepithelial, and glomerular mesangial lesions. Rapid cellular activation of endothelial cells and podocytes by IgA deposition may precede the events of hematuria in IgAN. The significant differences between human and murine IgAN limit the translation of these data to the human disease. Further, similar study using human GdIgA1 is needed. However, the present findings regarding the kinetics of IgA deposition may indicate that not only glomerular mesangial cells but also endothelial cells and podocytes are plausible targets of glomerular injury in IgAN.

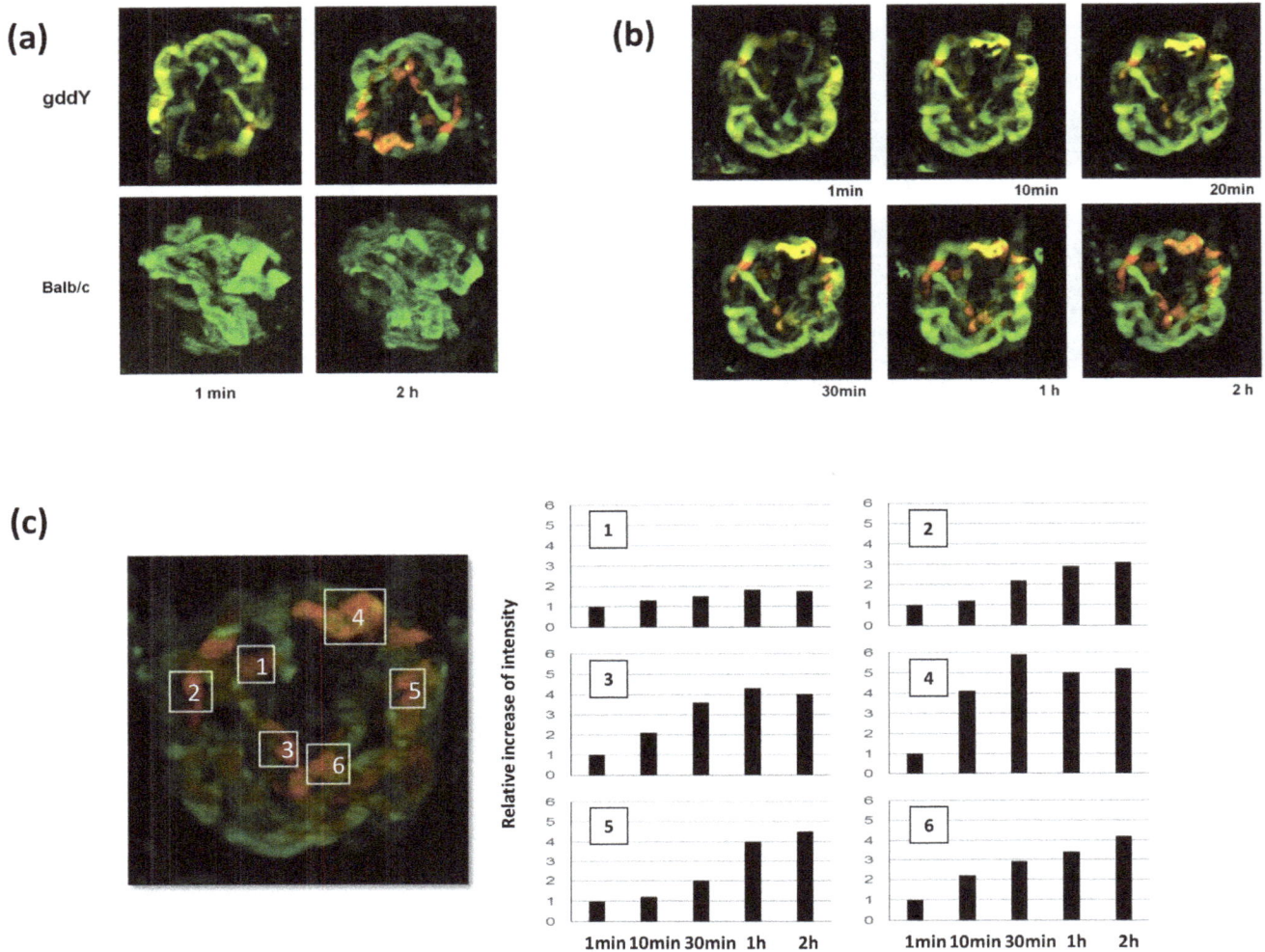

Figure 3. IgA from gddY mice is deposited along the glomerular capillary wall in a focal and segmental manner. Detailed kinetics of IgA deposition analyzed from 1 min to 2 h postinjection using confocal laser microscopy. Alexa Fluor 633-labeled IgA from gddY and Balb/c mice (red) and 500-kDa fluorescein-labeled dextran (green) were injected for analyzing kinetics of IgA deposition and visualizing blood vessel wall integrity, respectively. (a) IgA signals were detectable even after 1 min and accumulated up to 2 h in a focal and segmental manner in mice with IgA from gddY mice. In contrast, mice who received Balb/c IgA did not show a signal even after 2 h. (b)(c) Serial images of a glomerulus in mice with IgA from gddY mice showed that these IgA molecules accumulated on top of the initial aggregates along the glomerular capillaries. These aggregates were found in a focal and segmental manner but not in a diffuse and global manner.

Supporting Information

Video S1 *In vivo* **3D imaging of glomerulus after injection of nephritogenic IgA.** 3D images of glomeruli at 2 hours after single injection of purified IgA from gddY mice were evaluated by a confocal laser microscopy. Alexa Fluor 633-labeled IgA from gddY (red) and 500-kDa fluorescein-labeled dextran (green) were injected for analyzing kinetics of IgA deposition and visualizing blood vessel wall integrity, respectively. IgA signals were detectable after 2 h in a focal and segmental manner in mice with IgA from gddY mice.

Video S2 *In vivo* **3D imaging of glomerulus after injection of IgA from Balb/c mice.** 3D images of glomeruli at 2 hours after single injection of purified IgA from Balb/c mice were evaluated by a confocal laser microscopy. Alexa Fluor 633-labeled IgA from and Balb/c mice (red) and 500-kDa fluorescein-labeled dextran (green) were injected for analyzing kinetics of IgA

deposition and visualizing blood vessel wall integrity, respectively. IgA signals were detectable after 2 h in a focal and segmental manner in mice with IgA from gddY mice (Video images S1 and S3). In contrast, mice who received Balb/c IgA did not show clear signals after 2 h.

Video S3 *In vivo* **real-time imaging of glomerulus after injection of nephritogenic IgA.** Real-time images of glomeruli at 2 hours after single injection of purified IgA from gddY mice were evaluated by a confocal laser microscopy. Alexa Fluor 633-labeled IgA from gddY mice (red) and 500-kDa fluorescein-labeled dextran (green) were injected for analyzing kinetics of IgA deposition and visualizing blood vessel wall integrity, respectively. IgA signals were detectable after 2 h in a focal and segmental manner in mice with IgA from gddY mice.

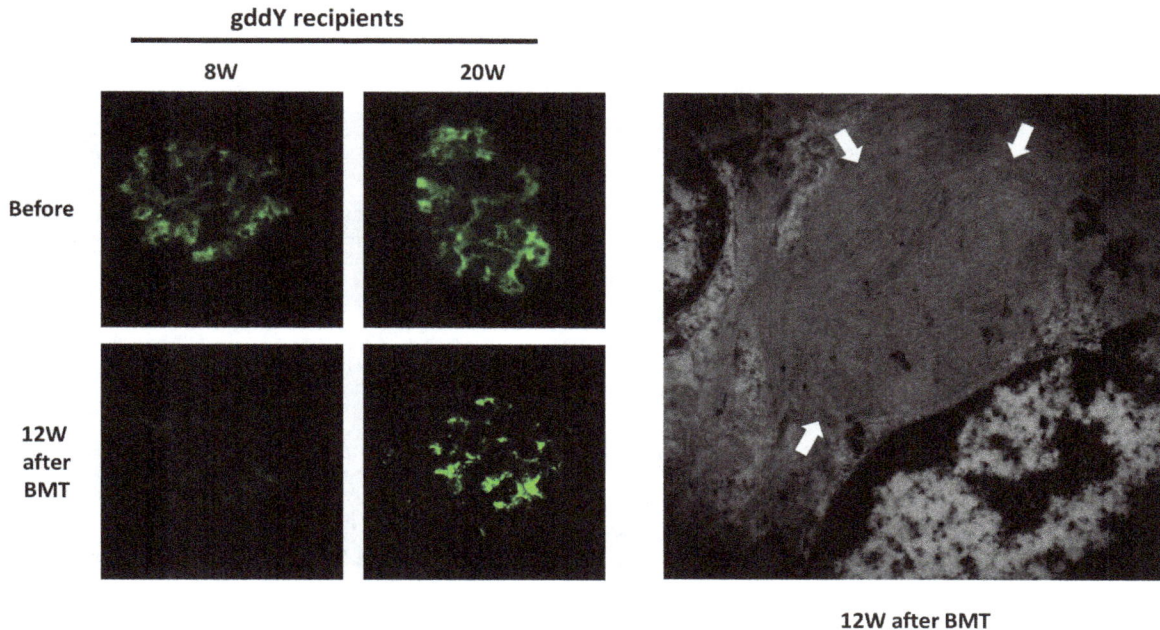

gddY recipients

Figure 4. Glomerular IgA deposits in old gddY mice did not disappear after bone marrow transplantation (BMT) despite improvement in proteinuria. BM cells from healthy Balb/c mice were transplanted into young (8 weeks) and old (20 weeks) gddY mice at an early stage of disease. Although proteinuria was present in the young and old recipients 12 weeks after BMT, fluorescence analysis still detected glomerular IgA deposition in old gddY recipients but not in young gddY recipients (left panels). Electron microscopy still detected paramesangial dense deposits showing fibrous and lattice structures in the old recipients (right panel).

Video S4 *In vivo* **real-time imaging of glomerulus after injection of IgA from Balb/c mice.** Real-time images of glomeruli at 2 hours after single injection of purified IgA from Balb/c mice were evaluated by a confocal laser microscopy. Alexa Fluor 633-labeled IgA from Balb/c mice (red) and 500-kDa fluorescein-labeled dextran (green) were injected for analyzing kinetics of IgA deposition and visualizing blood vessel wall integrity, respectively. IgA signals were detectable after 2 h in a focal and segmental manner in mice with IgA from gddY mice (Video images S1 and S3). In contrast, mice who received Balb/c IgA did not show clear signals after 2 h.

Acknowledgments

The authors thank T. Shibata, M. Yamada, and all members of the laboratory for technical support and helpful discussions.

Author Contributions

Conceived and designed the experiments: YT YS KY HS SH JN. Performed the experiments: KY YS HS KS. Analyzed the data: KY YS. Contributed reagents/materials/analysis tools: KY YS HS KS. Wrote the paper: KY YS.

References

1. Suzuki H, Moldoveanu Z, Hall S, Brown R, Vu HL, et al. (2008) IgA1-secreting cell lines from patients with IgA nephropathy produce aberrantly glycosylated IgA1. J Clin Invest. 118: 629–639.
2. Suzuki H, Kiryluk K, Novak J, Moldoveanu Z, Herr AB, et al. (2011) The pathophysiology of IgA nephropathy. J Am Soc Nephrol. 22: 1795–1803.
3. Wyatt RJ, Julian BA (2013) IgA nephropathy. N Engl J Med. 368: 2402–2414.
4. D'Amico G (1987) The commonest glomerulonephritis in the world: IgA nephropathy. Q J Med. 64: 709–727.
5. Donadio JV Jr, Grande JP (1997) Immunoglobulin A nephropathy: a clinical perspective. J Am Soc Nephrol. 8: 1324–1332.
6. Moreno JA, Martín-Cleary C, Gutiérrez E, Rubio-Navarro A, Ortiz A, et al. (2012) Haematuria: the forgotten CKD factor? Nephrol Dial Transplant. 27: 28–34.
7. Julian BA, Cannon VR, Waldo FB, Egido J (1991) Macroscopic hematuria and proteinuria preceding renal IgA deposition in patients with IgA nephropathy. Am J Kidney Dis. 17: 472–479.
8. Galla JH (1995) IgA nephropathy. Kidney Int. 47: 377–387.
9. Suzuki H, Fan R, Zhang Z, Brown R, Hall S, et al. (2009) Aberrantly glycosylated IgA1 in IgA nephropathy patients is recognized by IgG antibodies with restricted heterogeneity. J Clin Invest. 119: 1668–1677.
10. Hebert LA (1988) Disposition of IgA-containing circulating immune complexes. Am J Kidney Dis. 12: 388–392.
11. Suzuki H, Suzuki Y, Yamanaka T, Hirose S, Nishimura H, et al. (2005) Genome-wide scan in a novel IgA nephropathy model identifies a susceptibility

locus on murine chromosome 10, in a region syntenic to human IgAN1 on chromosome 6q22–23. J Am Soc Nephrol. 16: 1289–1299.
12. Okazaki K, Suzuki Y, Otsuji M, Suzuki H, Kihara M, et al. (2012) Development of a model of early-onset IgA nephropathy. J Am Soc Nephrol. 23: 1364–1374.
13. Suzuki Y, Tomino Y (2008) Potential immunopathogenic role of the mucosa-bone marrow axis in IgA nephropathy: Insights from animal model. Semin Nephrol. 28: 66–77.
14. Hashimoto A, Suzuki Y, Suzuki H, Ohsawa I, Brown R, et al. (2012) Determination of severity of murine IgA nephropathy by glomerular complement activation by aberrantly glycosylated IgA and immune complexes. Am J Pathol. 181: 1338–1347.
15. Suzuki H, Suzuki Y, Aizawa M, Yamanaka T, Kihara M, et al. (2007) Th1 polarization in murine IgA nephropathy directed by bone marrow-derived cells. Kidney Int. 72: 319–327.
16. Nakata J, Suzuki Y, Suzuki H, Sato D, Kano T, et al. (2013) Experimental evidence of cell dissemination playing a role in pathogenesis of IgA nephropathy in multiple lymphoid organs. Nephrol Dial Transplant. 28: 320–326.
17. Aizawa M, Suzuki Y, Suzuki H, Pang H, Kihara M, et al. (2007) Roles of bone marrow, mucosa and lymphoid tissues in pathogenesis of murine IgA nephropathy. Contrib Nephrol. 157: 164–168.
18. Aizawa M, Suzuki Y, Suzuki H, Pang H, Kihara M, et al. (2014) Uncoupling of glomerular IgA deposition and disease progression in alymphoplasia mice with IgA nephropathy. PLoS One. 9: e95365.

19. Suzuki H, Suzuki Y, Narita I, Aizawa M, Kihara M, et al. (2008) Toll-like receptor 9 affects severity of IgA nephropathy. J Am Soc Nephrol. 19: 2384–2395.

20. Kajiyama T, Suzuki Y, Kihara M, Suzuki H, Horikoshi S, Tomino Y. (2011) Different pathological roles of toll-like receptor 9 on mucosal B cells and dendritic cells in murine IgA nephropathy. Clin Dev Immunol. 2011: 819646.

21. Maiguma M, Suzuki Y, Suzuki H, Okazaki K, Aizawa M, et al. (2014) Dietary zinc is a key environmental modifier in the progression of IgA nephropathy. PLoS One. 9: e90558.

22. Sato D, Suzuki Y, Kano T, Suzuki H, Matsuoka J, et al. (2012) Tonsillar TLR9 expression and efficacy of tonsillectomy with steroid pulse therapy in IgA nephropathy patients. Nephrol Dial Transplant. 27: 1090–1097.

23. Nakata J, Suzuki Y, Suzuki H, Sato D, Kano T, Yanagawa H, et al. (2014) Changes in nephritogenic serum galactose-deficient IgA1 in IgA nephropathy following tonsillectomy and steroid therapy. PLoS One 9: e89707.

24. Cameron JS, Clark WF (1982) A role for insoluble antibody-antigen complexes in glomerulonephritis? Clin Nephrol. 18: 55–61.

25. Rifai A, Mannik M (1983) Clearance kinetics and fate of mouse IgA immune complexes prepared with monomeric or dimeric IgA. J Immunol. 130: 1826–32.

26. Rifai A, Mannik M (1984) Clearance of circulating IgA immune complexes is mediated by a specific receptor on Kupffer cells in mice. J Exp Med. 160: 125–137.

27. Rifai A (1987) Experimental models for IgA-associated nephritis.. Kidney Int 31: 1–7.

28. Ward DM, Lee S, Wilson CB (1986) Direct antigen binding to glomerular immune complex deposits. Kidney Int. 30: 706–711.

29. Roccatello D, Picciotto G, Ropolo R, Coppo R, Quattrocchio G, et al. (1992) Kinetics and fate of IgA-IgG aggregates as a model of naturally occurring immune complexes in IgA nephropathy. Lab Invest. 66: 86–95.

30. Monteiro RC, Halbwachs-Mecarelli L, Roque-Barreira MC, Noel LH, Berger J, et al. (1985) Charge and size of mesangial IgA in IgA nephropathy. Kidney Int. 28: 666–671.

31. Hiki Y, Kokubo T, Iwase H, Masaki Y, Sano T, et al. (1999) Underglycosylation of IgA1 hinge plays a certain role for its glomerular deposition in IgA nephropathy. J Am Soc Nephrol. 10: 760–769.

32. Nishie T, Miyaishi O, Azuma H, Kameyama A, Naruse C, et al. (2007) Development of immunoglobulin A nephropathy-like disease in β-1,4-galacto-syltransferase-I-deficient mice. Am J Pathol. 170: 447–456.

33. Kobayashi I, Nogaki F, Kusano H, Ono T, Miyawaki S, et al. (2002) Interleukin-12 alters the physicochemical characteristics of serum and glomerular IgA and modifies glycosylation in a ddY mouse strain having high IgA levels. Nephrol Dial Transplant. 17: 2108–2116.

34. Berthoux F, Suzuki H, Thibaudin L, Yanagawa H, Maillard N, et al. (2012) Autoantibodies targeting galactose-deficient IgA1 associate with progression of IgA nephropathy. J Am Soc Nephrol. 23: 1579–1587.

35. Suzuki Y, Matsuzaki K, Suzuki H, Okazaki K, Yanagawa H, et al. (2014) Serum levels of galactose deficient IgA1 and related immune complex are associated with disease activity of IgA nephropathy. Clin Exp Nephrol. Available: http://link.springer.com/content/pdf/10.1007%2Fs10157-013-0921-6.pdf Accessed 2014 July 13.

36. Barratt J, Smith AC, Molyneux K, Feehally J (2007) Immunopathogenesis of IgAN. Semin Immunopathol. 29: 427–443.

37. Iwata Y, Wada T, Uchiyama A, Miwa A, Nakaya I, et al. (2006) Remission of IgA nephropathy after allogeneic peripheral blood stem cell transplantation followed by immunosuppression for acute lymphocytic leukemia. Intern Med. 45: 1291–1295.

38. van den Wall Bake AW, Daha MR, van Es LA (1989) Immunopathogenetic aspects of IgA nephropathy. Nephrologie. 10: 141–145.

39. Suzuki Y, Tomino Y (2007) The mucosa-bone-marrow axis in IgA nephropathy. Contrib Nephrol. 2007; 157: 70–79.

40. Zuo N, Suzuki Y, Sugaya T, Osaki K, Kanaguchi Y, et al. (2011) Protective effects of tubular liver-type fatty acid-binding protein against glomerular damage in murine IgA nephropathy. Nephrol Dial Transplant. 26: 2127–2137.

41. Suzuki Y, Shirato I, Okumura K, Ravetch JV, Takai T, et al. (1998) Distinct contribution of Fc receptors and angiotensin II-dependent pathways in anti-GBM glomerulonephritis. Kidney Int. 54: 1166–1174.

42. Boyce NW, Holdsworth SR (1987) Intrarenal hemodynamic alterations induced by anti-GBM antibody. Kidney Int. 31: 8–14.

43. Suzuki Y, Gómez-Guerrero C, Shirato I, López-Franco O, Hernández-Vargas P, et al. (2002) Susceptibility to T cell-mediated injury in immune complex disease is linked to local activation of renin-angiotensin system: the role of NF-AT pathway. J Immunol. 169: 4136–4146.

44. Auffray C, Fogg D, Garfa M, Elain G, Join-Lambert O, et al. (2007) Monitoring of blood vessels and tissues by a population of monocytes with patrolling behavior. Science. 317: 666–670.

45. Devi S, Li A, Westhorpe CL, Lo CY, Abeynaike LD, et al. (2013) Multiphoton imaging reveals a new leukocyte recruitment paradigm in the glomerulus. Nat Med. 19: 107–112.

14

The Reduction of Regional Cerebral Blood Flow in Normal-Appearing White Matter Is Associated with the Severity of White Matter Lesions in Elderly

Jianhui Fu[1,2*◑¶], **Jie Tang**[1◑¶], **Jinghao Han**[3], **Zhen Hong**[1]

1 Department of Neurology, Huashan Hospital, Fudan University, Shanghai, China, **2** Department of Neurology, Shanghai Pudong Hospital, Fudan University Pudong Medical Center, Shanghai, China, **3** Departments of Medicine and Therapeutics, Chinese University of Hong Kong, Prince of Wales Hospital, Hong Kong, China

Abstract

White matter lesions (WMLs) in normal elderly are related to chronic ischemia, and progression of WML occurs mostly in moderate to severe disease. However, the mechanism is uncertain. Thus, we enrolled fifty-six normal elderly patients without large artery disease. The severity of WML on MRI was graded as grade 0, I, II and III using the modified Fazekas scale. Cerebral blood flow (CBF) was measured by Xenon-CT. We found that CBF (mL/100 g/min) within periventricular lesions and in the right and left centrum semiovales were 20.33, 21.27 and 21.03, respectively, in group I; 16.33, 15.55 and 15.91, respectively, in group II; and 14.05, 14.46 and 14.23, respectively, in group III. CBF of normal-appearing white matter (NAWM) around periventricular areas and in the right and left centrum semiovales were 20.79, 22.26 and 22.15, respectively, in group 0; 21.12, 22.17 and 22.25, respectively, in group I; 18.02, 19.45 and 19.62, respectively, in group II; and 16.38, 18.18 and 16.74, respectively, in group III. Significant reductions in CBF were observed not only within lesions but also in NAWM surrounding the lesions. In addition, CBF was reduced significantly within lesions compared to NAWM of the same grade. Furthermore, CBF was reduced significantly in NAWM in grades II and III when compared to grades 0 and I. Our finding indicates that ischemia may play a role in the pathogenesis of WML. Additionally, our finding provides an alternative explanation for finding that the progression of WML occurred more commonly in patients with moderate to severe WML.

Editor: Francisco J. Esteban, University of Jaén, Spain

Funding: This research was supported by grants form the Science and Technology Commission of Shanghai Municipality (Grant NO. 14ZR1437300). The funder had no role in study design, data collection and analysis, decision to publish, and preparation of the manuscript.

Competing Interests: The authors have declared that no competing interests exist.

* Email: jianhuifu@126.com

◑ These authors contributed equally to this work.

¶ These authors are co-first authors on this work.

Introduction

White matter lesions (WMLs) are frequently observed on Flair and T2-weighted brain MRI scans in clinically normal elderly patients and are strongly associated with increasing age [1,2]. Clinical evidence has shown that WMLs are related to a variety of neurological diseases, especially vascular cognitive impairment [3–5]. Anatomical and pathological studies have suggested that chronic ischemia caused by diffuse arteriolosclerosis may contribute to the presence of WML [6–9]. Many studies have found significant reduction in blood flow within the WMLs by measuring cerebral blood flow (CBF) using different technique [10–14]. However, whether a reduction of blood flow is the cause of WML or just a secondary response to the reduced demands of damaged tissue is still unknown.

Using Flair and T2-weighted brain MRI, O'Sullivan et al [11] were the first to report a reduction in CBF in both periventricular WMLs and normal–appearing white matter (NAWM) around periventricular areas. This finding further suggests that chronic ischemia may be the cause of WMLs. If this is the case, areas with NAWM with decreased CBF may develop into WML in long-term follow-up studies. However, there are some limitations in this study that may weaken these important findings. First, all participants had a history of clinical lacunar syndrome, which may be caused by a sudden disruption of blood supply in one of the perforating arteries. Diagnosis of intracranial large artery disease was based on the diameter of the acute infarct on MRI; hence, intracranial large artery disease cannot be completely ruled out. Second, the MMSE score of some participants was less than 24; thus, patients with dementia, including Alzheimer disease, may have been enrolled. Third, the relatively small sample size limited classification of participants by the severity of WML, and as a result, the relationship between the CBF in NAWM regions and WMLs and the severity of the WML is not clear.

More recent longitudinal studies [15–17] have shown that the progression of WML occurred mostly in moderate to severe WML during the following period. All those findings indicated that the severity of WML was associated with the progression of WML. However, the mechanism is uncertain.

Chronic ischemia is the underlying cause of WML; therefore, our hypothesis is that blood flow is decreased not only in white matter lesions but also in areas of NAWM around the lesions and that the reduction of the blood flow in both areas is associated with the severity of WML. To test this hypothesis, we measured CBF within white matter lesions and in normal-appearing white matter around the lesions by Xeon-CT in normal elderly subjects, which may provide further evidence regarding the role of chronic ischemia in the pathogenesis of WML.

Methods

Participants and Data collection

One hundred eighty-three consecutive subjects who visited the outpatient clinic of the neurological department for general health check at Huashan Hospital, Shanghai, China, between October 2006 and June 2007 were studied. All subjects underwent a careful neurological and general physical examination. A history of hypertension, diabetes mellitus, stroke or transient ischemic attack, ischemic heart disease, atrial fibrillation, smoking, and alcohol consumption were also noted. Detailed information on risk factors has been reported previously. This study and its methodology were approved by the Institutional Review Board of Huashan Hospital and by the ethics committee of Huashan Hospital.

Inclusion and Exclusion Criteria

Subjects were enrolled in this study if the following criteria were fulfilled: (1) no history of stroke and atrial fibrillation, (2) MMSE> 24, and (3) no signs or symptoms of neurological manifestations when examined by a neurologist. Subjects younger than 60 years of age or with a history of head trauma or neurosurgery were excluded. Carotid artery ultrasonography was performed in each individual using a color-flow B-mode Doppler ultra-sonography (ATL3000, USA) with a 7.5-MHz imaging transducer. Carotid artery stenosis was defined according to standardized criteria. Subjects with carotid stenosis of >50% lumen diameter reduction were excluded. MR angiography was performed for each individual to rule out intracranial artery stenosis that might interfere with the hemodynamic status. A total of 56 subjects were included in the study and underwent further neuroimaging examinations. The mean age of all participants was 67.4 ± 8.2 (range, 60–79) years, and 34 (60.7%) were men. Each subject signed an informed consent form.

MRI Examinations

Brain MRI examination was performed with a 1.5 T scanner (GE Signa Horizon) using a head coil with quadrature detection. The brain imaging protocol involved (1) T1- and T2-weighted spin-echo axial images (TR/TE 440/14 ms and TR/TE/3000/ 110 ms, respectively) and sagittal T1-weighted images (2) fluid attenuated inversion recovery (FLAIR) axial images (TR/TE 10002/126 ms). All axial images had a 5-mm slice thickness with a 0.5-mm slice gap and a matrix of 256×205.

WMLs were detected as hyperintensity on FLAIR sequence of MRI, without prominent hypointensity on T1-weighted scans, and they were 2 mm or more in diameter on hard copy film. The lesions were classified into four grades according to the modified Fazekas rating scale [18]: grade 0, no lesion (including symmetrical, well defined caps or bands); grade I, focal lesions >2 mm; grade II, beginning confluence of lesions; and grade III, diffuse involvement of the entire region, with or without involvement of U fibers.

Xenon Contrast CT Examinations

Xenon CT was performed within 30 days of the MRI examinations. To match the slices of CT and MR imaging, the

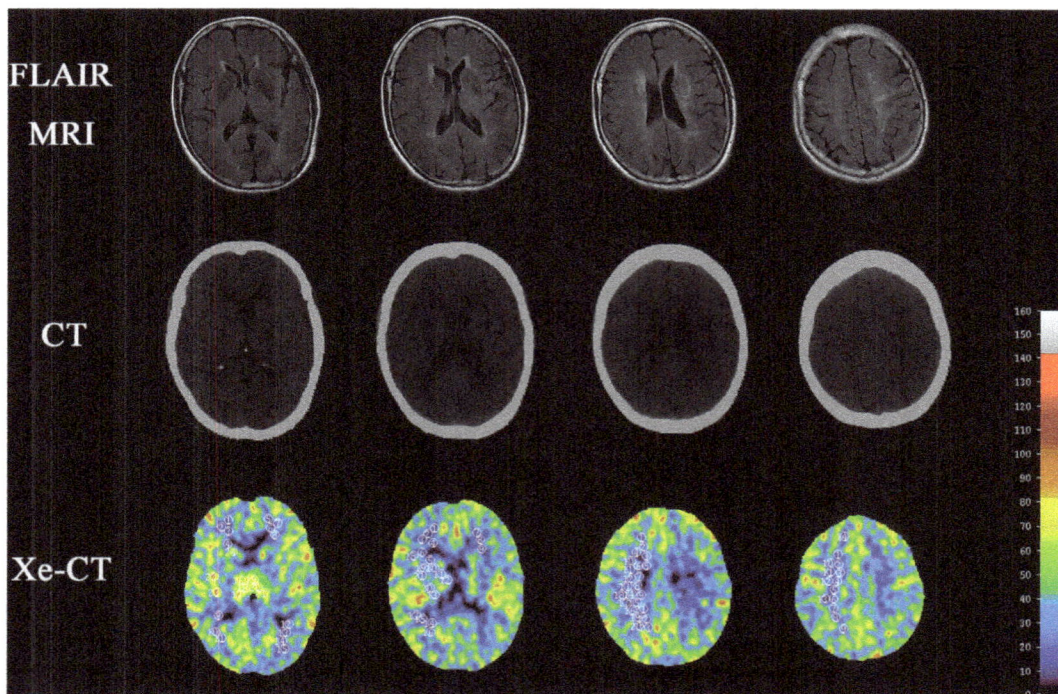

Figure 1. Flair imaging, normal CT and Xe-CT at different levels of subjects with WML.

Table 1. Clinical characteristics of all participants (n = 56) in each grade.

Clinical characteristics	Grade 0 (n = 10)	Grade I (n = 13)	Grade II (n = 17)	Grade III (n = 16)	P*
Age, years, Mean (SD)	65.3±6.3	64.5±5.8	68.9±7.7	68.1±8.1	0.310
Male, n	7	8	11	8	0.672
Hypertension, n	4	5	9	10	0.434
Diabetes mellitus, n	1	1	1	4	0.211
Ischemic heart disease, n	1	0	2	0	0.168
Smoking, n	0	1	1	3	0.269
Alcohol consumption, n	0	0	1	1	0.662

*Compared among the four groups.

CT table was adjusted to the same slice width as that of the MR imaging. An initial conventional CT scan was executed. We examined 4 CT sections that showed that WML matched with MRI on xenon contrast CT scan. Each participant inhaled a gas mixture containing 28% stable xenon, 25% oxygen, and 47% air for 4.3 minutes. For each section, CT scans were performed twice before the xenon inhalation and 4 times during the xenon inhalation. At the end of the study, the results were transferred to a workstation. Data analysis was performed with dedicated post-processing software (Xe-CT System 2; Diversified Diagnostic Products Inc, Houston, TX).

Analysis of Regional CBF

To analyze regional CBF, the whole brain was divided into cortex, white matter and basal ganglia. The cortex was then subdivided into frontal, parietal, occipital and temporal lobes. The white matter region was subdivided into centrum semiovale and periventricular regions (including anterior, lateral and posterior regions of ventricle). The basal ganglia were subdivided into caudate nucleus, lenticular nucleus and thalamus.

To calculate the values of CBF in each region of white matter and basal ganglia, a round ROI (region of interest) of 40 pixels was selected as a measurable unit. We placed the round ROI on each distinct WML or normal-appearing white matter region separately at each section level in each individual, and the mean value of CBF was then calculate for each region (Figure 1). The mean values of CBF in each region of the cortex were calculated automatically by the software. CBF measurement was carried out by the same radiologist.

Statistical Analysis

Statistical analysis software (SAS) 6.12 was used for the statistical analysis. Statistical significance for intergroup differences was assessed by the 2-tailed Fisher's exact test, chi-squared test for categorical variables and Student's t-test for continuous variables. A level of $P<0.05$ was considered statistically significant.

Results

Of the 56 cases, 10 had grade 0 WML, 13 had grade I lesions, 12 had grade II lesions and 16 had grade III lesions. The clinical characteristics of all participants with and without WML are shown in table 1. We did not find any significant differences in age, gender or other vascular risk factors among the different grades of WML.

The mean values of CBF within periventricular lesions and in the right and left centrum semiovales among different WML grades are shown in table 2. The mean CBF (mL/100 g/min)

within lesions in these areas were 20.33 (2.52), 21.27 (1.02) and 21.03 (1.83), respectively, in group I; 16.33 (2.03), 15.55 (1.71) and 15.91 (0.98), respectively, in group II; and 14.05 (2.63), 14.46 (2.17) and 14.23 (1.95), respectively, in group III. Group differences in terms of CBF between different severities of WML were significant ($P<0.05$) within most WML regions.

The mean values of CBF in the periventricular NAWM regions and in right and left centrum semiovales among different grades of WML are shown in table 2. The mean CBF (mL/100 g/min) of NAWM in these areas were 20.79 (2.78), 22.26 (1.9) and 22.15 (2.4), respectively, in group 0; 21.12 (1.50), 22.17 (1.50) and 22.25 (2.13), respectively, in group I; 18.02 (2.41), 19.45 (1.94) and 19.62 (1.54), respectively, in group II; and 16.38 (3.22), 18.18 (2.84) and 16.74 (2.97), respectively, in group III. There is no significant difference in CBF values of NAWM between grade 0 and I. but significant differences ($P<0.05$) in CBF were found in subjects with grade II and III WMLs when compared to those with grade 0 and I WMLs. And the differences in CBF of NAWM between grades II and III WMLs were also significant ($P<0.05$).

A comparison of CBF between NAWM and lesions in the same grade WML is shown in table 2. A significant reduction in CBF was noted in all regions with grade II and III WML when compared with the corresponding areas of NAWM ($P<0.05$). A significant reduction in CBF was also found in some regions with grade I WML when compared with that of NAWM.

A comparison of CBF between different regions in the same grade WML or in the NAWM around the same grade WML is shown in table 3. There were not significant differences ($P>0.05$) in CBF between right or left centrum semiovale area and periventricular area in each grade WML or in the NAWM around the grade I or III WML.

The mean CBF values in various grey matter regions are shown in table 4. Significant reductions in CBF of the bilateral temporal lobes and the lenticular nucleus were observed in grades II and III when compared with CBF of grades 0 and I ($P<0.05$). CBF in other grey matter regions and nuclei did not show significant differences when compared to the flow within WMLs of different severities.

Discussion

Our data showed that the regional cerebral blood flow in white matter lesions and in normal-appearing white matter was decreased in normal elderly with white matter lesions. Moreover, the degree of the decrease was related to the severity of the lesions.

Our study showed ischemia within WMLs, which is consistent with other studies using a variety of techniques to measure CBF [10–14,19]. Furthermore, reductions of CBF within lesions were

Table 2. Mean (SD) CBF (mL/100 g/min) of NAWM and lesions in each grade.

Region	Grade 0 (n = 10)	Grade I (n = 13)			Grade II (n = 17)			Grade III (n-16)		
	NAWM	NAWM	Lesions	P*	NAWM	Lesions	P*	NAWM	Lesions	P*
RLV	21.58±2.33	21.53±2.14	20.67±1.84	0.006	18.52±1.17[1]	17.18±2.42[3]	<0.001	16.80±2.48[1,2]	14.90±2.76[3,4]	<0.001
LLV	23.10±4.31	23.01±4.15	22.14±3.82	0.002	18.82±2.56[1]	16.72±1.84[3]	<0.001	17.21±5.93[1]	13.61±3.51[3,4]	<0.001
RAV	19.97±3.72	20.84±3.44	20.28±2.62	0.247	18.03±3.12[1]	16.52±2.24[3]	0.005	16.13±3.12[1]	13.97±2.19[3,4]	0.004
LAV	19.81±3.48	21.67±3.59	20.80±2.72	0.053	17.17±2.47[1]	15.19±1.91[3]	<0.001	16.08±2.96[1]	13.66±2.64[3]	<0.001
RPV	19.39±2.26	19.72±2.29	18.48±2.13	0.224	18.84±2.57	17.53±2.19	<0.001	16.83±2.45[1,2]	14.25±2.29[3,4]	<0.001
LPV	20.88±2.54	19.97±2.06	19.61±1.98	0.172	16.72±2.56[1]	14.86±1.55[3]	0.001	15.23±2.38[1]	13.90±2.40[3]	<0.001
WPV	20.79±2.78	21.12±2.95	20.33±2.52	0.106	18.02±2.41[1]	16.33±2.03[3]	<0.001	16.38±3.22[1,2]	14.05±2.63[3,4]	<0.001
RCS	22.26±1.9	22.17±1.50	21.27±1.02	0.017	19.45±1.94[1]	15.55±1.71[3]	<0.001	18.18±2.84[1]	14.46±2.17[3]	<0.001
LCS	22.15±2.4	22.25±2.13	21.03±1.83	0.003	19.62±1.54[1]	15.91±0.98[3]	<0.001	16.74±2.97[1,2]	14.23±1.95[3,4]	<0.001

P* refers to CBF within lesions compared to that in NAWM in the same group.
[1] Compared with grades 0 and I, CBF of NAWM in grades II and III, P value <0.05;
[2] compared with grade II, CBF of NAWM in grade III, P value <0.05.
[3] Compared with grade I, CBF within lesions in groups II and III, P value <0.05;
[4] compared with grade II, CBF within lesions in group III, P value <0.05.
NAWM means normal-appearing white matter. RLV means right lateral of ventricle, LLV means left lateral of ventricle; RAV means right anterior of ventricle, LAV means left anterior of ventricle; RPV means right posterior of ventricle, LPV means left posterior of ventricle; WPV means whole periventricular areas; RCS means right centrum semiovale, LCS means left centrum semiovale.

Table 3. Mean (SD) CBF values (mL/100 g/min) in different area in each grade.

	Region	RCS	WPV	P*	LCS	WPV	P*
Grade I (n=13)	NAWM	22.17±1.50	21.12±2.95	0.095	22.25±2.13	21.12±2.95	0.026
	Lesions	21.27±1.02	20.33±2.52	0.075	21.03±1.83	20.33±2.52	0.107
Grade II (n=17)	NAWM	19.45±1.94	18.02±2.41	0.004	19.62±1.54	18.02±2.41	0.007
	Lesions	15.55±1.71	16.33±2.03	0.067	15.91±0.98	16.33±2.03	0.242
Grade III (n=16)	NAWM	18.18±2.84	16.38±3.22	0.010	16.74±2.97	16.38±3.22	0.604
	Lesions	14.46±2.17	14.05±2.63	0.277	14.23±1.95	14.05±2.63	0.729

P* refers to CBF comparison between different areas in the same group. NAWM means normal-appearing white matter, WPV means whole periventricular areas; RCS means right centrum semiovale, LCS means left centrum semiovale.

associated with the severity of WMLs in both the centrum semiovale and the periventricular regions. Using xenon contrast CT methods, Miyazawa et al [10] found a similar reduction in CBF in the centrum semiovale in a group of neurological normal elderly without large artery disease. But they did not measure the CBF within WMLs in the periventricular regions because subjects with periventricular WMLs were excluded in their study. Hatazawa et al [13] found a reduction in blood flow within the WML using the positron emission tomographic (PET). However, there was no significant difference in CBF between subjects with severe and mild WML. The limitations of the study included a relatively small sample size and poor spatial resolution of PET to differentiate normal and abnormal white matter, which may underestimate the reduction of cerebral blood flow.

The most important finding of our study is that the reduction of CBF is not only in WML areas but also in NAWM areas around the lesion, and the CBF in WML is lower than in NAWM areas around it. Using 1.5 T MRI and 99 mTc single-photo emission computed tomography (SPECT), a recent study [19] found that the WMH perfusion was lower than NAWM perfusion in normal elderly, which is consistent of our results. Using Flair and T2-weighted brain MRI, O'Sullivan [11] also found a reduction of CBF in the periventricular lesions when compared to areas with normal-appearing white matter. However, a similar reduction in CBF was not observed in the centrum semiovale, and the reduction in CBF in NAWM regions was not associated with the severity of WML. Recent study found that microstructural deterioration within NAWM in cerebral small vessel diseases by DTI [20], and the decrease of CBF in NAWM exhibited in our results may be a possible explanation of this finding. Therefore, combining the DTI and flair images can better assess the white matter changes [21]. Our finding of reduced CBF in both WML and NAWM regions provides further evidence that chronic ischemia may play a role in the pathogenesis of WML in the centrum semiovale and periventricular regions.

Neuro-epidemiological studies showed that the progression of WMLs occurred mostly in moderate to severe WML but seldom in mild WML during the follow-up period [15–17]. In our study, The CBF in NAWM surrounding grades II and III WML areas was substantially lower than that surrounding grades 0 and I WML areas, which means that even look like normal form MRI imaging, in fact, the hypoperfusion in areas around WML in grades II and III is serious. Recently, a prospective study showed that the changes of NAWM precede visually appreciable WML that was only the tip of the iceberg of white matter alteration [22]. The significant decline of CBF in NAWM surrounding moderate or severe WML observed by us suggests the grade II or III WML may be more likely to develop than grade I WML. However, the relationship between the CBF in NAWM and the progression of WML needs to be evaluated in longitudinal studies.

Although there has been some controversy regarding whether WML in centrum semiovale and in periventricular regions represent distinct subcategories of WML or should be considered as a continuum [6,8,23–25], our data indicated that WMLs in the centrum semiovale and in the periventricular regions may share a common underlying chronic ischemic mechanism. We found that reduction of CBF is only associated with the severity but not the location of the lesions. Our results are consistent with evidence from anatomical and pathological studies [6–8,25]. Blood supply in the centrum semiovale and periventricular regions come from long perforating arterioles with few collateral compensation; thus, these areas are considered watershed areas, which are more vulnerable to the assault by hypoperfusion caused by the fluctuation in blood pressure [7]. Pathological studies [6,8] have

Table 4. Mean (SD) CBF values (mL/100 g/min) of grey matter regions in each grade.

Gray matter region	Grade 0 (n = 10)	Grade I (n = 13)	Grade II (n = 17)	Grade III (n = 16)	P
R frontal lobe	48.00±10.62	51.67±10.83	46.58±14.48	46.48±10.71	0.448
L frontal lobe	47.46±10.65	50.39±10.33	43.39±15.56	42.34±10.13	0.192
R temporal lobe	53.04±7.71	56.06±10.33	48.92±15.56[1]	47.21±10.13[1]	0.010
L temporal lobe	50.76±7.02	53.80±5.59	45.86±8.07[1]	43.29±9.86[1]	0.004
R parietal lobe	48.85±11.17	51.83±14.21	45.99±14.82	47.31±9.99	0.469
L parietal lobe	45.49±8.44	48.43±10.10	42.87±12.9	42.60±11.02	0.330
R occipital lobe	46.16±6.73	47.88±7.05	43.98±8.72	44.29±8.06	0.370
L occipital lobe	44.58±6.11	45.53±7.19	44.08±9.14	41.72±7.29	0.435
R caudate nucleus	71.99±12.16	74.66±9.29	68.92±10.75	66.78±17.89	0.283
L caudate nucleus	69.61±7.55	67.91±11.16	65.51±11.77	60.28±10.28	0.214
R lenticular nucleus	72.67±14.82	79.37±10.57	67.96±13.45[1]	67.54±11.15[1]	0.027
L lenticular nucleus	78.61±10.07	81.29±6.99	75.70±12.38[1]	72.17±11.62[1,2]	0.032
R thalamus	83.34±12.25	84.26±12.56	79.80±10.72	80.01±11.91	0.533
L thalamus	83.29±12.41	84.17±11.55	81.94±9.16	81.46±12.88	0.339

[1]Compared with grades 0 and I, CBF in grades II and III, P value <0.05;
[2]compared with grade II, CBF in grade III, P value <0.05. R means right side, L means left side.

also demonstrated that vascular fibrosis and lipohyalinosis were observed in the centrum semiovale and the periventricular regions. DeCarli et al [25] failed to identify distinct subcategories of lesions located in the centrum semiovale and the periventricular regions using a MRI 3D mapping technique. All the aforementioned studies suggest that categorical distinctions between these two regions may be arbitrary.

Notably, in our study, a higher severity of WMLs was associated with lower regional CBF in bilateral temporal lobes and the lenticular nucleus. Reductions of CBF in the basal ganglia have also been reported by a PET study with $H_2^{15}O$ and $^{15}O_2$ that was performed in subjects with or without WML [13], but we are the first to show an association between reduced CBF in the temporal lobe and the severity of WML. The values of CBF in each lobe were calculated automatically by the software to avoid methodological bias; thus, the results are reliable. Two points may help explain the association between the severity of WMLs and the decrease of CBF in temporal lobe and lenticular nucleus. First, WML is strongly associated with increasing age and arteriolosclerosis is a systemic disease, we believe that apart from white matter lesions, reduced blood supply in the vascular bed due to brain atrophy may also contribute to the relatively low blood flow. Second, the connectional diaschisis may also an alternative explanation of those results. The cortical-subcortical circuits go though the centrum semiovale and periventricular white matter, and the ischemia in whiter matter may lead to the dysfunction of brain network, which may contribute to connectional diaschisis [26,27] that further cause the reduction of CBF in remote areas by the impaired neurovascular coupling [28].

The spatial limitation of xenon-CT must be considered when interpreting our results. As the sensitivity of CT in detecting WML is lower than MRI, it is difficult to discriminate normal-appearing white matter from the white matter lesions on xenon-CT mapping completely. The drawing of ROI may be arbitrary to some extent even though we compared the lesions on MRI and CT carefully before calculating the values of CBF. To minimize the measurement error, all the ROI analyses were completed by the same radiologist.

In summary, we found that the reductions of CBF not only in WML but also in NAWM regions were associated with the severity of WML in the centrum semiovale and the periventricular regions in neurologically normal elderly subjects without large artery occlusive disease. The reduction of CBF in bilateral temporal lobes and the lenticular nucleus further support our hypothesis that chronic ischemia may play a major role in the pathogenesis of WML. Moreover, our findings might provide an alternative explanation for the phenomenon that progression of WML occurs more commonly in patients with moderate to severe WML. Long-term follow-up studies may help to know if NAWM regions with reduced CBF further develop into white matter lesions, and help to generate a causal relationship between chronic ischemia and WML.

Author Contributions

Conceived and designed the experiments: JF ZH. Performed the experiments: JF JT JH. Analyzed the data: JF JT JH. Contributed to the writing of the manuscript: JF JT JH ZH.

References

1. Grueter BE, Schulz UG (2012) Age-related cerebral white matter disease (leukoaraiosis): a review. Postgrad Med J 88: 79–87.
2. O'Sullivan M (2008) Leukoaraiosis. Pract Neurol 8: 26–38.
3. Nichtweiss M, Weidauer S, Treusch N, Hattingen E (2012) White matter lesions and vascular cognitive impairment: part 1: typical and unusual causes. Clin Neuroradiol 22: 193–210.
4. Poggesi A, Gouw A, van der Flier W, Pracucci G, Chabriat H, et al. (2013) Cerebral white matter changes are associated with abnormalities on neurological examination in non-disabled elderly: the LADIS study. J Neurol 260: 1014–1021.
5. Schmidt R, Ropele S, Ferro J, Madureira S, Verdelho A, et al. (2010) Diffusion-weighted imaging and cognition in the leukoariosis and disability in the elderly study. Stroke 41: e402–408.
6. Fazekas F, Kleinert R, Offenbacher H, Schmidt R, Kleinert G, et al. (1993) Pathologic correlates of incidental MRI white matter signal hyperintensities. Neurology 43: 1683–1689.

7. Pantoni L, Garcia JH (1997) Pathogenesis of leukoaraiosis: a review. Stroke 28: 652–659.

8. Auriel E, Bornstein NM, Berenyi E, Varkonyi I, Gabor M, et al. (2011) Clinical, radiological and pathological correlates of leukoaraiosis. Acta Neurol Scand 123: 41–47.

9. Brown WR, Thore CR (2011) Review: cerebral microvascular pathology in ageing and neurodegeneration. Neuropathol Appl Neurobiol 37: 56–74.

10. Miyazawa N, Satoh T, Hashizume K, Fukamachi A (1997) Xenon contrast CT-CBF measurements in high-intensity foci on T2-weighted MR images in centrum semiovale of asymptomatic individuals. Stroke 28: 984–987.

11. O'Sullivan M, Lythgoe DJ, Pereira AC, Summers PE, Jarosz JM, et al. (2002) Patterns of cerebral blood flow reduction in patients with ischemic leukoaraiosis. Neurology 59: 321–326.

12. Fu JH, Yuan J, Li S, Guo QH, Hong Z, et al. (2009) [Quantitative analysis of regional cerebral blood flow in elderly with white matter lesions]. Zhonghua Yi Xue Za Zhi 89: 1175–1178.

13. Hatazawa J, Shimosegawa E, Satoh T, Toyoshima H, Okudera T (1997) Subcortical hypoperfusion associated with asymptomatic white matter lesions on magnetic resonance imaging. Stroke 28: 1944–1947.

14. Uh J, Yezhuvath U, Cheng Y, Lu H (2010) In vivo vascular hallmarks of diffuse leukoaraiosis. J Magn Reson Imaging 32: 184–190.

15. Schmidt R, Enzinger C, Ropele S, Schmidt H, Fazekas F (2003) Progression of cerebral white matter lesions: 6-year results of the Austrian Stroke Prevention Study. Lancet 361: 2046–2048.

16. Firbank MJ, Teodorczuk A, van der Flier WM, Gouw AA, Wallin A, et al. (2012) Relationship between progression of brain white matter changes and late-life depression: 3-year results from the LADIS study. Br J Psychiatry 201: 40–45.

17. Kreisel SH, Blahak C, Bazner H, Inzitari D, Pantoni L, et al. (2013) Deterioration of gait and balance over time: the effects of age-related white matter change–the LADIS study. Cerebrovasc Dis 35: 544–553.

18. Wahlund LO, Barkhof F, Fazekas F, Bronge L, Augustin M, et al. (2001) A new rating scale for age-related white matter changes applicable to MRI and CT. Stroke 32: 1318–1322.

19. Makedonov I, Black SE, MacIntosh BJ (2013) Cerebral small vessel disease in aging and Alzheimer's disease: a comparative study using MRI and SPECT. Eur J Neurol 20: 243–250.

20. Papma JM, de Groot M, de Koning I, Mattace-Raso FU, van der Lugt A, et al. (2014) Cerebral small vessel disease affects white matter microstructure in mild cognitive impairment. Hum Brain Mapp 35: 2836–2851.

21. Zhan W, Zhang Y, Mueller SG, Lorenzen P, Hadjidemetriou S, et al. (2009) Characterization of white matter degeneration in elderly subjects by magnetic resonance diffusion and FLAIR imaging correlation. Neuroimage 47 Suppl 2: T58–65.

22. de Groot M, Verhaaren BF, de Boer R, Klein S, Hofman A, et al. (2013) Changes in normal-appearing white matter precede development of white matter lesions. Stroke 44: 1037–1042.

23. Sachdev P, Wen W, Chen X, Brodaty H (2007) Progression of white matter hyperintensities in elderly individuals over 3 years. Neurology 68: 214–222.

24. Gouw AA, Seewann A, van der Flier WM, Barkhof F, Rozemuller AM, et al. (2011) Heterogeneity of small vessel disease: a systematic review of MRI and histopathology correlations. J Neurol Neurosurg Psychiatry 82: 126–135.

25. DeCarli C, Fletcher E, Ramey V, Harvey D, Jagust WJ (2005) Anatomical mapping of white matter hyperintensities (WMH): exploring the relationships between periventricular WMH, deep WMH, and total WMH burden. Stroke 36: 50–55.

26. Carrera E, Tononi G (2014) Diaschisis: past, present, future. Brain.

27. Lawrence AJ, Chung AW, Morris RG, Markus HS, Barrick TR (2014) Structural network efficiency is associated with cognitive impairment in small-vessel disease. Neurology.

28. Hall CN, Reynell C, Gesslein B, Hamilton NB, Mishra A, et al. (2014) Capillary pericytes regulate cerebral blood flow in health and disease. Nature 508: 55–60.

15

Variation of Densitometry on Computed Tomography in COPD – Influence of Different Software Tools

Mark O. Wielpütz[1,2,3,4]*, **Diana Bardarova**[1,2,3], **Oliver Weinheimer**[1,2], **Hans-Ulrich Kauczor**[1,2,3], **Monika Eichinger**[1,2,3], **Bertram J. Jobst**[1,2,3], **Ralf Eberhardt**[5], **Marcel Koenigkam-Santos**[1,2,3,4], **Michael Puderbach**[1,2,3,4], **Claus P. Heussel**[1,2,3]

1 Department of Diagnostic and Interventional Radiology, University Hospital of Heidelberg, Heidelberg, Germany, 2 Translational Lung Research Center Heidelberg (TLRC), Member of the German Center for Lung Research (DZL), Heidelberg, Germany, 3 Department of Diagnostic and Interventional Radiology with Nuclear Medicine, Thoraxklinik at University of Heidelberg, Heidelberg, Germany, 4 Department of Radiology, German Cancer Research Center (dkfz), Heidelberg, Germany, 5 Department of Pneumology and Respiratory Critical Care Medicine, Thoraxklinik at University of Heidelberg, Heidelberg, Germany

Abstract

Objectives: Quantitative multidetector computed tomography (MDCT) as a potential biomarker is increasingly used for severity assessment of emphysema in chronic obstructive pulmonary disease (COPD). Aim of this study was to evaluate the user-independent measurement variability between five different fully-automatic densitometry software tools.

Material and Methods: MDCT and full-body plethysmography incl. forced expiratory volume in 1s and total lung capacity were available for 49 patients with advanced COPD (age = 64 ± 9 years, forced expiratory volume in 1s = $31 \pm 6\%$ predicted). Measurement variation regarding lung volume, emphysema volume, emphysema index, and mean lung density was evaluated for two scientific and three commercially available lung densitometry software tools designed to analyze MDCT from different scanner types.

Results: One scientific tool and one commercial tool failed to process most or all datasets, respectively, and were excluded. One scientific and another commercial tool analyzed 49, the remaining commercial tool 30 datasets. Lung volume, emphysema volume, emphysema index and mean lung density were significantly different amongst these three tools ($p < 0.001$). Limits of agreement for lung volume were [−0.195, −0.052l], [−0.305, −0.131l], and [−0.123, −0.052l] with correlation coefficients of $r = 1.00$ each. Limits of agreement for emphysema index were [−6.2, 2.9%], [−27.0, 16.9%], and [−25.5, 18.8%], with $r = 0.79$ to 0.98. Correlation of lung volume with total lung capacity was good to excellent ($r = 0.77$ to 0.91, $p < 0.001$), but segmented lung volume (6.7 ± 1.3 – $6.8 \pm 1.3l$) were significantly lower than total lung capacity ($7.7 \pm 1.7l$, $p < 0.001$).

Conclusions: Technical incompatibilities hindered evaluation of two of five tools. The remaining three showed significant measurement variation for emphysema, hampering quantitative MDCT as a biomarker in COPD. Follow-up studies should currently use identical software, and standardization efforts should encompass software as well.

Editor: Heinz Fehrenbach, Research Center Borstel, Germany

Funding: This study was supported by grants from the Bundesministerium für Bildung und Forschung (www.bmbf.de) to the German Center for Lung Research (DZL) (82DZL00401, 82DZL00402, 82DZL00404). The funders had no role in study design, data collection and analysis, decision to publish, or preparation of the manuscript.

Competing Interests: The authors have declared that no competing interests exist.

* Email: mark.wielpuetz@med.uni-heidelberg.de

Introduction

Chest multidetector computed tomography (MDCT) remains the gold standard for imaging-based phenotyping of cigarette smoke-induced chronic obstructive pulmonary disease (COPD) [1,2]. Two main features, related to distinct clinical phenotypes, may be assessed: airway remodeling and emphysema [3–7]. Densitometry of the lung parenchyma based on Hounsfield units (HU) is currently the method of choice for non-invasive objective emphysema quantification [1,8,9]. As such it has been implemented in various clinical trials including the COPDGene study

[10,11]. Its acceptance in clinical routine is rapidly broadening, leading to an implementation into the workflow of interventional emphysema therapy in many specialized centers [12]. Usually, lung volumes with a density lower than the commonly used threshold of −950 HU are accepted as emphysema [3]. Densitometry of emphysema varies with inspiration depth [13,14], exposure parameters incl. low-dose scans [15,16], and reconstruction settings incl. kernel, iterative algorithms vs. filtered back-projection, and slice thickness [17–20]. Between different scanner manufacturers variation of lung density and emphysema is

thought to be reproducible within close margins using similar scanning and reconstruction parameters [16]. For a large multicenter trial (COPDGene), a dedicated lung phantom was employed to allow for inter-center quality control aimed at standardized examination parameters [10]. A broad standardization of densitometry including repeat calibration of the individual setup at each site encompassing the individual scanner, reconstruction and the post-processing software with dedicated emphysema phantoms is currently missing. However, these steps are essential in the implementation of densitometry as a routine imaging-derived biomarker across different centers, comparable to efforts undertaken for laboratory testing of biomarkers, e.g. for blood samples [21]. In a previous report more than seven years ago, we compared different software tools, which needed user-interaction to complete lung segmentation and implied processing times around 59–105 minutes per patient [22]. Since then, development in software algorithms and computer performance has led to the introduction of several scientific and also commercially available tools, which warrant automatic lung segmentation and densitometry within the work-up of a routine diagnostic chest MDCT scan, delivering emphysema quantification without user-interaction. At present, there is also no clear consensus on which parameters should be measured, and how the respective software algorithms should work in emphysema quantification. This leads to an often confusing usage of different terminology between different software. None of these tools, have been validated against each other, and measurement variation between different software tools is not known. Therefore, the present study was conducted to determine the measurement variation between two commercially available state-of-the-art products and an in-house scientific tool for emphysema quantification based on the identical MDCT examinations of advanced COPD patients suffering from emphysema.

Materials and Methods

Ethics Statement

The study was carried out as a retrospective analysis of clinically indicated MDCT performed in July 2012, and has been approved by the Ethics Committee of the Medical Faculty of the University of Heidelberg. Informed written consent for examination and further data processing was obtained from patients or legal guardians.

Patient Population

49 COPD patients referred to MDCT for the evaluation of endoscopic lung volume reduction procedures were enrolled into the study. Table 1 shows a summary of the patients' clinical characteristics.

Pulmonary Function Testing

Whole-body plethysmography (MasterScreen Body, E. Jaeger, Hoechberg, Germany) was performed according to the guidelines of the European Respiratory Society and the standards of the American Thoracic Society (ATS) [23], and the European Coal and Steal Community (ECSC) predicted values served as the standard of reference [24]. The following lung function parameters (absolute and percent predicted values) were used for further analysis: forced expiratory volume in 1s (FEV1), residual volume (RV), and total lung capacity (TLC). To estimate the degree of hyperinflation, the RV to TLC ratio was calculated (RV/TLC).

Multidetector Computed Tomography

Exclusively non-enhanced thin-section MDCT was routinely performed in supine position as recommended for COPD [4,25]. Before scanning, all patients received an instructed training to achieve full end-inspiratory breath-hold. All patients were examined with a 4-slice Volume Zoom helical computer tomograph (Siemens Medical Solutions AG, Forchheim, Germany) with a dose-modulated protocol at 120 kV, 70 mAs effective, a collimation of 1.25 mm, and pitch 2 leading to a typical breath-hold length of 19 s. Reconstruction was performed with a slice thickness of 1.25 mm and 1.0 mm increment in a medium soft B40f algorithm as recommended for densitometry [3,6]. The scale of attenuation coefficients with this system ranges from −1,024 to +3,072 HU. The system was calibrated for water quarterly and after major maintenance, and for air daily. All examinations were visually inspected by a reader with more than 5 years of experience in chest radiology for adequate inspiration, absence of significant motion artifacts and inclusion of all parts of the chest, similar to the inclusion criteria of the COPDGene study [10]. Minor respiratory artifacts were accepted, if they did not impair diagnostic image quality, e.g. slight diaphragmatic motion. The examination protocol and equipment were kept constant during the study period.

Quantitative MDCT Densitometry Tools

YACTA. YACTA ("yet another CT analyzer") (version 1.1, programming by O. W.) analyzed each stack of around 300 images per patient fully automatically, as employed in previous studies [6,25–27]. YACTA operates in a server-mode and may receive DICOM data directly from the PACS system. Because it is an in-house software, the exact steps of lung and airway segmentation, and emphysema quantification are controlled for and described in detail elsewhere [28,29]. Neither user interaction nor manual correction of the segmentation were carried out. A lung voxel was assigned to emphysema if its density equaled or was below the threshold of −950 HU [1,3], with a noise correction for voxels with −910 to −949HU that needed at least 4 adjacent voxels with a density of < −950 HU. The following variables were computed and exported as a structured report and to an in-house scientific data-base for further analysis: lung volume (LV), lung weight, trachea volume, emphysema volume (EV), emphysema surface, emphysema index (EI), mean lung density (MLD), and 15th percentile of lung density histogram. Transfer of the results sheet into the PACS was not available. Measurement results and processing time were recorded for further analysis.

LowATT. Aquarius is a commercially available visualization software package (version 4.4.7, TeraRecon, Foster City, California, USA). For emphysema quantification the integrated semi-automated tool LowATT was employed. The MDCT datasets were sent from the PACS to the respective post-processing server. Then each patient was loaded manually into the software surface on a dedicated workstation. A pre-selection of the emphysema threshold is possible, and the interval from −1024 to −950 HU was used for the present study. Results are presented as a color-coded emphysema visualization in multiplanar reformats (MPR) and a results sheet, which may be sent back to the PACS. The following parameters were calculated by lowATT: lung volume (equals LV), low attenuation volume (equals EV) and low attenuation volume in percent (equals EI). Mean lung density was not available. Measurement results and processing time were thus recorded for further analysis.

Pulmo 3D. Syngo.Via (version VA20B, Siemens Medical Solutions, Forchheim, Germany) is a commercial post-processing software environment for routine diagnostics. The MDCT

Table 1. Patient characteristics.

Number of subjects	49
Age (years)	64±9
Male/female	24/25
Pack years	39±22
Weight (kg)	66.2±13.3
BMI (kg/m²)	23.3±2.6
GOLD I/II/III/IV	1/1/26/21
FEV1 (l/s)	0.8±0.3
FEV1 (%)	31±6
TLC (l)	7.7±1.7
TLC (%)	128±11
RV (l)	5.3±1.4
RV (%)	230±31

BMI = body mass index, FEV1 = forced expiratory volume in 1 s, TLC = total lung capacity, RV = residual volume. Percentage values refer to the predicted volumes.

datasets were sent from the PACS to the respective post-processing server. Then each patient was loaded manually into the integrated tool Pulmo 3D for densitometry. The emphysema threshold can be selected manually, and −950 HU was chosen as for the other software. Densitometry results are displayed as color-coded emphysema maps in MPR and a results sheet, which may be sent back to the PACS. Parameters measured were: lung volume (equals LV), mean lung density (equals MLD), full width at half maximum of lung density histogram, and low attenuation volume in percent (equals EI). The EV needed to be calculated manually by multiplying low attenuation volume in percent with lung volume. Measurement results and processing time were thus recorded for further analysis.

Software excluded from analysis. Initially, we intended to study another free open-source scientific tool as well as a commercial product platform by a large vendor. The open-source tool could interpret 11 from 49 (22%) datasets only, with an unexpected halt during the segmentation process of the remaining 38 datasets. Adequate error management possibilities were not available to the average user. The commercial tool loaded all datasets into the viewer, but halted during segmentation in all datasets. There was no possibility to correct the error by the user. Thus, both tools were excluded from further analysis.

Statistical Analysis

Computational results were reviewed by a reader with more than 5 years of expertise in chest radiology, preceding their statistical evaluation. All data were recorded in a dedicated database (Excel, Microsoft Corp., Redmond, USA) and analyzed using SigmaPlot (Systat Software GmbH, Erkrath, Germany) software. Parametric data are displayed as mean ± standard deviation, non-parametric data as median ± median average deviation. Measurement results with similar meaning provided all three software tools are segmented LV (l), segmented EV (l) and EI (%), which were used for statistical comparison by repeated measures analysis of variance (RM ANOVA) (LV, EV) or RM ANOVA on ranks (EI) with post-hoc tests as appropriate. MLD in HU was computed by YACTA and Pulmo 3D only, and compared by Wilcoxon signed rank test. In a tandem analysis differences were plotted against the mean of two methods by using the approach described by Bland and Altman [30]. We also

calculated coefficients of variation as the ratio of the standard deviation of the mean inter-software difference to the mean difference of both measurements. LV, EV and EI were correlated with lung function tests, and Pearson correlation coefficient or Spearman rank order correlation coefficient r were computed as appropriate. A p-value of<0.05, corrected with the Bonferroni-Holm method in case of multiple comparisons, was considered statistically significant [31].

Results

Data processing

All 49 (100%) datasets were evaluated by YACTA without user interaction within a runtime of around 3 minutes per patient, depending on the amount of emphysema. No obvious segmentation errors regarding airways or lung volume were observed upon inspection of the results in the three-dimensional MPR mode. LowATT completely evaluated all 49 (100%) datasets also, without any unexpected halt during data processing. Mean runtime was below 3 minutes per patient from sending the patient to the server to completion of the results. A review of the segmentation results by color-coded MPR revealed, that in 17 cases (35%) central airways were segmented as emphysema; in a single case the left lung was segmented as belonging to the airway tree (Figure 1). These cases first remained in the analysis, because the intention of our study was an user-independent approach. Pulmo 3D could process 30 of the 49 (61%) datasets loaded into the viewer in less than 3 minutes, but failed to generate results for the remaining 19 datasets, without providing a specific error protocol or management. The 30 datasets processed were included into the analysis and did not show obvious errors in airways or lung segmentation upon inspection of the color-coded MPR. In 9 out of 17 cases in which lowATT delivered erroneous results segmenting central airways as emphysema, Pulmo 3D did not process the dataset at all. Only 21 (43%) datasets altogether were processed without obvious segmentation errors by all of the three software tools.

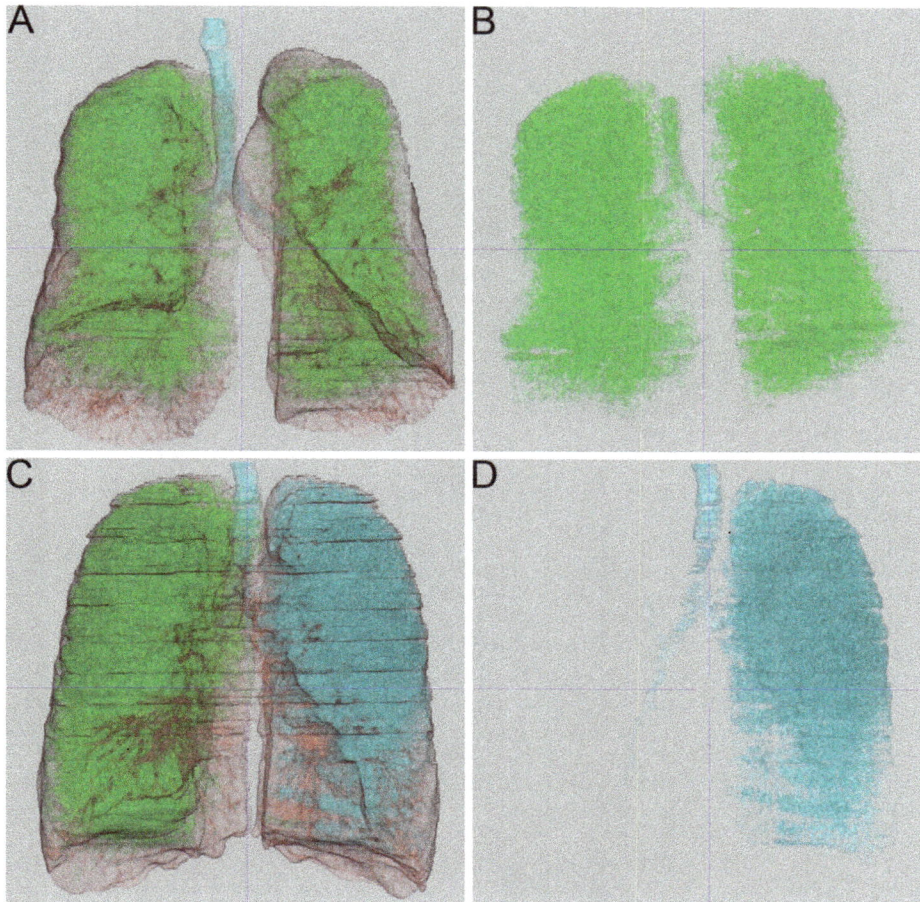

Figure 1. Emphysema visualization by density maps. Every software offered volume-rendering of segmented central airways (highlighted in blue), lung (brown) and emphysema (green). Leakage of the segmentation algorithms from airways into the parenchyma and vice versa are frequent sources of error in densitometry on computed tomography datasets, which results in faulty results or unexpected halt of the software tool. A, B 73–year-old patient, FEV1 = 43%, emphysema index calculated with 37% and 40%, not processed by the third software tool. A suggests correct segmentation of airways and emphysema, whereas isolated display of emphysema in B demonstrates that the software has assigned the airway tree actually also to the emphysema volume. C, D 52–year-old patient, FEV1 = 20%, emphysema index calculated with 41% and 45%, not processed by the third software tool. Visualization of the segmented airways and emphysema in C, and selective display of the segmented airways in D show that airway segmentation leaked into the left lung. Respiratory artifacts can be appreciated in C, which have obscured the airway wall of segmental airways on the left side.

Variation of lung volume, emphysema volume and emphysema index

To test whether the software tools deliver similar measurements, we compared the output variables LV, EV and EI. The means of these were significantly different amongst all three tools (p<0.001) (Table 2). Figure 2 and Table 3 summarize the results of a tandem comparison of the three tools. For LV, the largest differences were seen for Pulmo 3D vs. YACTA with a mean difference of -0.218 l and limits of agreement as wide as -0.305 to -0.131 l. For EV, Pulmo 3D vs. lowATT had a low mean difference of -0.051 l, but the widest limits of agreement from -0.575 to 0.473 l. In the case of EI, which is computed from LV and EV, differences ranged from -5.0 to -1.7%. The limits of agreement were max. -25.5 to 18.8% again for Pulmo 3D vs. lowATT. MLD could be compared for Pulmo 3D vs. YACTA only, delivering a difference of -21 HU and limits of agreement from -28 to -16 HU (Table 3).

We repeated the comparison of the measurement results with the remaining 21 datasets after removal of those with obvious segmentation errors (Tables S1 and S2). Importantly, even after this manual interaction densitometry results for LV, EV, EI and MLD remained significantly different between the three tools (Table S1). The mean differences, limits of agreement and coefficients of variation between the software tools for LV, EV and MLD were not changed substantially. Only regarding EI, differences were now lower than 2%, and limits of agreement did not exceed $\pm 8\%$ (Table S2).

Correlation with lung function testing

A previous study in patients with COPD suggested that plethysmography may overestimate TLC in obstructive lung disease [32]. In the absence of another standard of reference, we compared segmented lung volumes derived from the three softwares to TLC measured by lung function testing. Usually, this is done to validate whether MDCT was performed at full inspiratory breath hold. We found that segmented LV (6.7 ± 1.3–6.8 ± 1.3 l) were significantly lower than TLC (7.7 ± 1.7 l) (p< 0.001) as expected (Table 1 and 2). Correlation of lung volumes

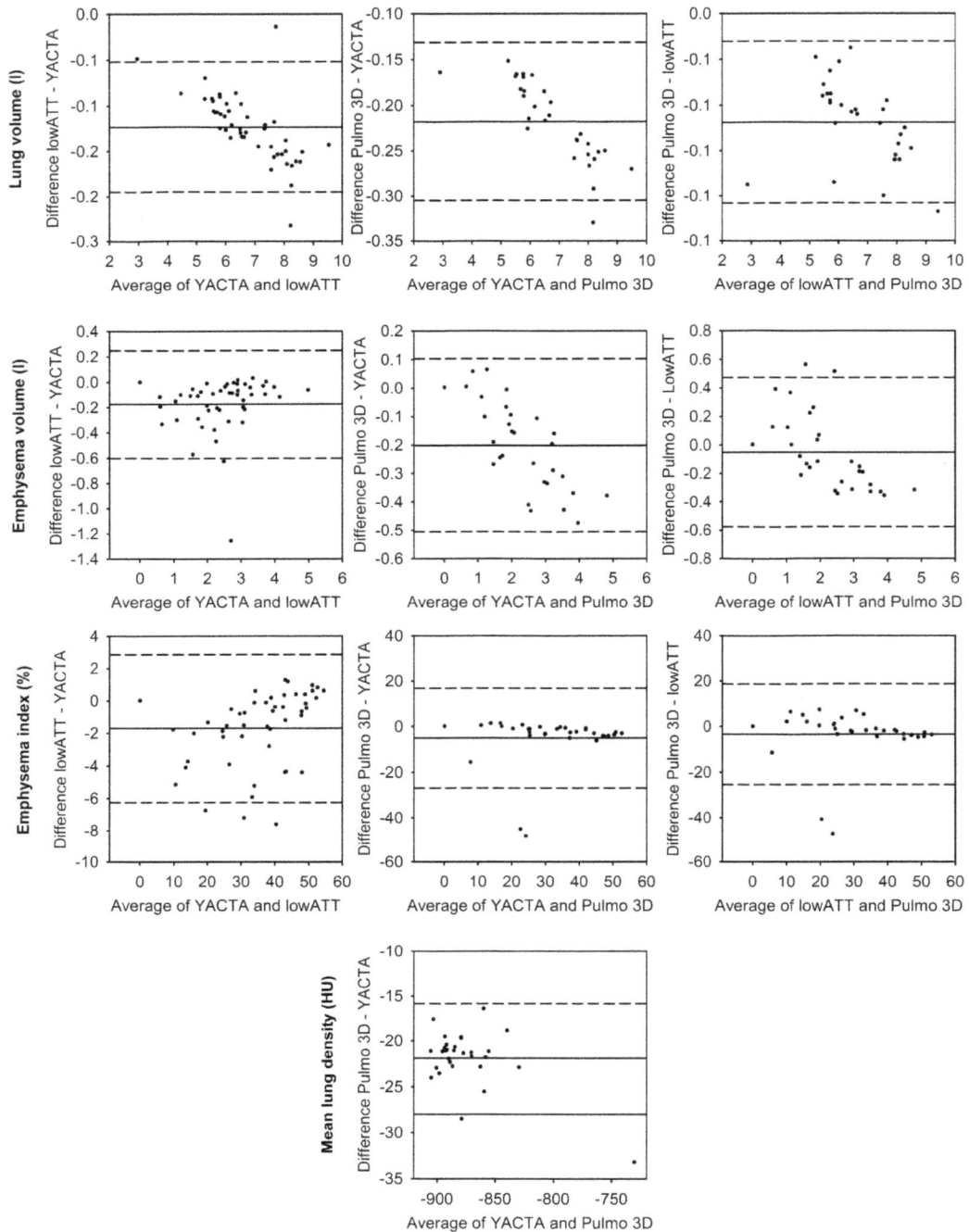

Figure 2. Variation of densitometry. Bland-Altman-plots are given for each inter-software comparison for lung volume, emphysema volume, emphysema index and mean lung density. The central line indicates the mean difference and the dashed lines indicate upper and lower limits of agreement.

with TLC was good to excellent for all three softwares, and the correlation coefficient was highest for Pulmo 3D (r = 0.91) (Figure 3, Table S3). However, there was no relevant correlation of EV or EI with other lung function parameters (Table S3 and S4).

Discussion

In order to introduce quantitative MDCT into routine patient work-up in emphysema and COPD care, it is necessary to agree on and strictly control for examination protocols, post-processing, measurement parameters and parameter interpretation [21]. These parameters must thus have a high reproducibility among different sites covering different CT scanners and software equipment. The present study sought to investigate the measure-

Table 2. Overview of the densitometry results.

	YACTA	lowATT	Pulmo 3D	p
LV (l)	6.824±1.255	6.657±1.251	6.689±1.356	<0.001
EV (l)	2.514±0.991	2.339±1.025	2.195±1.043	<0.001
EI (%)	38.8±8.8	37.0±9.4	33.5±9.5	<0.001
MLD (HU)	−877±8		−895±13	<0.001

LV = lung volume, EV = emphysema volume, EI = emphysema index, MLD = mean lung density, HU = Hounsfield units.

ment variability of densitometry among different software tools on a predefined set of thin-section MDCT from COPD patients. Measurement results for segmented lung volumes, emphysema volumes and, consecutively, emphysema index were significantly different between one in-house scientific tool and two up-to-date commercially available tools from major vendors. Not all tools were able to process the standard DICOM datasets, even commercially available tools failed to process 39–100% of scheduled data. Only in-house scientific software (YACTA) and a single commercial tool (lowATT) analyzed all data successfully.

In 1979 Harris proposed that the desirable imprecision of two laboratory tests assessing the same parameter should be equal or less than half of the intra-individual biological variation [33]. Reference normal values for emphysema have not been established [34]. The true intra-individual variability of emphysema on quantitative densitometry of repeated MDCT examinations has little been studied. Shaker and colleagues reported a short-term coefficient of variation of 6.8% for emphysema volume with a threshold of −910 HU for repeated examination with the identical scanner and post-processing software in a 2-week interval [35]. For repeated low-dose scans in a 3-month interval Gietema and colleagues found coefficients of variation for the emphysema score (equals EI in our study) of 34% with a limits of agreement

(95% confidence interval) from −13.4 to 12.6% at −910 HU, and 58% with a limits of agreement from −1.3 to 1.1% at −950 HU [36]. Hence, the short-term inter-scan intra-individual variability at −950 HU is low. Soejima et al. reported an annual change of relative low attenuation areas (equals EI in our study) between 0.7% and 2.3% (95% confidence interval) in 47 current or former smokers with a threshold of −912 HU [37]. In a more recent study Hoesein et al. reported a mean annual increase of emphysema of 1.07% (confidence interval 1.06–1.09%) in 3,670 former and current smokers at −950 HU [38]. Interestingly, the reported long-term data showed a variability that is within the limits of reported short-term variability. Hence, a clear definition of a tolerable variance in emphysema quantification cannot be given. A more practical approach would be oriented at the clinical consequences of measurement variability. Following Harris' proposal and considering the previously published data, variability of the EI measured with two different software tools in the present study should be approximately less than 1%. However, the inter-software variability in our study is much higher than the recent reports on emphysema progression with median differences from −5.0 to −1.7% and limits of agreement as wide as −25.5 to 18.8% for EI (Table 3). As currently, there is insufficient data available on the impact of MDCT-derived quantitative parame-

Table 3. Variation of densitometry.

		lowATT - YACTA	Pulmo 3D - YACTA	Pulmo 3D - lowATT	p-value
LV (l)	r	1.00	1.00	1.00	<0.001
	ΔLV	−0.124	−0.218	−0.088	<0.001
	Limits of agreement	−0.195, −0.052	−0.305, −0.131	−0.123; −0.052	
	Coefficient of variation	0.3	0.2	0.2	
EV (l)	r	0.98	0.99	0.98	<0.001
	ΔEV	−0.175	−0.201	−0.051	<0.001
	Limits of agreement	−0.600, 0.250	−0.505, 0.103	−0.575, 0.473	
	Coefficient of variation	1.2	0.8	5.2	
EI (%)	r	0.98	0.79	0.80	<0.001
	ΔEI	−1.7	−5.0	−3.4	<0.05
	Limits of agreement	−6.2, 2.9	−27.0, 16.9	−25.5, 18.8	
	Coefficient of variation	1.4	2.2	3.3	
MLD (HU)	r		0.99		<0.001
	ΔMLD		−21		<0.001
	Limits of agreement		−28, −16		
	Coefficient of variation		0.1		

LV = lung volume, EV = emphysema volume, EI = emphysema index, MLD = mean lung density, HU = Hounsfield units. Differences (Δ) and limits of agreement were calculated in accordance with the approach of Bland and Altman.

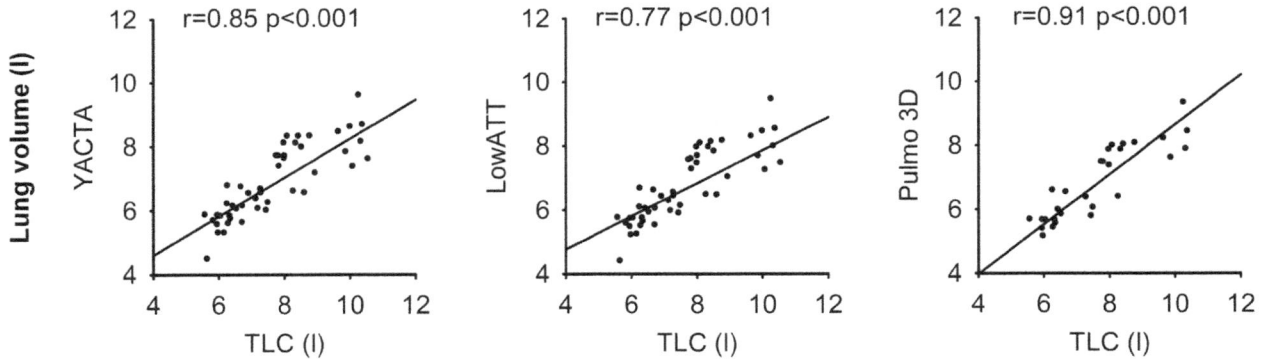

Figure 3. Correlation with lung function testing. The segmented lung volume provided by each individual software showed a good correlation with the total lung capacity (TLC) as measured by lung function testing. Pearson correlation coefficient r and respective p-value are indicated for each plot.

ters on treatment decisions, we are currently unable to give exact margins of tolerable inter-software differences. It is however conceivable, that a measurement variability beyond approx. 10% is relevant for identifying patients suitable for lung volume reduction strategies considering the selection criteria of the VENT Study for example [12]. For this study threshold values for the emphysema index for performing therapy have been postulated, but our results show that these threshold values must be defined for each software used for quantification separately. The inter-software variation may otherwise lead to erroneous exclusion or inclusion for therapy.

Potential sources of error are the steps of lung segmentation, airway segmentation and subsequent emphysema segmentation. A frequently observed problem is the "leakage" of mostly region growing-based algorithms from airways into lung parenchyma, or from segmented emphysema into the airway tree (Figure 1). This leads to substantial miscalculations of the respective volumes, and warrants a validation step by a radiologist before the results are used clinically. Apparently, lowATT provided segmentation results with errors in separating airways from emphysema in some cases. These were not observed with YACTA and Pulmo 3D, but the latter did not provide results for 19 cases at all, some of which showed errors with lowATT also. In total, only 21 datasets could be processed by all three software tools without major segmentation errors. Even in this reduced set of MDCT exams, measurement variability was similar compared to the full patient population. Maximal limits of agreement still were as wide as -7.9 to 7.4% for EI (Table S2). More minor variations in segmentation and noise correction between software are very likely and a source of different densitometry results. A more subtle reason for measurement variation is the extent of airway segmentation into the periphery of the airway tree. Currently, there is no consensus on to which airway generation the airway tree needs to be segmented in order to exclude these airways from lung parenchyma, and thus emphysema. The scope of this study was to evaluate the softwares' potential for fully-automatic lung densitometry, meaning that neither user-interaction nor correction of the results would be necessary. Moreover, only YACTA provided a tool for manual correction of the computational segmentation results with the software version evaluated for this study.

Similar studies in other important fields of quantitative MDCT have brought up results similar to our study: For example, our study compares well to research by de Hoop et al. who compared six different software tools for automated lung nodule volumetry. The authors found a variation between 16.4–22.3%, which they

concluded were unacceptably large with regard to therapy decision in serial exams [39]. A subsequent study by this group revealed similar results [40]. Oberoi et al. investigated the inter-software variation of non-calcified coronary artery plaque quantification. They concluded that inter-platform reproducibility was poor and that serial studies need to use identical software in a research setting [41].

Some limitations of our study need to be addressed. In the absence of a standard of reference in vivo, it is impossible to validate the true EV and thus EI. TLC measured by plethysmography may also be inappropriate as a reference for MDCT-derived LV in the setting of severe COPD [32]. Furthermore, acquisition conditions for plethysmography and MDCT are completely different (prone position, trained technician giving prompt instructions etc.), probably leading to lower segmented LV than TLC also in our study. Thus, we may not evaluate accuracy of the different software tools. The fact that there was no apparent correlation between EV or EI with FEV1, RV or RV/TLC (Table S3 and S4) in contrast to previously published results should not confuse the reader [3,6]. This is explained by the selection of our patient cohort, mainly consisting of end-stage COPD patients. Thus, there is little variation in lung function impairment and densitometry results, which diminished statistical correlation analysis. It is problematic that two of the tools initially investigated for this study could not process most of the datasets provided although their intended use is vendor-independent. This still may be explained as a conflict of different platforms from different vendors. Furthermore, the examinations were performed on a relatively old 4-slice MDCT system. Other densitometry parameters of emphysema currently subject to debate such as the 15th percentile of the lung histogram were not delivered by the commercial software tools and could not be evaluated in this study [42,43]. The fact that we compared three out of many other scientific and medical class product tools does not pose a limitation. It is conceivable, that inter-software variability for other tools will range within the same order of magnitude. The in-house scientific software YACTA has not been certified as a medical class product, and may thus not be used in clinical routine.

Following our results we conclude that inter-software variation of densitometry is greater than the natural intra-individual variability of emphysema and beyond acceptable margins for longitudinal studies and identifying patients for lung volume reduction procedures, hampering its broad introduction as a reproducible biomarker. Computational results need to be validated by an experienced radiologist to rule out obvious sources of error. As a perspective, efforts currently undertaken to standardize scanning parameters and quality checks with dedicated attenuation phantoms such as used for the COPDGene study [44] should encompass densitometry software also, to control for all possible factors along the measurement setup from acquisition to computational measurements. Measuring reference emphysema phantoms regularly at each site, similar to quality assurance in laboratories, would foster the acceptance of densitometry as an endpoint in interventional trials, and potentially in clinical routine in the future. Until then, longitudinal studies should be performed using the identical software.

Supporting Information

Table S1 Results of densitometry after user interaction. N = 21, LV = lung volume, EV = emphysema volume, EI = emphysema index, MLD = mean lung density, HU = Hounsfield units.

Table S2 Variation of densitometry after user interaction. N = 21, LV = lung volume, EV = emphysema volume, EI = emphysema index, MLD = mean lung density, HU = Hounsfield units. Mean differences (Δ) and limits of agreement were calculated in accordance with the approach of Bland and Altman.

Table S3 Correlation of quantitative MDCT with lung function. Correlation coefficients were calculated for lung volume (LV), emphysema volume (EV), emphysema index (EI), and mean lung density (MLD) with with forced expiratory volume within 1 s (FEV1, FEV1%), vital capacity (VC), Tiffeneau index (FEV1/VC), residual volume (RV), total lung capacity (TLC), and RV/TLC ratio. *$p < 0.05$.

Table S4 Correlation of quantitative MDCT with lung function after user interaction. Correlation coefficients were calculated for lung volume (LV), emphysema volume (EV), emphysema index (EI), and mean lung density (MLD) with with forced expiratory volume within 1 s (FEV1, FEV1%), vital capacity (VC), Tiffeneau index (FEV1/VC), residual volume (RV), total lung capacity (TLC), and RV/TLC ratio. *$p < 0.05$.

Acknowledgments

We thank all patients for their willingness to contribute to this study. This work contains parts of the doctoral thesis of cand. med. Diana Bardarova, Heidelberg, Germany. The expert technical assistance of Melanie Segovic is gratefully appreciated.

Author Contributions

Conceived and designed the experiments: MOW DB OW HUK ME BJJ RE MKS MP CPH. Performed the experiments: MOW DB OW BJJ. Analyzed the data: MOW DB OW BJJ CPH. Contributed reagents/materials/analysis tools: MOW DB OW HUK CPH. Contributed to the writing of the manuscript: MOW DB OW HUK ME BJJ RE MKS MP CPH.

References

1. Coxson HO, Mayo J, Lam S, Santyr G, Parraga G, et al. (2009) New and current clinical imaging techniques to study chronic obstructive pulmonary disease. Am J Respir Crit Care Med 180: 588–597.
2. Rabe KF, Hurd S, Anzueto A, Barnes PJ, Buist SA, et al. (2007) Global strategy for the diagnosis, management, and prevention of chronic obstructive pulmonary disease: GOLD executive summary. Am J Respir Crit Care Med 176: 532–555.
3. Coxson HO, Rogers RM (2005) Quantitative computed tomography of chronic obstructive pulmonary disease. Acad Radiol 12: 1457–1463.
4. Kauczor HU, Wielpütz MO, Owsijewitsch M, Ley-Zaporozhan J (2011) Computed Tomographic Imaging of the Airways in COPD and Asthma. J Thorac Imaging 26: 290–300.
5. Ley-Zaporozhan J, van Beek EJ (2010) Imaging phenotypes of chronic obstructive pulmonary disease. J Magn Reson Imaging 32: 1340–1352.
6. Heussel CP, Herth FJ, Kappes J, Hantusch R, Hartlieb S, et al. (2009) Fully automatic quantitative assessment of emphysema in computed tomography: comparison with pulmonary function testing and normal values. Eur Radiol 19: 2391–2402.
7. Hoffman EA, Simon BA, McLennan G (2006) State of the Art. A structural and functional assessment of the lung via multidetector-row computed tomography: phenotyping chronic obstructive pulmonary disease. Proc Am Thorac Soc 3: 519–532.
8. Gevenois PA, De Vuyst P, de Maertelaer V, Zanen J, Jacobovitz D, et al. (1996) Comparison of computed density and microscopic morphometry in pulmonary emphysema. Am J Respir Crit Care Med 154: 187–192.
9. Coxson HO, Rogers RM, Whittall KP, D'Yachkova Y, Pare PD, et al. (1999) A quantification of the lung surface area in emphysema using computed tomography. Am J Respir Crit Care Med 159: 851–856.
10. Regan EA, Hokanson JE, Murphy JR, Make B, Lynch DA, et al. (2010) Genetic epidemiology of COPD (COPDGene) study design. COPD 7: 32–43.
11. Han MK, Kazerooni EA, Lynch DA, Liu LX, Murray S, et al. (2011) Chronic obstructive pulmonary disease exacerbations in the COPDGene study: associated radiologic phenotypes. Radiology 261: 274–282.
12. Sciurba FC, Ernst A, Herth FJ, Strange C, Criner GJ, et al. (2010) A randomized study of endobronchial valves for advanced emphysema. N Engl J Med 363: 1233–1244.
13. Stoel BC, Putter H, Bakker ME, Dirksen A, Stockley RA, et al. (2008) Volume correction in computed tomography densitometry for follow-up studies on pulmonary emphysema. Proc Am Thorac Soc 5: 919–924.
14. Madani A, Van Muylem A, Gevenois PA (2010) Pulmonary emphysema: effect of lung volume on objective quantification at thin-section CT. Radiology 257: 260–268.
15. Zaporozhan J, Ley S, Weinheimer O, Eberhardt R, Tsakiris I, et al. (2006) Multi-detector CT of the chest: influence of dose onto quantitative evaluation of severe emphysema: a simulation study. J Comput Assist Tomogr 30: 460–468.
16. Yuan R, Mayo JR, Hogg JC, Pare PD, McWilliams AM, et al. (2007) The effects of radiation dose and CT manufacturer on measurements of lung densitometry. Chest 132: 617–623.
17. Ley-Zaporozhan J, Ley S, Weinheimer O, Iliyushenko S, Erdugan S, et al. (2008) Quantitative analysis of emphysema in 3D using MDCT: influence of different reconstruction algorithms. Eur J Radiol 65: 228–234.
18. Gierada DS, Bierhals AJ, Choong CK, Bartel ST, Ritter JH, et al. (2010) Effects of CT section thickness and reconstruction kernel on emphysema quantification relationship to the magnitude of the CT emphysema index. Acad Radiol 17: 146–156.
19. Mets OM, Willemink MJ, de Kort FP, Mol CP, Leiner T, et al. (2012) The effect of iterative reconstruction on computed tomography assessment of emphysema, air trapping and airway dimensions. Eur Radiol 22: 2103–2109.
20. Choo JY, Goo JM, Lee CH, Park CM, Park SJ, et al. (2014) Quantitative analysis of emphysema and airway measurements according to iterative reconstruction algorithms: comparison of filtered back projection, adaptive statistical iterative reconstruction and model-based iterative reconstruction. Eur Radiol 24: 799–806.
21. Kauczor HU, Heussel CP, Herth FJ (2013) Longitudinal quantitative low-dose CT in COPD: ready for use? Lancet Respir Med 1: 95–96.
22. Heussel CP, Achenbach T, Buschsieweke C, Kuhnigk J, Weinheimer O, et al. (2006) [Quantification of pulmonary emphysema in multislice-CT using different software tools]. Rofo 178: 987–998.
23. Miller MR, Hankinson J, Brusasco V, Burgos F, Casaburi R, et al. (2005) Standardisation of spirometry. Eur Respir J 26: 319–338.
24. Quanjer PH, Tammeling GJ, Cotes JE, Pedersen OF, Peslin R, et al. (1993) Lung volumes and forced ventilatory flows. Report Working Party Standardization of Lung Function Tests, European Community for Steel and Coal. Official Statement of the European Respiratory Society. Eur Respir J Suppl 16: 5–40.
25. Heussel CP, Kappes J, Hantusch R, Hartlieb S, Weinheimer O, et al. (2009) Contrast enhanced CT-scans are not comparable to non-enhanced scans in emphysema quantification. Eur J Radiol 74: 473–478.
26. Wielpütz MO, Eichinger M, Weinheimer O, Ley S, Mall MA, et al. (2013) Automatic airway analysis on multidetector computed tomography in cystic fibrosis: correlation with pulmonary function testing. J Thorac Imaging 28: 104–113.
27. Wielpütz MO, Weinheimer O, Eichinger M, Wiebel M, Biederer J, et al. (2013) Pulmonary emphysema in cystic fibrosis detected by densitometry on chest multidetector computed tomography. PLoS One 8: e73142.

28. Weinheimer O, Achenbach T, Bletz C, Duber C, Kauczor HU, et al. (2008) About objective 3-d analysis of airway geometry in computerized tomography. IEEE Trans Med Imaging 27: 64–74.

29. Weinheimer O, Achenbach T, Heussel CP, Düber C (2011) Automatic Lung Segmentation in MDCT Images. In: Proceedings of the Fourth International Workshop on Pulmonary Image Analysis. Toronto. 241–255.

30. Bland JM, Altman DG (1986) Statistical methods for assessing agreement between two methods of clinical measurement. Lancet 1: 307–310.

31. Holm S (1979) A simple sequentially rejective multiple test procedure. Scandinavian Journal of Statistics 6: 65–70.

32. Garfield JL, Marchetti N, Gaughan JP, Steiner RM, Criner GJ (2012) Total lung capacity by plethysmography and high-resolution computed tomography in COPD. Int J Chron Obstruct Pulmon Dis 7: 119–126.

33. Harris EK (1979) Statistical principles underlying analytic goal-setting in clinical chemistry. Am J Clin Pathol 72: 374–382.

34. Smith BM, Barr RG (2013) Establishing normal reference values in quantitative computed tomography of emphysema. J Thorac Imaging 28: 280–283.

35. Shaker S, Dirksen A, Laursen L, Maltbaek N, Christensen L, et al. (2004) Short-term reproducibility of computed tomography-based lung density measurements in alpha-1 antitrypsin deficiency and smokers with emphysema. Acta Radiologica 45: 424–430.

36. Gietema HA, Schilham AM, van Ginneken B, van Klaveren RJ, Lammers JW, et al. (2007) Monitoring of smoking-induced emphysema with CT in a lung cancer screening setting: detection of real increase in extent of emphysema. Radiology 244: 890–897.

37. Soejima K, Yamaguchi K, Kohda E, Takeshita K, Ito Y, et al. (2000) Longitudinal follow-up study of smoking-induced lung density changes by high-resolution computed tomography. Am J Respir Crit Care Med 161: 1264–1273.

38. Mohamed Hoesein FA, Zanen P, de Jong PA, van Ginneken B, Boezen HM, et al. (2013) Rate of progression of CT-quantified emphysema in male current and ex-smokers: a follow-up study. Respir Res 14: 55.

39. de Hoop B, Gietema H, van Ginneken B, Zanen P, Groenewegen G, et al. (2009) A comparison of six software packages for evaluation of solid lung nodules using semi-automated volumetry: what is the minimum increase in size to detect growth in repeated CT examinations. Eur Radiol 19: 800–808.

40. Ashraf H, de Hoop B, Shaker SB, Dirksen A, Bach KS, et al. (2010) Lung nodule volumetry: segmentation algorithms within the same software package cannot be used interchangeably. Eur Radiol 20: 1878–1885.

41. Oberoi S, Meinel FG, Schoepf UJ, Nance JW, De Cecco CN, et al. (2014) Reproducibility of noncalcified coronary artery plaque burden quantification from coronary CT angiography across different image analysis platforms. AJR Am J Roentgenol 202: W43–49.

42. Diciotti S, Sverzellati N, Kauczor HU, Lombardo S, Falchini M, et al. (2011) Defining the intra-subject variability of whole-lung CT densitometry in two lung cancer screening trials. Acad Radiol 18: 1403–1411.

43. Coxson HO, Dirksen A, Edwards LD, Yates JC, Agusti A, et al. (2013) The presence and progression of emphysema in COPD as determined by CT scanning and biomarker expression: a prospective analysis from the ECLIPSE study. Lancet Respir Med 1: 129–136.

44. Sieren JP, Newell JD, Judy PF, Lynch DA, Chan KS, et al. (2012) Reference standard and statistical model for intersite and temporal comparisons of CT attenuation in a multicenter quantitative lung study. Med Phys 39: 5757–5767.

16

⁶⁴Cu-DOTA-Anti-CTLA-4 mAb Enabled PET Visualization of CTLA-4 on the T-Cell Infiltrating Tumor Tissues

Kei Higashikawa[1,2], **Katsuharu Yagi**[1], **Keiko Watanabe**[1], **Shinichiro Kamino**[3], **Masashi Ueda**[1], **Makoto Hiromura**[3], **Shuichi Enomoto**[1,3]*

1 Graduate School of Medicine, Dentistry, and Pharmaceutical Sciences, Okayama University, Okayama, Japan, **2** Japan Society for the Promotion of Science, Tokyo, Japan, **3** Next-generation Imaging Team, RIKEN Center for Life Science Technologies, Kobe, Japan

Abstract

Cytotoxic T lymphocyte-associated antigen-4 (CTLA-4) targeted therapy by anti-CTLA-4 monoclonal antibody (mAb) is highly effective in cancer patients. However, it is extremely expensive and potentially produces autoimmune-related adverse effects. Therefore, the development of a method to evaluate CTLA-4 expression prior to CTLA-4-targeted therapy is expected to open doors to evidence-based and cost-efficient medical care and to avoid adverse effects brought about by ineffective therapy. In this study, we aimed to develop a molecular imaging probe for CTLA-4 visualization in tumor. First, we examined CTLA-4 expression in normal colon tissues, cultured CT26 cells, and CT26 tumor tissues from tumor-bearing BALB/c mice and BALB/c nude mice by reverse transcription polymerase chain reaction (RT-PCR) analysis and confirmed whether CTLA-4 is strongly expressed in CT26 tumor tissues. Second, we newly synthesized ⁶⁴Cu-1,4,7,10-tetraazacyclo-dodecane-N,N',N'',N'''-tetraacetic acid-anti-mouse CTLA-4 mAb (⁶⁴Cu-DOTA-anti-CTLA-4 mAb) and evaluated its usefulness in positron emission tomography (PET) and ex-vivo biodistribution analysis in CT26-bearing BALB/c mice. High CTLA-4 expression was confirmed in the CT26 tumor tissues of tumor-bearing BALB/c mice. However, CTLA-4 expression was extremely low in the cultured CT26 cells and the CT26 tumor tissues of tumor-bearing BALB/c nude mice. The results suggested that T cells were responsible for the high CTLA-4 expression. Furthermore, ⁶⁴Cu-DOTA-anti-CTLA-4 mAb displayed significantly high accumulation in the CT26 tumor, thereby realizing non-invasive CTLA-4 visualization in the tumor. Together, the results indicate that ⁶⁴Cu-DOTA-anti-CTLA-4 mAb would be useful for the evaluation of CTLA-4 expression in tumor.

Editor: Gabriele Multhoff, Technische Universitaet Muenchen, Germany

Funding: This work was supported by a grant-in-aid for COE projects by MEXT, Japan, titled "Center of excellence for molecular and gene targeting therapies with micro-doze molecular imaging modalities.", a grant from Japan Society for the Promotion of Science (grant number: 12J06885, URL: http://www.jsps.go.jp/english/index.html), and a grant form the Ministry of Education, Culture, Sports, Science and Technology (URL: http://www.pref.okayama.jp/page/287673.html). The funders had no role in study design, data collection and analysis, decision to publish or preparation of the manuscript.

Competing Interests: The authors have declared that no competing interests exist.

* Email: semo@riken.jp

Introduction

Cancer is a complex mixture of host and tumor cells. Whereas the human body has the ability to produce an anti-tumor immune response, cancers develop multiple strategies to evade the host immune system [1]. Cytotoxic T lymphocyte-associated antigen-4 (CTLA-4), also known as cluster of differentiation 152 (CD152), is one of the most important molecules that are involved in the downregulation of the immune system and the anti-tumor response. CTLA-4 is expressed predominantly on the surface of two major subsets of CD4+ T cells: regulatory T cells (Tregs) and activated CD4+ effector cells, and activated CD8+ effector T cells [2,3]. In addition, recent research showed that various tumor cells also express CTLA-4 [4].

CTLA-4 targeted therapy augments endogenous response to tumor cells, thereby leading to tumor cell death when utilized on its own or with other therapeutic interventions [3]. It is for this reason that CTLA-4 has attracted attention as a target molecule of cancer immunotherapy [5]. Fully human anti-CTLA-4 monoclo-

nal antibodies (mAbs), ipilimumab and tremelimumab, were developed for the treatment of cancer patients. Ipilimumab is the first drug to demonstrate survival benefits in metastatic melanoma patients, and was approved by the US Food and Drug Administration (FDA) for the treatment of advanced melanoma in 2011. Pre-clinical and clinical trials of anti-CTLA-4 mAbs have been conducted for the treatment of other cancers, including colon, breast, lung, ovarian, and prostate cancers [3,6].

Although CTLA-4-targeted therapy is an attractive method for the treatment of various cancers, the therapy is beset by several problems. First, the enhanced T cell response by the CTLA-4 blockade frequently produces autoimmune-related adverse effects, such as rash, diarrhea, colitis, hepatitis, and hypophysitis [7,8]. A superagonist antibody for CD28 (TGN1412), which directly stimulates T cells, caused life-threatening inflammatory reactions in a London clinical trial [9]. Extreme precaution must be taken when CTLA-4-targeted antibodies are used for the treatment because CTLA-4 is an antagonist of CD28–ligand interactions [10]. Second, antibody drugs are extremely expensive. One treatment course of ipilimumab in the United States consists of four doses at US$30,000 per dose [2,11]. Clearly, there is an urgent need to develop a method to screen patients for sensitivity to the CTLA-4-targeted therapy, to eliminate adverse effects brought about by ineffective therapy and reduce unnecessary financial burden in non-sensitive patients. The identification of CTLA-4 expression in tumor prior to molecular targeted therapy would lead to evidence-based and cost-efficient medical care.

Biopsy is principally conducted to evaluate the expression of molecules of interest. However, it is an invasive and stressful procedure. Moreover, biopsy evaluates the expression of target molecules only in a localized region of the tumor. Thus, it is difficult to acquire information of a patient's sensitivity to a molecular targeted drug for tumors existing in whole body.

Molecular imaging can provide molecular information of the whole body in a noninvasive manner and be used for the determination of sensitivity to antibody drugs. Tumor imaging probes for human epidermal growth factor receptor 2 (HER2) [12–14], epidermal growth factor receptor (EGFR) [15–18], and vascular endothelial growth factor (VEGF) [19,20], which are the target molecules of trastuzumab, cetuximab/panitumumab, and bevacizumab, respectively, have been developed. The expression of those molecules in tumor was detected with their respective probes by positron emission tomography (PET) or single photon emission computed tomography (SPECT). However, to our knowledge, a molecular imaging probe that targets CTLA-4 has yet to be developed.

In this study, we aimed to develop a molecular imaging probe for CTLA-4 visualization in tumor. First, CTLA-4 expression was examined in CT26 tumor tissues and cultured CT26 cells by reverse transcription polymerase chain reaction (RT-PCR) analysis. Second, we newly developed ^{64}Cu-1,4,7,10-tetraazacyclododecane-N,N',N'',N'''-tetraacetic acid (DOTA)-anti-mouse CTLA-4 mAb by introducing DOTA groups to anti-mouse CTLA-4 mAb and subsequent radiolabeling with ^{64}Cu. The utility of ^{64}Cu-DOTA-anti-CTLA-4 mAb as an imaging probe was assessed by PET imaging and ex-vivo biodistribution analysis. We prepared tumor-bearing mice by syngeneic implantation of CT26 cells (mouse colon tumor cell line) to BALB/c mice for PET imaging. Immune-deprived mice bearing human tumor cell lines were not used because T cells might be responsible for the CTLA-4 expression in the tumor tissues.

Materials and Methods

Cell culture

CT26 was purchased from American Type Culture Collection and cultured in RPMI 1640 medium supplemented with 10% fetal bovine serum, 4 mM L-glutamine, 10 U/mL penicillin, and 10 mg/mL streptomycin at 37°C in a humidified atmosphere containing 5% CO_2.

Preparation of subcutaneous tumor model mice

Female BALB/c and BALB/c (nu/nu) nude mice (4–6 weeks old) were purchased from CLEA Japan Inc. Tumor-bearing BALB/c and BALB/c nude mice were prepared by subcutaneously implanting CT26 cells ($1–4\times10^6$ cells). Investigations were initiated after receiving approval from the committee on animal experiments of Okayama University.

RT-PCR analysis

RNA extraction and cDNA synthesis were conducted by using the same methods as our previous report [21]. Total RNA was isolated from cultured cells and tissues with TRIZOL reagent (Life

Technologies Co., Ltd.) and a PureLink RNA Mini Kit (Life Technologies Co., Ltd.). One microgram of total RNA was used as the template for single-strand cDNA synthesis with a Transcriptor First Strand cDNA Synthesis Kit (Roche Co., Ltd.). Analysis of mRNA expression levels was carried out with RT-PCR using TaKaRa Ex Taq (TaKaRa Co., Ltd.). The amplification of β-actin is shown as internal control. Primer sequences are listed in Table S1. The amplicons were separated on agarose gel (AGAROSE I, Amresco, Inc.), stained with ethidium bromide, and visualized with a Benchtop 2UV Transilluminator (UVP, Inc.).

^{64}Cu-DOTA-anti-CTLA-4 mAb production

Anti-mouse CTLA-4 mAb (200–500 μg) (R&D Systems, Inc.) was conjugated to DOTA-mono-N-hydroxysuccinimide ester (DOTA-mono-NHS ester; Macrocyclics, Inc.) in phosphate-buffered saline without calcium and magnesium (pH 7.5) (PBS (−)), by using a 100-fold molar excess of DOTA-mono-NHS ester. The mixture was stirred at room temperature (RT) for three hours to give the DOTA-anti-CTLA-4 antibody. The DOTA-anti-CTLA-4 antibody was purified with a PD-10 column (GE Healthcare Co., Ltd.) and an Amicon-Ultra 50 K device (Millipore Co., Ltd.). The DOTA-anti-CTLA-4 antibody was analyzed by size-exclusion high-performance liquid chromatography (SE-HPLC) using TSK-GEL Super SW3000 (Tosoh Co., Ltd.). The mobile phase of 10 mM PBS (−) containing 0.3 M NaCl was used and the flow rate was 0.35 mL/min.

^{64}Cu was produced by irradiating a 99.6% ^{64}Ni-enriched nickel target with 12 MeV protons using a cyclotron (CYPRIS-HM12, Sumitomo Heavy Industries, Ltd.). Then, ^{64}Cu was purified with a Muromac column (Muromachi Technos Co., Ltd.). The buffer solution of DOTA-anti-CTLA-4 mAb was replaced with 0.1 M acetate buffer (pH 6.5) three times by using an Amicon-Ultra 50 K device (Millipore Co., Ltd.). DOTA-anti-CTLA-4 mAb was radiolabeled with ^{64}Cu by incubating at 40°C for one hour. To remove excess ^{64}Cu, the buffer was replaced with 0.2 M glycine buffer by using the Amicon-Ultra 50 K device. Buffer of the purified antibody solution was replaced with PBS (−) by using the Amicon-Ultra 50 K device. The resultant solution was used for injection.

The radiochemical purity of ^{64}Cu-DOTA-antibodies in PBS (−) was confirmed by reversed phase radio-thin layer chromatography (TLC). This analysis was performed with a TLC aluminum sheet, RP-18 F254 S (Merck Chemicals Co., Ltd.) and methanol:water:acetic acid (4:1:1) was used as the mobile phase. TLC chromatograms were obtained by autoradiography (FLA-7000IR; GE Healthcare Co., Ltd.). ^{64}Cu-DOTA-isotype IgG$_{2A}$ (^{64}Cu-DOTA-Control IgG) was produced in the same way as that for negative control by using rat IgG$_{2A}$ isotype control (R&D Systems, Inc.).

Assay for CTLA-4 binding activity

The CTLA-4 binding activity of DOTA-anti-CTLA-4 mAb and DOTA-Control IgG was examined by enzyme-linked immunosorbent assay (ELISA) and compared with that of original anti-CTLA-4 mAb and DOTA-Control IgG. Twenty ng of recombinant mouse CTLA-4 (R&D Systems, Inc.) in 50 mM carbonate buffer (pH 9.6) per well was added into a 96-well ELISA plate (R&D Systems, Inc.). After blocking with 3% bovine serum albumin (BSA) and 1% Tween 20 in PBS (−) containing 0.05% Tween 20, 5 ng of the antibodies in PBS (−) containing 1% BSA and 0.05% Tween 20 was added to each well and incubated for one hour. After incubation, each well was treated with 50 uL of HRP-conjugated anti-rat IgG (R&D Systems, Inc.) diluted 1:6000 with PBS (−) containing 1% BSA and 0.05% Tween 20.

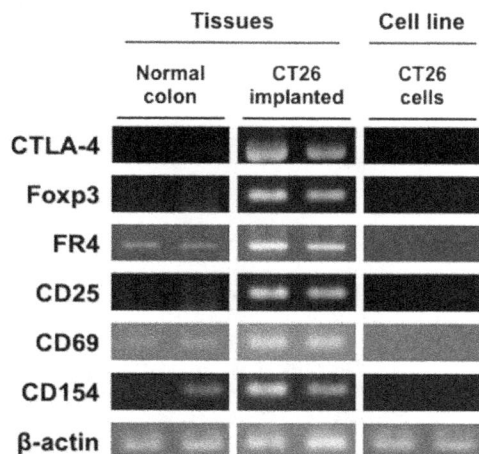

Figure 1. RT-PCR in normal colon tissues, CT26 tumor tissues, and cultured CT26 cells. Expression of CTLA-4, Treg markers, and T cell activation markers in normal colon tissues, CT26 tumor tissues, and cultured CT26 cells.

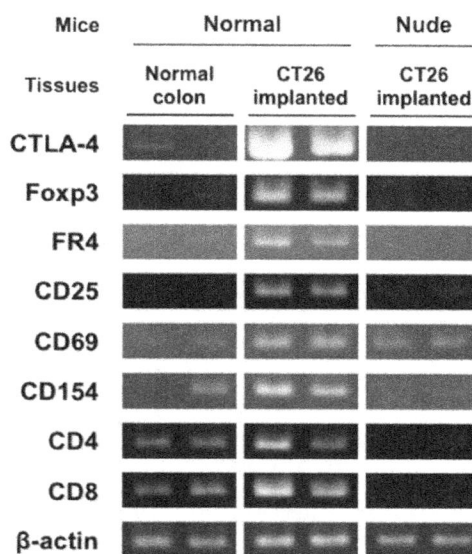

Figure 2. Gene expression analyses in tissues from tumor-bearing BALB/c and BALB/c nude mice. CTLA-4 and T cell marker expression in normal colon tissues from normal BALB/c mice, CT26 tumor tissues from tumor-bearing BALB/c mice, and CT26 tumor tissues from tumor-bearing BALB/c nude mice.

Peroxidase activity was visualized with a TMB Microwell Peroxidase Substrate System (Kirkegaard & Perry Laboratories, Inc.) and the absorbance at 450 nm was measured. The absorbance was corrected by performing a blank trial. The corrected absorbance values of DOTA-anti-CTLA-4 mAb and DOTA-Control IgG were respectively divided by the absorbance of anti-CTLA-4 mAb, and relative immunoreactivities were calculated.

Matrix-assisted laser desorption-ionization time-of-flight mass spectrometry (MALDI-TOF-MS) analysis

MALDI-TOF-MS was conducted to determine the extent of DOTA conjugation to antibodies using a method similar to that reported by Lu et al. [22]. MALDI-TOF-MS was performed by using an Ultraflex III MALDI TOF/TOF (Bruker Daltonics Co., Ltd.). Non- and DOTA-conjugated antibodies were desalted with PD Spin Trap G-25 (GE Healthcare Co., Ltd.). Sinapinic acid (Nacalai Tesque, Inc.) at 20 mg/mL in 2:1 acetonitrile/H_2O with 0.1% trifluoroacetic acid (Wako Pure Chemical Industries, Co., Ltd.) was used as the MALDI matrix.

PET imaging study

^{64}Cu-DOTA-anti-CTLA-4 mAb (4 μg, approximately 16 MBq) or ^{64}Cu-DOTA-Control IgG (4 μg, approximately 14 MBq) was intravenously administered to CT26-bearing BALB/c mice via the tail vein. Forty-eight hours after administration of the radiolabeled antibodies, probe uptake in the CT26-bearing mice was measured with a small-animal PET scanner (microPET Focus220; Siemens Medical Solutions Inc.). During PET imaging, the mice were anesthetized with 1.5% isoflurane and 1.5% N_2O gas, and placed in the prone position. Emission data were acquired for 60 min. The acquired data were summed into sinograms and three-dimensional images were reconstructed by maximum a posteriori (MAP). Coronal and sagittal images were displayed in 918×760 and 550×760 pixel formats, respectively, with a pixel size of 0.053 mm×0.053 mm. The image intensity was expressed by standardized uptake value (SUV). SUV$_{max}$ was calculated by ASIPRO software package (Concorde Microsystems, Inc.).

Biodistribution study

Forty-eight hours after administration of ^{64}Cu-DOTA-anti-CTLA-4 mAb (4 μg, 1 MBq) or ^{64}Cu-DOTA-Control IgG (4 μg, 1 MBq), the animals were immediately sacrificed and the organs and blood were removed. The organs and blood were weighed and radioactivities were counted with a gamma counter (ARC-7001B, ALOKA Co., Ltd.). Decay-corrected uptake was expressed as the percentage of injected dose per gram and calculated as the ratio to blood or muscle for comparison of the accumulation abilities in the CT26 tumor between ^{64}Cu-DOTA-anti-CTLA-4 antibody and ^{64}Cu-DOTA-Control IgG.

Immunohistological staining

Tumor-bearing BALB/c mice were sacrificed and CT26 tumor tissues including the normal tissues around them were resected and embedded in Optimal Cutting Temperature (O.C.T.) compound (Sakura Finetek Japan Co., Ltd.). Ten-μm-thick frozen tissue sections were prepared and mounted on MAS-coated glass slides (Matsunami Glass Ind., Co., Ltd.). The tissue sections were fixed with 4% paraformaldehyde in PBS (−), blocked with 5% goat serum in PBS (−), and incubated with anti-CTLA-4 antibody (R&D Systems, Inc.). Then, the tissue sections were subjected to endogenous peroxidase inactivation with 0.19% H_2O_2/methanol (Wako Pure Chemical Industries, Ltd.), followed by incubation with horseradish peroxidase conjugated anti-rat IgG antibody (R&D Systems, Inc.). Immunocomplexes were visualized with a DAB substrate kit (Dako Co., Ltd.).

Statistical analysis

SUV$_{max}$ data are expressed as means ± standard deviation (SD) and other data are expressed as means ± standard error of mean (SEM). Statistical significance was determined using the Student's t-test. The level of significance was taken as $p < 0.01$. The tests were performed using GraphPad Prism software (GraphPad Software, Inc.).

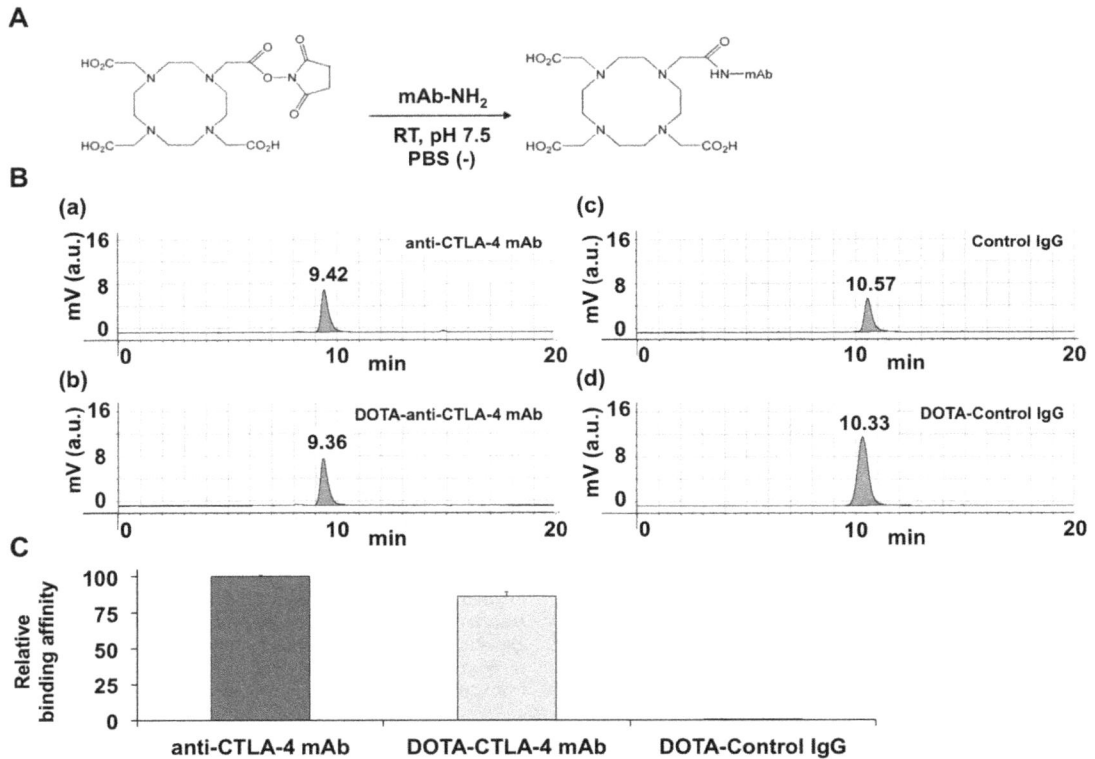

Figure 3. Preparation of DOTA-conjugated mAb. A. Scheme of the synthesis of DOTA-conjugated mAb. B. HPLC analysis of original and DOTA-conjugated mAbs. C. Evaluation of CTLA-4 binding activity of DOTA-anti-CTLA-4 mAb. Data are expressed as means ± SEM.

Results

CTLA-4 was strongly expressed in CT26 tumor tissues but not cultured CT26 cells

First, RT-PCR was carried out to examine CTLA-4 expression in CT26 tumor tissues and cultured CT26 cells, and the results were compared to those obtained with normal colon tissues (Fig. 1). CTLA-4 (amplicon length: 920 base pairs (bp)) was strongly expressed in CT26 tumor tissues compared with normal colon tissues.

On the other hand, CTLA-4 expression was extremely low in cultured CT26 cells. Moreover, Treg markers, such as forkhead box P3 (Foxp3) and folate receptor 4 (FR4) [23,24], were more strongly expressed in the tumor tissues than the normal colon tissues and the cultured CT26 cells. The expression of CD25 and CD69, which are molecules expressed on regulatory and activated

T cells [23–25], was also increased in the tumor tissues compared to the normal colon tissues and the cultured CT26 cells. CD154, which is induced on T cells by T cell activation [26], was also more strongly expressed in the tumor tissues than the normal colon tissues and the cultured CT26 cells.

CTLA-4 and T cell marker expression was low in CT26 tumor tissues from tumor-bearing BALB/c nude mice

From the results of Fig. 1, we assumed that T cells were involved in CTLA-4 expression in the CT26 tumor tissues from the tumor-bearing BALB/c mice, and CT26 tumor tissues from the tumor-bearing BALB/c nude mice did not express CTLA-4 due to a marked decrease of T cells in those mice. Thus, we prepared two subcutaneous tumor models by syngeneic subcutaneous transplantation of CT26 into normal BALB/c mice or BALB/c nude mice, and compared CTLA-4 and T cell marker

Table 1. Average molecular weights of original and DOTA-conjugated antibodies, and estimated numbers of DOTA chelators per unit antibody.

Antibody	Average molecular weight	Mass difference	The number of DOTA per antibody
anti-CTLA-4 mAb	150097	1634	4.2
DOTA-anti-CTLA-4 mAb	151731		
Control IgG	147870	1686	4.4
DOTA-Control IgG	149557		

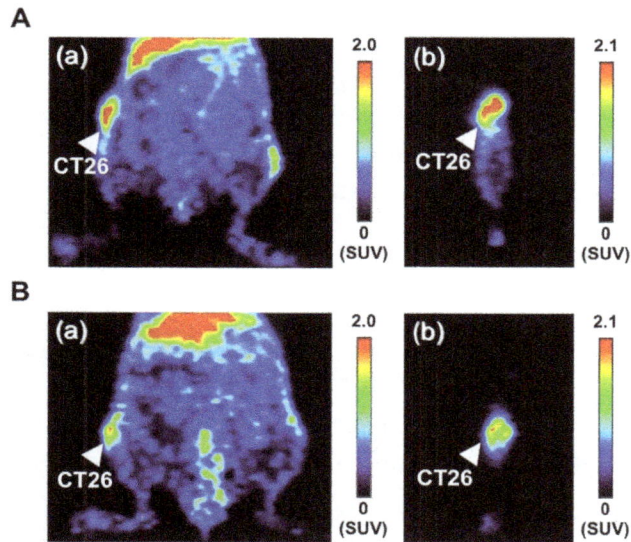

Figure 4. PET images of ^{64}Cu-DOTA-anti-CTLA-4 mAb and ^{64}Cu-DOTA-Control IgG. A. Representative coronal (a) and sagittal (b) PET images of ^{64}Cu-DOTA-anti-CTLA-4 mAb in CT26-bearing mice. B. Representative coronal (a) and sagittal (b) PET images of ^{64}Cu-DOTA-Control IgG in CT26-bearing mice.

expression in the CT26 tumor tissues from the tumor-bearing BALB/c mice with those from the tumor-bearing BALB/c nude mice by RT-PCR analysis (Fig. 2).

RT-PCR showed that CTLA-4 expression was dramatically decreased in the CT26 tumor tissues from the tumor-bearing BALB/c nude mice, compared with those from the tumor-bearing BALB/c mice. Furthermore, we confirmed that the expression of CD4 and CD8 as well as Foxp3, FR4, CD69, CD154, and CD25 was markedly decreased in the tumor tissues from the tumor-bearing BALB/c nude mice.

DOTA-conjugated antibody probe was synthesized

DOTA chelators were conjugated to each mAb, as shown in Figure 3A. The chromatograms of all the mAbs showed a single peak. In addition, the retention times of anti-CTLA-4 mAb, DOTA-anti-CTLA-4 mAb, Control IgG, and DOTA-Control IgG were 9.42, 9.36, 10.57, and 10.33, respectively (Fig. 3B). The retention times of DOTA-conjugated antibodies were slightly shorter than those of the original antibodies, suggesting that anti-CTLA-4 mAb or Control IgG conjugated to DOTA and was well purified. Furthermore, MALDI-TOF-MS analysis was carried out to measure the average number of DOTA chelators that were conjugated to anti-CTLA-4 mAb or Control IgG (Table 1). The mass differences between anti-CTLA-4 mAb and DOTA-anti-CTLA-4 mAb, and between Control IgG and DOTA-Control IgG were 1634 and 1686, respectively. The mass differences were divided by the mass value of single DOTA conjugation (386 mass units), and the resulting values represented the average number of DOTA chelators that were conjugated to anti-CTLA-4 mAb or Control IgG. From the calculations, 4.2 or 4.4 DOTA chelators on average were conjugated into a single molecule of anti-CTLA-4 mAb or Control IgG.

Then, the binding activity of DOTA-anti-CTLA-4 mAb to CTLA-4 was measured by ELISA (Figure 3C). The binding activity of DOTA-anti-CTLA-4 mAb to CTLA-4 was 86.3±2.8%

of that of the original anti-CTLA-4 mAb. The binding activity of DOTA-Control IgG was 0.3±0.1%.

^{64}Cu-DOTA-anti-CTLA-4 mAb enabled clear visualization of CTLA-4-positive tumor by PET

^{64}Cu-DOTA-anti-CTLA-4 mAb and ^{64}Cu-DOTA-Control IgG were obtained in radiochemical yields of 94% and 97%, respectively. The radiochemical purities of both probes were higher than 94%. To evaluate the ^{64}Cu-DOTA-anti-CTLA-4 mAb uptake by CTLA-4 positive tumor (CT26), we performed PET and ex-vivo biodistribution analysis. Representative coronal and sagittal images are shown in Figure 4. At 48 hours after administration of the probes, ^{64}Cu-DOTA-anti-CTLA-4 mAb clearly visualized the CT26 tumors and ^{64}Cu-DOTA-anti-CTLA-4 mAb showed higher accumulation in the tumors than ^{64}Cu-DOTA-Control IgG (^{64}Cu-DOTA-anti-CTLA-4 mAb: SUV-max = 2.65±0.01, n = 2; ^{64}Cu-DOTA-Control IgG: SUV-max = 2.06±0.32, n = 2).

The results were consistent with those of the ex-vivo biodistribution study (Fig. 5). ^{64}Cu-DOTA-anti-CTLA-4 mAb showed significantly higher accumulation in the CT26 tumors than ^{64}Cu-DOTA-Control IgG (7.49±0.32%ID/g vs. 5.84±0.38%ID/g, p<0.01). Moreover, ^{64}Cu-DOTA-anti-CTLA-4 mAb showed higher tumor-to-blood and tumor-to-muscle ratios than ^{64}Cu-DOTA-Control IgG (tumor-to-blood ratio: 0.58±0.03 vs. 0.40±0.02, p<0.001; tumor-to-muscle ratio: 8.48±0.63 and 5.31±0.35, p<0.01).

In addition, CTLA-4 protein expression in the CT26 tumor was confirmed by immunohistochemical staining (Fig. S1A). CTLA-4 was weakly expressed in the normal tissues surrounding the tumor (Fig. S1B).

Discussion

CT26 is a N-nitroso-N-methylurethane-induced, undifferentiated colon carcinoma cell line and recent cancer immunotherapy studies have shown that CTLA-4 blockade reduced CT26 colon tumor size and was effective in CT26 tumor models [27,28]. Therefore, in this study, we used the CT26 cell line to prepare subcutaneous tumor models for PET imaging.

First, we compared CTLA-4 expression in CT26 tumor tissues, normal colon tissues, and/or cultured CT26 cells by RT-PCR analyses and confirmed that CTLA-4 was strongly expressed in the CT26 tumor tissues compared to the normal colon tissues. There are four functionally different forms of CTLA-4: the full-length form (containing exons 1–4), the soluble form (exons 1, 2, and 4), the ligand-independent form (exons 1, 3, and 4), and the form containing only exons 1 and 4 [29–34]. In our experiments, the full-length form of CTLA-4 (amplicon length: 920 bp), which is a representative immunosuppressive form of CTLA-4, was expressed in the CT26 tumor tissues.

On the other hand, we found that CTLA-4 was not expressed in the cultured CT26 cells, although it was strongly expressed in the CT26 tumor tissues. Contardi et al. reported some human tumor cell lines that expressed CTLA-4 [4]. On the other hand, CTLA-4 is expressed also on CD25[+] (and/or) Foxp3[+] (and/or) FR4[+] CD4[+] Tregs, activated CD4[+] effector T cells, and activated CD8[+] effector T cells [2,3,24]. In addition, flow cytometry analysis by Valzasina et al. revealed that almost all CD4[+] T cells in the CT26 tumor tissues expressed CD25 [35]. From those reports, we hypothesized that CTLA-4 expression in the CT26 tumor tissues regulated by T cells. To prove our hypothesis, we examined the expression of several T cell markers in normal colon tissues, CT26 tumor tissues, and cultured CT26 cells. RT-PCR analysis showed

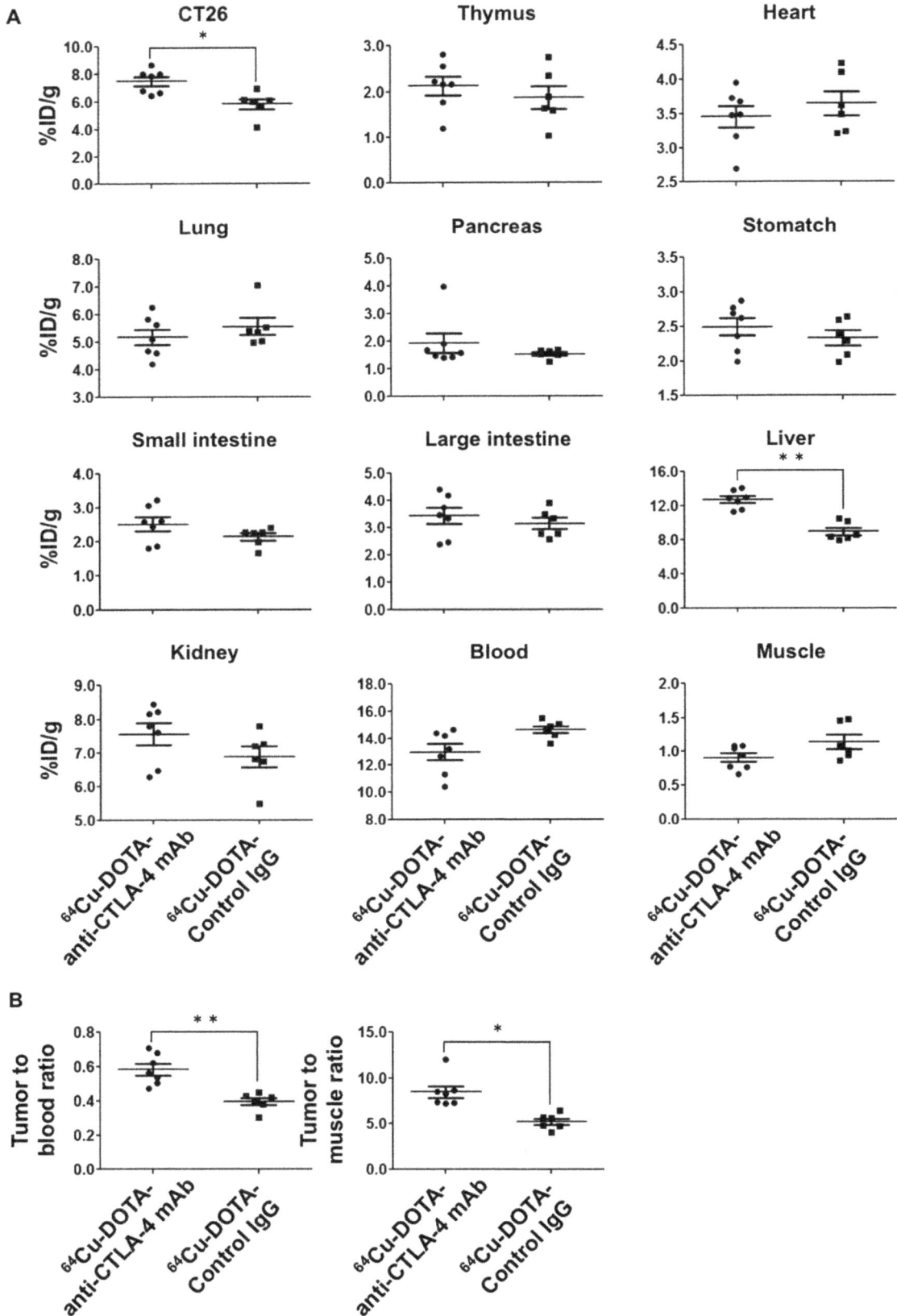

Figure 5. Biodistribution analysis of ^{64}Cu-labeled antibody probes. A. %ID/g of ^{64}Cu-DOTA-anti-CTLA-4 mAb (n = 7) and ^{64}Cu-DOTA-Control IgG (n = 6). B. Tumor-to-blood and tumor-to-muscle ratios of ^{64}Cu-DOTA-anti-CTLA-4 mAb (n = 7) and ^{64}Cu-DOTA-Control IgG (n = 6). Data are expressed as means ± SEM. Symbols* and ** denote p<0.01 and p<0.001 vs. ^{64}Cu-DOTA-Control IgG, respectively.

that Treg markers and T cell activation markers were strongly expressed in the CT26 tumor tissues but not the normal colon tissues or cultured CT26 cells. Therefore, we assumed that the T cells were responsible for CTLA-4 expression in the CT26 tumor tissues. Then, we used RT-PCR to compare the expression of CTLA-4 and T cell markers in the CT26 tumor tissues of tumor-bearing BALB/c mice with those of tumor-bearing BALB/c nude mice in hopes of elucidating the relationship between CTLA-4 expression in the CT26 tumor tissues and T cells. BALB/c nude mice are thymus-deficient and thus, the number of T cells is greatly reduced in those mice. Interestingly, we found that the expression of CTLA-4 as well as T cell markers was quite low in the CT26 tumor tissues from the BALB/c nude mice. The results indicated that T cells were responsible for the CTLA-4 expression.

Second, we developed a molecular imaging probe that targets CTLA-4 and examined its utility in mice bearing CTLA-4-expressing CT26 tumor. The anti-CTLA-4 mAb for the imaging probe synthesis was made by using recombinant mouse CTLA-4 representing an extracellular domain of mouse CTLA-4 (Ala36-Phe161) as the immunogen. We selected this mAb for CTLA-4 imaging probe synthesis because clinically used anti-CTLA-4 mAb (ipilimumab) also recognizes the extracellular domain of CTLA-4 and a mAb probe that recognizes the extracellular domain of CTLA-4 is suited for the prediction of the efficacy and drug disposition of ipilimumab.

For CTLA-4 imaging, we conjugated anti-CTLA-4 mAb to DOTA. DOTA-conjugated mAb was prepared by reacting the nucleophilic amino group in the amino acid residue (particularly in lysine) of mAb with the electrophilic DOTA-mono-NHS ester. The binding activity of antibodies to CTLA-4 may be reduced, particularly when DOTA conjugates to lysine residues critical for mAb binding to CTLA-4 [36]. Therefore, it is necessary to check in advance the binding activities of the antibodies. We examined the binding activity of DOTA-conjugated anti-CTLA-4 mAb and compared it with that of control IgG. ELISA confirmed that the binding activity of DOTA-anti-CTLA-4 mAb was preserved for use in CTLA-4 imaging although a slight reduction ($86.3 \pm 2.8\%$) was observed relative to the binding activity of the original anti-CTLA-4 mAb. The binding activity of DOTA-Control IgG was extremely low ($0.3 \pm 0.1\%$) compared with that of DOTA-anti-CTLA-4 mAb. The results indicate the successful preparation of metal-chelator-conjugated anti-CTLA-4 mAb having CTLA-4 binding activity.

The choice of the positron emitter is an important factor for successful PET imaging. In our study, ^{64}Cu was used for labeling mAbs. ^{64}Cu decay generates positron emissions applicable to PET and the half-life of ^{64}Cu ($T_{1/2} = 12.7$ h) is sufficiently long for imaging up to 24 to 48 h after administration to accommodate the mAb localization time. Therefore, ^{64}Cu has been used for the development of mAb-based radiopharmaceuticals [13,15,19]. In our preliminary biodistribution analyses, tumor uptake on ^{64}Cu-DOTA-anti-CTLA-4 mAb was not significantly higher than that on ^{64}Cu-DOTA-Control IgG at 24 h after administration of the probes (data was not shown). Therefore, we chose later time point (48 h) for PET imaging and ex-vivo biodistribution analysis.

The utility of ^{64}Cu-DOTA-anti-CTLA-4 mAb was examined by PET and ex-vivo biodistribution analysis. We were able to visualize CTLA-4-positive tumor by PET with ^{64}Cu-DOTA-anti-CTLA-4 mAb as the probe. Ex-vivo biodistribution analysis also revealed that ^{64}Cu-DOTA-anti-CTLA-4 mAb showed significant accumulation in the CT26 tumor compared to ^{64}Cu-DOTA-Control IgG. The results indicated that ^{64}Cu-DOTA-anti-CTLA-4 mAb is useful for the noninvasive imaging of CTLA-4 expression in tumor. Furthermore, we quantified PET images and calculated ^{64}Cu-DOTA-anti-CTLA-4 mAb/^{64}Cu-DOTA-Control IgG ratio in the CT26. The mean ratio of SUV_{max} values in CT26 was 1.29 in the PET image and that in CT26 was 1.28 in the ex-vivo biodistribution analysis; further, the quantitative value of PET was similar to the ex-vivo biodistribution data. Thus, quantitativity was ensured in our PET experiment. In addition, although further investigation is needed, ^{64}Cu-DOTA-anti-CTLA-4 mAb could be used in the diagnosis of other types of tumor invaded by T cells, regardless of CTLA-4 expression in the tumor cells.

In conclusion, we have developed ^{64}Cu-DOTA-anti-CTLA-4 mAb and evaluated its potential as a new radiotracer for the noninvasive evaluation of CTLA-4 expression in tumor. Our results demonstrated that ^{64}Cu-DOTA-anti-CTLA-4 mAb visualized CTLA-4 expression in CT26 tumor in a noninvasive manner. Therefore, ^{64}Cu-DOTA-anti-CTLA-4 mAb is useful for evaluating CTLA-4 expression in the tumor. The evaluation of CTLA-4 expression in tumors using ^{64}Cu-DOTA-anti-CTLA-4 mAb would enable selection of patients sensitive to CTLA-4-targeted therapy, thereby eliminating the adverse effects brought about by ineffective therapy and reducing unnecessary financial burden in non-sensitive patients.

Supporting Information

Figure S1 Immunohistochemically stained images of CTLA-4 in representative CT26 tumor and normal tissue sections. A. CT26 tumor tissue section. B. Normal tissue section surrounding CT26 tumor tissue. Scale bar = 50 ?m.

Acknowledgments

The authors thank Dr. Yasuhiro Wada and Dr. Emi Hayashinaka for technical support in the reconstitution of PET images; Dr. Yousuke Kanayama, Dr. Takanori Sasaki, and Mr. Fumiaki Takenaka for helpful discussions and technical assistance in PET or ex-vivo biodistribution experiments; and Professor Dr. Satoshi Tanaka for relevant suggestions.

Author Contributions

Conceived and designed the experiments: KH KY MH SE. Performed the experiments: KH KY KW. Analyzed the data: KH KY. Contributed reagents/materials/analysis tools: SE. Wrote the paper: KH SK MU MH SE.

References

1. Yaguchi T, Sumimoto H, Kudo-Saito C, Tsukamoto N, Ueda R, et al. (2011) The mechanisms of cancer immunoescape and development of overcoming strategies. Int J Hematol 93: 294–300.

2. Pardoll DM (2012) The blockade of immune checkpoints in cancer immunotherapy. Nat Rev Cancer 12: 252–264.

3. Grosso JF, Jure-Kunkel MN (2013) CTLA-4 blockade in tumor models: an overview of preclinical and translational research. Cancer Immun 13: 5.

4. Contardi E, Palmisano GL, Tazzari PL, Martelli AM, Fala F, et al. (2005) CTLA-4 is constitutively expressed on tumor cells and can trigger apoptosis upon ligand interaction. Int J Cancer 117: 538–550.

5. Lesterhuis WJ, Haanen JBAG, Punt CJA (2011) Cancer immunotherapy - revisited. Nat Rev Drug Discov 10: 591–600.

6. Ribas A, Hanson DC, Noe DA, Millham R, Guyot DJ, et al. (2007) Tremelimumab (CP-675,206), a cytotoxic T lymphocyte-associated antigen 4

blocking monoclonal antibody in clinical development for patients with cancer. Oncologist 12: 873–883.

7. Torino F, Barnabei A, De Vecchis L, Salvatori R, Corsello SM (2012) Hypophysitis induced by monoclonal antibodies to cytotoxic T lymphocyte antigen 4: challenges from a new cause of a rare disease. Oncologist 17: 525–535.

8. Weber JS, Kahler KC, Hauschild A (2012) Management of immune-related adverse events and kinetics of response with ipilimumab. J Clin Oncol 30: 2691–2697.

9. Suntharalingam G, Perry MR, Ward S, Brett SJ, Castello-Cortes A, et al. (2006) Cytokine storm in a phase 1 trial of the anti-CD28 monoclonal antibody TGN1412. N Engl J Med 355: 1018–1028.

10. Walker LSK, Sansom DM (2011) The emerging role of CTLA4 as a cell-extrinsic regulator of T cell responses. Nat Rev Immunol 11: 852–863.

11. Sondak VK, Smalley KS, Kudchadkar R, Grippon S, Kirkpatrick P (2011) Ipilimumab. Nat Rev Drug Discov 10: 411–412.

12. Dijkers EC, Oude Munnink TH, Kosterink JG, Brouwers AH, Jager PL, et al. (2010) Biodistribution of 89Zr-trastuzumab and PET imaging of HER2-positive lesions in patients with metastatic breast cancer. Clin Pharmacol Ther 87: 586–592.

13. ClinicalTrials.gov website. Available: http://clinicaltrials.gov/ct2/show/NCT00605397. Accessed 2014 Sep 20.

14. ClinicalTrials.gov website. Available: http://clinicaltrials.gov/ct2/show/NCT00474578. Accessed 2014 Sep 20.

15. Cai WB, Chen K, He LN, Cao QH, Koong A, et al. (2007) Quantitative PET of EGFR expression in xenograft-bearing mice using Cu-64-labeled cetuximab, a chimeric anti-EGFR monoclonal antibody. Eur J Nucl Med Mol Imaging 34: 850–858.

16. Niu G, Li Z, Xie J, Le QT, Chen X (2009) PET of EGFR antibody distribution in head and neck squamous cell carcinoma models. J Nucl Med 50: 1116–1123.

17. Bhattacharyya S, Kurdziel K, Wei L, Riffle L, Kaur G, et al. (2013) Zirconium-89 labeled panitumumab: a potential immuno-PET probe for HER1-expressing carcinomas. Nucl Med Biol 40: 451–457.

18. ClinicalTrials.gov website. Available: http://clinicaltrials.gov/show/NCT00691548. Accessed 2014 Sep 20.

19. Paudyal B, Paudyal P, Oriuchi N, Hanaoka H, Tominaga H, et al. (2011) Positron emission tomography imaging and biodistribution of vascular endothelial growth factor with 64Cu-labeled bevacizumab in colorectal cancer xenografts. Cancer Sci 102: 117–121.

20. Nagengast WB, de Korte MA, Oude Munnink TH, Timmer-Bosscha H, den Dunnen WF, et al. (2010) 89Zr-bevacizumab PET of early antiangiogenic tumor response to treatment with HSP90 inhibitor NVP-AUY922. J Nucl Med 51: 761–767.

21. Higashikawa K, Akada N, Yagi K, Watanabe K, Kamino S, et al. (2011) Exploration of target molecules for molecular imaging of inflammatory bowel disease. Biochem Biophys Res Commun 410(3): 416–21.

22. Lu SX, Takach EJ, Solomon M, Zhu Q, Law SJ, et al. (2005) Mass spectral analyses of labile DOTA-NHS and heterogeneity determination of DOTA or DM1 conjugated anti-PSMA antibody for prostate cancer therapy. J Pharm Sci 94: 788–797.

23. Sakaguchi S, Miyara M, Costantino CM, Hafler DA (2010) FOXP3+ regulatory T cells in the human immune system. Nat Rev Immunol 10: 490–500.

24. Yamaguchi T, Hirota K, Nagahama K, Ohkawa K, Takahashi T, et al. (2007) Control of immune responses by antigen-specific regulatory T cells expressing the folate receptor. Immunity 27: 145–159.

25. Simms PE, Ellis TM (1996) Utility of flow cytometric detection of CD69 expression as a rapid method for determining poly- and oligoclonal lymphocyte activation. Clin Diagn Lab Immunol 3: 301–304.

26. Elgueta R, Benson MJ, de Vries VC, Wasiuk A, Guo Y, et al. (2009) Molecular mechanism and function of CD40/CD40L engagement in the immune system. Immunol Rev 229: 152–172.

27. Selby MJ, Engelhardt JJ, Quigley M, Henning KA, Chen T, et al. (2013) Anti-CTLA-4 Antibodies of IgG2a Isotype Enhance Antitumor Activity through Reduction of Intratumoral Regulatory T Cells. Cancer Immunol Res 1: 32–42.

28. Mitsui J, Nishikawa H, Muraoka D, Wang L, Noguchi T, et al. (2010) Two distinct mechanisms of augmented antitumor activity by modulation of immunostimulatory/inhibitory signals. Clin Cancer Res 16: 2781–2791.

29. Teft WA, Kirchhof MG, Madrenas J (2006) A molecular perspective of CTLA-4 function. Annu Rev Immunol 24: 65–97.

30. Ueda H, Howson JM, Esposito L, Heward J, Snook H, et al. (2003) Association of the T-cell regulatory gene CTLA4 with susceptibility to autoimmune disease. Nature 423: 506–511.

31. Vijayakrishnan L, Slavik JM, Illes Z, Greenwald RJ, Rainbow D, et al. (2004) An autoimmune disease-associated CTLA-4 splice variant lacking the B7 binding domain signals negatively in T cells. Immunity 20: 563–575.

32. Araki M, Chung D, Liu S, Rainbow DB, Chamberlain G, et al. (2009) Genetic Evidence That the Differential Expression of the Ligand-Independent Isoform of CTLA-4 Is the Molecular Basis of the Idd5.1 Type 1 Diabetes Region in Nonobese Diabetic Mice. J Immunol 183: 5146–5157.

33. Liu SM, Sutherland APR, Zhang Z, Rainbow DB, Quintana FJ, et al. (2012) Overexpression of the CTLA-4 Isoform Lacking Exons 2 and 3 Causes Autoimmunity. J Immunol 188: 155–162.

34. Gerold KD, Zheng PL, Rainbow DB, Zernecke A, Wicker LS, et al. (2011) The Soluble CTLA-4 Splice Variant Protects From Type 1 Diabetes and Potentiates Regulatory T-Cell Function. Diabetes 60: 1955–1963.

35. Valzasina B, Piconese S, Guiducci C, Colombo MP (2006) Tumor-induced expansion of regulatory T cells by conversion of CD4(+)CD25(−) lymphocytes is thymus and proliferation independent. Cancer Res 66: 4488–4495.

36. Knowles SM, Wu AM (2012) Advances in immuno-positron emission tomography: antibodies for molecular imaging in oncology. J Clin Oncol 30: 3884–3892.

17

Stochastic Tracking of Infection in a CF Lung

Sara Zarei[1]*, Ali Mirtar[2], Forest Rohwer[3], Peter Salamon[4]

1 Computational Science Research Center, San Diego State University, San Diego, California, United States of America, **2** Electrical and Computer Eng. Dep/University of California San Diego, San Diego, California, United States of America, **3** Department of Biology, San Diego State University, San Diego, California, United States of America, **4** Department of Mathematics and Statistics, San Diego State University, San Diego, California, United States of America

Abstract

Magnetic Resonance Imaging (MRI) and Computed Tomography (CT) scan are the two ubiquitous imaging sources that physicians use to diagnose patients with Cystic Fibrosis (CF) or any other Chronic Obstructive Pulmonary Disease (COPD). Unfortunately the cost constraints limit the frequent usage of these medical imaging procedures. In addition, even though both CT scan and MRI provide mesoscopic details of a lung, in order to obtain microscopic information a very high resolution is required. Neither MRI nor CT scans provide micro level information about the location of infection in a binary tree structure the binary tree structure of the human lung. In this paper we present an algorithm that enhances the current imaging results by providing estimated micro level information concerning the location of the infection. The estimate is based on a calculation of the distribution of possible mucus blockages consistent with available information using an offline Metropolis-Hastings algorithm in combination with a real-time interpolation scheme. When supplemented with growth rates for the pockets of mucus, the algorithm can also be used to estimate how lung functionality as manifested in spirometric tests will change in patients with CF or COPD.

Editor: Wayne Iwan Lee Davies, University of Western Australia, Australia

Funding: This material is based upon work supported by the National Institutes of Health under Grant no. 56586B. The funders had no role in study design, data collection and analysis, decision to publish, or preparation of the manuscript.

Competing Interests: The authors have declared that no competing interests exist.

* Email: sara.zarei@alumni.ucsd.edu

Introduction

Patients with chronic obstructive pulmonary disease (COPD) or cystic fibrosis (CF) have chronic lung inflammation which causes airflow limitation and the scarring of lung tissues. Their airways are generally inflamed and produce excess amounts of mucus that impair the flow of air into and out of their lungs.

Our hypothesis is that the scarring, and ultimate remodeling of a CF lung is mostly due to the contact between the lung lining and the mucus. Inflammatory cytokines induce scars in lung tissue [1]. This contact between mucous biofilm and lung tissue facilitates virulent microbes that also play a role in remodeling a CF lung. In comparison with a normal lung, the airway fluids of CF patients contain large amounts of neutrophils as a result of the inflammatory response [2]. Thus our hypothesis is that mucus accumulation is primarily responsible for damage to the lung and therefore tracking its propagation is a crucial task for better diagnosis and treatment.

Spirometry, the measurement of a patient's breathing, is the standard clinical tool for monitoring lung disease. The two most common spirometric indicators are the forced expiratory volume in one second, FEV_1, and the forced vital capacity, FVC. FEV_1 measures the volume of air that can forcibly be blown out in one second while FVC measures the volume of air that can forcibly be blown out after a full inspiration maneuver. Although these tests provide a global measure of airflow obstruction and restriction, they do not give detailed information about the location of mucus blockage. Additional information is available from the repeated imaging of CF patients' lungs. This is usually in the form of chest x-ray, computed tomography (CT) or magnetic resonance imaging (MRI). Despite the fact that CT is an optimal morphological assessment of CF lung changes, the associated exposure to ionizing radiation is a serious obstacle. Therefore, MRI might be the appropriate method for imaging CF patient's lungs [3,4].

MRI was first introduced as an alternative imaging tool for patients with CF in 1987 [5]. There are numerous methods for the analysis of chest MRI. Theilmann et al. proposed a new MRI imaging method that can spatially locate the pockets of infection and measure the amount of mucus located within each pocket. This information is obtained with a resolution of approximately 1.0 cm^3 [6]. This resolution is equivalent to the last 10 generations of airways combined. Despite the accuracy level of MRI images, they do not contain any micro-level information on smaller airways. Hence the precise location of infection cannot be obtained from the MRI data.

There have been research studies on mesoscopic modeling of Cystic Fibrosis [7]. Such studies however did not address the micro level information about mucus propagation through the airways. The goal of this research is to provide the clinician with an algorithm that can track the location and propagation of mucus in a CF patient's lungs. Tracking the growth, or shrinkage of these pockets can be correlated to the efficacy of different treatment regimens on each pocket. Assuming further progress in metagenomic and transcriptomic analyses of sputum samples, tracking may allow also correlating the growth or shrinkage of these pockets and the composition of the local microbial community structure within the pocket.

The central tool introduced in the present article for tracking pockets of inflammation is based on using our airflow model [8] in reverse, i.e., as the main ingredient in an inverse problem. Our airflow model can calculate the flow and the total resistance corresponding to a given distribution of mucus obstructions in respiratory airways. The solution of the inverse problem is achieved by randomly sampling the many possible mucus configurations consistent with the current information regarding a patient. Many micro-scale distributions match any observed MRI and spirometric data. The fortuitous finding in the calculations described below is that a large majority of the possible distributions fall within narrow ranges of certain parameters such as which generations of airways contain how much mucus. Can we be certain of these most likely locations being the actual mucus distribution? The fact that most of the distributions consistent with the spirometric and MRI data have these features makes them a good bet while not giving us certainty that any *one* configuration is of this form. In fact, however, repeated MRI measurements separated by small challenges such as coughing or even just taking a few deep breaths reveal that mucus inside the lungs of CF patients show small but discernible movements in response to such challenges. Given this dynamic picture, the possibility that all of the configurations of mucus would avoid the configurations that can be realized the largest number of ways is extremely unlikely. We describe below how to construct such distributions that best represent the state of airways corresponding to the patients lung functionality test values (FEV$_1$ and FVC) and any available MRI or CT data. We use a maximum entropy approach to construct such estimates by sampling all consistent distributions and choosing the one that can be realized the largest number of ways. We find that the predicted microscopic distribution of mucus is generally sharply peaked, allowing us to estimate the distribution of mucus as the one that appears the most frequently in our simulation. The entire computation process can take a long time and would require enormous computational space to run the simulation for the entire 2^{23} airways in a lung. However after running the simulation once for a patient, we can store most of the data so the next simulations only take a few minutes to complete.

Given the micro-scale distribution obtained from our inverse problem, we can use our physiological model [9] to predict the growth and propagation of this distribution, thereby predicting the progression of the disease. This second model requires a rate for the growth of the mucus volume at each location. Currently only one overall average growth rate is available, a growth rate that was estimated based on a forty year CF population average [9]. Predictions of this model with the average growth rate can nonetheless be compared to actual observed disease progression between exacerbations. For predictions during exacerbations, a database of treatment and community specific growth rates are needed and in-principle available from multiple MRI and metagenomic/transcriptomic analyses. Two such datasets allow the extraction of pocket specific growth rates and corresponding linear extrapolation for the mucus volume in each pocket. This can at least lengthen the times between imaging sessions.

Methods

Inverse Problem Using Metropolis-Hastings Algorithm

Our algorithm uses CF patients' spirometry test values of FVC, FEV$_1$ and any available mucus distribution data from CT scans or MRI as its input. It then identifies the distribution of mucus obstructed bronchioles throughout different airway generations. The model assumes the lung airways to be binary branching trees [10] extending over 23 generations from the bronchus down to the alveoli. It further assumes a fractal structure [11–13] for the parameters of the binary airway tree.

Considering the fact that there are 2^{23} bronchioles in a human lung, there are astronomically many possible configurations for a certain amount of mucus distributed in an airway tree, even given the mucus in each voxel. In fact many of these configurations will result in the same FEV$_1$ and FVC values. Since exhaustive sampling of these configurations is impossible, we use the Metropolis-Hastings Markov chain Monte Carlo algorithm to sample a few hundred million and base our estimates on such a sample. The goal of this section is to introduce this method.

Our algorithm proceeds from an assumed amount of mucus to be distributed into the 2^{23} airways. It starts from a random distribution and obtains an unbiased sample of configurations satisfying certain requirements. These requirements are implemented as soft constraints via an energy function

$$E = (\alpha)(\text{Calculated FEV}_1 - \text{Patient FEV}_1)^2 + \\ (1-\alpha)(\text{Calculated FVC} - \text{Patient FVC})^2 \quad (1)$$

where (α) and $(1-\alpha)$ are weight factors. In our algorithm we set $\alpha = 0.5$. The energy function is used as a way to force the sampling to stay near values with low energy, i.e. configurations with approximately correct spirometric readings.

We then examine successive samples by performing a random walk on the space of mucus configurations. Each move in our random walk reallocates the location of some of the mucus. The resulting distribution of mucus configurations turns out to be sharply peaked in certain natural parameters, a fact exploited by our algorithm.

The Metropolis algorithm is a widely used procedure for sampling a sequence from a specified distribution on a large finite set. It describes equilibrium for systems whose configurations have probability proportional to the Boltzmann factor $(e^{-E/T})$. This is a weighting factor which determines the relative probability that the system will be found in a particular configuration at energy E when the temperature of the environment is T [14]. We used a constant temperature, $T = 1$, making the probability of a configuration with energy E proportional to $\exp(-E)$.

The following steps describe the Metropolis algorithm [15].

- Initiate the sampling from an arbitrary configuration A, with known energy E_A.
- Define a new neighbor configuration B from configuration A.
- Calculate the new configuration energy, E_B. This trial move is then either accepted or rejected according to the following simple probabilistic rule.
- If $E_B < E_A$ we accept the new configuration.
- if $E_B > E_A$, we may accept configuration B with the following probability.

$$p = e^{-(E_B - E_A)/T} \quad (2)$$

- Repeat until sufficient number of configurations have been collected.

To apply the Metropolis algorithm to our model, we need to define neighboring configurations. Our definition moves a certain amount of mucus between a few chosen bronchioles. This keeps the energy re-evaluation step computationally cheap and, provided we allow such rearrangement between all types of airways, we avoid the problems created by local minima. This assures that the system settles into and stays near the lowest energy configurations as the simulation proceeds [16].

Two-Dimensional Probability Density Function Estimation (PDFE-2D) of Mucus Obstructions

Imaging provides us with the data that corresponds to the spatial location of infection pockets and the amount of mucus within each pocket. Both MRI and CT images can have various resolutions and our approach is scalable to any resolution. For concreteness below we work with a resolution of 1 cm^3 and refer to this smallest volume as a voxel - a volume element.

Since on average the total lung capacity of an adult human is about 6 liters [17], an image will have about 6000 voxels. Using the binary tree structure of the lung airway, we set these voxels at the end of the 13th generation to approximately match the number of these elements to the number of subtrees that remain. Since $2^{13} = 8192 \approx 6000$, we can identify the mucus in the voxel with the mucus in the subtree of $2^{23-13} = 2^{10}$ bronchioles terminating in the alveoli. Thus each voxel in our lung model represents a binary tree structure that has a total of 10 bifurcations, from generation 13 to 23, with a known total amount of mucus obtained from imaging data.

Using a three-dimensional model of the human airway tree that was developed by [18], we are able to map each MRI or CT scan voxel into our lung model's voxels with their corresponding mucus content. The main task of our algorithm is to locate the infection in the airway tree structure of a CF lung. To achieve this goal, we use two summary features for each voxel: (1) the percent of alveoli that are accessible, i.e., not totally blocked and (2) the total resistance to flow from the alveoli to the 13th generation brochiole bronchiole assigned to the voxel. These two microscopic features correspond loosely to the spirometric indicators FVC and FEV$_1$, respectively.

In order for us to calculate each voxel's resistance and the percent of accessible alveoli (for simplicity, we refer to this as the AA%), we first have to define how mucus is distributed in a voxel's binary tree structure. There is an astronomical number of configurations for filling a binary tree of 10 generations with a given amount of mucus. Approximately, it is given by $(2^{10})^{M/m}$ where M is the total mucus volume and m is the volume of the smallest bronchiole. Thus even at this level, we used Metropolis-Hastings to sample many mucus configurations, recording the values of AA% and resistance for each configuration. We set the amount of mucus within each voxel and calculate the distribution of AA% and resistance: our PDFE-2D distribution.

Hence if a voxel contains 5% mucus, the first step is randomly filling up the voxel's airway tree with the specified mucus amount. Then using the Metropolis algorithm, at each state we move only a fraction of the mucus within a bronchiole that is equivalent to the smallest bronchiole's volume in a lung airway tree. We refer to this as the "unit volume". Once a unit volume is moved to a different location, the corresponding voxel's parameters (AA% and resistance) are recalculated.

In order to expedite the computational process; Dulcinea computing clusters from the Computational Science Research Center at San Diego State University were used for collecting almost 54 million samples. The Dulcinea computing clusters contains 12 workstations each with Dual-Quad Xeon central processing unit (CPU) (E5520 2.27GHz) and Dual Tesla graphic processing unit (GPU) (M1060) which provides the total of 96 CPU cores. The cluster system utilizes 3GB of memory per CPU core for nodes 1 to 10 and utilizes 6GB of memory per CPU core

for nodes 11 and 12. After obtaining these samples the probability distributions for different amount of mucus are calculated. Figure 1A to Figure 1D illustrate the probability density function for (5%, 30%, 65%, and 75%) mucus respectively. As shown in Figure 1A, when there is only 5% mucus in a voxel, the most likely configuration has 86% of its alveoli accessible and the voxel's resistance increases by a factor of almost 1.1. When the mucus level reaches almost 30% there are only 27% accessible alveoli and the voxel resistance is almost 2.2 times a healthy voxel with no mucus. On the other hand in Figure 1C and 1D the number of accessible alveoli value approaches zero while the resistance value reaches infinity. This refers to a case that a voxel is almost completely filled with mucus to an extent that no more air can pass through and therefore blocks all the corresponding alveoli at the end of the branching tree.

Figure 2 displays the maximum likelihood combinations of AA% and resistance ratio for different amount of mucus in a voxel. As the mucus reaches almost 60% of the available airway volume in the voxel, there is no remaining access to the alveoli and as a result there is no gas exchange taking place in that particular part of the airway tree. After collecting these distributions, the model can initiate the prediction steps as well as providing the microlevel information about the location of obstructed bronchioles. We will discuss each outcome in the next two sections. Please note that all data underlying the findings of this section have been discussed in the manuscript. Other than the massive computing power needed to produce the findings in Figure 1 and Figure 2, all the relevant data have been shared.

Results

Micro-Level Information on Obstructed Bronchioles

In order to spatially locate each bronchiole in a human airway tree we used Kitaoka et al.'s three-dimensional model [18]. Once we receive the imaging data for each voxel, we need to map the values to our model's voxel using spatial location coordinates. Next we use the probability density function that we found in the previous section to determine the corresponding voxel parameters, AA% and resistance ratio, sampled according to the PDFE-2D distributions. The model randomly select a combination of percent accessible alveoli and resistance for each voxel in a way that the total resistance and number of accessible alveoli from these voxels provide the same value as the patient's FEV$_1$ and FVC. There is a complex calculation taking place in parallel to obtain the rate of flow (FEV$_1$) from the total resistance of all the voxels. To find the distribution of voxel parameters we use the Metropolis algorithm to focus the Markov chain to sample many configurations meeting our constraints. This is achieved by choosing the configuration energy provided in Eq(1).

At this stage we have mapped the voxels from imaging data into our model in a way that the total rate of airflow and the accessible alveoli of the lung model resemble the corresponding patient's FEV$_1$ and FVC values respectively. Once the current state of a CF lung is implemented we can obtain clinically useful information, such as mucus distribution within each voxel or predicted future states of each voxel and associated FEV$_1$ and FVC values as described in the next section.

Figure 3 displays the flowchart of this process. As shown in this flowchart, once we have all the voxels' parameters, we can select certain voxels for further analysis. We again apply the Metropolis algorithm on the selected voxel in order to visualize the distribution of mucus in its airway tree structure. For the chosen voxel, we have its mucus volume, its resistance and its AA%. We randomly fill out the voxels' airway tree to reach their

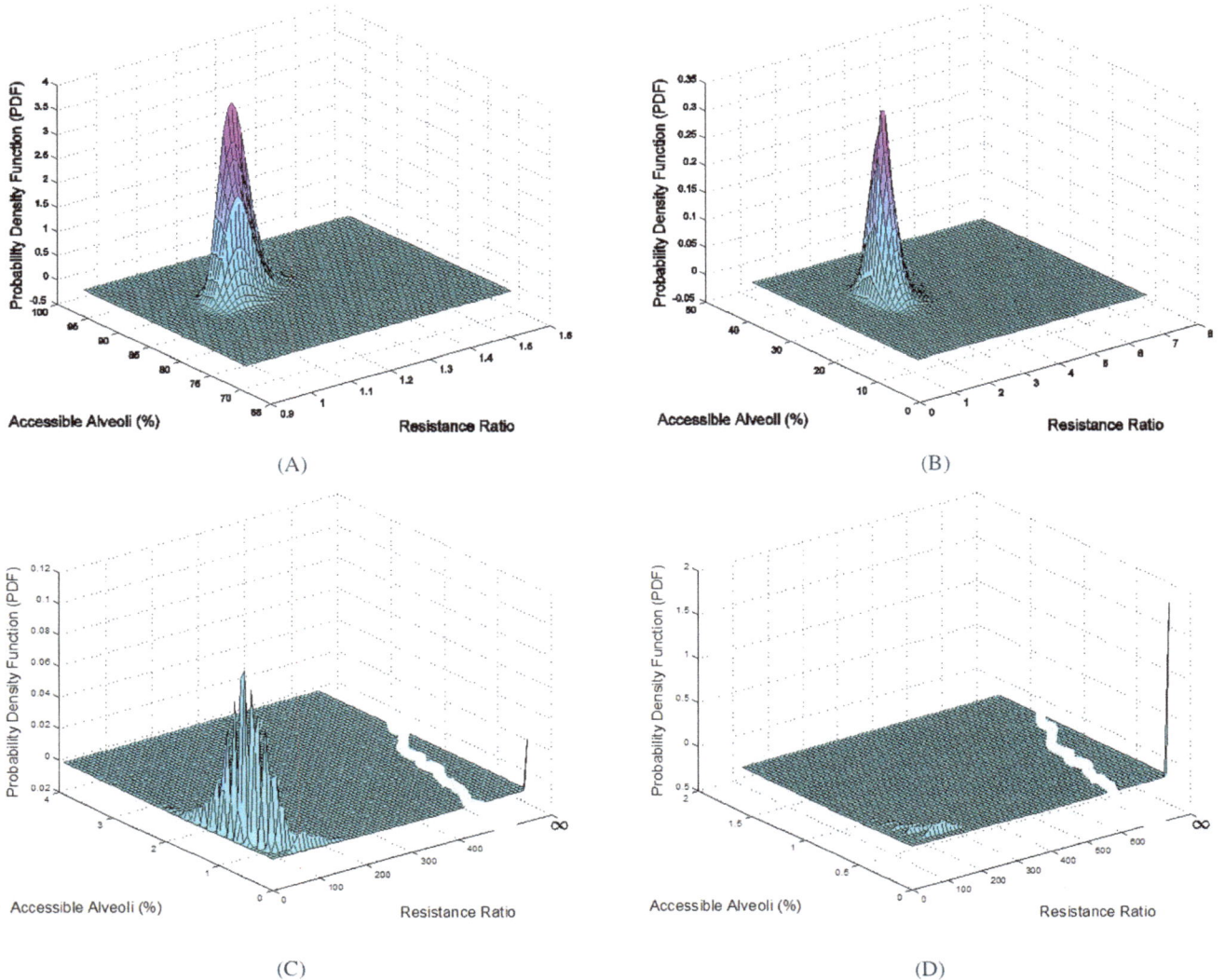

Figure 1. Probability density function for different percent volume of mucus in a small voxel of the lung. (A) 5%, **(B)** 30%, **(C)** 65% **and (D)** 75% Each voxel represents a subtree from generation 13 to 23 of the binary tree structure of lung. The x-axis is the corresponding airflow resistance and the y-axis shows the percent accessible alveoli.

corresponding mucus volume. At each iteration the new resistance and AA% are collected. To move to the neighbor configuration we move a unit volume of mucus in a bronchiole to keep the total mucus volume of the voxel fixed. The state energy we use for this step is as follows:

$$E = (\alpha)(\text{Resistance of the current state} -$$

$$\text{Target voxel's resistance})^2 + (1 - \alpha) \qquad (3)$$

$$(\text{AA\% of the current state} - \text{Target voxel's AA\%})^2$$

where $\alpha = 0.5$. After we obtained enough samples we constructed the corresponding mucus distribution for the selected voxels. Figures 4 displays two examples of the mucus distribution for voxels that contained (5%) and (30%) mucus. As shown in these figures, as the percent mucus increases, the dominantly filled generation moves to bigger bronchioles. The y axis repressnts represents % normalized mucus where:

Normalized mucus in generation n

$$= \frac{(\dfrac{\text{Mucus Volume in generation } n}{\text{Total mucus volume in voxel}})}{(\dfrac{\text{Airway volume in generation } n}{\text{Total airway volume in voxel}})} \qquad (4)$$

Predicting future values of FEV$_1$ and FVC

In this section we use the mucus distribution and growth model presented in [9] to make predictions about the lung functionality of a CF patient. As can be seen in Figure 5 we use the imaging voxels' data and the constant mucus growth rate from [9], or, if available, infection and treatment specific growth rates specific to each voxel to predict the mucus growth in each pocket of infection. The model again resorts to the Monte Carlo method to randomly select the AA% and resistance from our model described in the

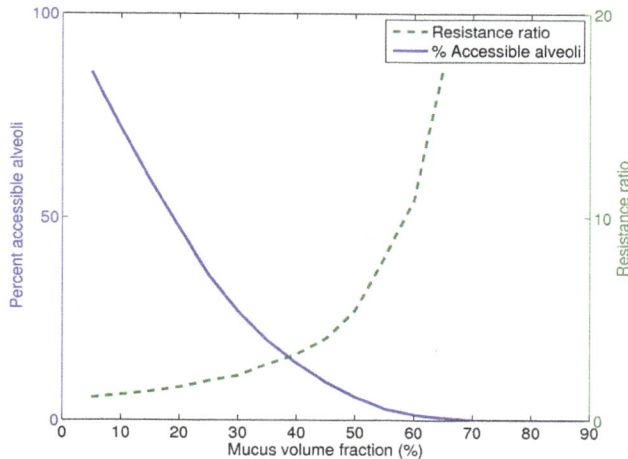

Figure 2. Maximum likelihood of percent of accessible alveoli AA% and airflow resistance for a given mucus volume fraction inside a voxel. The x-axis is mucus volume% and the two y-axes show the most probable combination of the airflow resistance ratio and percent of accessible alveoli. The resistance value increases as the mucus amount rises. Number of accessible alveoli decreases as the mucus volume grows, which leads to a lower lung functionality test value or FVC value.

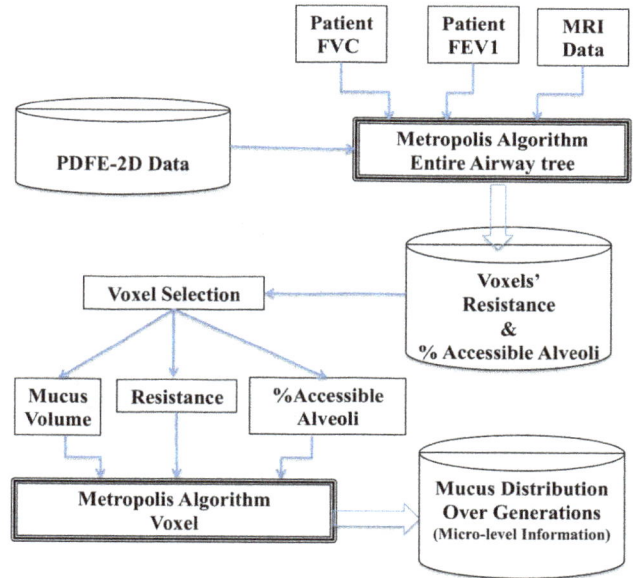

Figure 3. Generating the Micro-level information on obstructed bronchioles. This flowchart shows how the algorithm produces the mucus distribution of a selected voxel. Using the lung functionality test values: FEV1 and FVC and the data obtained from MRI lung imaging we can obtain the corresponding mucus distributions among the different generations of lung.

PDFE-2D section and calculates the new FEV_1 and FVC at each iteration and stores their values. After collecting enough samples we can predict the FEV_1 and FVC distributions for a patient after the indicated time period. For example, Figure 6 displays the probability density function of the predicted FEV_1 and FVC. As shown in the figure it is predicted that FEV_1 and FVC of our CF patient are approximately 61% and 78% respectively.

This method can even be applied to follow a patient's progress with out fewer imaging tests. Since most CF patients take spirometry test more often than any imaging tests, we can use our model without recourse to imaging data. This time the model takes only the FEV_1 and the FVC values of a patient as input. After applying the Metropolis algorithm (using additional rearrangements of mucus between voxels) the model can still provide an estimate of the distribution of mucus throughout the airway tree. This can be propagated using the constant any hypothetical growth rates to predict the next spirometric test. We have created a Matlab GUI version of the algorithm; its sample output is shown in Figures 7, 8 and 9.

Since the mean mucus growth rate was estimated based on years of data from many CF patients, such predictions should work reasonably well for a patient between exacerbations. Our model can also be used to predict the progression during exacerbations, albeit with voxel specific growth rates informed by much more data than we currently possess. Using one mean mucus growth rate is a shortcoming not of our algorithm but rather of the paucity of data to which our predictions have been applied. There is every indication that soon we will have reasonable metagenomic [19–22] and metabolomic [23] tools to assess the microbial composition present in a CF lung and will be able to infer growth rates that are specific to the community composition as well as the antibiotic administered. Entering voxel specific growth rates based on more information than we at present possess and using our program to test predictions can move our understanding of the patient's state to a new and quantitative level.

We can improve the accuracy level of the model by extending the resolution of our PDFE-2D distributions. The current PDFEs

were constructed with 5% bins as described in PDFE-2D model section.

Discussion

With current research studies about cystic fibrosis, CF treatment is poised for great strides. Non-genetic treatments such as Ivacaftor (trade name Kalydeco, developed as VX-770) only works on patients with a certain mutation of cystic fibrosis which accounts for 4–5% of cystic fibrosis cases [24].

While an eventual cure for the disease by replacement of the defective gene is likely, we expect such treatment not to be available anytime soon. Rather we anticipate that new observational tools such as metagenomics, transcriptomics, metabolomics and MRI imaging coupled with our modeling approach will give the clinician unprecedented ability to follow and treat the disease. The models will provide quantitative predictions of responses to various drug regimens and prescribe adaptively implemented optimal controls for treatment. Predicting the impact of mucus growth on lung functionality will correlate the current stage of the disease with how infection has been propagating throughout different generations of lung. This will enable the physician with a tool to track this propagation of infection.

The various sub-models required here will soon be informed by data characterizing the microbial communities present. Such data comes from metagenomic and transcriptomics analyses of sputum samples and metabolomic analyses of exhaled air. In our current model we predict the dynamic distribution of mucus in a CF lung in the absence of treatment as a stepping stone for eventually eventual treatment and microbial community specific modeling of the treatment response.

According to a research study done by Willner et al. [25] microbial diversity in a CF lung is much higher than suggested by culturing alone. They were able to characterize the diversity of

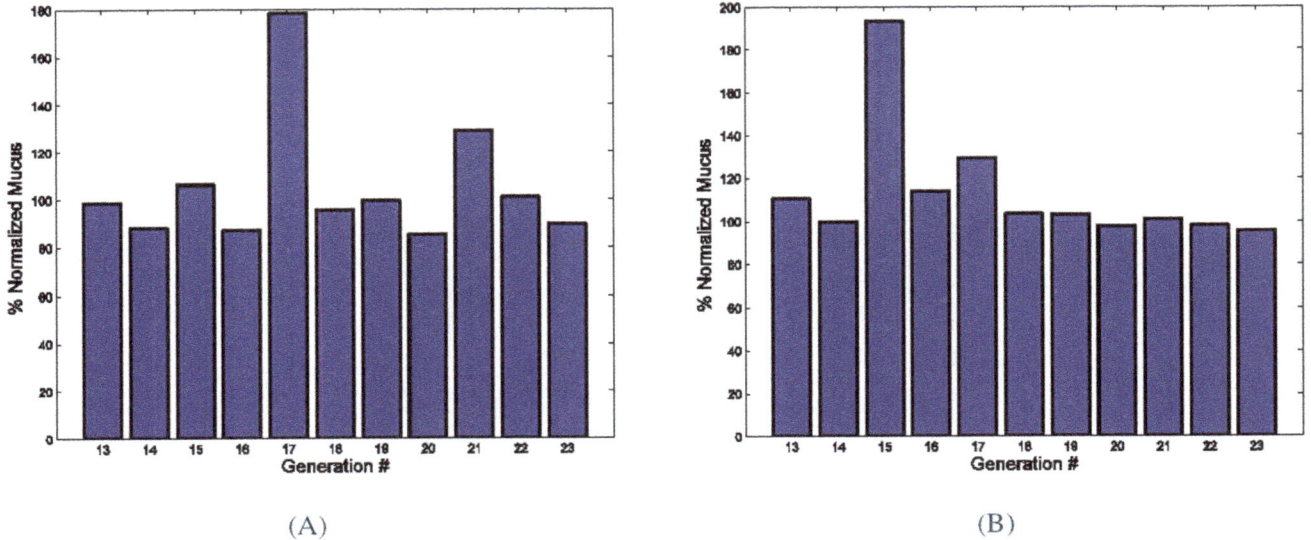

(A)   (B)

Figure 4. Mucus distribution among different generations of lung for two selected voxels. Figure (A) represents a voxel with 5% mucus volume that has 78% accessible alveoli: AA and resistance ratio of 1.22. Figure (B) repsresents represents a voxel with 30% mucus that has 19.45% AA and resistance ratio of 4.2. The x-axis is the generation number of the corresponding bronchioles in the selected voxel. The y-axis shows the normalized mucus present, which is equal to the ratio of the mucus amount in a generation to the total mucus volume in a voxel, divided by the ratio of the air volume in that generation to the total voxel volume.

microbial communities in tissue sections from anatomically distinct regions of the CF lung. Their result indicated that microbial communities in the Cystic Fibrosis lung are spatially heterogeneous. This Spatial heterogeneity will cause regional differences in microbial biomass and antibiotic resistance. The next version of the model, can use their results to adjust the parameters according to the microbial communities found and the treatment administered (e.g., timing of antibiotic administration, types of antibiotics, steroids, etc). The present model should be taken as a proof-of-concept step toward that goal. This will provide an opportunity for

the researcher, and eventually the clinician, to access a framework for accurate quantitative predictions.

Our methods are completely scalable – the 1.0 cm^3 for the size of one voxel was for illustration. Any resolution scale however forces estimation of the distribution on spatial scales below this resolution. Since estimation of the distribution on finer spatial scales would perforce need the solution of an inverse problem with many possible solutions and since the movement of mucus hinted that the "right answer" would in any case not be a unique distribution, we were led naturally to using Monte Carlo

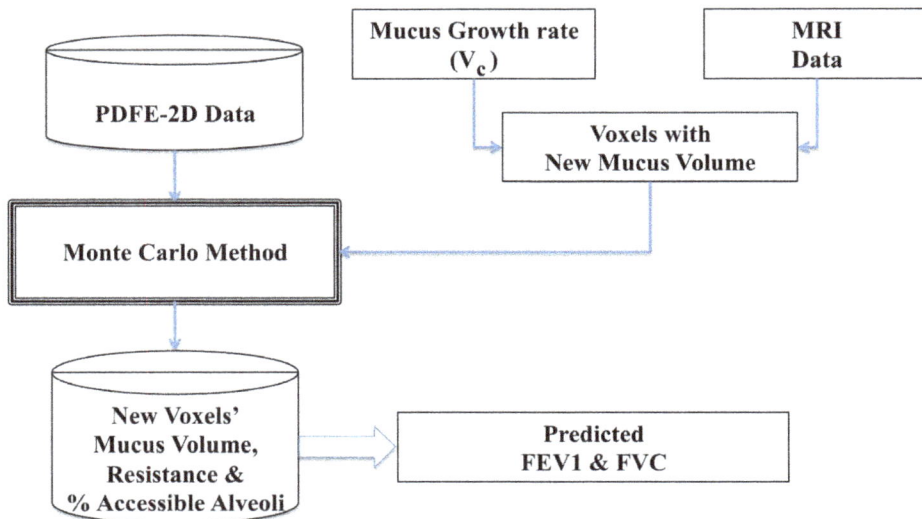

Figure 5. FEV$_1$ and FVC values predictions predicted from the lung model. This flowchart illustrates the process of how our lung model predicts the FVC and FEV$_1$ of a CF patient given the previous mucus content of each voxel along with a mucus growth rate.

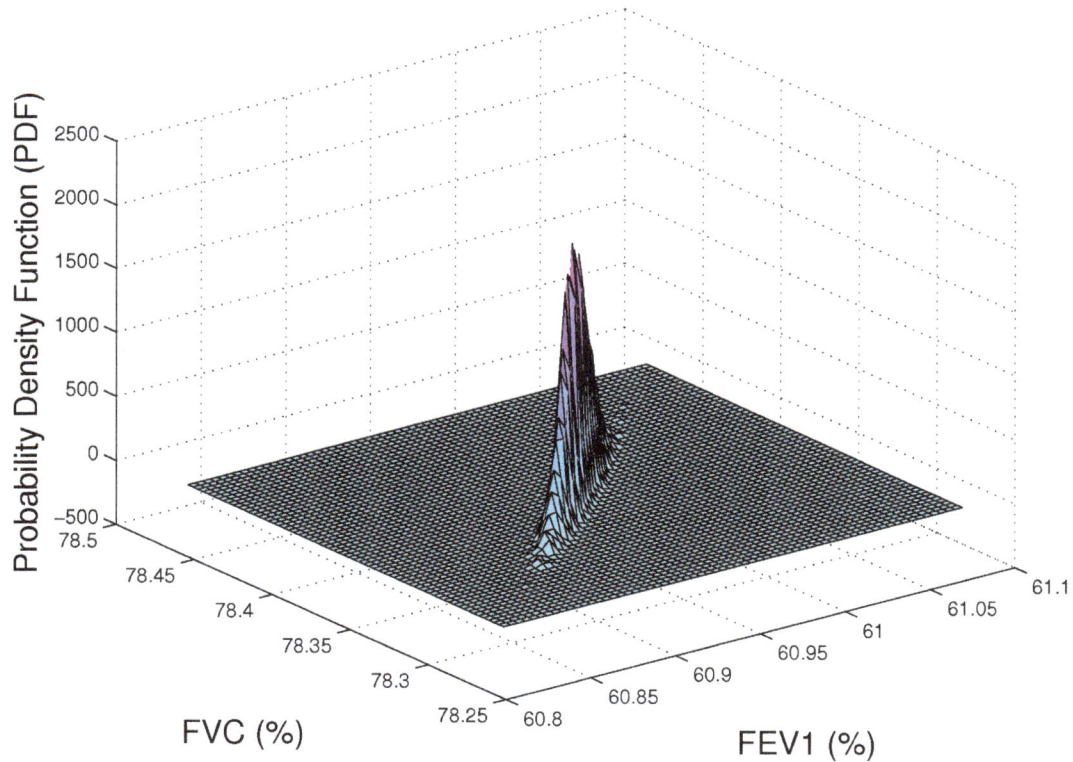

Figure 6. FEV$_1$ and FVC probability density function estimation. The x-axis shows the predicted FEV$_1$ values and the y-axis is the predicted FVC values for a hypothetical the synthetic lung example described in the text.

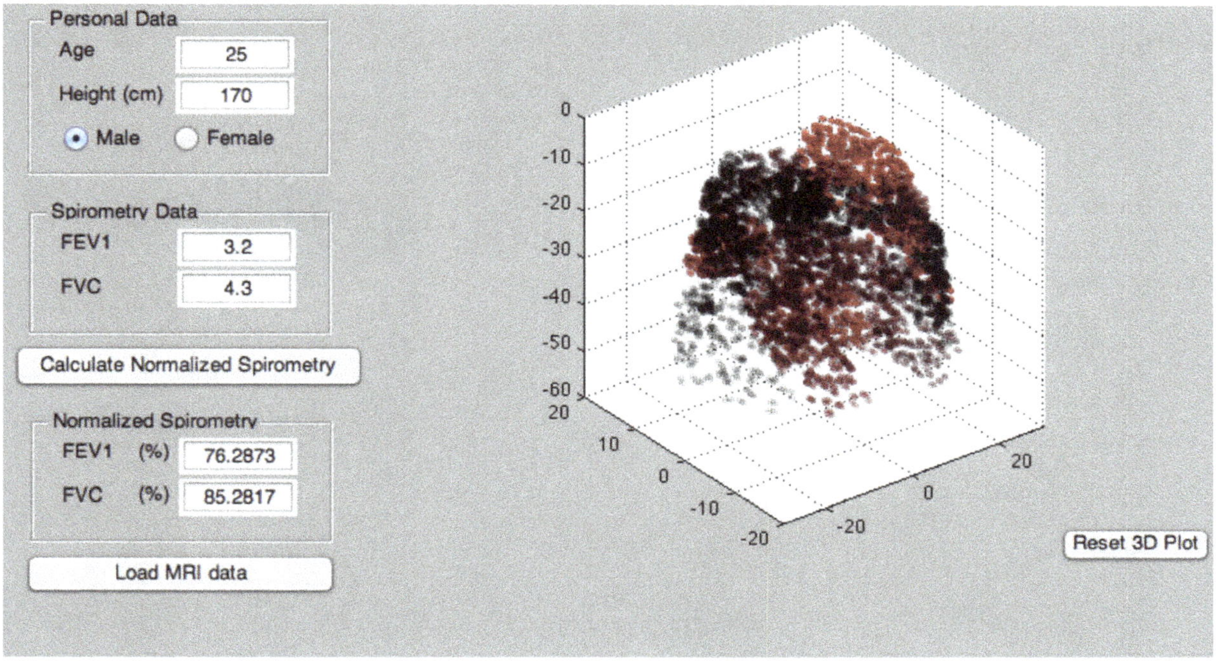

Figure 7. In this window user can enter the input parameters: patient's age, height, sex and Imaging data. The Model displays a 3D-lung that contains all the MRI/CT scan voxels.

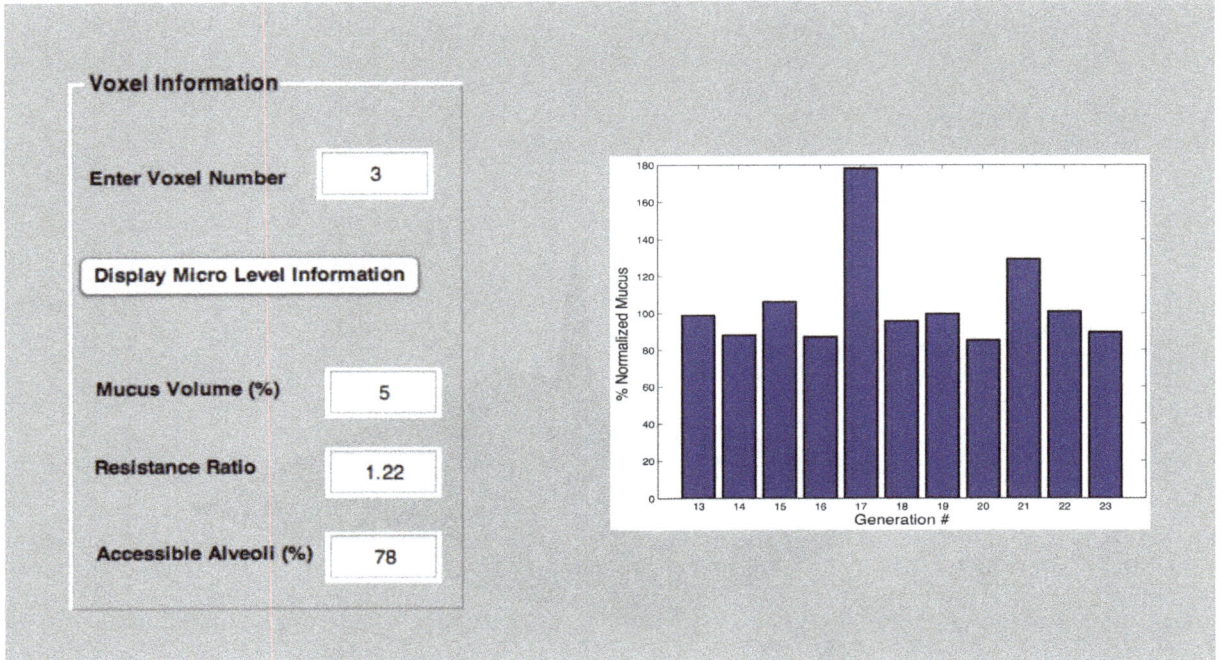

Figure 8. This window shows the mucus distribution among generations. The user selects a voxel and the model displays its corresponding parameters along with the micro-level information.

estimation methods for the most likely distribution and the corresponding spirometric observables. The resulting models and algorithms form a clinically useful tool with which to reassess the various simplest possible sub-models and assumptions used in our work so far. These models can play a crucial role in future treatments of the disease.

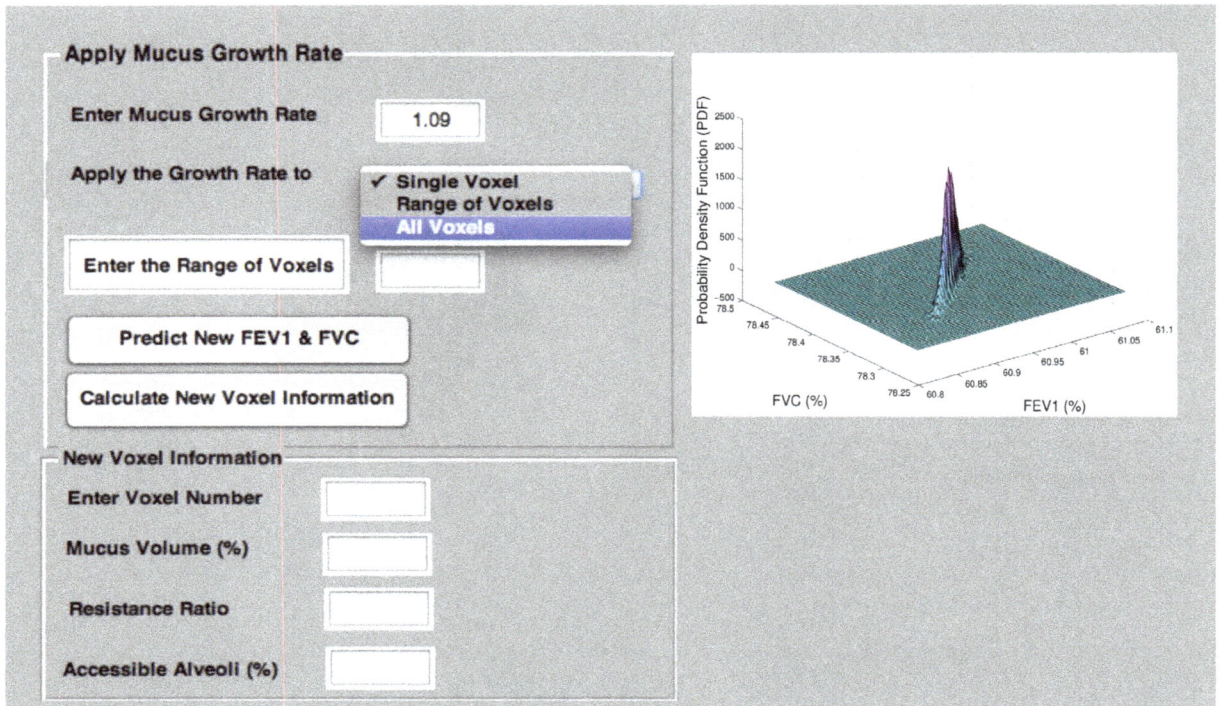

Figure 9. This window provides the user with a probability density function of the predicted FEV$_1$ and FVC. User can enter a specific mucus growth rate for different voxels and the new FEV$_1$ and FVC will be calculated.

Acknowledgments

This material is based upon work supported by the National Institutes of Health under Grant no. 56586B.

The funders had no role in study design, data collection and analysis, decision to publish, or preparation of the manuscript.

Author Contributions

Conceived and designed the experiments: SZ AM FR PS. Performed the experiments: SZ AM FR PS. Analyzed the data: SZ AM FR PS. Contributed reagents/materials/analysis tools: SZ AM FR PS. Wrote the paper: SZ AM FR PS.

References

1. Tirouvanziam R (2006) Neutrophilic inflammation as a major determinant in the progression of cystic fibrosis. Drug News Perspect 19: 609–614.
2. Koehler DR, Downey GP, Sweezey NB, Tanswell AK, Hu J (2004) Lung inflammation as a therapeutic target in cystic fibrosis. Amer J of Resp Cell and Mol Biol 31: 377–381.
3. Eichinger M, Puderbach M, Heussel CP, Kauczor HU (2006) Mri in mucoviscidosis (cystic fibrosis). Radiologe, German 46 (4): 275–276.
4. Hopkins SR, Levin DL, Emami K, Kadlecek S, Yu J, et al. (2007) Advances in magnetic resonance imaging of lung physiology. J of App Physiol 102 (3): 1244–1254.
5. Fiel SB, Friedman AC, Caroline DF, Radecki PD, Faerber E, et al. (1987) Magnetic resonance imaging in young adults with cystic fibrosis. Chest 91: 181–184.
6. Theilmann RJ, Arai TJ, Samiee A, Dubowitz DJ, Hopkins SR, et al. (2009) Quantitative mri measurement of lung density must account for the change in t(2) (*) with lung inflation. J of MRI 30: 527–534.
7. Voit EO (2014) Mesoscopic modeling as a starting point for computational analyses of cystic fibrosis as a systemic disease. Biochim et Biophy Acta 1844 (1): 258–270.
8. Zarei S, Mirtar A, Andresen B, Salamon P (2013) Modeling the airflow in a lung with cystic fibrosis. J of Non-Equil Thermodyn 38 (2): 119–140.
9. Zarei S, Mirtar A, Rohwer F, Conrad DJ, Theilmann RJ, et al. (2012) Mucus distribution model in a lung with cystic fibrosis. J of Comp and Math Meth in Med.
10. Weibel ER (1991) Design of airways and blood vessels considered as branching trees. Lung: Sci Found 1: 1061–1071.
11. Altemeier WA, McKinney S, Glenny RW (2005) A fractal analysis of the radial distribution of bronchial capillaries around large airways. J of App Physiol 98: 850–855.
12. Glenny RW, Bernard SL, Robertson HT (2000) Pulmonary blood flow remains fractal down to the level of gas exchange. J of App Physiol 89: 742–748.
13. West BJ (1990) Physiology in fractal dimensions: error tolerance. Anna of Biomed Engi 18 (2): 135–149.
14. Richey M (2010) The evolution of markov chain monte carlo methods. Amer Math Mon 117 (5): 383–413.
15. Saeta PN (2004). The metropolis algorithm: Statistical systems and simulated annealing. URL http://saeta.physics.hmc.edu/courses/p170/Metropolis.pdf.
16. Salamon P, Sibani P, Frost R (2002) Facts, Conjecture, and Improvements for Simulated Annealing. Philadelphia: Society for Industrial and Applied Mathematics.
17. Marieb E, Hoehn K (2010) Human Anatomy and Physiology. Prentice Hall PTR. 8th ED.
18. Kitaoka H, Suk B (1997) Branching design of the bronchial tree based on a diameter-flow relationship. J of App Physiol 82: 968–976.
19. Willner D, Furlan M, Haynes M, Schmieder R, Angly FE, et al. (2009) Metagenomic analysis of respiratory tract dna viral communities in cystic fibrosis and non-cystic fibrosis individuals. PLoS One 4 (10): e7370.
20. Lim YW, Evangelista JS, Schmieder R, Bailey B, Haynes M, et al. (2014) Clinical insights from metagenomic analysis of sputum samples from patients with cystic fibrosis. J of Clin Microbi 52 (2): 425–437.
21. Lim YW, Schmieder R, Haynes M, Furlan M, Matthews TD, et al. (2013) Mechanistic model of rothia mucilaginosa adaptation toward persistence in the cf lung, based on a genome reconstructed from metagenomic data. PloS one 8 (5): e64285.
22. Lim YW, Schmiederb R, Haynesa M, Willnerd D, Furlana M, et al. (2013) Metagenomics and metatranscriptomics: Windows on cf-associated viral and microbial communities. J of Cystic Fibrosis 12 (2): 154–164.
23. Whiteson KL, Meinardi S, Lim YW, Schmieder R, Maughan H, et al. (2014) Breath gas metabolites and bacterial metagenomes from cystic fibrosis airways indicate active ph neutral 2, 3-butanedione fermentation. ISME J.
24. McPhail G, Clancy J (2013) Ivacaftor: The first therapy acting on the primary cause of cystic fibrosis. Drugs of today 49: 253–260.
25. Willner D, Furlan M, Haynes M, Schmieder R, Lim YW, et al. (2011) Spatial distribution of microbial communities in the cystic fibrosis lung. ISME J 6: 471–747.

18

Meningiomas: A Comparative Study of ^{68}Ga-DOTATOC, ^{68}Ga-DOTANOC and ^{68}Ga-DOTATATE for Molecular Imaging in Mice

María Luisa Soto-Montenegro[1,2]*, Santiago Peña-Zalbidea[1], Jose María Mateos-Pérez[1], Marta Oteo[4], Eduardo Romero[4], Miguel Ángel Morcillo[4], Manuel Desco[1,3]

1 Unidad de Medicina y Cirugía Experimental, Instituto de Investigación Sanitaria Gregorio Marañón, Madrid, Spain, **2** Centro de Investigación Biomédica en Red de Salud Mental (CIBERSAM), Madrid, Spain, **3** Departamento de Bioingeniería e Ingeniería Aeroespacial, Universidad Carlos III, Madrid, Spain, **4** Unidad de Aplicaciones Biomédicas y Farmacocinética, Centro de Investigaciones Energéticas, Medioambientales y Tecnológicas (CIEMAT), Madrid, Spain

Abstract

Purpose: The goal of this study was to compare the tumor uptake kinetics and diagnostic value of three ^{68}Ga-DOTA-labeled somatostatin analogues (^{68}Ga-DOTATOC, ^{68}Ga-DOTANOC, and ^{68}Ga-DOTATATE) using PET/CT in a murine model with subcutaneous meningioma xenografts.

Methods: The experiment was performed with 16 male NUDE NU/NU mice bearing xenografts of a human meningioma cell line (CH-157MN). ^{68}Ga-DOTATOC, ^{68}Ga-DOTANOC, and ^{68}Ga-DOTATATE were produced in a FASTLab automated platform. Imaging was performed on an Argus small-animal PET/CT scanner. The SUV_{max} of the liver and muscle, and the tumor-to-liver (T/L) and tumor-to-muscle (T/M) SUV ratios were computed. Kinetic analysis was performed using Logan graphical analysis for a two-tissue reversible compartmental model, and the volume of distribution (V_t) was determined.

Results: Hepatic SUV_{max} and V_t were significantly higher with ^{68}Ga-DOTANOC than with ^{68}Ga-DOTATOC and ^{68}Ga-DOTATATE. No significant differences between tracers were found for SUV_{max} in tumor or muscle. No differences were found in the T/L SUV ratio between ^{68}Ga-DOTATATE and ^{68}Ga-DOTATOC, both of which had a higher fraction than ^{68}Ga-DOTANOC. The T/M SUV ratio was significantly higher with ^{68}Ga-DOTATATE than with ^{68}Ga-DOTATOC and ^{68}Ga-DOTANOC. The V_t for tumor was higher with ^{68}Ga-DOTATATE than with ^{68}Ga-DOTANOC and relatively similar to that of ^{68}Ga-DOTATOC.

Conclusions: This study demonstrates, for the first time, the ability of the three radiolabeled somatostatin analogues tested to image a human meningioma cell line. Although V_t was relatively similar with ^{68}Ga-DOTATATE and ^{68}Ga-DOTATOC, uptake was higher with ^{68}Ga-DOTATATE in the tumor than with ^{68}Ga-DOTANOC and ^{68}Ga-DOTATOC, suggesting a higher diagnostic value of ^{68}Ga-DOTATATE for detecting meningiomas.

Editor: C. Andrew Boswell, Genentech, United States of America

Funding: This research was supported by Ministerio de Ciencia e Innovación (PI11/00616, PI10/02986, CEN-20101014) and Comunidad de Madrid (ARTEMIS S2009/DPI-1802). The funders had no role in study design, data collection and analysis, decision to publish, or preparation of the manuscript.

Competing Interests: The authors have declared that no competing interests exist.

* Email: marisa@mce.hggm.es

Introduction

Meningiomas arise from the meningothelial cells of the arachnoid membranes, which are attached to the inner layer of the dura mater [1]. With a yearly incidence of approximately 7.44/100,000, they account for 35% of primary intracranial tumors [2]. Meningiomas are usually diagnosed using morphologic imaging methods such as computed tomography (CT) and magnetic resonance imaging (MRI). However, meningiomas located near the base of the skull may be difficult to distinguish from other lesions, such as lymphomas, metastases, or neurinomas. Consequently, management of meningiomas at these sites requires a specific therapeutic approach [3]. Functional imaging techniques could be advantageous for detecting meningiomas in cases where

biopsy is risky (eg, location near critical intracranial structures) and for tumors located at the skull base, with possible infiltration of bone structures.

Meningiomas express a large variety of receptors, including progesterone, androgens, growth factor, prolactin, dopamine, and somatostatin receptor subtype 2 (SSTR2) [4,5]. Abundant expression of SSTRs is a characteristic of many types of tumors, mainly neuroendocrine tumors (NETs), lung cancer, lymphomas, and meningiomas. To date, five different SSTR subtypes have been identified (SSTR1–5). Meningiomas express relatively high levels of SSTR2, thus making them ideal targets for functional imaging and radionuclide therapy with radiolabeled somatostatin analogues [5,6]. These receptors can be visualized *in vivo* by targeted positron emission tomography (PET) tracers.

^{68}Ga-DOTA–labeled somatostatin analogues are PET tracers that bind specifically to somatostatin receptors (SSTRs). [68]Ga has clear advantages: it has a short half-life (68 minutes), which facilitates its application in clinical practice, and can be produced with a [68]Ge/^{68}Ga radionuclide generator. The 3 compounds most widely used in PET functional imaging are ^{68}Ga-DOTATOC (^{68}Ga-DOTA -Tyr[3]-octreotide), ^{68}Ga-DOTANOC (^{68}Ga-DOTA-Nal[3]-octreotide), and ^{68}Ga-DOTATATE (^{68}Ga-DOTA-Tyr[3]-octreotate). ^{68}Ga-DOTATOC and ^{68}Ga-DOTATATE are commonly used for PET/CT imaging of SSTRs. Their high affinity has been demonstrated for SSTR2, which is one of the most common SSTR subtypes found in tumors [7]. ^{68}Ga-DOTANOC targets a broader range of somatostatin subtype receptors, including SSTR2, SSTR3, and SSTR5 [8]. Preliminary results in humans suggest that this new radiopeptide identifies more metastases than SSTR2-specific tracers [9]. However, it is not yet clear which of these somatostatin analogues provides better results in the case of meningiomas.

^{68}Ga-DOTATOC is the most commonly used radiotracer for imaging meningioma [10,11,12]. The ability of ^{68}Ga-DOTATOC to adequately detect this tumor has proven useful for planning radiation therapy. Moreover, ^{68}Ga-DOTATOC-PET data can complement anatomical data from MRI and CT to improve target volume definition, especially in cases with complex infiltration and recurrent disease after surgery [13,14]. In fact, recent progress in the development of PET radiotracers has enabled PET/CT imaging of various SSTRs, and ^{68}Ga-DOTA–labeled somatostatin analogues have been reported to show higher sensitivity for the detection of NETs and other types of tumors than the most widely used radiotracer, 2-deoxy-2-[^{18}F] fluoro-D-glucose, which measures glucose metabolism [15,16].

To our knowledge, the PET radiotracers ^{68}Ga-DOTATOC, ^{68}Ga-DOTANOC, and ^{68}Ga-DOTATATE have not been directly compared in terms of tumor uptake and ability to detect meningiomas. Therefore, the goal of this study was to compare the tumor uptake kinetics and diagnostic value of these three ^{68}Ga-DOTA-labeled somatostatin analogues in a PET/CT animal model with subcutaneous human meningioma xenografts.

Materials and Methods

1. Cell culture

CH-157MN tumor cells were provided by Randy Jensen, from the Department of Neurosurgery of the University of Utah Health Care. This human malignant meningioma cell line exhibits microscopic, immunohistochemical, and ultrastructural features of meningioma [17,18]. Cells were grown in Dulbecco's Modified Eagle's Medium (DMEM) (from Sigma-Aldrich) containing 10% fetal bovine serum (FBS), 2 mM L-glutamine, 50 units/ml penicillin, and 50 μg/ml streptomycin. Cultures were maintained at 37°C and in 5% CO_2. Cell viability was over 90%, as determined by trypan-blue staining.

2. Meningioma mouse flank xenograft model

The experiment was performed with 16 male NUDE NU/NU mice. The animals were purchased from Charles River Laboratories (Spain), maintained at a constant temperature (24±0.5°C) under a 12 hour light/dark cycle, and permitted free access to commercial rodent laboratory chow and water. All experimental procedures were conducted in conformity with European Communities Council Directive 2010/63/EU and approved by the Ethics Committee for Animal Experimentation of our hospital (Comité de Ética de Experimentación Animal, CEEA; number ES280790000087).

A CH-157MN tumor cell suspension containing 1.5×10^6 cells in a volume of 0.1 ml was injected subcutaneously into both flanks using a 30-gauge needle to increase the probability of growth.

The tumor size threshold to start PET/CT imaging was 0.1 cc.

3. Synthesis of ^{68}Ga-DOTA-peptides

The precursors were obtained from BCN Peptides (Barcelona, Spain) (DOTATOC) and ABX GmbH (Radeberg, Germany) (DOTATATE and DOTANOC). The reagents HCl 30%, ethanol, acetonitrile, and HEPES were obtained from Merck; NaCl was obtained from Sigma Aldrich.

Most of the synthesis was performed using an automated process programmed in a FastLab module (General Electric Healthcare). Before synthesis was started, the precursor (11.37, 11.13, and 10.98 nmols of DOTATOC, DOTATATE, and DOTANOC, respectively) and HEPES were introduced into the needle of the reactor. [68]Ga was obtained from a 50-mCi Obninsk [68]Ge/^{68}Ga radionuclide generator (Eckert & Ziegler) by elution with HCl 0.1N.

In this step, we applied a fractionation method, keeping only the middle (most active) part of the eluate. The effluent containing the ^{68}Ga was stored in a reservoir, and HCl 30% was added. The mixture was passed through a SAX cartridge (SPE-Spezialkartuschen Chromafix PS-HCO3, Macherey-Nagel) for purification and concentration of ^{68}Ga, which was eluted from the cartridge to the reactor using 200 μL of ultrapure water. The mixture was heated at 95°C for 10 minutes for labeling. Once the reaction had finished, the reactor was washed with ultrapure water to obtain the ^{68}Ga-DOTA-peptide, which was purified by passing it through a C18 cartridge (Sep-Pak SPE Waters). The product was eluted from the Sep-Pak with ethanol and heated at 120°C for evaporation of ethanol and sterilization. The radiotracer was finally formulated in phosphate-buffered saline (PBS)/NaCl (1/3).

The protocol used for the synthesis of ^{68}Ga-DOTATATE and ^{68}Ga-DOTANOC was slightly different from that of ^{68}Ga-DOTATOC. Changes included a second elution of the anion exchange cartridge that duplicated the volume in the reactor, thus increasing acidity (pH = 4.5 for ^{68}Ga-DOTATOC and pH = 4.0 for ^{68}Ga-DOTATATE and ^{68}Ga-DOTANOC). Also, the reactor was washed twice to recover more activity. The reason for these changes was to improve the radiochemical yield that increased from 37.8% to 67.8% for ^{68}Ga-DOTATATE and from 43% to 66.1% for ^{68}Ga-DOTANOC.

Quality controls were carried out before administration of the tracer. The products were clear and colorless. pH was measured using pH paper strips, which consistently yielded values of around 7. The purity of the radiochemical was measured in a 1200 Agilent HPLC system, the average of all tracers being greater than 98%. Radiosynthesis values are expressed as mean ± SEM (standard error of mean).

4. Determination of SSTR affinity

Affinity was determined from three independent experiments performed in triplicate and was measured by means of a homologous competitive binding experiment according to Motulsky and Neubig [19]. The IC_{50} (concentration of cold ligand [somatostatin-28] that reduces specific binding of radioligand by 50%) was determined by competitive binding assays with [^{125}I]-somatostatin-28 (Amersham Pharmacia Biotech, UK) in CH-157MN meningioma cells. Briefly, cells were incubated into a 24-well cell culture plate ($2-2.5 \times 10^5$ cells/well) at 37°C for 1 hour in a CO_2 incubator with 0.5 nM [^{125}I]-somatostatin-28 (Amersham Pharmacia Biotech, UK) in the presence of increasing concentrations of somatostatin-28 (0.1 nM-10 μM) in 0.25 ml of binding

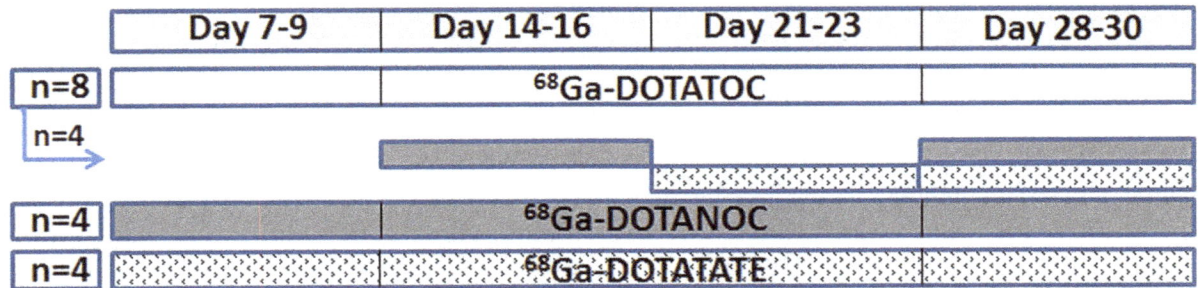

Figure 1. Experimental protocol. Animals were imaged with ^{68}Ga-DOTATOC (white line), ^{68}Ga-DOTANOC (gray line) and/or ^{68}Ga-DOTATATE (dotted line). Half of the animals imaged with ^{68}Ga-DOTATOC were also imaged with the other two radiotracers in alternate days with respect to ^{68}Ga-DOTATOC (n represents the number of animals).

media (DMEM, 2 mM L-glutamine, 50 units/ml penicillin and 50 μg/ml streptomycin). The reaction medium was aspirated after incubation. Cells were rinsed with 0.5 ml of ice-cold PBS twice and lysed in 0.5 ml of 1 N NaOH for five minutes. The activity in cells was measured in a Packard Cobra II gamma counter. The competitive binding curves were obtained by plotting the [^{125}I]-somatostatin-28 bound to cells against concentrations of cold ligand. IC_{50} and maximum numbers of binding sites (B_{max}) were calculated using Origin 7.5 software (OriginLab Corporation, Northampton, Massachusetts, USA).

5. PET imaging studies

Animals were scanned on a small-animal PET scanner (ARGUS PET-CT, SEDECAL, Madrid, Spain) under anesthesia (isoflurane, 3% induction and 1.5% maintenance in 100% O_2). Imaging was performed 7–28 days after tumor cell inoculation. Animals were imaged over four consecutive weeks (at days 7, 14, 21 & 28 after cell inoculation) with one radiotracer (n = 8 with ^{68}Ga-DOTATOC; n = 4 with ^{68}Ga-DOTANOC and n = 4 with ^{68}Ga-DOTATATE). Half of the animals imaged with ^{68}Ga-DOTATOC were also imaged with the other two radiotracers in alternate days with respect to ^{68}Ga-DOTATOC (Figure 1). Overall, n values for the PET study were: 27 for ^{68}Ga-DOTATOC, 20 for ^{68}Ga-DOTANOC and 21 for ^{68}Ga-DOTATATE.

The tracers (^{68}Ga-DOTATOC, ^{68}Ga-DOTANOC, or ^{68}Ga-DOTATATE) were injected into the tail vein (mean, 11.47 MBq; range, 9.25–20.35 MBq) and a dynamic study centered in the tumor was acquired for 90.3 minutes (112 frames: 20×10 s, 10×30 s, and 82×60 s). Frames corresponding to the last 60 minutes of the study were summed to form a static image. Images were reconstructed using the 2D–OSEM (Ordered Subset Expectation Maximization) algorithm (16 subsets and two iterations), which yields a spatial resolution for this scanner of 1.45 mm Full Width at Half Maximum (FWHM), with a voxel size of 0.3875×0.3875×0.7750 mm^3. The energy window was 400–700 keV. Decay and deadtime corrections were applied.

6. CT imaging study

CT images were acquired using the PET/CT scanner with the following parameters: 320 mA, 45 KV, 360 projections, eight shots, resulting in 200 μm of resolution. CT images were reconstructed using a Feldkamp algorithm after obtaining an isotropic voxel size of 0.125 mm [20]. Thanks to the intrinsic

alignment of the PET/CT device, these anatomical images did not require any registration with their corresponding PET scans and were used to draw the various regions of interest (ROIs) used in this study.

7. Analysis of PET-CT data

Three 3D ROIs were drawn manually on the CT image, one for each tissue of interest (tumor, liver, and muscle), plus a background ROI outside the body area. Since the CT images are intrinsically registered to the PET images, the ROIs drawn on the CT image were directly overlaid on the PET image after correction for the different image sizes. The assessment of PET data included calculation of the maximum standard uptake value (SUV_{max}) on the static tomographic study and computation of the volume of distribution (V_t) from the dynamic study.

a) Static study. Tumor, muscle, and liver SUV_{max} values at 30–90 minutes post-injection were recorded. As our field of view did not include the brain, the usual localization of this type of tumor, we selected two reference tissues: the liver, which consistently shows a slight to moderate physiologic SSTR density, and muscle, with low SSTR expression, similar to that of the brain [21]. The SUV_{max} of the tumor lesions was normalized to the SUV_{max} of the liver (T/L) and muscle (T/M) [21]. The T/L and T/M SUV ratios were considered markers of the ability of the radiopharmaceutical to localize in the tumor.

b) Dynamic study. V_t was calculated from dynamic PET data using standard Logan graphical analysis for a two-tissue reversible compartmental model [22]. Image-derived input functions and tissue time-activity curves were obtained by manually drawing ROIs over the static PET image (artery) or CT image (liver, muscle, and tumor). The artery used was the descending aorta, because the spillover from other organs is low and the descending aorta extends from the upper chest to the lower abdomen [23]. The model was resolved using the tracer kinetic modeling library [24].

8. Immunohistochemistry

The animals were sacrificed in a CO_2 chamber. Tumors were extracted and fixed in 10% formalin solution. Five-micrometer paraffin sections were used for immunohistochemical analysis. High temperature antigen unmasking (microwaving of slides in 0.01-M citrate buffer for 10 minutes) was used after deparaffinization to enhance staining. Sections were incubated with 5% horse serum for 30 minutes to block the Fc receptor in tissue and then

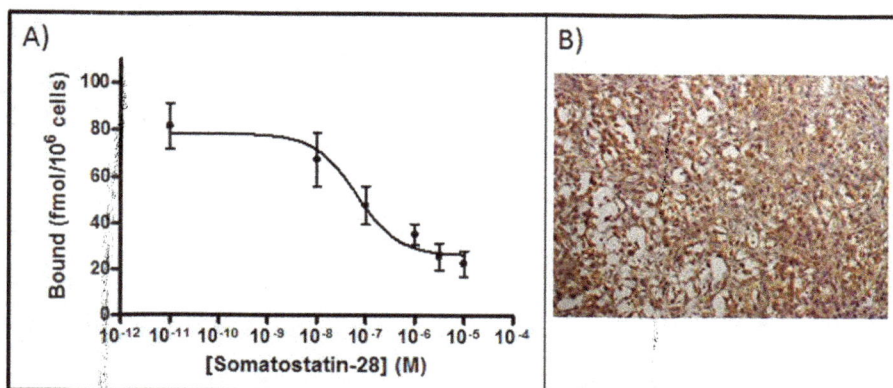

Figure 2. SSTR affinity and immunohistochemistry studies. A) Competitive binding of [^{125}I]-Somatostatin-28 to CH-57MN cells incubated at 37°C. IC_{50} and maximum numbers of binding sites (B_{max}) were calculated using Origin 7.5 software. Data are from three independent experiments performed in triplicate (Mean $\pm$ SEM). B) Immunohistochemistry using SSTR2 antibody (original magnification, x20). Tumor obtained from the CH-157MN cell line.

washed three times with sterile PBS (pH 7.5) before incubation with polyclonal antibody IgG anti-SSTR2 (Sigma-Aldrich, St. Louis, Missouri, USA) and dilution (1/50) in PBS/bovine serum albumin [25]. Goat anti-rabbit IgG-peroxidase secondary antibody was purchased from Sigma-Aldrich (St. Louis, Missouri, USA). For immunohistochemistry, peroxidase was visualized using diaminobenzidine as a substrate (Vector Laboratories, Burlingame, CA, USA). The sections were counterstained with hematoxylin.

9. Statistical analysis

The data analysis only included tumors grown in the left flank. SUV_{max} and V_t are presented as mean $\pm$ standard error of mean (SEM). Homogeneity of variance was assessed using Levene's test. Data were analyzed using one-way analysis of variance (ANOVA) followed by post hoc tests (Tukey's HSD) when statistical significance was reached ($p < 0.05$).

Results

Radiosynthesis

Radiosynthesis was successfully performed with the three somatostatin analogues. For ^{68}Ga-DOTATOC, ^{68}Ga-DOTA-NOC and ^{68}Ga-DOTATATE respectively, the mean activity (MBq) was 232.73 ± 14.06, 275.28 ± 14.80 and 274.90 ± 10.36; the decay-corrected radiochemical yield (%) was 54.03 ± 2.45, 66.13 ± 3.35 and 67.81 ± 3.12; the radiochemical purity (%) was 97.86 ± 0.51, 99.38 ± 0.31 and 99.68 ± 0.13 and the injected specific activity (MBq/nmol) was 11.07 ± 1.09, 12.45 ± 1.29 and 12.33 ± 1.32.

Tumor growth

All animals developed tumors on both flanks, although only left side tumors were included in the data analysis. Tumor volumes were 0.13 ± 0.01 cc (7–9 days), 0.73 ± 0.10 cc (14–16 days), 1.55 ± 0.21 cc (21–23 days) and 1.55 ± 0.32 cc (28–30 days). Tumor growth showed a second grade polynomial trend with an $R^2 = 0.9619$.

In vitro binding study

Figure 2A shows the high binding affinity of SSTR in CH-157MN cells for the universal ligand somatostatin-28. The IC_{50} was 63.7 ± 32.3 nM and the B_{max} was 78.4 ± 6.5 fmol/10^6 cells.

Immunohistochemistry

Immunohistochemical analysis showed that the tumor expressed SSTR2 (Figure 2B); staining was more intense on the periphery of the cells and showed weaker reactivity inside them.

Static imaging study: SUV_{max} analysis

Figure 3 shows the mean SUV_{max} for tumor, muscle, and liver, as well as the T/L and T/M SUV ratios for each radiotracer. The ANOVA revealed significant differences in liver uptake between radiotracers ($p < 0.001$, $F = 9.164$), with ^{68}Ga-DOTANOC showing higher uptake than ^{68}Ga-DOTATOC or ^{68}Ga-DOTATATE ($p < 0.001$). No significant differences between tracers were found for SUV_{max} in tumor and muscle tissue.

The ANOVA also revealed significant differences in T/L SUV ratio between radiotracers ($p < 0.001$, $F = 19.646$), with ^{68}Ga-DOTANOC showing lower uptake than ^{68}Ga-DOTATOC and ^{68}Ga-DOTATATE ($p < 0.001$). No differences were found between ^{68}Ga-DOTATATE and ^{68}Ga-DOTATOC.

As for differences in the T/M SUV ratio, ANOVA revealed significant differences between the radiotracers ($p < 0.01$, $F = 5.560$), with ^{68}Ga-DOTATATE uptake proving to be higher than that of ^{68}Ga-DOTATOC ($p < 0.01$) and ^{68}Ga-DOTANOC ($p < 0.05$).

Figure 3 shows comparative PET/CT images of the same animal for the three radiotracers. The tumors in the flank were better visualized with 68Ga-DOTATOC and 68Ga-DOTATATE than with 68Ga-DOTANOC.

Dynamic study: V_t analysis

ANOVA revealed significant differences in V_t between radiotracers in the tumor ($p = 0.0132$, $F = 5.349$) and radiotracers in the liver ($p = 0.0013$, $F = 10.706$). Post hoc tests revealed significant differences between ^{68}Ga-DOTANOC and ^{68}Ga-DOTATOC

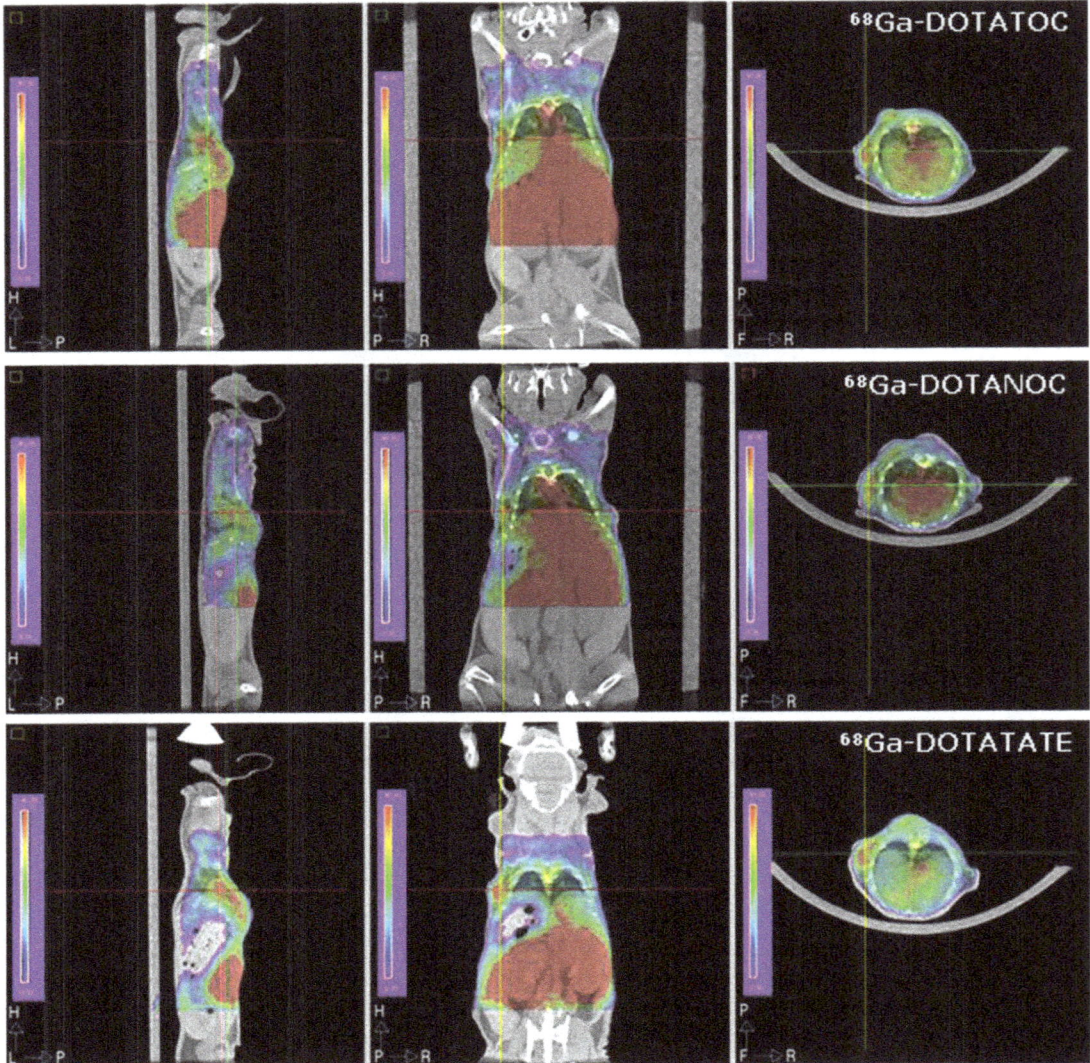

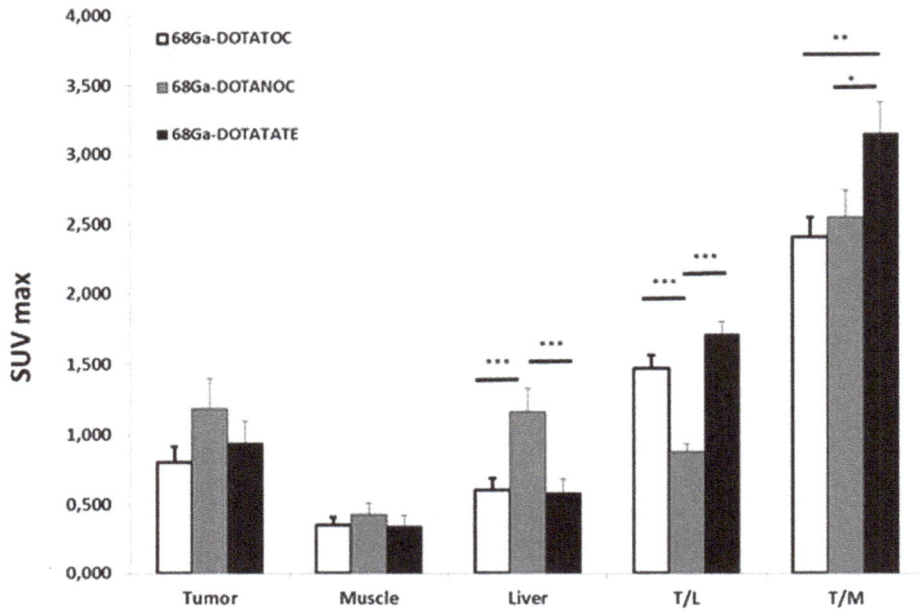

Figure 3. Tumor uptake visualized by PET. From top to bottom (^{68}Ga-DOTATOC, ^{68}Ga-DOTANOC, and ^{68}Ga-DOTATATE), PET/CT images show radiotracer uptake in the tumor of the same animal. The graph shows the mean SUV_{max} for muscle, liver, T/L, and T/M ratios for each radiotracer. Values are expressed as mean ± SEM (***$p<0.001$, ^{68}Ga-DOTATOC and ^{68}Ga-DOTANOC; $^{$$$}p<0.001$, ^{68}Ga-DOTATOC and ^{68}Ga-DOTATATE; $^{&&&}p<0.001$, ^{68}Ga-DOTANOC and ^{68}Ga-DOTATATE) (n = 20–27 images per group).

($p<0.01$ for tumor and $p<0.05$ for liver). Statistically significant differences were also found between ^{68}Ga-DOTANOC and ^{68}Ga-DOTATATE ($p<0.05$ for tumor and $p<0.05$ for liver).

No significant differences were found for V_t in muscle. Figure 4 shows the V_t (liver, muscle, and tumor) for each radiotracer.

Discussion

To our knowledge, this is the first report to compare the tumor uptake and diagnostic value of the three ^{68}Ga-DOTA-labeled somatostatin analogues ^{68}Ga-DOTATOC, ^{68}Ga-DOTANOC, and ^{68}Ga-DOTATATE using PET/CT in an animal model with a subcutaneous meningioma xenograft. Our study demonstrates the ability of the three radiolabeled somatostatin analogues to image mice bearing human meningioma xenografts.

Only three papers have evaluated the kinetics of ^{68}Ga-DOTA-labeled somatostatin analogues by PET in humans. The first focused on meningiomas located near the skull base [26]. The kinetics of ^{68}Ga-DOTATOC was analyzed using a two-tissue compartmental model, which revealed significant differences between meningiomas and the reference tissue, with high values in the tumor for vascular fraction, receptor binding, and K_1/k_2 and k_3/k_4 ratios. These data highlight that the main mechanisms responsible for tracer accumulation are receptor binding and trapping by internalization. The second and third studies compared the kinetics of ^{68}Ga-DOTATOC and ^{68}Ga-DOTATATE in NETs [27,28] and did not reveal significant differences in kinetic behavior between the tracers. Our results are consistent with those of these studies: no significant differences in V_t were found between the two tracers, suggesting that the human meningioma cell line used had predominantly SSTR2, since both radiotracers exhibit mostly SSTR2-selective binding. Moreover, our binding and immunohistochemical studies showed that the CH-157MN meningioma cells expressed SSTR2 and, consequently, suggest that both radiotracers could be equally used for imaging and staging patients with meningioma. On the contrary, V_t in the tumor was lower for ^{68}Ga-DOTANOC than for the other two tracers, and although ^{68}Ga-DOTANOC has higher affinity for SSTR2 than ^{68}Ga-DOTATOC, it also has affinity for SSTR3 and SSTR5 [29]. Consequently, there seems to be no advantage to using a tracer that targets a broader range of somatostatin subtype receptors when imaging meningioma.

We recorded significant differences between radiotracers in the SUV of the liver and the T/L and T/M SUV ratios. Uptake of ^{68}Ga-DOTANOC in the liver was greater than that of the other tracers, probably because ^{68}Ga-DOTANOC is more lipophilic than ^{68}Ga-DOTATATE and ^{68}Ga-DOTATOC, resulting in increased accumulation of tracer in the liver [8]. The T/L SUV ratio was similar for both ^{68}Ga-DOTATOC and ^{68}Ga-DOTATATE and higher than that of ^{68}Ga-DOTANOC, presumably because of the lower uptake of these tracers than of ^{68}Ga-DOTANOC in the liver. This finding must be taken into account if the tumor is located in the liver. On the other hand, the T/M SUV ratio for ^{68}Ga-DOTATATE was significantly higher than that obtained with ^{68}Ga-DOTATOC or ^{68}Ga-DOTANOC. Normalization to a tissue with moderate SSTR expression (liver) or to a tissue with low SSTR expression (muscle) yields slightly different results, indicating that the organ distribution of these somatostatin analogues differs depending on the peptide used in the radiotracer. Since expression of SSTR is similar in both muscle and brain tissue, muscle was the tissue chosen for normalization in our study. In this respect, uptake of ^{68}Ga-DOTATATE in the tumor was greater than that of the other two tracers, suggesting that ^{68}Ga-DOTATATE might be considered the radiotracer of choice for detection of meningioma in the brain.

Few authors have compared the SUV_{max} of [^{68}Ga]-labeled somatostatin analogues, and none were assessed in meningiomas. Poeppel et al. showed that the SUV_{max} of ^{68}Ga-DOTATOC tended to be higher than that of ^{68}Ga-DOTATATE [7,21]. Velikyan et al. found no statistically significant differences in tumor uptake between ^{68}Ga-DOTATOC and ^{68}Ga-DOTATATE, but suggested that the slight difference in healthy organ distribution may render ^{68}Ga-DOTATATE preferable for planning of peptide receptor radionuclide therapy [28,30]. Yang et al. suggested that ^{68}Ga-DOTATATE may be more sensitive and specific than ^{68}Ga-DOTATOC [31]. Our results are in line with those of previous works with NETs, and the organ distribution for ^{68}Ga-DOTATATE and ^{68}Ga-DOTATOC is also very similar. Only two studies have compared tumor detection rates of ^{68}Ga-DOTATATE and ^{68}Ga-DOTANOC in patients with NETs [32,33]. Wild et al. detected significantly more lesions with ^{68}Ga-DOTANOC than with ^{68}Ga-DOTATATE [33], probably owing to its broader somatostatin receptor binding profile [29]. On the contrary, Kabasakal et al. demonstrated that images obtained with ^{68}Ga-DOTATATE and ^{68}Ga-DOTANOC could have comparable diagnostic accuracy for NETs, although ^{68}Ga-DOTATATE showed a higher uptake and may have a potential advantage over ^{68}Ga-DOTANOC [32]. Our results agree with those of Kabasakal et al. and provide further evidence in favor of ^{68}Ga-DOTATATE as the first-choice radiotracer or of ^{68}Ga-DOTATOC as the second choice in the case of meningiomas.

Our study has several limitations. The first is the low anatomical resolution of the PET images. Measurements of metabolic activity by this technique in small regions may not be entirely accurate, since the activity of the ROI could be contaminated by that of surrounding regions. However, partial volume effects were minimized by defining the ROI on a registered CT scan of the same animal. Second, although partial volume effects were not corrected in the kinetic analysis, we were not measuring absolute values of V_t but merely comparing the relative volumes of distribution between the three tracers. Since each tracer was studied using the same tumor, with only a short time interval between studies, and with CT-defined ROIs, it is likely that the partial volume effects would be similar for all tracers. Finally, SUV was normalized using liver (with moderate-high SSTR expression) and muscle (with low SSTR expression), whereas it would also be advisable to have used brain tissue, as the tumor/brain ratio could be more informative about uptake differences with this tumor type in practice. In any case, with the current normalized values and the result of the kinetic analysis, it can be assumed that at least ^{68}Ga-DOTATATE shows increased uptake with regards to the other two tracers, assuming that the tumor/muscle ratio would be considered similar to that of the tumor/brain ratio.

In conclusion, this study demonstrates the ability of the three radiolabeled somatostatin analogues tested to image a human meningioma cell line. Although the V_t was relatively similar for

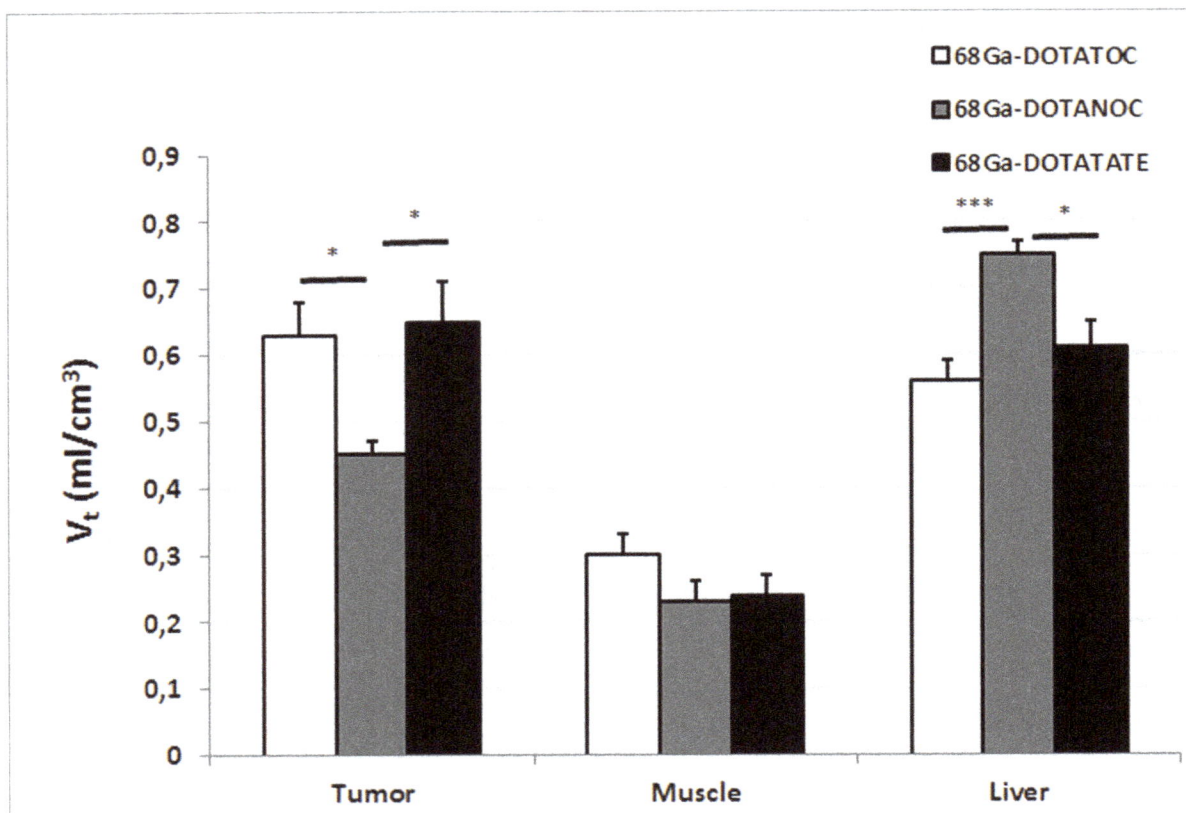

Figure 4. Plots of volume of distribution (V_t) (ml/cm^3) for liver, muscle and tumor for each radiotracer. Values are expressed as mean $\pm$ SEM (*$p < 0.05$; **$p < 0.01$; ***$p < 0.001$) (n = 7–10 images per group).

^{68}Ga-DOTATATE and ^{68}Ga-DOTATOC, ^{68}Ga-DOTATATE showed a higher tumor to muscle ratio uptake than the other radiotracers, suggesting that it should be the preferred option for detecting meningiomas.

Acknowledgments

We thank Alexandra de Francisco and Yolanda Sierra for their support in animal handling and PET/CT imaging, Randy Jenssen of the University of Utah for providing the CH-157MN cells, and BCN Peptides for providing DOTATOC. We also thank the General Electric Healthcare Gallea Project.

Author Contributions

Conceived and designed the experiments: MLSM MD. Performed the experiments: MLSM SP MO ER. Analyzed the data: MLSM MO JMMP MAM MD. Contributed reagents/materials/analysis tools: MLSM SP MO ER MAM MD. Contributed to the writing of the manuscript: MLSM JMMP MAM MD. Obtained permission for use of cell line: MLSM.

References

1. Mawrin C, Perry A (2010) Pathological classification and molecular genetics of meningiomas. J Neurooncol 99: 379–391.
2. Ostrom QT, Gittleman H, Farah P, Ondracek A, Chen Y, et al. (2013) CBTRUS statistical report: Primary brain and central nervous system tumors diagnosed in the United States in 2006–2010. Neuro Oncol 15 Suppl 2: ii1–56.
3. Guermazi A, Lafitte F, Miaux Y, Adem C, Bonneville JF, et al. (2005) The dural tail sign–beyond meningioma. Clin Radiol 60: 171–188.
4. Dutour A, Kumar U, Panetta R, Ouafik L, Fina F, et al. (1998) Expression of somatostatin receptor subtypes in human brain tumors. Int J Cancer 76: 620–627.
5. Schulz S, Pauli SU, Handel M, Dietzmann K, Firsching R, et al. (2000) Immunohistochemical determination of five somatostatin receptors in meningioma reveals frequent overexpression of somatostatin receptor subtype sst2A. Clin Cancer Res 6: 1865–1874.
6. Arena S, Barbieri F, Thellung S, Pirani P, Corsaro A, et al. (2004) Expression of somatostatin receptor mRNA in human meningiomas and their implication in in vitro antiproliferative activity. J Neurooncol 66: 155–166.
7. Poeppel TD, Binse I, Petersenn S, Lahner H, Schott M, et al. (2013) Differential uptake of (68)Ga-DOTATOC and (68)Ga-DOTATATE in PET/CT of gastroenteropancreatic neuroendocrine tumors. Recent Results Cancer Res 194: 353–371.
8. Wild D, Schmitt JS, Ginj M, Macke HR, Bernard BF, et al. (2003) DOTA-NOC, a high-affinity ligand of somatostatin receptor subtypes 2, 3 and 5 for labelling with various radiometals. Eur J Nucl Med Mol Imaging 30: 1338–1347.
9. Wild D, Macke HR, Waser B, Reubi JC, Ginj M, et al. (2005) 68Ga-DOTANOC: a first compound for PET imaging with high affinity for somatostatin receptor subtypes 2 and 5. Eur J Nucl Med Mol Imaging 32: 724.
10. Combs SE, Welzel T, Habermehl D, Rieken S, Dittmar JO, et al. (2013) Prospective evaluation of early treatment outcome in patients with meningiomas treated with particle therapy based on target volume definition with MRI and 68Ga-DOTATOC-PET. Acta Oncol 52: 514–520.
11. Yilmaz S, Ocak M, Asa S, Gulsen F, Halac M, et al. (2013) Appearance of intracranial meningioma in FDG and 68Ga-DOTATOC PET/CT. Rev Esp Med Nucl Imagen Mol 32: 60–61.
12. Graf R, Nyuyki F, Steffen IG, Michel R, Fahdt D, et al. (2013) Contribution of 68Ga-DOTATOC PET/CT to target volume delineation of skull base meningiomas treated with stereotactic radiation therapy. Int J Radiat Oncol Biol Phys 85: 68–73.
13. Milker-Zabel S, Zabel-du Bois A, Henze M, Huber P, Schulz-Ertner D, et al. (2006) Improved target volume definition for fractionated stereotactic radiotherapy in patients with intracranial meningiomas by correlation of CT, MRI, and [68Ga]-DOTATOC-PET. Int J Radiat Oncol Biol Phys 65: 222–227.

14. Afshar-Oromieh A, Giesel FL, Linhart HG, Haberkorn U, Haufe S, et al. (2012) Detection of cranial meningiomas: comparison of (6)(8)Ga-DOTATOC PET/CT and contrast-enhanced MRI. Eur J Nucl Med Mol Imaging 39: 1409–1415.

15. Kuyumcu S, Ozkan ZG, Sanli Y, Yilmaz E, Mudun A, et al. (2013) Physiological and tumoral uptake of (68)Ga-DOTATATE: standardized uptake values and challenges in interpretation. Ann Nucl Med 27: 538–545.

16. Prasad V, Baum RP (2010) Biodistribution of the Ga-68 labeled somatostatin analogue DOTA-NOC in patients with neuroendocrine tumors: characterization of uptake in normal organs and tumor lesions. Q J Nucl Med Mol Imaging 54: 61–67.

17. Ragel BT, Couldwell WT, Gillespie DL, Wendland MM, Whang K, et al. (2008) A comparison of the cell lines used in meningioma research. Surg Neurol 70: 295–307; discussion 307.

18. Ragel BT, Elam IL, Gillespie DL, Flynn JR, Kelly DA, et al. (2008) A novel model of intracranial meningioma in mice using luciferase-expressing meningioma cells. Laboratory investigation. J Neurosurg 108: 304–310.

19. Motulsky H, Neubig R (2002) Analyzing radioligand binding data. Curr Protoc Neurosci Chapter 7: Unit 7 5.

20. Abella M, Vaquero JJ, Sisniega A, Pascau J, Udías A, et al. (2012) Software architecture for multi-bed FDK-based reconstruction in X-ray CT scanners. Comput Meth Prog Bio 107: 218–232.

21. Poeppel TD, Binse I, Petersenn S, Lahner H, Schott M, et al. (2011) 68Ga-DOTATOC versus 68Ga-DOTATATE PET/CT in functional imaging of neuroendocrine tumors. J Nucl Med 52: 1864–1870.

22. Logan J, Fowler JS, Volkow ND, Wolf AP, Dewey SL, et al. (1990) Graphical analysis of reversible radioligand binding from time-activity measurements applied to [N-11C-methyl]-(−)-cocaine PET studies in human subjects. J Cereb Blood Flow Metab 10: 740–747.

23. Dimitrakopoulou-Strauss A, Georgoulias V, Eisenhut M, Herth F, Koukouraki S, et al. (2006) Quantitative assessment of SSTR2 expression in patients with non-small cell lung cancer using (68)Ga-DOTATOC PET and comparison with (18)F-FDG PET. Eur J Nucl Med Mol Imaging 33: 823–830.

24. Mateos-Pérez JM, Desco M, Vaquero JJ (2014) Tracer Kinetic Modeling with R for Batch Processing of Dynamic PET Studies. In: ILMRR, editor. Springer International Publishing. doi:10.1007/978-3-319-00846-2_75. pp. 301–304.

25. Martinez-Cruz AB, Santos M, Lara MF, Segrelles C, Ruiz S, et al. (2008) Spontaneous squamous cell carcinoma induced by the somatic inactivation of retinoblastoma and Trp53 tumor suppressors. Cancer Res 68: 683–692.

26. Henze M, Dimitrakopoulou-Strauss A, Milker-Zabel S, Schuhmacher J, Strauss LG, et al. (2005) Characterization of 68Ga-DOTA-D-Phe1-Tyr3-octreotide kinetics in patients with meningiomas. J Nucl Med 46: 763–769.

27. Lubberink M, Sandstrom M, Sörensen J, Granberg D, Garske-Román U, et al. (2013) Tracer kinetic analysis of 68Ga-DOTATATE and 68Ga-DOTATOC in neuroendocrine tumours. Society of Nuclear Medicine & Molecular Imaging 2013. Vancouver, BC, Canada: J Nucl Med. pp. P200.

28. Velikyan I, Sundin A, Sorensen J, Lubberink M, Sandstrom M, et al. (2014) Quantitative and Qualitative Intrapatient Comparison of 68Ga-DOTATOC and 68Ga-DOTATATE: Net Uptake Rate for Accurate Quantification. J Nucl Med 55: 204–210.

29. Antunes P, Ginj M, Zhang H, Waser B, Baum RP, et al. (2007) Are radiogallium-labelled DOTA-conjugated somatostatin analogues superior to those labelled with other radiometals? Eur J Nucl Med Mol Imaging 34: 982–993.

30. Sandstrom M, Velikyan I, Garske-Roman U, Sorensen J, Eriksson B, et al. (2013) Biodistribution and radiation dosimetry of 68Ga-DOTATOC and 68Ga-DOTATATE in patients with neuroendocrine tumors. J Nucl Med 54: 1755–1759.

31. Yang J, Kan Y, Ge BH, Yuan L, Li C, et al. (2013) Diagnostic role of Gallium-68 DOTATOC and Gallium-68 DOTATATE PET in patients with neuroendocrine tumors: a meta-analysis. Acta Radiol.

32. Kabasakal L, Demirci E, Ocak M, Decristoforo C, Araman A, et al. (2012) Comparison of (6)(8)Ga-DOTATATE and (6)(8)Ga-DOTANOC PET/CT imaging in the same patient group with neuroendocrine tumours. Eur J Nucl Med Mol Imaging 39: 1271–1277.

33. Wild D, Bomanji JB, Benkert P, Maecke H, Ell PJ, et al. (2013) Comparison of 68Ga-DOTANOC and 68Ga-DOTATATE PET/CT within patients with gastroenteropancreatic neuroendocrine tumors. J Nucl Med 54: 364–372.

19

Is 3-Tesla Gd-EOB-DTPA-Enhanced MRI with Diffusion-Weighted Imaging Superior to 64-Slice Contrast-Enhanced CT for the Diagnosis of Hepatocellular Carcinoma?

Bettina Maiwald*, Donald Lobsien, Thomas Kahn, Patrick Stumpp

Department of Diagnostic and Interventional Radiology, University of Leipzig, Leipzig, Germany

Abstract

Objectives: To compare 64-slice contrast-enhanced computed tomography (CT) with 3-Tesla magnetic resonance imaging (MRI) using Gd-EOB-DTPA for the diagnosis of hepatocellular carcinoma (HCC) and evaluate the utility of diffusion-weighted imaging (DWI) in this setting.

Methods: 3-phase-liver-CT was performed in fifty patients (42 male, 8 female) with suspected or proven HCC. The patients were subjected to a 3-Tesla-MRI-examination with Gd-EOB-DTPA and diffusion weighted imaging (DWI) at b-values of 0, 50 and 400 s/mm^2. The apparent diffusion coefficient (ADC)-value was determined for each lesion detected in DWI. The histopathological report after resection or biopsy of a lesion served as the gold standard, and a surrogate of follow-up or complementary imaging techniques in combination with clinical and paraclinical parameters was used in unresected lesions. Diagnostic accuracy, sensitivity, specificity, and positive and negative predictive values were evaluated for each technique.

Results: MRI detected slightly more lesions that were considered suspicious for HCC per patient compared to CT (2.7 versus 2.3, respectively). ADC-measurements in HCC showed notably heterogeneous values with a median of $1.2 \pm 0.5 \times 10^{-3}$ mm^2/s (range from 0.07 ± 0.1 to $3.0 \pm 0.1 \times 10^{-3}$ mm^2/s). MRI showed similar diagnostic accuracy, sensitivity, and positive and negative predictive values compared to CT (AUC 0.837, sensitivity 92%, PPV 80% and NPV 90% for MRI vs. AUC 0.798, sensitivity 85%, PPV 79% and NPV 82% for CT; not significant). Specificity was 75% for both techniques.

Conclusions: Our study did not show a statistically significant difference in detection in detection of HCC between MRI and CT. Gd-EOB-DTPA-enhanced MRI tended to detect more lesions per patient compared to contrast-enhanced CT; therefore, we would recommend this modality as the first-choice imaging method for the detection of HCC and therapeutic decisions. However, contrast-enhanced CT was not inferior in our study, so that it can be a useful image modality for follow-up examinations.

Editor: Andreas-Claudius Hoffmann, West German Cancer Center, Germany

Funding: This work was supported by a research grant from Bayer Vital, Leverkusen, Germany. This was used to buy contrast media for the MRI-examination. The funders had no role in study design, data collection and analysis, decision to publish, or preparation of the manuscript. None of the author received specific funding for this work. www.bayerpharma.com.

Competing Interests: The study was supported by a research grant from Bayer Vital, Leverkusen, Germany but this did not modify the authors' results and conclusion in any way. It was used to buy contrast media (Gd-EOB-DTPA (Primovist®)) for the MRI-examination of the patients. This contrast medium is a specific tool in imaging liver lesions since it is metabolized by the hepatocytes. It is officially approved by the European Medicines Agency (EMA) as well as by the Food and Drug Administration (FDA) in the USA and the authors currently use it daily in clinical routine. The funders had no role in study design, data collection and analysis, decision to publish or preparation of the manuscript. The authors' employments were not paid by the research grant. None of the authors received personal funding for this work and therefore no personal competing interests exist.

* Email: bettina.maiwald@medizin.uni-leipzig.de

Introduction

Hepatocellular carcinoma (HCC) is one of the most common malignancies worldwide. Liver cirrhosis is a precancerous condition associated with the development of HCC. Other important risk factors include chronic hepatitis B and C, as well as alcohol abuse. The sequential carcinogenesis from regenerative nodules to overt HCC has been described previously, and the *de novo* development of HCC without prior liver cirrhosis has also been delineated [1–5].

HCC can be diagnosed by various imaging modalities, including ultrasound, multidetector computed tomography (CT) and magnetic resonance imaging (MRI). Despite these versatile imaging modalities, correct characterization of HCC versus other liver lesions remains a challenging task, and a definite diagnosis often cannot be made based on imaging alone [6]. However, in cancer patients, a precise diagnosis is important for optimal treatment planning [2,7].

Concerning advanced magnetic resonance techniques, diffusion weighted imaging (DWI) has the ability to differentiate between malignant and benign liver lesions [8–12]. A recently developed liver-specific contrast medium, Gd-EOB-DTPA (Gadolinium-ethoxybenzyl-diethylene-triamine-pentaacetic-acid), is a paramagnetic contrast agent with properties of extracellular and hepatobiliary contrast media for use in MR imaging of the liver. This reagent allows for dynamic perfusion imaging and the evaluation of liver function. Gd-EOB-DTPA is taken up in hepatocytes to approximately 50% via OATP-1 (organic anion transporter protein-1), increasing the signal intensity of the liver parenchyma approximately 20 min after injection [13–16]. Several studies have demonstrated that this reagent improved the detection and characterization of focal liver lesions [17–19].

High field-strength MRI at 3.0 Tesla provides better tissue contrast compared to 1.5 Tesla due to a greater signal-to-noise ratio, improved image quality, higher resolution imaging and faster scanning times [20].

The aim of this study was to compare the diagnostic power of CT with 3 Tesla MRI using Gd-EOB-DTPA for the diagnosis of HCC and to evaluate the diagnostic impact of DWI with apparent diffusion coefficient (ADC) quantification in this setting.

Material and Methods

Patient Selection

Fifty patients (mean age 60.6 years, range 29–84 years, mean body weight 79,8 kg, range 45–120 kg, 42 male, 8 female, Table 1) with suspected or proven HCC were included in this prospective single-centre study to evaluate the diagnostic performance of contrast-enhanced CT and Gd-EOB-DTPA-enhanced MRI in terms of lesion detection. Inclusion criteria were suspicious findings in the US or/and increased laboratory parameters (e.g., alpha-fetoprotein). Exclusion criteria were renal failure, allergy to contrast agents, hyperthyreoidism, pregnancy and, especially for the MRI-examination, pacemaker or other non-compatible implants and claustrophobia. The aetiology of liver cirrhosis in the patient cohort was as follows: 26 patients with alcohol induced liver cirrhosis, 2 with Hepatitis B- and 3 with Hepatitis C-related chronic liver disease, 3 patients with hemochromatosis, one with Budd-Chiari-Syndrome and one with non-alcoholic steatohepatitis. 14 patients had cryptogenic liver cirrhosis. Based on the Child-Pugh-Classification, the severity of liver cirrhosis was classified as class A in 27 patients, class B in 16 patients and class C in 7 patients [Table 1].

The histopathological report after resection or biopsy of a lesion served as the gold standard for diagnosis, whereas a surrogate of follow-up (after 6 months) or complementary imaging technique (ultrasound, digital subtraction angiography) in combination with clinical (loss of weight, general state) and paraclinical parameters (especially alpha-fetoprotein) was used in unresected lesions.

This study was approved by the ethics committee of the medical faculty of the University of Leipzig, and all patients provided written informed consent.

Imaging technique

Multiphase-CT was performed using two different scanners (Brilliance 64/iCT; Philips Healthcare, Eindhoven, Netherlands) with identical parameters to prevent bias within the CT: collimation of 0.625 mm, rotation time of 0.75 s, tube voltage of 120 kV, tube current 200 mAs and adjusted with automatic dose modulation, reconstructed slice thickness of 3 mm, matrix 512*512). The contrast agent (Iopromide Ultravist 370, Bayer Vital GmbH, Leverkusen, Germany) was applied at a constant volume of 100 ml at a rate of 3 ml/s (Power injector mississippi, Ulrich Medical, Ulm, Germany). The unenhanced phase, early arterial phase 10 s after bolustracking (positioning the respective region of interest in the abdominal aorta just above the coeliac trunk, threshold 150 HU) and portal venous phase 60 s after reaching the threshold were acquired.

Subsequent MRI (median time: 2.2 days, range 0–30d) was performed in all subjects using a 3.0 Tesla scanner (TrioTim, Siemens Medical Solutions, Erlangen, Germany). The study protocol consisted of the following sequences:

(1) T2w-HASTE (half-fourier acquisition single-shot turbo spin echo) coronal and axial

(2) T1w-VIBE (volume-interpolated breath-hold examination) coronal unenhanced, axial unenhanced and dynamic after contrast medium was applied (Gd-EOB-DTPA (Primovist), Bayer Vital GmbH, Leverkusen, Germany) at 0.1 ml/kg bodyweight at a rate of 2 ml/s using a power injector (Spectris solaris EP, Medrad, Dusseldorf, Germany), followed by a 30 ml saline flush. Scanning times were as follows: arterial phase, 2 s; portalvenous phase, 30–40, equilibrium phase, 2–3 min; and hepatobiliary phase, 20 min after the contrast bolus reached the abdominal aorta.

(3) Diffusion-weighted sequence coronal and axial (b-value 0, 50 and 400 s/mm^2)

(4) T2w TSE (turbo spin echo) with fat saturation coronal

(5) T1w in phase and opposed phase axial

See Table 2 for more details concerning the sequences.

Imaging analysis

Image analysis focused on the number, size and detectability of liver lesions, as well as image quality. A radiologist with 10 years of experience in abdominal imaging performed the analysis using a picture archiving and communication system workstation (Magic-View 1000, Siemens Medical Solutions, Erlangen, Germany). The observer was aware of the patients being at risk of HCC, but otherwise blinded to all patient data. Diagnosis of HCC was based on hypervascularization in the arterial phase and washout in the portal venous phase or delayed phase, as suggested by the European Association for the Study of the Liver and the American Association for the Study of Liver Disease for MRI and CT [1]. In addition, focal areas with a suspicious hypointense signal in the hepatobiliary phase were used to detect HCC [21] (Figure 1). The radiologist recorded the presence and anatomical location of lesions, as well as diagnostic confidence using the following 5-point scale: 1 = definitely not HCC, 2 = probably not HCC, 3 = equivocal, 4 = probably HCC, 5 = definitely HCC.

Lesion detectability and image quality were evaluated using a 5-point rating-scale (1 = excellent, 2 = good, 3 = fair, 4 = poor, 5 = unacceptable). The average largest tumour diameter was determined using a measuring tool integrated in the workstation software.

ADC-values were measured for each clearly demarcated lesion in ADC-map by drawing a circular region of interest into the tumour that encompassed as much of the lesion as possible while excluding vascular structures and necrotic tissue.

Imaging analysis was accomplished according to the following settings:

Table 1. Demographics, aetiology of liver cirrhosis and patients clinical condition.

Gender	
Male	42
Female	8
Mean age (years)	60.6 (range 29–84)
Mean weight (kg)	79.8 (range 45–120)
Aetiology of liver cirrhosis	
Alcoholic disease	26
Hepatitis B	2
Hepatitis C	3
Haemochromatosis	3
Budd-Chiari-Syndrome	1
Non-alcoholic steatohepatosis	1
Cryptogenic	14
Child Pugh Status	
A (5–6)	27
B (7–9)	16
C (10–15)	7

1) In general, CT-scans were compared with

2) complete MRI-examinations (including conventional dynamic MRI with hepatobiliary phase and DWI).

To estimate the impact of the hepatobiliary phase and diffusion-weighted imaging, MRI-data were subdivided into three sets:

3) conventional dynamic MRI without the hepatobiliary phase and DWI

4) dynamic MRI including the hepatobiliary phase

5) MRI including diffusion-weighted sequences.

In addition, the observer evaluated the reading time.

Statistical analysis

Statistical analysis was performed using SPSS 20.0 for Windows (statistical package for social sciences 20.0, Chicago, IL, USA) and Microsoft Excel (Microsoft, Redmond, WA, USA). The diagnostic performance of each technique was assessed by measuring the area under the curve (AUC) of the free-response receiver operating characteristic analysis (ROC-curve) on a lesion-per-patient-basis.

Sensitivity, specificity, and positive and negative predictive values were calculated for patients assigned a diagnostic confidence level of 4 and 5 (probably and definitely HCC). In addition, we included patients with a confidence level of 3, because in clinical routine, a suspicious lesion must be clarified (e.g., by further imaging or biopsy). The differences in the ROC-curves, sensitivities, specificities, positive predictive value (PPV) and negative predictive value (NPV) were statistically analysed using a binomial test. Student's t-test was used to calculate significant differences for image quality, detectability and reading time between the image modalities, P-values <0.05 were considered significantly different.

Table 2. MR Imaging Parameters.

Parameter	T2-weighted (HASTE)	T1-weighted (VIBE)	DWI	T2-weighted TSE	T1-weighted in and out of phase
Imaging plane	Coronal and axial	Coronal and axial unenhanced, axial enhanced	Coronal and axial	Coronal	Axial
Fat saturation	No	Yes	Yes	Yes	No
Respiratory triggering	Breath-hold (12 s)	Breath-hold (16 s)	Respiratory-triggered	Respiratory-triggered	Breath-hold (18 s)
Repetition time (TR)	800 ms	2.92 ms	2000 ms	2000 ms	212 ms
Echo time (TE)	83 s	0.86 ms	60 ms	81 ms	2.32 ms
Flip angle	160°	10°	-	120°	65°
Bandwidth	781 Hz/Px	540 Hz/Px	1736 Hz/Px	260 Hz/Px	930 Hz/Px
Field of view (FOV)	450 mm	400 mm	380 mm	400 mm	380 mm
Slice thickness	5 mm	3 mm	5 mm	5 mm	5 mm
Matrix	320*256	256*200	192*154	320*224	256*200

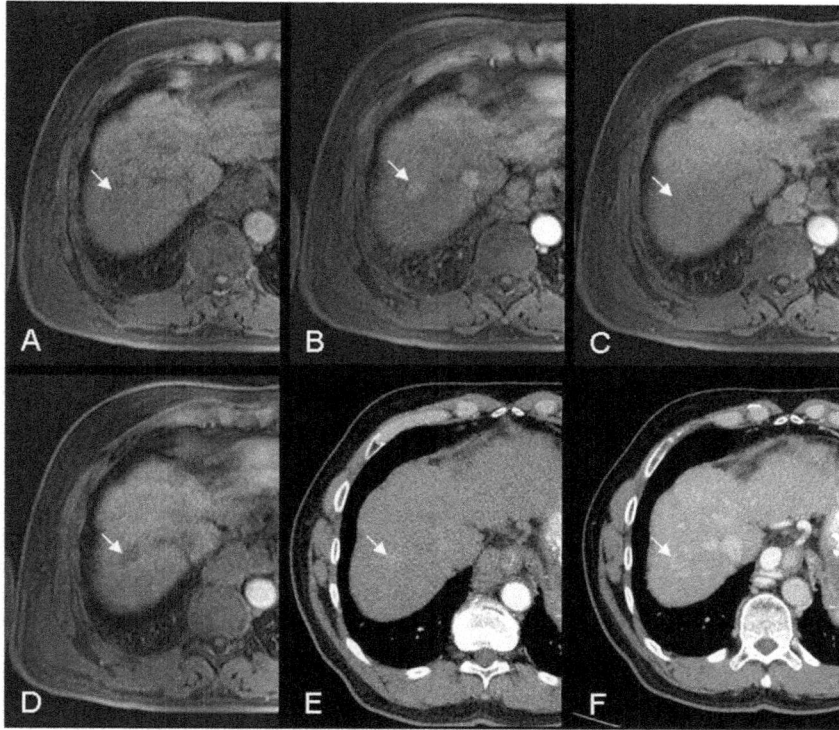

Figure 1. A 59-year-old male patient with liver cirrhosis (Child A) and HCC (arrow) in segment 7. Axial images: A) lesion is barely visible using unenhanced T1w-VIBE, B) marked arterial enhancement in T1w-VIBE following i.v. administration of contrast medium, C) typical washout of the lesion in the equilibrium phase (T1w-VIBE), and D) a clear hypointense lesion in the hepatobiliary phase (20 min after contrast agent injection, T1w-VIBE). Similar behaviour was observed with typical contrast medium enhancement in CT: E) early arterial phase after bolus tracking and F) washout in the portal venous phase with pseudocapsule.

Results

In 35 of 50 patients, the histopathological report after resection or biopsy of a lesion served as the gold standard for diagnosis, and in 24 of these 35 patients, the diagnosis of HCC was proven histopathologically. In 2 additional cases, HCC was diagnosed at follow-up (after 6 months) via clinical and paraclinical parameters.

In our study, 26 of 50 patients were positive for HCC (MRI-related: 9 patients with one lesion, 4 patients with 2 lesions, 3 patients with 3 lesions and 10 patients with 4 or more lesions).

ROC-curves for MRI displayed similar AUCs as observed for CT (0.837 vs. 0.798, p = 0.48). Sensitivity and positive and negative predictive values were measured for both methods (sensitivity 92%, PPV 80% and NPV 90% for MRI vs. sensitivity 85%, PPV 79% and NPV 82% for CT). Specificity was 75% for both techniques (see Table 3 and Figure 2). False positives resulted from numerous metastases of a neuroendocrine carcinoma, one adenoma and regenerative nodules. Because we calculated sensitivity, specificity, and positive and negative predictive values on a per-patient-basis, our subset analyses revealed no differences.

On a *liver-lesion-per-patient basis*, we detected slightly more lesions that were suspicious for HCC using MRI compared to CT, but this value did not reach statistical significance (mean, 2.7 for MRI versus 2.3 for CT, p = 0.256, Figure 3). One additional HCC was identified with aid of the hepatobiliary phase compared to conventional dynamic MRI; this lesion measured 8 mm in diameter (Figure 4). Compared to Gadolinium-EOB-DTPA-enhanced MRI-images evaluated with the hepatobiliary phase, no additional lesions were detected by DWI. However, DWI identified one additional malignant lesion compared to conventional dynamic MRI-scan. This was the same 8 mm diameter lesion that was observed with the hepatobiliary phase, and this finding impacted patient treatment (Figure 4).

Lesion size was similar using both methods, with an average greatest diameter of 33 mm for CT and 32 mm for MRI (measured in the arterial phase T1w VIBE; p = 0.195). Twenty malignant neoplasms were >3 cm, 16 lesions were 2–3 cm and 35 lesions were <2 cm, as determined by MRI-scans.

ADC-measurements in 32 lesions showed extremely heterogeneous values, with a mean of $1.2 \pm 0.5 \times 10^{-3}$ mm^2/s (range, 0.07 ± 0.1 to $3.0 \pm 0.1 \times 10^{-3}$ mm^2/s; Figure 5).

The radiologist reported that the *detectability* of lesions was similar using both methods using a 5-point rating scale (2.6 for CT and 2.7 for MRI, p = 0.807; range from 2.6 to 4.0 between sequences, 1 = excellent, 5 = unacceptable). The ability of MRI to detect lesions was significantly better using the hepatobiliary phase (2.2, range from 1 to 4) compared to conventional dynamic MRI (2.9, p = 0.005), but the difference was not significantly different compared to DWI (2.6, p = 0.125).

Image quality (2.2 for CT vs. 2.3 for MRI, p = 0.249, 2 = good, 3 = fair) was more scattered within MR sequences (1.8 in T1w HASTE and 2.9 in T2w TSE). Image quality was rated better for the hepatobiliary phase and conventional dynamic MRI than for DWI (2.0 for hepatobiliary phase, 2.1 for dynamic MRI without hepatobiliary phase and 2.7 for DWI, p<0.001). No significant disparity was noted between conventional dynamic MRI and the hepatobiliary phase (p = 0.342).

Table 3. Diagnostic accuracy, sensitivity, specificity, PPV and NPV for MRI and CT (binomial test, p<0.05 = significant).

	MRI	CT	P-value
Diagnostic accuracy (AUC)	0.837	0.798	0.4795
Sensitivity	0.92	0.85	0.4795
Specificity	0.75	0.75	1.000
PPV	0.80	0.79	0.500
NPV	0.90	0.82	1.000

The average *reading time* for MR-images was16.9 min and significantly longer than the reading time for CT-scans, which averaged 4.5 min. (p<0.001).

Discussion

Accuracy

In our study, MRI showed similar diagnostic accuracy for the detection of HCC compared to CT. Reports by Akai et al. and Lee et al. demonstrated similar results with a tendency to higher diagnostic accuracy for MRI, but also without statistically significant differences [22,23]. One explanation for this discrepancy might be the high number of suspicious lesions with a diameter greater than 3 cm in our study population. Haradome et al. also showed no difference in diagnostic accuracy between conventional dynamic MRI and CT. However, using the hepatobiliary phase, MRI displayed significantly higher accuracy than CT, especially for lesions smaller than 1.5 cm [24]. Kim demonstrated that MRI has better sensitivity for the detection of HCCs due to an increased delineation of hypointensity of HCC at a three-minute late phase and a hepatocyte phase [25], supporting previous reports [26–28]. While these studies report that CT is inferior to MRI, the use of different contrast agents, older scanner technology and different scanning parameters of the CTs must be taken into account. Similar to our study parameters, several groups used an early arterial phase [25,27]. For example, Chan et al. described better conspicuity for hepatocellular carcinomas using a bolus tracking delay of 6s for achieving the arterial phase [29]. Other studies state that the late arterial phase (e.g., approximately 14–30 s from 100 HU-threshold) is the optimal scan window for the detection of HCC [30]. Moreover, differences in histopathological subtypes of HCC might also yield different enhancement patterns [31], making it difficult to clearly specify standard examination protocols.

Detectability and number of lesions

Although the reader rated the subjective detectability of liver lesions similarly for MRI and CT, slightly more liver lesions per patient were detected using 3T MRI. Although this did not reach statistical significance, it is important for therapeutic decisions because liver transplantation can achieve excellent results in patients with HCC according to the benchmark defined by the Milan criteria (solitary HCC of less than 5 cm or with up to three nodules of less than 3 cm) [32–34]. Furthermore, decision to surgically resect tumours or use minimally invasive therapies (i.e., radiofrequency ablation (RFA), laser-induced interstitial thermotherapy (LITT), microwave ablation (MWA), cryoablation and transarterial chemoembolisation (TACE), etc.) depends on number and size of hepatocellular carcinomas, as visualised using CT or MRI [35,36].

In our study, the detectability of lesions using MRI with the hepatobiliary phase 20 min after i.v. injection of Gd-EOB-DTPA was significantly better than conventional dynamic MRI. In one patient a suspicious lesion with a diameter of 8 mm was only observed with the hepatobiliary phase and DWI, but not with conventional dynamic MRI (Figure 4). This lesion changed the therapeutic management of the patient because it was the 4th HCC suspicious lesion in his liver, which excluded him from the liver transplantation list according to the Milan criteria [32]. These data support several studies reporting that Gd-EOB-DTPA enhanced MRI is superior to conventional dynamic MRI [17,21,24].

Gd-EOB-DTPA is a gadolinium-based, liver specific MRI contrast medium that allows diagnosis derived from haemodynamics during the extracellular phase and measures hepatocellular function during the hepatobiliary phase. Information regarding the degree of cellular differentiation might also be possible [18]. Concerning the timing of hepatobiliary phase imaging, Motosugi

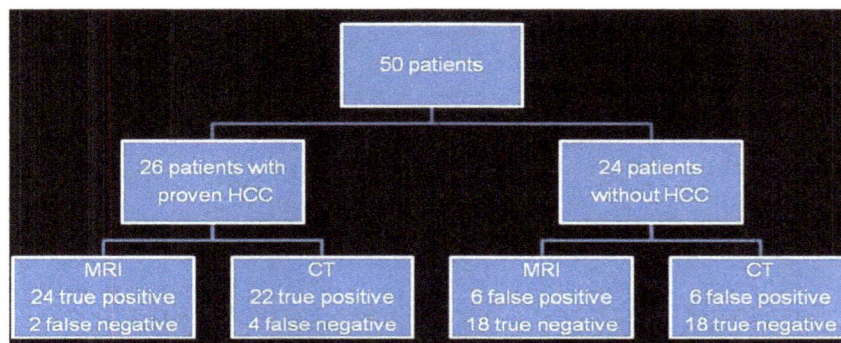

Figure 2. Flow chart for identification of patients with HCC in MRI and CT.

Is 3-Tesla Gd-EOB-DTPA-Enhanced MRI with Diffusion-Weighted Imaging Superior to 64-Slice...

169

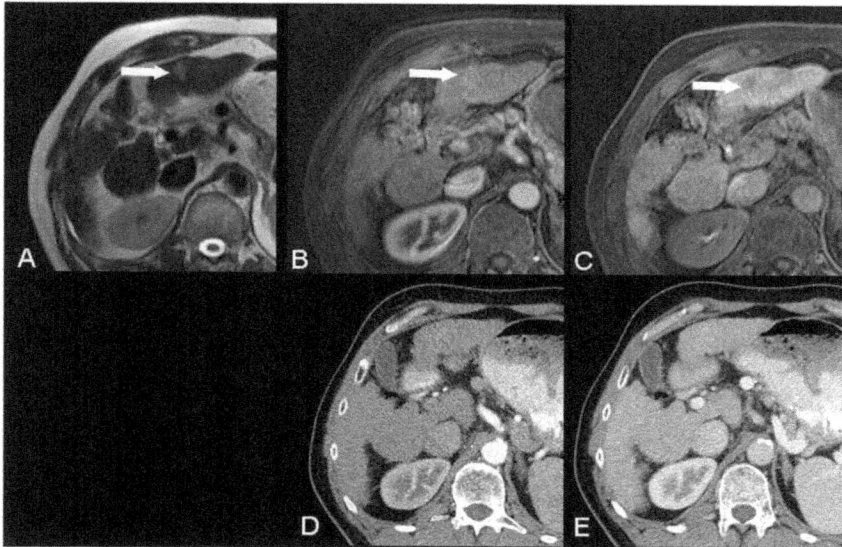

Figure 3. A 59-year-old male patient with liver cirrhosis and HCC (arrow) in S3 was only observed using MRI: *A)* **markedly hyperintense HCC in T2w-HASTE axial,** *B)* **typical arterial enhancement in T1w-VIBE, and** *C)* **hypointense lesion in the hepatobiliary phase.** No lesion was detected using CT: *D)* early arterial phase and *E)* portal venous phase.

et al. described that if the liver parenchyma is sufficiently enhanced 10 min after injection, no further imaging is necessary to detect focal liver lesions. However, the visual liver to spleen contrast scores 20 min after injection were frequently higher than 10 min images in patients with chronic liver diseases. These data indicate that a longer delay of 20 min might be more useful for patients with chronic liver diseases [37]. Because all of our patients suffered from chronic liver disease, we acquired hepatobiliary phase images 20 min after contrast application.

DWI

DWI is commonly used in liver imaging to assess various focal lesions. In particular, DWI has a higher detection rate and diagnostic performance for small, malignant liver lesions com-

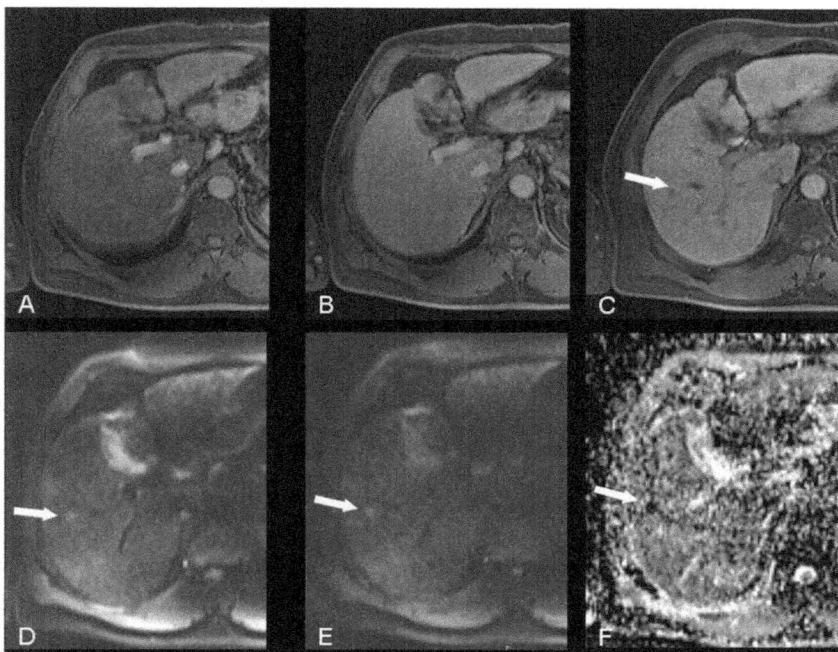

Figure 4. MRI of a 53-years-old male patient with HCC (arrow) in Segment 5: no lesion was identified in the arterial (A) and equilibrium phases (B), a small hypointense lesion was only observed in the hepatobiliary phase (C) and in DWI, where it is seen as a hyperintense lesion in b 50- (D) and b 400-images (E) and hypointense in the ADC-map (F).

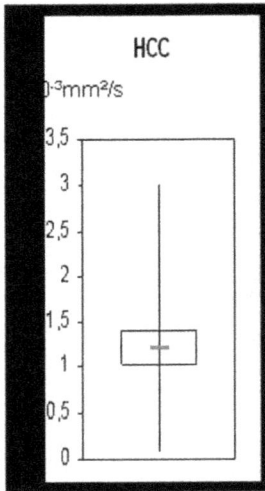

Figure 5. Range of ADC-values (10^{-3} mm^2/s) in lesions suspicious for HCC.

pared to conventional dynamic MRI with different contrast agents; however, these results are not always significant [38–40]. A recent study by Holzapfel et al. reported no significant difference in diagnostic accuracy and sensitivity between diffusion weighted imaging, Gd-EOB-DTPA-enhanced imaging and combined imaging for the detection of focal liver lesions. However, for lesions smaller than 10 mm, a combination of DWI and Gd-EOB-DTPA significantly increased the overall detection rate. Similar to our findings regarding HCC-related diagnostic accuracy, Gadolinium-enhanced MRI and the combination of DWI and Gd-EOB-DTPA enhanced MRI demonstrated equal results [41]. In our 50 patients, just one additional HCC suspicious lesion was detected with DWI compared to conventional dynamic MRI, an 8 mm lesion that was also detected with hepatobiliary phase imaging. Therefore, DWI did not improve the detection of HCC compared to imaging with Gd-EOB-DTPA in our study.

Park et al. also demonstrated that DWI was outperformed by contrast enhanced T1-weighted imaging for the detection of HCC, but it represents a reasonable alternative [42]. However, if Gd-EOB-DTPA is used in the hepatic imaging, a time gap occurs between the equilibrium phase and the hepatobiliary phase, and because there is no significant impact of contrast media on achieving diffusion-weighted imaging and ADC-maps [43–45]. This gap can easily be filled with respiratory-triggered, diffusion-weighted imaging, which can provide additional information for the characterization of focal liver lesions. An important advantage of DWI is that no contrast agent is necessary, a property that is especially valuable for patients with poor renal function [39]. In our department, diffusion-weighted MR imaging is part of the routine liver protocol for all patients.

The potential to differentiate between benign and malignant liver lesions using ADC-quantification was previously reported in the literature [8–12]. Several thresholds have been proposed to accomplish this task, but there is still considerable overlap between benign and malignant liver lesions [9]. Vandecavaeye confirmed

that there is no significant difference in ADC between malignant and benign lesions in patients with cirrhotic liver disease [46]. In our study, the mean ADC-value of HCC lesions was $1.2\pm0.5\times10^{-3}$ mm^2/s, which is similar to values reported in the literature. For example, Naoto measured an ADC-value of $1.31\pm0.28\times10^{-3}$ mm^2/s [12], and Holzapfel reported an ADC-value of $1.12\pm0.28\times10^{-3}$ mm^2/s for a small number of HCC samples [9]. These variances are likely due to differential cellularity of the tumours [47]. Another influential factor are the b-values chosen for DWI. In our study, we used relatively low b-values (b = 0, 50 and 400 s/mm^2), which have the disadvantage of being influenced by perfusion effects. Measured ADC-values tend to decrease as the b-value increases [48]. However, the use of low (perfusion-sensitive) b-values has several advantages: it provides a higher signal-to-noise ratio and more anatomical information of the liver, it is less sensitive to eddy current-induced distortions and it suppresses signals from the hepatic vasculature, which improves the detectability of perivascular lesions [49–51]. Further investigations are needed to determine the best b-values for liver imaging.

Our study has some limitations. First, there was a bias in patient recruitment because we included patients with proven or suspected HCC. This stipulation might result in an overestimation of specificity. Second, we could not achieve a histological proof for every detected lesion due to ethical reasons, so we had to use follow-up examinations and surrogates of clinical and paraclinical findings to confirm the presence of lesions. For this reason, we calculated sensitivity, specificity, and positive and negative predictive values on a patient basis. Third, our study group was relatively small, and further studies with more patients might yield statistically significant results. Fourth, we used a first generation MR-scanner with 3 Tesla, which can suffer from B0 artefacts within the liver parenchyma. Newer MR-Scanners with different coil and RF impulse designs (i.e., the TrueForm and Multi-Transmit) reduce these artefacts and can increase the diagnostic ability for liver imaging. Finally, we only determined ADC-values for suspicious lesions that were clearly visible in the ADC-map. However, our ADC-values were comparable to the values given in literature.

Conclusions

Our study did not show a statistically significant difference in detection of HCC between 3-Tesla Gd-EOB-DTPA-enhanced MRI with diffusion-weighted imaging and 64-slice contrast-enhanced CT.

As we detected slightly more lesions per patient using MRI, we recommend this imaging modality as the first-choice imaging method for the detection of HCC and individual therapeutic decisions. However, contrast-enhanced CT was not inferior in our study, indicating that it represents a useful image modality when MRI is not available or for follow-up examinations.

Author Contributions

Conceived and designed the experiments: BM PS. Performed the experiments: BM. Analyzed the data: PS DL BM. Contributed reagents/materials/analysis tools: BM PS TK. Wrote the paper: BM DL TK PS.

References

1. Bruix J, Sherman M (2005) Management of hepatocellular carcinoma. Hepatology 42: 1208–36

2. Kudo M (2010) The 2008 Okuda lecture: Management of hepatocellular carcinoma: from surveillance to molecular targeted therapy. J Gastroenterol Hepatol 25: 439–52

3. El-Serag HB (2007) Epidemiology of hepatocellular carcinoma in USA. Hepatol Res 37: S88–94

4. Tannapfel A, Wittekind C (2003) Pathology of hepatocellular carcinoma. Chir Gastroenterol 19: 225–230.

5. Tanimoto A, Lee JM, Murakami T, Huppertz A, Kudo M, et al. (2009) Consensus report of the 2nd International Forum for Liver MRI. Eur Radiol 19: S975–89

6. Zech CJ, Reiser MF, Herrmann KA (2009) Imaging of hepatocellular carcinoma by computed tomography and magnetic resonance imaging: state of art. Dig Dis 27: 114–24

7. Rempp H, Boss A, Helmberger T, Pereira P (2011) The current role of minimally invasive therapies in the management of liver tumors. Abdom Imaging 36: 635–47

8. Bruegel M, Holzapfel K, Gaa J, Woertler K, Waldt S, et al. (2008) Characterization of focal liver lesions by ADC measurements using a respiratory triggered diffusion-weighted single-shot echo-planar MR imaging technique. Eur Radiol 18: 477–85

9. Holzapfel K, Bruegel M, Eiber M, Ganter C, Schuster T, et al. (2010) Characterization of small (≤10 mm) focal liver lesions: value of respiratory-triggered echo-planar diffusion-weighted MR imaging. Eur J Radiol 76: 89–95

10. Moteki T, Ishizaka H, Horikoshi H, Matsumoto M (1995) Differentiation between hemangiomas and hepatocellular carcinomas with the apparent diffusion coefficient calculated from turboFLASH MR images. J Magn Reson Imaging 5: 187–91

11. Kim T, Murakami T, Takahashi S, Hori M, Tsuda K, et al. (1995) Diffusion-weighted single-shot echoplanar MR imaging for liver disease. AJR Am J -Roentgenol 173: 393–8

12. Koike N, Cho A, Nasu K, Seto K, Nagaya S, et al. (2009) Role of diffusion-weighted magnetic resonance imaging in the differential diagnosis of focal hepatic lesions. World J Gastroenterol 14; 15: 5805–12

13. Hamm B, Staks T, Mühler A, Bollow M, Taupitz M, et al. (1995) Phase I clinical evaluation of Gd-EOB-DTPA as a hepatobiliary MR contrast agent: safety, pharmacokinetics, and MR imaging. Radiology 195: 785–92

14. Clément O, Mühler A, Vexler V, Berthezène Y, Brasch RC (1992) Gadolinium-ethoxybenzyl-DTPA, a new liver-specific magnetic resonance contrast agent. Kinetic and enhancement patterns in normal and cholestatic rats. Invest Radiol 27: 612–9

15. Schuhmann-Giampieri G, Schmitt-Willich H, Press WR, Negishi C, Weinmann HJ, et al. (1992) Preclinical evaluation of Gd-EOB-DTPA as a contrast agent in MR imaging of the hepatobiliary system. Radiology 183: 59–64

16. Weinmann HJ, Schuhmann-Giampieri G, Schmitt-Willich H, Vogler H, Frenzel T, et al. (1991) A new lipophilic gadolinium chelate as a tissue-specific contrast medium for MRI. Magn Reson Med 22: 233–7

17. Huppertz A, Balzer T, Blakeborough A, Breuer J, Giovagnoni A, et al. (2004) Improved detection of focal liver lesions at MR imaging: multicenter comparison of gadoxetic acid-enhanced MR images with intraoperative findings. Radiology 230: 266–75

18. Huppertz A, Haraida S, Kraus A, Zech CJ, Scheidler J, et al. (2005) Enhancement of focal liver lesions at gadoxetic acid-enhanced MR imaging: correlation with histopathologic findings and spiral CT—initial observations. Radiology 234: 468–78

19. Reimer P, Rummeny EJ, Shamsi K, Balzer T, Daldrup HE, et al. (1996) Phase II clinical evaluation of Gd-EOB-DTPA: dose, safety aspects, and pulse sequence. Radiology 199: 177–83

20. Low RN (2007) Abdominal MRI advances in the detection of liver tumours and characterisation. Lancet Oncol 8: 525–35

21. Ahn SS, Kim MJ, Lim JS, Hong HS, Chung YE, et al. (2010) Added value of gadoxeticacid-enhanced hepatobiliary phase MR imaging in the diagnosis of hepatocellular carcinoma. Radiology 255: 459–66

22. Akai H, Kiryu S, Matsuda I, Satou J, Takao H, et al. (2011) Detection of hepatocellular carcinoma by Gd-EOB-DTPA-enhanced liver MRI: Comparison with triple phase 64 detector row helical CT. Eur J Radiol 80: 310–5

23. Lee CH, Kim KA, Lee J, Park YS, Choi JW, et al. (2012) Using low tube voltage (80kVp) quadruple phase liver CT for the detection of hepatocellular carcinoma: Two-year experience and comparison with Gd-EOB-DTPA enhanced liver MRI. Eur J Radiol 81: e605–11

24. Haradome H, Grazioli L, Tinti R, Morone M, Motosugi U, et al. (2011) Additional value of gadoxetic acid-DTPA-enhanced hepatobiliary phase MR imaging in the diagnosis of early-stage hepatocellular carcinoma: comparison with dynamic triple-phase multidetector CT imaging. J Magn Reson Imaging 34: 69–78

25. Kim YK, Kim CS, Han YM, Kwak HS, Jin GY, et al. (2009) Detection of hepatocellular carcinoma: gadoxetic acid-enhanced 3-dimensional magnetic resonance imaging versus multi-detector row computed tomography. J Comput Assist Tomogr 33: 844–50

26. Di Martino M, Marin D, Guerrisi A, Baski M, Galati F, et al. (2010) Intraindividual comparison of gadoxetate disodium-enhanced MR imaging and 64-section multidetector CT in the Detection of hepatocellular carcinoma in patients with cirrhosis. Radiology 256: 806–16

27. Pitton MB, Kloeckner R, Herber S, Otto G, Kreitner KF, et al. (2009) MRI versus 64-row MDCT for diagnosis of hepatocellular carcinoma. World J Gastroenterol 15: 6044–51

28. Sano K, Ichikawa T, Motosugi U, Sou H, Muhi AM, et al. (2011) Imaging study of early hepatocellular carcinoma: usefulness of gadoxetic acid-enhanced MR imaging. Radiology 261: 834–44

29. Chan R, Kumar G, Abdullah B, Ng Kh, Vijayananthan A, et al. (2011) Optimising the scan delay for arterial phase imaging of the liver using the bolus tracking technique. Biomed Imaging Interv J 7: e12

30. Kim MJ, Choi JY, Lim JS, Kim JY, Kim JH, et al. (2006) Optimal scan window for detection of hypervascular hepatocellular carcinomas during MDCT examination. AJR Am J Roentgenol 187: 198–206

31. Lee JH, Lee JM, Kim SJ, Baek JH, Yun SH, et al. (2012) Enhancement patterns of hepatocellular carcinomas on multiphasicmultidetector row CT: comparison with pathological differentiation. Br J Radiol 85: e573–83

32. Mazzaferro V, Bhoori S, Sposito C, Bongini M, Langer M, et al. (2011) Milan criteria in liver transplantation for hepatocellular carcinoma: an evidence-based analysis of 15 years of experience. Liver Transpl 17: S44–57

33. Cauchy F, Fuks D, Belghiti J (2012) HCC: current surgical treatment concepts. Langenbecks Arch Surg 397: 681–95

34. Mazzaferro V, Regalia E, Doci R, Andreola S, Pulvirenti A, et al. (1996) Liver transplantation for the treatment of small hepatocellular carcinomas in patients with cirrhosis. N Engl J Med 334: 693–699

35. Llovet JM (2005) Updated treatment approach to hepatocellular carcinoma. J Gastroenterol 40: 225–35

36. Kudo M, Okanoue T (2007) Japan Society of Hepatology. Management of hepatocellular carcinoma in Japan: consensus-based clinical practice manual proposed by the Japan Society of Hepatology. Oncology 72: S2–15

37. Motosugi U, Ichikawa T, Tominaga L, Sou H, Sano K, et al. (2009) Delay before the hepatocyte phase of Gd-EOB-DTPA-enhanced MR imaging: is it possible to shorten the examination time? Eur Radiol 19: 2623–9

38. Kim YK, Lee MW, Lee WJ, Kim SH, Rhim H, et al. (2012) Diagnostic accuracy and sensitivity of diffusion-weighted and of gdoxetic acid-enhanced 3-T MR Imaging alone or in combination in the detection of small liver metastasis (≤ 1.5 cm in diameter). Invest Radiol 47: 159–66

39. Yu JS, Chung JJ, Kim JH, Cho ES, Kim DJ, et al. (2011) Detection of small intrahepatic metastases of hepatocellular carcinomas using diffusion-weighted imaging: comparison with conventional dynamic MRI. Magn Reson Imaging 29: 985–92

40. Chung J, Yu JS, Kim DJ, Chung JJ, Kim JH, et al. (2011) Hypervascular hepatocellular carcinoma in the cirrhotic liver: diffusion-weighted imaging versus superparamagnetic iron oxide-enhanced MRI. Magn Reson Imaging 29: 1235–43

41. Holzapfel K, Eiber MJ, Fingerie AA, Bruegel M, Rummeny EJ, et al. (2012) Detection, classification, and characterization of focal liver lesions: value of diffusion-weighted MR imaging, gadoxetic acid-enhanced MR imaging and the combination of both methods. Abdom Imaging 37: 74–82

42. Park MS, Kim S, Patel J, Hajdu CH, Do RK, et al. (2012) Hepatocellular carcinoma: Detection with diffusion-weighted vs. contrast-enhanced MRI in pre-transplant patients. Hepatology 56: 140–8

43. Kinner S, Umutlu L, Blex S, Maderwald S, Antoch G, et al. (2012) Diffusion weighted MR imaging in patients with HCC and liver cirrhosis after administration of different gadolinium contrast agents: Is it still reliable? Eur J Radiol 81: 625–8

44. Choi JS, Kim MJ, Choi JY, Park MS, Lim JS, et al. (2010) Diffusion-weighted MR imaging of liver on 3.0-Tesla system: effect of intravenous administration of gadoxetic acid disodium. Eur Radiol 20: 1052–60

45. Chiu FY, Jao JC, Chen CY, Liu GC, Jaw TS, et al. (2005) Effect of intravenous gadolinium-DTPA on diffusion-weighted magnetic resonance images for evaluation of focal hepatic lesions. J Comput Assist Tomogr 29: 176–80

46. Vandecaveye V, De Keyzer F, Verslype C, Op de Beeck K, Komuta M, et al. (2009) Diffusion-weighted MRI provides additional value to conventional dynamic contrast-enhanced MRI for detection of hepatocellular carcinoma. Eur Radiol 19: 2456–66

47. Koike N, Cho A, Nasu K, Seto K, Nagaya S, et al. (2009) Role of diffusion-weighted magnetic resonance imaging in the differential diagnosis of focal hepatic lesions. World J Gastroenterol 15: 5805–12

48. Hollingsworth KG, Lomas DJ (2006) Influence of perfusion on hepatic MR diffusion measurement. NMR Biomed 19: 231–5

49. Nasu K, Kuroki Y, Nawano S, Kuroki S, Tsukamoto T, et al. (2006) Hepatic metastases: diffusion-weighted sensitivity-encoding versus SPIO-enhanced MR imaging. Radiology 239: 122–30

50. Goshima S, Kanematsu M, Kondo H, Yokoyama R, Kajita K, et al. (2008) Diffusion-weighted imaging of the liver: optimizing b value for the detection and characterization of benign and malignant hepatic lesions. J Magn Reson Imaging 28: 691–7

51. Takahara T, Kwee TC (2012) Low b-value diffusion-weighted imaging: Emerging applications in the body. J Magn Reson Imaging 35: 1266–73

20

Hydrogel-Forming Microneedles Prepared from "Super Swelling" Polymers Combined with Lyophilised Wafers for Transdermal Drug Delivery

Ryan F. Donnelly[1]*, Maelíosa T. C. McCrudden[1], Ahlam Zaid Alkilani[1,2], Eneko Larrañeta[1], Emma McAlister[1], Aaron J. Courtenay[1], Mary-Carmel Kearney[1], Thakur Raghu Raj Singh[1], Helen O. McCarthy[1], Victoria L. Kett[1], Ester Caffarel-Salvador[1], Sharifa Al-Zahrani[1], A. David Woolfson[1]

1 School of Pharmacy, Queen's University Belfast, Belfast, Co. Antrim, United Kingdom, 2 School of Pharmacy, Zarqa University, Zarqa, Jordan

Abstract

We describe, for the first time, hydrogel-forming microneedle arrays prepared from "super swelling" polymeric compositions. We produced a microneedle formulation with enhanced swelling capabilities from aqueous blends containing 20% w/w Gantrez S-97, 7.5% w/w PEG 10,000 and 3% w/w Na_2CO_3 and utilised a drug reservoir of a lyophilised wafer-like design. These microneedle-lyophilised wafer compositions were robust and effectively penetrated skin, swelling extensively, but being removed intact. In in vitro delivery experiments across excised neonatal porcine skin, approximately 44 mg of the model high dose small molecule drug ibuprofen sodium was delivered in 24 h, equating to 37% of the loading in the lyophilised reservoir. The super swelling microneedles delivered approximately 1.24 mg of the model protein ovalbumin over 24 h, equivalent to a delivery efficiency of approximately 49%. The integrated microneedle-lyophilised wafer delivery system produced a progressive increase in plasma concentrations of ibuprofen sodium in rats over 6 h, with a maximal concentration of approximately 179 µg/ml achieved in this time. The plasma concentration had fallen to 71±6.7 µg/ml by 24 h. Ovalbumin levels peaked in rat plasma after only 1 hour at 42.36±17.01 ng/ml. Ovalbumin plasma levels then remained almost constant up to 6 h, dropping somewhat at 24 h, when 23.61±4.84 ng/ml was detected. This work represents a significant advancement on conventional microneedle systems, which are presently only suitable for bolus delivery of very potent drugs and vaccines. Once fully developed, such technology may greatly expand the range of drugs that can be delivered transdermally, to the benefit of patients and industry. Accordingly, we are currently progressing towards clinical evaluations with a range of candidate molecules.

Editor: Masaya Yamamoto, Institute for Frontier Medical Sciences, Kyoto University, Japan

Funding: This study was supported by Biotechnology and Biological Sciences Research Council grant numbers BB/FOF/287 and BB/E020534/1 (http://www.bbsrc.ac.uk/) and Wellcome Trust grant number WT094085MA (http://www.wellcome.ac.uk/). The funders had no role in study design, data collection and analysis, decision to publish, or preparation of the manuscript.

Competing Interests: Ryan Donnelly and David Woolfson are named inventors on a patent application related to hydrogel-forming microneedle arrays (details below). They are working with a number of companies with a view to commercialisation of this technology. They provide advice, through consultancy, to these companies. None of the other authors have any competing interests. Donnelly, R.F., Woolfson A.D., McCarron, P.A., Morrow, D.I.J., Morrissey, A. (2007). Microneedles/Delivery Device and Method. British Patent Application No 0718996.2. Filed September 28th 2007. International publication No WO2009040548. Approved for grant in Japan and China. US, Europe, India and Australia pending.

* Email: r.donnelly@qub.ac.uk

Introduction

Microneedle (MN) arrays, micron scale, minimally-invasive devices that painlessly by-pass the skin's *stratum corneum* barrier, have been shown to be extremely effective in enhancing transdermal delivery of water soluble drugs, biomolecular therapeutics and vaccines [1–3]. The compounds delivered to date have typically been of high potency, meaning only a low dose is required to achieve a therapeutic affect (e.g. insulin) [4,5] or elicit the required immune response [6,7]. Clearly, the majority of marketed drug substances, including many antibodies, are not low dose, high potency molecules. Indeed, many drugs require doses of several hundred milligrams per day in order to achieve therapeutic plasma concentrations in man. Until now, such high doses could

not be delivered transdermally from a patch of reasonable size, even for molecules whose physicochemical properties are ideal for passive diffusion across the skin's *stratum corneum* barrier. Therefore, transdermal delivery has traditionally been limited to fairly lipophilic, low molecular weight, high potency drug substances. Since most drugs do not possess these properties, the transdermal delivery market has not expanded beyond around 20 drugs. Marketed MN-based patches are likely to increase this number of drugs in the coming years. However, this increase will only be maximised if high dose molecules can be delivered in therapeutic doses using MN. We have previously shown that suitably-formulated dissolving MN platforms can deliver therapeutic doses of a low potency, high dose drug substance [8]. However, deposition of polymer in skin from a dissolving MN system may be undesirable if the system is to be used on an ongoing basis. The dissolving MN system employed in this previous study would deposit approximately 5–10 mg of polymer per cm^2 in skin [8]. If the patch size were 10 cm^2, then 50–100 mg of polymer would be deposited in the patient's skin every time the product is applied. While vaccines are used infrequently, most therapeutic agents need to be administered regularly. Accordingly, dissolving MN systems may be most appropriate to rapid delivery of low dose vaccines [6,9].

We have recently described novel hydrogel-forming MN arrays, prepared under ambient conditions that contain no drug themselves [10]. Instead, they rapidly imbibe skin interstitial fluid upon insertion to form continuous, unblockable conduits between the dermal microcirculation and an attached patch-type drug reservoir. Such hydrogel-forming MN initially act simply as a tool to pierce the *stratum corneum* barrier. Upon insertion, they function as a rate-controlling membrane, allowing sustained drug delivery at a rate controllable by adjustment of crosslink density, which dictates swelling rate [10,11]. Importantly, such MN are removed intact from skin, leaving no measurable polymer residue behind, but are sufficiently softened, even after 1 minute of skin insertion to preclude reinsertion, thus further reducing the risk of transmission of infection [12]. In the present study, we substantially modified this novel system to facilitate delivery of clinically-relevant doses of a low potency, high dose drug substance and rapid delivery of a model protein by using a modifying agent to increase swelling capabilities [13] and using a hygroscopic lyophilised drug reservoir (**Figure 1**).

Methods and Materials

2.1. Chemicals

Polyethylene glycol (PEG, MW 10,000 Da), ibuprofen-sodium, chicken ovalbumin (OVA, albumin from chicken egg, grade IIV), mouse monoclonal anti-chicken ovalbumin antibody (moAb), Ph. Eur. Gelatin, D-mannitol and tetramethylbenzidine (TMB) substrate were purchased from Sigma-Aldrich, Dorset, UK. Phosphate buffered saline tablets, pH 7.4 (PBS) were obtained from Oxoid Ltd., Hampshire, UK. Rabbit anti-ovalbumin horse-radish peroxidase (HRP) conjugated-polyclonal antibody was purchased from Gene Tex Inc Alton Pkwy, Irvine, USA. SuperBlock T20 was purchased from Thermo Scientific, Rockford, Illinois, USA. 50C-Mannitol was supplied by Roquette, Lestrem, France. Gantrez AN-139 and S-97, copolymers of methyl vinyl ether and maleic anhydride and methyl vinyl ether and maleic acid, respectively (PMVE/MAH and PMVE/MA, with molecular masses of 1,080,000 and 1,500,000 respectively) were gifts from Ashland, Kidderminster, UK. Unless otherwise stated, all other chemicals and materials were supplied by Sigma-Aldrich (Dorset, UK) or Fisher Scientific (Loughborough, UK).

2.2. Preparation of hydrogel films

The aim here was to investigate various polymeric compositions in order to find a material capable of rapid swelling, but which would be sufficiently hard in the dry state to penetrate the skin. Importantly, once swollen, the material should maintain structural integrity and be reasonably robust during handling.

Stock solutions of Gantrez S-97 (40% w/w) or AN-139 (30% w/w) [13,14] were prepared using deionised water (**Figure 2A**). Hydrogel films were then prepared using varying concentrations of the co-polymer, PEG 10,000 and the modifying agent, sodium carbonate (Na$_2$CO$_3$). The blends were centrifuged at 3,500 rpm for 15 minutes in order to remove any air bubbles. The aqueous blends (30 g) were then slowly poured into moulds consisting of a

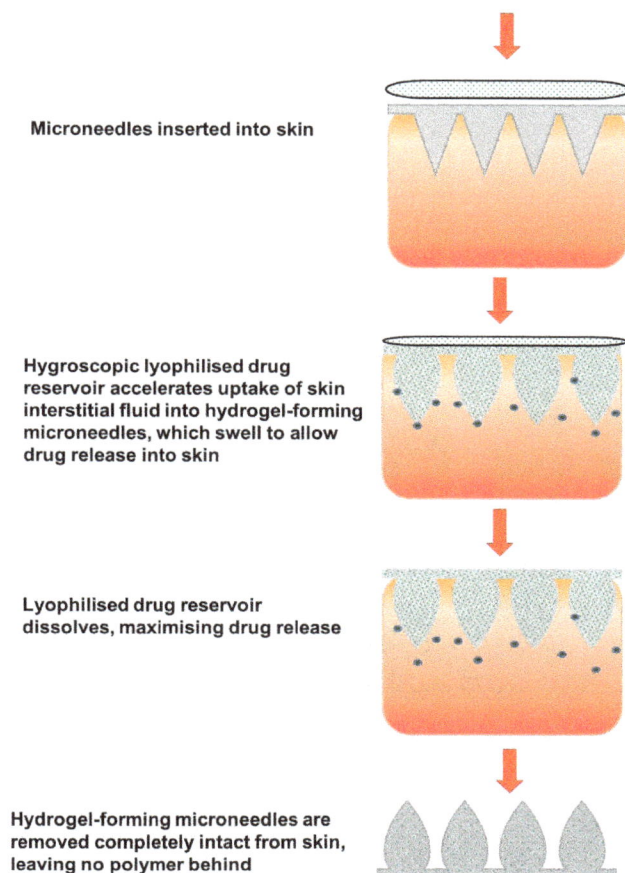

Microneedles inserted into skin

Hygroscopic lyophilised drug reservoir accelerates uptake of skin interstitial fluid into hydrogel-forming microneedles, which swell to allow drug release into skin

Lyophilised drug reservoir dissolves, maximising drug release

Hydrogel-forming microneedles are removed completely intact from skin, leaving no polymer behind

Figure 1. Schematic representation of the concept of combining hydrogel-forming microneedles prepared from super swelling polymers and lyophilised wafer-type drug reservoirs for enhanced transdermal delivery of proteins and high dose low potency drug substances.

release liner with the siliconised surface facing upwards (Rayven, Inc., Saint Paul, MN, USA) secured to a Perspex base plate with stainless steel clamps. Once assembled, the internal dimensions available for casting were 100 mm×100 mm. The aqueous blends were spread evenly across the moulds and these were placed onto a level surface. The cast blend was dried for 48 hours at room temperature. After drying, the films were cured at 80°C for 24 h to induce chemical crosslinking between the PMVE/MA and PEG by ester formation [14,15]. Films were then removed from the mould by simply peeling the release liner, with attached film, off the base.

2.3. Swelling of hydrogel films in phosphate-buffered saline (PBS)

For swelling studies, individual film portions (1 cm^2) were weighed at the zero time point in the dry state (m$_0$) and then placed into a volume of PBS (pH 7.4). The film portions were removed at specific time points, surface fluid was removed between pieces of filter paper and the mass of the swollen film was recorded (m$_t$). PBS was selected as the swelling medium, as it was deemed to closely resemble/simulate skin interstitial fluid and has been used as the swelling medium in other similar studies [14]. The percentage swelling of the film was determined using

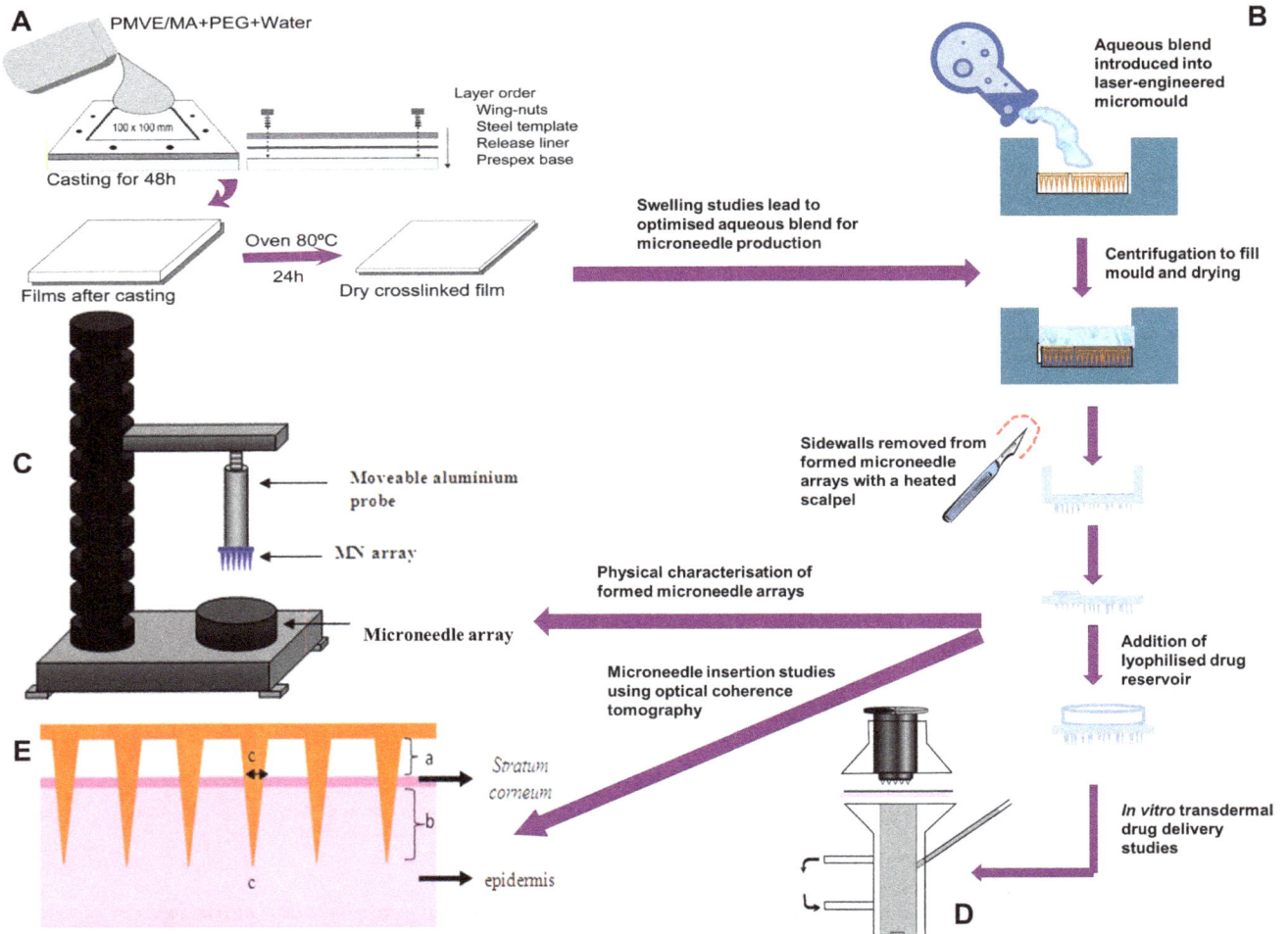

Figure 2. Schematic representation of casting and crosslinking of the super swelling hydrogel films (A), microneedle preparation (B), Texture Analyser set-up for investigation of physical properties of microneedles (C) and Franz cell set-up for *in vitro* transdermal drug release studies (D). Panel (**E**) shows a diagrammatic representation of the measurements recorded from the optical coherence tomographic images of microneedle penetration into excised neonatal porcine skin *in vitro*, namely; (a) the distance between the lower microneedle base plate and the *stratum corneum*, (b) the depth of microneedle penetration into the skin and (c) the width of the micropore created in the skin.

Equation 1.

$$\% \text{ Swelling} = \left(\frac{m_t - m_o}{m_o} \right) x \ 100\% \qquad (1)$$

To examine the controlled swelling mechanism of the PEG-crosslinked PMVE/MA hydrogels, a second order kinetic model was used to process the experimental data, as outlined in **Equation 2**, where A is the reciprocal of the initial swelling rate of the hydrogel, r_o, or $1/(k_s S_{eq}^2)$, where k_s is the swelling rate constant and B is the inverse of the degree of swelling at equilibrium, S_{eq} [16].

$$\% \text{EWC} = \frac{m_e - m_d}{m_d} x \ 100\% \qquad (2)$$

To analyse the kinetic model, t/S versus t graphs were plotted and respective swelling rate parameters were determined [14]. The dynamics of the water sorption process are usually investigated either by monitoring the change in physical dimensions of the

swelling hydrogel or by knowing the amounts of water imbibed by the hydrogel at various time points. In the current study, the latter procedure was engaged. Analysis of the swelling kinetics of the various films was carried out using **Equation 3** [14]. The portion of the water absorption curve with a fractional water uptake (M_t/M_∞) less than 0.60 was analyzed with **Equation 4**, where M_t is the mass of water absorbed at time t, M_∞ is the water uptake at equilibrium. k is a gel characteristic constant, which depends on the structural characteristics of the polymer and its interaction with the solvent and n is the swelling exponent, describing the mechanism of penetrant transport into the hydrogel. The constants n and k may be calculated from the slopes and intercepts of the plots of $\ln(M_t/M_\infty)$ versus $\ln t$ from the experimental data. The value of n provides an indication of the water transport mechanism. When n = 0.5, the swelling process is of Fickian nature and is diffusion controlled while the value of n between 0.5 and 1 suggests non-Fickian diffusion or more specifically anomalous diffusion. When n becomes exactly equal to unity, then the diffusion is termed case II diffusion. In some cases, the value for n has been found to exceed unity and this represents super case II transport [17–19].

$$t/S = A + Bt \qquad (3)$$

$$\frac{M_t}{M} = kt^n \qquad (4)$$

Hydrogel network structure characterization is a complex procedure because of the many types of possible networks, including, regular, irregular, loosely/highly cross-linked and imperfect networks. As a result of these variations in the network structure, only average values for the cross-linking density and molecular weight (MW) between crosslinks are represented using different experimental or theoretical methods [13,16–19]. In the present study, the number average MW between cross-links, $\bar{M}_C$, was determined using equilibrium swelling theory, $\bar{M}_C$ (Equi), rather than glass transition temperature. The magnitude of $\bar{M}_C$ affected the mechanical and physical properties of crosslinked polymers. The volume fraction of a polymer, ϕ, in the swollen state describes the amount of liquid that can be imbibed into a hydrogel and is described as a ratio of the polymer volume to the swollen gel volume (**Equation 5 and 6**).

$$\bar{M}_C (Equi) = \frac{-d_p V_s \phi^{1/3}}{[In(1-\phi) + \phi + \chi\phi^2]} \qquad (5)$$

$$\phi = \left[1 + \frac{d_p}{d_s}\left(\frac{m_a}{m_b}\right) - \frac{d_p}{d_s}\right]^{-1} \qquad (6)$$

Here, V_s is the molar volume of water (18 cm^3/mol), ϕ is volume fraction of polymer in the hydrogel, χ is the Flory-Huggins polymer-solvent interaction parameter; In the above Equation, m_a and m_b are the mass of polymer before and after swelling and d_p and d_s are the densities of polymer and solvent, respectively. The density of the polymeric films was calculated using the following formula; $d_p = w/SX$, where; X is the average thickness of the film, S is the cross-sectional area and w weight of the film. The polymer water interaction parameter (χ) reflects the thermodynamic interaction in hydrogels, which in turn indicates the change of interaction energy when polymer and solvent mix together. The χ parameters of hydrogels can be obtained experimentally *via* **Equation 7** [13,16–19].

$$\chi = \frac{1}{2} + \frac{\phi}{3} \qquad (7)$$

Equation 7 neglects the M_c dependence of the χ parameter, and therefore, this equation indicates that the χ values are always $\geq$ 0.50. In the present study, crosslink density, V_e, was determined using **Equation 8**. V_e represents the number of elastically effective chains, totally induced in a perfect network, per unit volume. Where, N_A is Avagadro's number (6.023×10^{23} mole^{-1}) [13,16–19].

$$V_e = d_p N_A / M_c \qquad (8)$$

2.4. Fabrication of hydrogel forming MN arrays

Formulations used to prepare MN were based upon the preceding swelling studies. Aqueous blends containing 15% w/w Gantrez AN-139 and 7.5% w/w PEG, 10,000 (control formulation) [14] were utilized to fabricate MN arrays as previously described [10,11]. The blend (500 mg) was poured into MN moulds (361 (19×19) needles perpendicular to the base and of conical shape, 600 μm high with base width of 300 μm and 50 μm interspacing on a 0.49 cm^2 patch) and these were centrifuged at 3,500 rpm for 15 min and dried at room temperature for 48 h. MN were crosslinked (esterification reaction) by heating at 80°C for 24 hours [10,11,14] and the sidewalls formed by the moulding process were removed using a heated blade (**Figure 2B**). MN arrays were also prepared from a so-called "super swelling" hydrogel formulation containing 20% w/w Gantrez S-97, 7.5% w/w PEG 10,000 and 3% w/w Na_2CO_3.

2.5. Mechanical characterisation of super swelling microneedle arrays

MN were subjected to standard mechanical tests using a TA-XT2 Texture Analyser (Stable Microsystems, Haslemere, UK) in compression mode, as described previously [10,11,20]. Briefly, MN arrays were visualised before testing using a light microscope (GXMGE-5 digital microscope, Laboratory Analysis Ltd, Devon, UK). MN arrays were then carefully placed on the flat stainless steel baseplate of the Texture Analyser with the needles pointing upwards. A flat-faced probe with a diameter of 11.0 mm was lowered at a speed of 0.5 mm s^{-1}. Upon contact with the MN array, the probe continued to travel at a speed of 0.5 mm s^{-1} until the required force had been exerted. Once the target force was reached, the probe was moved upwards at a speed of 0.5 mm s^{-1}. MN arrays were then viewed again under the light microscope.

2.6. Skin insertion studies

Neonatal porcine skin, a good model for human skin [21,22], was obtained from stillborn piglets and immediately (<24 hours after birth) excised, trimmed to a thickness of 700 μm using a dermatome (Integra Life Sciences, Padgett Instruments, NJ, USA) and frozen in liquid nitrogen vapour, as previously described [10,11,20]. Skin was then stored in aluminium foil at −20°C for no more than 7 days prior to use.

Skin was mounted on the baseplate of the Texture Analyser using cyanoacrylate adhesive (Loctite Ltd, Dublin, Ireland) while the MN were this time attached to the probe using double-sided tape (3M, Carrickmines, Ireland). The probe then moved downwards as described above until the required force had been exerted. Once the target force was reached, the probe was moved upwards at a speed of 0.5 mm s^{-1}. The number of MN in an array that had penetrated the skin's *stratum corneum* barrier was counted following visualisation of the pores formed in skin using methylene blue solution (1 mg/ml in PBS pH 7.4).

Optical coherence tomography (OCT), as described previously [23] allowed measurement of the depth of MN insertion for each application force, since the MN are transparent and accordingly can be left in place during OCT studies to mimic their intended use (EX1301 OCT microscope, Michelson Diagnostics, Kent, UK). OCT was also used to visualise the *in situ* swelling of the MN in real time skin at varying time intervals over a 3 h period. OCT data files were exported to Image J (National Institutes of Health, Bethesda, MD, USA) for measurement of insertion depth and false colours were applied using Ability Photopaint (Ability Software International, Horley, UK) for presentation purposes.

2.7. Preparation and characterisation of lyophilised drug reservoirs

A range of lyophilised wafer-type reservoirs loaded with the model compounds ovalbumin (OVA) or ibuprofen sodium were prepared containing varying concentrations of gelatin, mannitol and, in some instances, sodium chloride (NaCl) and sucrose. In the case of the ibuprofen sodium wafers, a variety of different gelatin sources, all at loadings of 10% w/w, were tested in combination with 3% w/w mannitol and 40% w/w ibuprofen sodium in deionised water.

To prepare OVA-containing reservoirs, the protein (0.5% w/w) was dissolved in distilled water, followed by the addition of gelatin, mannitol, NaCl and sucrose. It was then mixed by speed mixer at 3,000 rpm for 60 s and sonicated at 37°C for 60 min. To prepare the ibuprofen sodium-loaded reservoirs, the individual components were mixed by speed mixer at 3,000 rpm for 60 s and sonicated at 37°C for 60 min. The resulting OVA or ibuprofen-sodium formulations were then cast (500 mg in the case of OVA-loaded wafers and 250 mg in the case of ibuprofen sodium-loaded wafers) into cylindrical moulds with one open end moulds (diameter 15 mm, depth 5 mm), frozen at −80°C for a minimum of 60 min and then lyophilised in the freeze-drier (Virtis Advantage Bench top Freeze Drier System, SP Scientific, Warminster PA, USA), according to the following regime: primary drying for forty eight hours at a shelf temperature of −40°C, secondary drying for ten hours at a shelf temperature of 20°C and vacuum pressure of 50 mTorr.

Dried reservoirs were characterised using standard pharmacopoeial tests. Twenty reservoirs were selected randomly, weighed individually and their average weight was calculated to determine the weight uniformity. The percentage deviation of each reservoir from the average weight was determined. The thickness of the reservoirs was determined with a digital micrometer (Digital Calliper, 0–150 mm, Jade Products Rugby Limited, Warwickshire, UK). Five reservoirs were used and average values were calculated. Hardness was determined using a Copley Hardness Tester (Copley Scientific, Nottingham, UK). Twenty reservoirs were weighed (W_0) and then placed in the Friabilitor (Copley Scientific, Nottingham, UK). This was operated at 25 rpm for 4 min. The reservoirs were then weighed again (W). The % friability was then calculated using **Equation 9**. OVA and ibuprofen sodium contents were determined using the ELISA and HPLC methods described below following dissolution of the reservoirs in PBS pH 7.4.

$$\% \text{ Friability} = (W\text{-}W_0/W_0) * 100\% \qquad (9)$$

2.8. In vitro release studies

The diffusion of ibuprofen sodium (MW 228.26 g/mol) and OVA (MW 45,000 g/mol) from lyophilised active-loaded tablets through hydrogel MN arrays and across neonatal porcine skin was investigated in vitro using modified Franz diffusion cells (FDC-400 flat flange, 15 mm orifice diameter, mounted on an FDCD diffusion drive console providing synchronous stirring at 600 rpm and thermostated at 37 ± 1°C, Crown Glass Co. Inc., Sommerville, NJ, USA), as described previously [4]. Briefly, neonatal porcine skin was obtained from stillborn piglets and immediately (< 24 hours after birth) excised and trimmed to a thickness of 350 μm using an electric dermatome. Skin was then stored in aluminium foil at −20°C until required. Skin barrier function integrity was confirmed in all cases using standard transepidermal water loss

measurements (VapoMeter, Delfin Technologies Ltd, Kuopio, Finland), with any damaged skin immediately discarded. Neonatal porcine skin samples were then shaved carefully so as not to damage the skin (again confirmed by TEWL) and were then pre-equilibrated in phosphate buffered saline (PBS), pH 7.4, for 15 minutes prior to the commencement of experimentation. A circular specimen of the skin was secured to the donor compartment of the diffusion cell using cynoacrylate glue (Loctite, Dublin, Ireland) with the *stratum corneum* facing towards the donor compartment. This was then placed on top of dental wax, to give the skin support, and MN arrays inserted into the centre of the skin section, using a spring activated applicator at a force of 11 N/array. The lyophilised active-loaded wafers (which had been trimmed to size using a heated scalpel blade) were placed on the top of the MN, with 20 μl water used to initiate adhesion. A tubular stainless steel weight (diameter 11.0 mm, 3.5 g mass) was then placed on top of this. The donor compartments were mounted onto the receptor compartments and the Franz cell donor compartments covered with laboratory film (Parafilm, Pechiney Plastic Packaging, WI, USA) so as to avoid evaporation of PBS over the course of experimentation. At predetermined time intervals, a 200 μl sample was collected *via* the side arm of the Franz cell and the receiver compartment immediately replenished with an equivalent volume of release medium. OVA was quantified again using ELISA, while ibuprofen sodium was determined using HPLC.

2.9. In vivo evaluation of OVA and ibuprofen sodium delivery through super swelling MN

Prior to experimentation, rats were acclimatised to laboratory conditions for a 7 day period. Super swelling hydrogel MN arrays were manually inserted into the skin at a site on the rats' backs. An aliquot of water (20 μl) was applied to the centre of the array and the lyophilised reservoir (again trimmed to size) was placed on top of this. A bespoke adhesive film (Scotchpak 9732, 3M, Carrickmines, Ireland, coated with a 1.0 mm layer of DuroTak 34-416A, National Starch & Chemical Company, Bridgewater, NJ, USA) was applied on top of, and around the edges of, the lyophilised reservoirs to aid retention and provide occlusion. Following application of this integrated system, blood samples were collected at pre-defined time points over 24 h for analysis.

All animal experiments throughout this study were conducted according to the policy of the federation of European Laboratory Animal Science Associations and the European Convention for the protection of vertebrate animals used for experimental and other scientific purposes, with implementation of the principles of the 3R's (replacement, reduction, refinement). Ethical permission specifically for the experiments described here was obtained from the Queen's University Animal Welfare and Ethics Review Board and all researchers carrying out the work had Personal Licences from the UK Home Office. To anaesthetise the animals, isoflurane was used and carbon dioxide was used for euthanisation.

2.10. Extraction of plasma and drug

The following procedure was carried out in the case of ibuprofen sodium-containing samples only. Control rat blood for method development was obtained from healthy Sprague dawley rats. Blood from culled rats was collected via heart puncture with a heparinised syringe into ethylenediaminetetraacetic acid (EDTA)-coated tubes. Plasma separation was performed by centrifuging the blood at 500× g for 10 min in a refrigerated centrifuge (4°C). The plasma was then aliquoted into microtubes and stored at −80°C until required. In the case of standards used in assay development, 10 μl of ibuprofen-sodium working standard solutions were added to 190 µl blank plasma. In the case of plasma samples from MN-treated rats, the drug was extracted from the samples without the addition of any endogenous drug. Samples were then vortex mixed for 10 s in a poly(propylene) microtube and 500 µl each acetonitrile (ACN) was added. The samples were vortex mixed for 10 min and centrifuged at 14,000× g for 10 min at 4°C. The ACN extraction procedure was then repeated to ensure optimum extraction of the drug. The sample mixture was placed in a disposable glass culture tube and the extract dried under a stream of nitrogen at 35°C for 50 min using a Zymark TurboVap LV Evaporator Workstation (McKinley Scientific, Sparta, NJ, USA). The residue was then reconstituted in 200 µl PBS (pH 7.4) and collected into a microtube. This was then vortex mixed for 30 s and centrifuged at 14,000× g for 10 min at room temperature. The supernatant was transferred into an auto sampler vial and 50 µl was injected onto the HPLC column and detection carried out as outlined below. In the case of blood samples collected from OVA- treated rats, plasma was separated from whole blood as outlined and this was then quantified by ELISA experiments.

2.11. Pharmaceutical analysis of ibuprofen sodium

Ibuprofen sodium quantification in PBS (pH 7.4) and rat plasma was performed using reverse-phase high performance liquid chromatography (RP-HPLC) (Agilent 1200 Binary Pump, Agilent 1200, Standard Autosampler, Agilent 1200 Variable Wavelength Detector, Agilent Technologies UK Ltd., Stockport, UK) with UV detection at 220 nm. Gradient separation was achieved using an Agilent Eclipse XDB-C18 (5 µm pore size, 4.6×150 mm) analytical column fitted with a guard cartridge of matching chemistry. The mobile phase was 60%:40% methanol:10 mM potassium phosphate (pH 4.6), with a flow rate of 1 ml min^{-1}, and a run time of 30 min per sample. The injection volume was 50 µl. The chromatograms obtained were analysed using Agilent ChemStation Software B.02.01. Least squares linear regression analysis and correlation analysis were performed on the calibration curves produced, enabling determination of the equation of the line, its coefficient of determination and the residual sum of squares (RSS). To determine the limit of detection (LoD) and limit of quantification (LoQ), an approach based on the standard deviation of the response and the slope of the representative calibration curve was employed, as described in the guidelines from the International Conference on Harmonisation (ICH) [24]. Ibuprofen sodium, either dissolved in PBS (pH 7.4) (standards), or samples collected from the Franz cell apparatus (unknowns), was quantified by injection of the sample, following filter sterilisation through 0.2 µm filters, directly onto the HPLC column. In the case of plasma samples, the drug was first extracted from the plasma as described above and then the resulting sample, which had been reconstituted in PBS (pH 7.4) and filtered through a 0.2 µm filter, was injected onto the column. The method parameters for detection of ibuprofen sodium in PBS (pH 7.4) and plasma were identical.

2.12. Enzyme-linked immunosorbent assay (ELISA) for detection of OVA

An OVA ELISA, developed as described previously [25], was used to detect OVA in samples collected in both *in vitro* and *in vivo* experiments. Briefly, monoclonal anti-chicken egg albumin (ovalbumin) antibody produced in mouse (moAb) was diluted in 0.1 M bicarbonate buffer, pH 9.6 to the optimized concentration of 2.5 µg/ml. An aliquot (50 µl) of anti-ovalbumin was dispensed into the plate and incubated overnight at 4°C. The plate was filled with washing buffer 0.05% v/v Tween-PBS and soaked for 30 seconds before discarded. This process was repeated 5 times.

Then, the plate was turned onto absorbance paper to remove any remaining buffer. The plate was blocked with SuperBlock T20 buffer (150 µl/well) and incubated for 2 hours at room temperature. For the calibration curve, OVA solutions were freshly prepared at a concentration of 1 mg/ml in PBS produced concentrations of 1 µg/ml to 10 ng/ml. A 50 µl of sample was dispensed into wells, each sample was analysed in triplicate. The plate was covered and incubated for 1 hour at room temperature. The plate was washed and incubated with rabbit anti chicken OVA polyclonal antibody conjugate with horse-radish peroxidase (HRP) at the optimized concentration of 5 µg/ml in SuperBlock T20 buffer for 1 hour at room temperature. After the plate was washed, 50 µl of TMP was added to each well to detect antibody binding and incubated for 15 min. Colour development was ended using 50 µl/well of 4.0 M HCl and optical density was measured at 450 nm using a microplate reader spectrophotometer (EnSpire Multimode Plate Reader, PerkinElmer, Waltham, MA, USA). In terms of the analysis of blood samples collected during *in vivo* experiments, plasma was separated from whole blood as outlined below and this plasma was then subjected to the ELISA protocol outlined above.

2.13. Statistical analysis

Data was analysed, where appropriate, using the Student's t-test, one-way analysis of variance ANOVA, Mann-Whitney U-test or Wilcoxon test. In each case, a *p*-value less than 0.05 was considered to denote significance.

Results and Discussion

Microneedles (MN) prepared from hydrogel-forming materials have a range of advantageous characteristics. Firstly, the delivered dose is not limited by what can be loaded into, or onto the surface of the needles themselves, since the drug is contained within an attached patch-type drug reservoir. Secondly, controlled administration is possible for the first time with MN. Finally, since the MN are removed intact, no polymer is deposited in skin, while the inherent antimicrobial properties of the polymer composition used and the fact that the needles are soft upon removal mean transmission of infection from patient to patient is unlikely. To date, we have employed such systems in the effective *in vivo* delivery of potent biomolecules, such as insulin, and for sustained administration of proteins and small molecules over hours or days [10–12]. In order to take this technology to the next stage of development, we must now move beyond simply controlling transdermal permeation to demonstrate its utility in administration of clinically-relevant doses of non-potent drugs and in rapid delivery of large molecules with physicochemical properties similar to vaccine antigens. Accordingly, in the present study, we used our previous experience with hydrogels [13] to alter the MN formulation to enhance its swelling capabilities and changed the drug reservoir from a flexible polymeric patch to a lyophilised wafer-like design. Using a hygroscopic reservoir is likely to have two principal effects. Firstly, its high solid content and porous nature will attract water from skin interstitial fluid by osmosis through the hydrogel-forming MN, whose swelling rate will be enhanced. Secondly, since such lyophilised systems are rapidly soluble in water, the rate of drug dissolution and its subsequent availability for diffusion will also be increased. These theories were examined for the first time here using ibuprofen sodium and ovalbumin as model compounds. Importantly, we also examined MN arrays post removal, since it was possible that excessive swelling would reduce mechanical integrity.

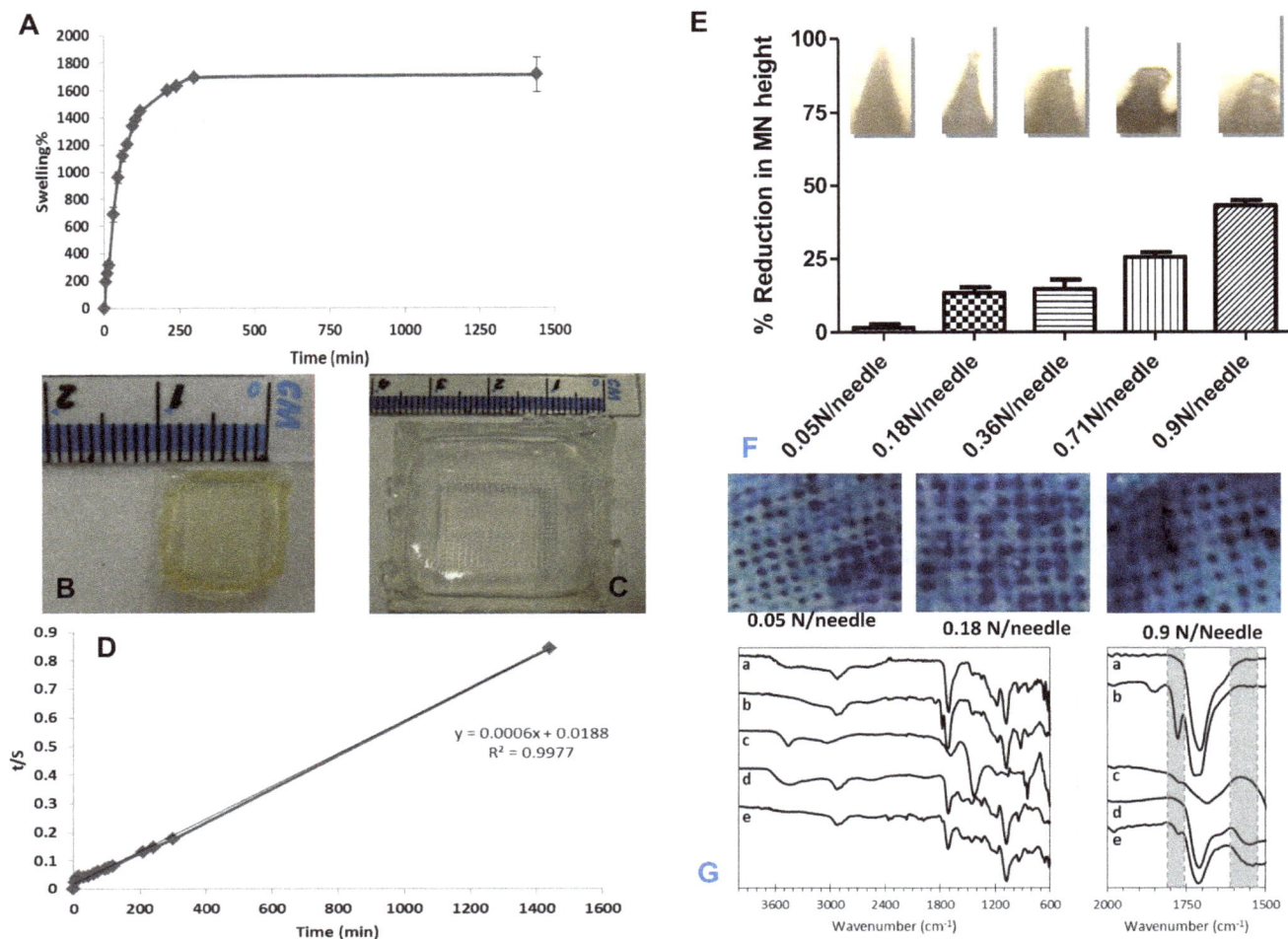

Figure 3. Swelling curve for crosslinked hydrogel films prepared from aqueous blends containing 20% w/w PMVE/MA, 7.5% w/w PEG and 3% Na₂CO₃ based on the increasing mass of the swelling array expressed as a percentage of the mass of a dry array (Means ± SD, n = 3) (A). Super swelling microneedle arrays prepared from aqueous blends containing 20% w/w PMVE/MA, 7.5% w/w PEG and 3% Na₂CO₃ as (**B**) xerogel and (**C**) post-swelling for 3 hours in PBS pH 7.4. t/S versus t swelling curves of super swelling hydrogel prepared from aqueous blends containing 20% w/w PMVE/MA, 7.5% PEG 10,000 and 3% Na₂CO₃ (Mean ± SD, n = 3) (**D**). Digital microscope images of super swelling hydrogel-forming MN (prepared from aqueous blends containing 20% w/w PMVE/MA and 3% Na₂CO₃) following the application of different forces (0.05, 0.18, 0.36, 0.71 and 0.9 N/needle). These images are representative of the percentage reduction in the heights of needles on the MN arrays observed following the application of the different forces (Means+SD, n = 3) (**E**). Digital images showing micropores in excised neonatal porcine skin following application of different forces and subsequent staining with methylene blue solution post microneedle removal (**F**). Attenuated total reflectance (ATR)-Fourier transform infrared (FTIR) spectra of dry hydrogels prepared from aqueous blends containing: 20% w/w Gantrez S-97, 7.5% w/w PEG 10.000 non crosslinked (a) and crosslinked (b) materials; Na₂CO₃ (c) and 20% w/w Gantrez S-97, 7.5% w/w PEG 10.000 and 3% w/w Na₂CO₃ non crosslinked (d) and crosslinked (e) materials. The left panel shows a closer view of the carbonyl region for the same materials. A FTIR Accutrac FT/IR-4100 Series (Jasco, Essex, UK) equipped with MIRacle diamond ATR was used at room temperature. Samples were scanned and recorded in the region of 4000–400 cm⁻¹ at a resolution of 4.0 cm⁻¹. The obtained spectra were an average of 64 scans. A standard smoothing process was applied to all the spectra using the equipment software (**G**).

Table 1. Aqueous blends used to prepare hydrogel formulations tested in the current study and the equilibrium swelling of the formed hydrogels (Means ± SD, n = 3).

Formulation no.	Ingredients (pH value of Gantrez gel prior to addition of other ingredients and making up to volume with deionised water)	Percentage swelling at equilibrium
Control formulation	15% w/w Gantrez AN-139 (pH 2) 7.5% w/w PEG 10,000	1071±106
1	15% w/w Gantrez S-97, (pH 2) 7.5% w/w PEG 10,000	918±13
2	20% w/w Gantrez S-97, (pH 2) 7.5% w/w PEG 10,000, 3% w/w Na₂CO₃	1708±125
3	15% w/w Gantrez AN-139, (adjusted to pH 4) 7.5% w/w PEG 10,000, 3% w/w Na₂CO₃	Dissolved
4	16% w/w Gantrez AN-139, (adjusted to pH 4) 6% w/w PEG 10,000, 3% w/w Na₂CO₃	Dissolved

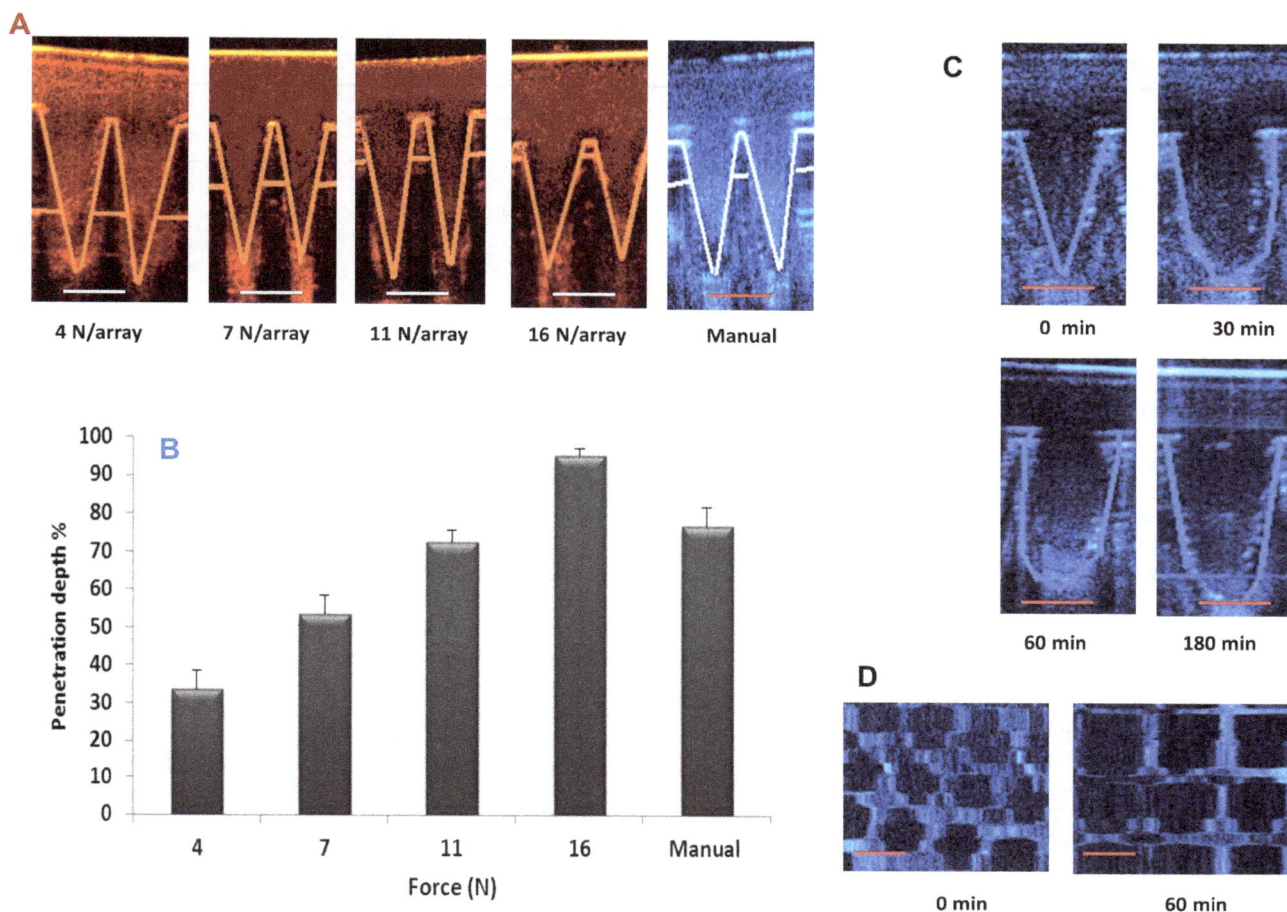

Figure 4. False colour 2D still images of super swelling MN arrays immediately following insertion into excised neonatal porcine skin at application forces of 4, 7, 11 or 16 N/array or using manual application. (Scale bar represents 300 μm in each case) (A). The effect of application force (N/array) upon the resultant penetration depth of super swelling MN arrays in neonatal porcine skin *in vitro*, expressed as a p [percentage of MN height (Means+S.D., n = 10)]. The penetration parameters of the MN arrays were quantified using optical coherence tomography (B). False colour images of the *in vitro* swelling profile of MN arrays in excised neonatal porcine skin recorded over a 3 h period, as assessed by optical coherence tomography (Scale bar represents 300 μm in each case) (C). OCT visualisation of the micropores residing within the skin immediately following MN array insertion (0 min) and following 60 min in skin (Scale bar represents 300 μm. in each case) (D).

3.1. Swelling studies

The results outlined in **Figure 3A** display the percentage swelling in PBS pH 7.4 of super swelling hydrogel films cast from aqueous blends of 20% w/w Gantrez S-97, 7.5% w/w PEG 10,000 and 3% w/w Na_2CO_3. The hydrogel formulation incorporating Na_2CO_3 as a modifying agent showed greater initial swelling and reached equilibrium more quickly than the control formula (15% Gantrez AN-139, 7.5% PEG). For example, after 1 hour, the percentage swelling of super swelling hydrogels (20% w/w Gantrez S-97, 7.5% w/w PEG and 3% w/w Na_2CO_3) was 1119%, compared to only 250% for the control formulation. Hydrogels prepared from aqueous blends containing 3% w/w

Table 2. The effect of force of application upon the resultant penetration characteristics of MN arrays cast from 20% w/w Gantrez S-97, 7.5% w/w PEG 10,000 and 3% w/w Na_2CO_3, in the geometry 19×19 with height 600 μm, width 300 μm and interspacing at base 50 μm into neonatal porcine skin, (Means ± SD, n = 10).

Force (N/array)	MN penetration depth (μm)	Pore width (μm)	Base plate/*Stratum corneum* distance (μm)
4	201±31	209±10	398±31
7	322±35	214±17	277±35
11	430±20	219±8	169±20
16	571±8	228±12	29±8
Manual	465±28	211±7	134±28

Table 3. *In vitro* swelling of MN arrays (19×19 MN, 600 μm height, 300 μm width at base, 50 μm interspacing at base) upon insertion into neonatal porcine skin, (Means ± SD, n = 15).

Time (min)	MN depth in skin (μm)
0	465.25±28.25
30	578.08±22.74
60	609.50±35.13
180	697.27±41.63

Na_2CO_3 showed a significant ($p<0.05$) increase in percentage swelling. The percentage swelling at equilibrium was 1071% and 1708% for the control and super swelling formulations, respectively (**Table 1**). **Figure 3** also illustrates the morphology of the MN array as a xerogel (B) and post-swelling in PBS (C). **Figure 3D** is representative of the liner regression plots derived from swelling curves using Equation 3.

Using attenuated total reflectance (ATR)-Fourier transform infrared (FTIR) spectroscopy, the mechanism of action of the modifying agent was confirmed to be due to sodium salt formation on free acid groups on the copolymer, thus reducing ester-based crosslinking (**Figure 3G**). The main difference that can be seen in the spectra of the crosslinked films in contrast with the non crosslinked ones, is the presence of a new band between 1800 and 1750 cm^{-1}. This band can be attributed to the new ester bonds formed between the Gantrez S-97 acid groups and the hydroxyl groups of the PEG molecules. In addition a new band between 1500 and 1600 cm^{-1} can be observed for super-swelling hydrogels that is not present in the other hydrogels. This band is characteristic for the salts of carboxyilic acids [26].

To examine the controlling mechanism of swelling of the super swelling hydrogel materials prepared from aqueous blends of 20% w/w Gantrez S-97, 7.5% w/w PEG and 3% w/w Na_2CO_3, the second order kinetic model (**Equation 4**) was used to process the experimental data. To analyse the kinetic model, t/S versus t graphs were plotted and respective swelling rate parameters were determined. **Figure 3D** shows representative linear regression plots of the swelling curves derived from **Equation 4**. The diffusional exponent, n, was determined to be 0.76, indicating an anomalous mechanism of water uptake. In addition, the diffusion coefficient (D_i) was 2.47×10^{-6} cm^2 min^{-1}. The volume fraction of polymer, ϕ, determined using **Equation 6** was 0.045, the

number average molecular weight between crosslinks, M_c, determined using **Equation 5**, was 6,793,627 g/mol. The crosslink density, V_e, determined using **Equation 8** was 1.08×10^{19}. Due to dissolution of other candidates, the formulation which was selected for continued investigation was that containing 20% w/w Gantrez S-97, 7.5% w/w PEG and 3% w/w Na_2CO_3.

3.2. Mechanical testing

MN arrays formulated using the super swelling formulation (20% w/w Gantrez S-97, 7.5% w/w PEG and 3% w/w Na_2CO_3) and in the geometry, 19×19 (height = 600 μm, width = 300 μm, interspacing = 50 μm) were used to investigate the effects of compression tests on the heights of individual needles on the MN array. The digital microscope images presented in **Figure 3E** are illustrative of the effects, on individual needles of the MN array, of the fracture forces applied by axial load. It is important to note that regardless of the force applied, none of the needles on the MN array broke or shattered upon application into the skin, rather bending. **Figure 3E** also shows the percentage reduction in the height of individual needles on the MN array upon application of increasing fracture forces. The reduction in MN height increased progressively with increases in the force applied. These MN deformed when applied to a stainless steel plate, but were not brittle, which is important from a patient safety point of view. This is especially true considering the relatively high forces applied here (>300 N was the maximal force applied over the 361 MN) and the much softer nature of skin.

Skin penetration of super swelling MN arrays was investigated using dermatomed neonatal porcine skin (approximately 350–450 μm thicknesses) and the percentage of holes (micro-conduits) created by the MN arrays was determined after staining of the skin

Table 4. Physical properties of lyophilised drug reservoirs.

Parameter	Means ± S.D.
Ovalbumin	
Weight (g)	0.32±0.01
Hardness (N)	119.7±5.0
Thickness (mm)	4.12±0.3
Friability	0.47% mass loss
Ibuprofen sodium	
Weight (g)	0.26±0.02
Hardness (N)	178±3
Thickness (mm)	4.96±0.6
Friability	0% mass loss

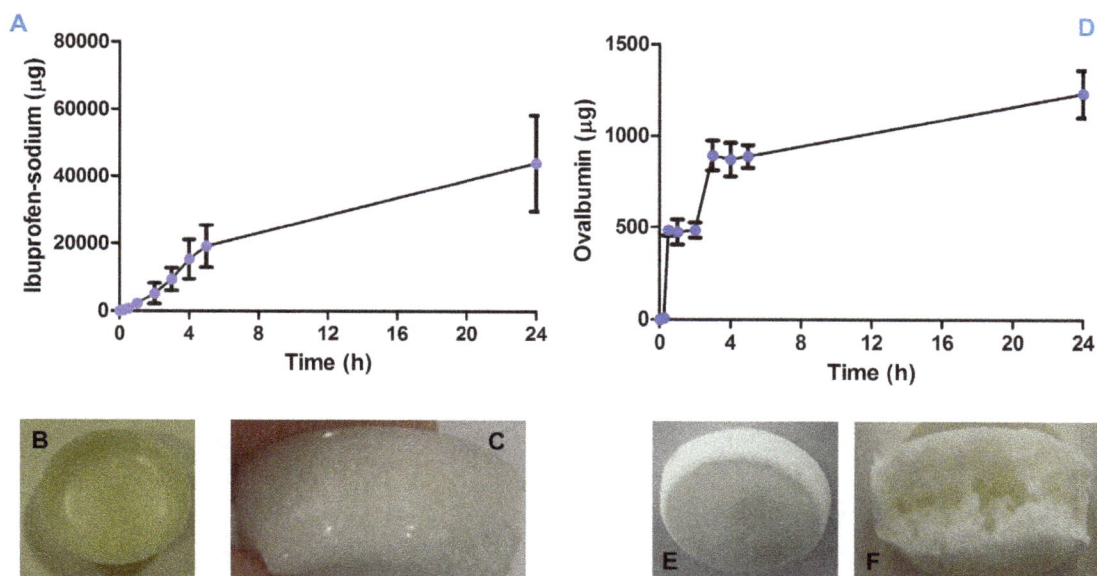

Figure 5. The *in vitro* cumulative permeation profile of ibuprofen sodium across dermatomed 350 μm neonatal porcine skin when delivered using in-dwelling super swelling MN arrays combined with lyophilised drug reservoirs (Means ± S.D., n = 9) (**A**). Digital images of the ibuprofen sodium-loaded lyophilised wafers used in *in vitro* and *in vivo* experiments and prepared from aqueous blends containing 10% w/w gelatin, 3% w/w mannitol and 40% w/w ibuprofen sodium (**B**, **C**). The *in vitro* cumulative permeation profile of OVA across dermatomed 350 μm neonatal porcine skin when delivered using in-dwelling super swelling MN arrays combined with lyophilised drug reservoirs (Means ± S.D., n = 5) (**D**). Digital images (**E**, **F**)of the OVA-loaded lyophilised wafers used in *in vitro* and *in vivo* experiments and prepared from aqueous blends containing 10% w/w gelatin, 40% w/w mannitol, 10% w/w NaCl, 1% w/w sucrose and 0.5% w/w OVA. These active-loaded tablets exhibited high porosities as exemplified in (**G**).

with methylene blue solution. Regardless of force applied, >85% of the MN in each array penetrated the *stratum corneum*, as evidenced by staining of the formed aqueous microconduits by the hydrophilic marker compound. However, with increasing applied forces, the penetration efficiency of the MN also increased (**Figure 3F**). In the case of the 0.9 N/needle applied force, the microconduits created could be traced onto the surface of the laboratory film (Parafilm) placed beneath the skin. This indicated that, at this highest insertion force, which equates to 324.9 N/ array as there are 361 needles in each array, the depth of penetration of the needles into the skin was at its greatest. In order to accurately measure miroconduit depth, optical coherence tomography was utilised. The penetration characteristics of MN arrays inserted into neonatal porcine skin using an applicator set to defined forces of 4, 7, 11 or 16 N/array are presented in **Table 2** and **Figure 4B**. Manual force (defined as "gentle finger pressure") was also used to insert the MN arrays and the penetration characteristics are very similar to those quoted when a force of 11 N/array was employed. Increasing force increased penetration depth and decreased distance between the lower MN baseplate and the *stratum corneum*, but microconduit width was largely unaffected.

3.3. In skin swelling

The swelling of the MN arrays upon application into skin was then investigated *in vitro* over 3 hours and in real time. Individual needles on the arrays exhibited an increase in height of approximately 40% by the end of the three-hour testing period (**Figure 4C** and **Table 3**). The microconduits residing within the skin immediately and 60 min post-MN array application were visualised (**Figure 4D**). Importantly, these images confirm that skin under occlusion swells and relaxes with the MN, meaning

their increase in volume does not result in the extravasation of the swollen MN from the skin.

3.4. Lyophilised drug reservoirs

Different OVA-loaded and ibuprofen sodium-loaded formulations were prepared and lyophilised. An OVA-loaded formulation containing 10% w/w gelatin (Sigma-Aldrich, Dorset, UK), 40% w/w mannitol (Sigma-Aldrich, Dorset, UK), 10% w/w NaCl, 1% w/w sucrose and 0.5% w/w OVA was determined to be the most suitable, in terms of morphology, strength and dissolution profile of the formed wafers and, hence, was chosen for further characterisation studies. In terms of the ibuprofen sodium, those wafers which were prepared from blends containing 10% w/w gelatin (Cryogel SG3, PB Gelatins, Pontypridd, UK), 3% w/w mannitol (Pearlitol 50C-Mannitol, Roquette, Lestrem, France) and 40% w/w ibuprofen sodium (Sigma-Aldrich, Dorset, UK) were chosen for subsequent investigation, as they were the most homogeneous. There was no loss of active in either case, with recoveries of 100% for ibuprofen sodium and 98±18% for OVA. In addition, the wafers all complied with pharmacopoeial standards [27] for hardness, weight variation, thickness and friability (**Table 4**).

3.5. *In vitro* drug release studies

Ibuprofen sodium exhibited an almost typical first order release profile across excised neonatal porcine skin *in vitro* (**Figure 5A**), with approximately 44 mg delivered in 24 h (range from 9 replicates: 35.2–68.9 mg over 24 h). As the ibuprofen sodium-loaded reservoirs were known to contain a mean loading of 124 mg approximately 37% of this was delivered in 24 h. OVA exhibited a tri-phasic release profile (**Figure 5D**), possibly due to the very different composition and morphology of the lyophilised

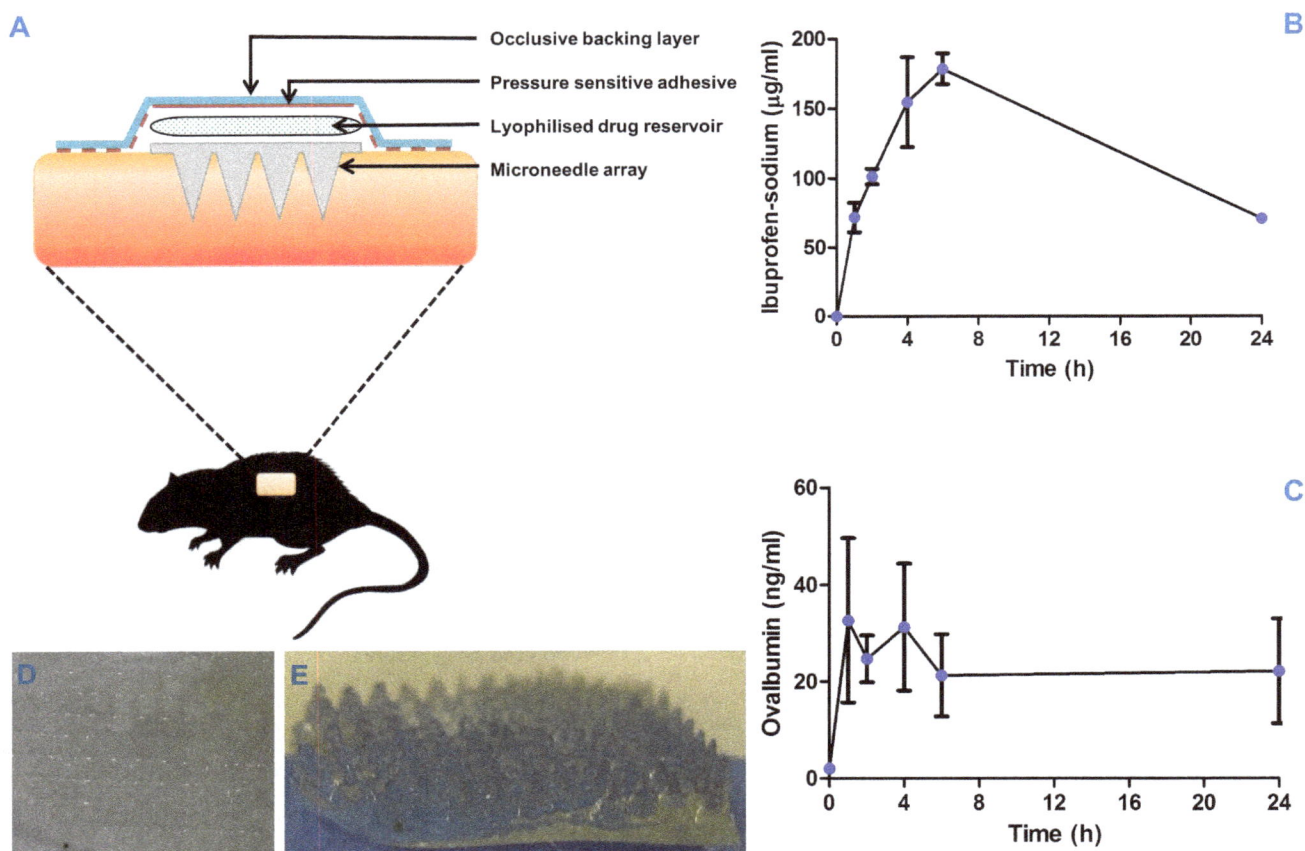

Figure 6. Schematic representation of application and retention strategies for rat experiments designed to evaluate *in vivo* **performance of super swelling microneedle arrays (A).** The *in vivo* plasma profiles of ibuprofen sodium (**B**) (Means ± S.D., n = 4) and OVA (**C**) (Means ± S.D., n = 3) following transdermal delivery using super swelling microneedle arrays with lyophilised drug reservoirs. Typical morphology of super swelling microneedles upon removal from rat skin *in vivo* after 24 hours insertion indicating that, despite extensive swelling, the microneedles are removed intact (**D, E**).

wafers (**Figure 5F**) and the much greater molecular weight and more complex molecular structure, as compared to ibuprofen sodium. The average total OVA content of the lyophilised wafers was 2.5±0.15 mg and it was found that the super swelling MN arrays delivered approximately 1.24 mg OVA over the 24 h experimental period (range from 5 replicates: 1.09–1.36 mg over 24 h). This equates to transdermal delivery of approximately 49% of the OVA loaded into the wafers on average. This is interesting to note, since such effective *in vitro* transdermal delivery has not been seen previously for either high dose low potency molecules or proteins. However, it is unsurprising, given the high molecular weight between crosslinks of the super swelling hydrogel calculated at equilibrium (6,793,627 g/mol) compared to the molecular weights of ibuprofen sodium (229.29 g/mol) and even ovalbumin (44,300 g/mol). Drug permeation is thus likely to be affected more by the dissolution rate of the lyophilised wafers than the hydrogel material, assuming in-skin swelling is complete.

3.6. *In vivo* experiments

In the case of experiments carried out using OVA-loaded reservoirs, two super swelling MN arrays and active-loaded wafers were applied to the backs of the animals (**Figure 6A**). In contrast, four MN arrays and their respective ibuprofen sodium-loaded reservoirs were applied to the backs of the animals in parallel drug delivery experiments. Plasma profiles in the case of both model

compounds differed from the patterns of drug permeation profiles seen *in vitro*. This is unsurprising, given that the two experiments are distinct from one another, since the *in vitro* experiments do not have biodistribution, metabolism or excretion components as we have *in vivo*.

For ibuprofen sodium (**Figure 6B**), the integrated MN array delivery system produced a progressive increase in plasma concentrations over 6 h, with a maximal concentration of approximately 179 µg/ml achieved in this time. The plasma concentration had fallen to 71+6.7 µg/ml by 24 h. Therapeutic plasma levels of ibuprofen in humans range between 10 and 15 µg/ml [28] and these levels were achieved within the first hour of MN application. Based on this knowledge and the *in vivo* results, we can approximate the patch size necessary for use in human volunteer studies. An average human male weighs approximately 60 kg [29], which is 286 times greater than the weight of a 210 g rat (the average weight of rat used in these experiments). The peak plasma ibuprofen sodium concentration achieved in the rats at 6 h (179±19 µg/ml) is approximately 18 times greater than the human therapeutic blood levels [28] and this was achieved with MN arrays of total approximate area of 2 cm^2 (4×0.5 cm^2). By this rationale, a MN patch design of no greater than 32 cm^2 could potentially deliver therapeutically-relevant doses of ibuprofen sodium in healthy volunteer studies. Typical commercialised transdermal patches can be as large as 30 or 40 cm^2 (Novartis make Nicotinell nicotine patches of 30 cm^2 [30]; Janssen make Duragesic CII (fentanyl) patches of 32 and 42 cm^2 [31]). Accordingly, it is very reasonable to suggest that a MN product could be successfully developed based on the technology and data presented here. Indeed, we have previously shown that scaling up MN patch size is a relatively straightforward process [8,10].

OVA levels peaked in plasma after only 1 hour (**Figure 6C**) at 42.36±17.01 ng/ml. This represents a significant finding, since macromolecules are normally absorbed quite slowly when administered intradermally [4,5] OVA plasma levels then remained almost constant up to 6 h, dropping somewhat at 24 h, when 23.61±4.84 ng/ml was detected.

Importantly, the super swelling hydrogel MN arrays remained intact over the 24 h application period in all cases, thus allowing their removal as an intact unit at the end of the experiment (**Figure 6D, E**). As can be appreciated, the MN array extensively absorbed interstitial fluid to form a swollen hydrogel matrix, thus enabling delivery of OVA and ibuprofen sodium across the skin and into the systemic circulation. However, the system was sufficiently robust when swollen to ensure that the MN were removed intact.

Conclusions

The work presented here shows, for the first time, that exploitation of so-called "super swelling" hydrogel materials in microneedle-enhanced transdermal drug delivery is a highly promising approach to increasing the range of drugs that can be delivered transdermally. Using such systems in combination with lyophilised wafer-type drug reservoirs facilitated delivery of doses of ibuprofen sodium that could be extrapolated to a useful and usable product for human treatment. Rapid protein delivery using ovalbumin as the model indicated that this technology may also find use in macromolecular drug delivery and vaccine administration. The value to industry is likely to be considerable, since this technology is distinctly different from conventional microneedle systems, which are presently only suitable for bolus delivery of very potent drugs and vaccines. Accordingly, we are currently progressing towards clinical evaluations with a range of candidate molecules.

Author Contributions

Conceived and designed the experiments: RFD MTCM AZA ADW. Performed the experiments: MTCM AZA EM ECS SAZ EL. Analyzed the data: MTCM AZA EM ECS SAZ. Contributed reagents/materials/analysis tools: RFD TRRS HOM VLK ADW. Wrote the paper: RFD MTCM AZA EL EM AJC MCK ECS SAZ ADW.

References

1. Chandrasekhar S, Iyer LK, Panchal JP, Topp EM, Cannon JB, et al. (2013) Microarrays and microneedle arrays for delivery of peptides, proteins, vaccines and other applications. Expert Opin Drug Deliv 10: 1155–1170.
2. Pierre MB, Rossetti FC (2014) Microneedle-based drug delivery systems for transdermal route. Curr Drug Targets 15: 281–291.
3. Gratieri T, Alberti I, Lapteva M, Kalia YN (2013) Next generation intra- and transdermal therapeutic systems: using non- and minimally-invasive technologies to increase drug delivery into and across the skin. Eur J Pharm Sci 50: 609–622.
4. Migalska K, Morrow DIJ., Garland MJ, Thakur RRS, Woolfson AD, et al. (2011) Laser-engineered dissolving microneedle arrays for transdermal macro-molecular drug delivery. Pharm Res 28: 1919–1930.
5. Ito Y, Hirono M, Fukushima K, Sugioka N, Takada K (2012) Two-layered dissolving microneedles formulated with intermediate-acting insulin. In-t J Pharm 436: 387–393
6. Hong X, Wei L, Wu F, Wu Z, Chen L, et al. (2013) Dissolving and biodegradable microneedle technologies for transdermal sustained delivery of drug and vaccine. Drug Des Devel Ther 7: 945–952.
7. Koutsonanos DG, Compans RW, Skountzou I (2013) Targeting the skin for microneedle delivery of influenza vaccine. Adv Exp Med Biol 785: 121–32.
8. McCrudden MTC, McCrudden C, McAlister E, Zaid Alkilani A, Woolfson AD, et al. (2014) Dissolving microneedle arrays for enhanced transdermal delivery of high dose low potency drug substances. J Cont Rel 180: 71–80.
9. Hirobe S, Azukizawa H, Matsuo K, Zhai Y, Quan YS, et al (2013) Development and clinical study of a self-dissolving microneedle patch for transcutaneous immunization device. Pharm Res 30: 2664–2674
10. Donnelly RF, Thakur RRS, Garland MJ, Migalska K, Majithiya R, et al. (2012) Hydrogel-forming microneedle arrays for enhanced transdermal drug delivery. Adv Funct Mat 22: 4879–4890.
11. Donnelly RF, Morrow DI, McCrudden MT, Alkilani AZ, Vicente-Pérez EM, et al. (2014) Hydrogel-forming and dissolving microneedles for enhanced delivery of photosensitizers and precursors. Photochem Photobiol doi: 10.1111/php.12209.
12. Donnelly RF, Thakur RRS., McCrudden MTC., Zaid-Alkilani A, O'Mahony C, et al. (2013) Hydrogel-forming microneedle arrays exhibit antimicrobial properties: Potential for enhanced patient safety. Int J Pharm 451: 76–91.
13. Thakur RRS, McCarron PA, Woolfson AD, Donnelly RF (2009) Investigation of swelling and network parameters of poly (ethylene glycol)-crosslinked poly (methyl vinyl ether-co-maleic acid) hydrogels. Eur Polym J 45: 1239–1249.
14. Mikolajewska P, Donnelly RF, Garland MJ, Morrow DIJ, Iani V, et al. (2010) Microneedle pre-treatment of human skin improves 5-aminolevulininc acid (ALA) and 5-aminolevulinic acid methyl ester (MAL) induced PpIX production for topical photodynamic therapy without increase in pain or erythema. Pharm Res 27: 2213–2220.
15. McCarron PA, Woolfson AD, Donnelly RF, Andrews GP, Zawislak A, et al. (2004) Influence of plasticiser type and storage conditions on the properties of poly(methyl vinyl ether-co-maleic anhydride) bioadhesive films. J App Polym Sci 91: 1576–1589.
16. Peniche C, Cohen ME, Vázquez B, San Román J (1997) Water sorption of flexible networks based on 2-hydroxyethyl methacrylate-triethylenglycol dimethacrylate copolymers. Polymer 38: 5977–5982.
17. Peppas NA, Korsmeyer RW (1987) Dynamically swelling hydrogels in controlled release applications Hydrogels in Medicine and Pharmacy. Boca Raton, Florida: CRC Press Inc. 109–136 p.
18. Ritger PL, Peppas NA (1987) A simple equation for description of solute release II: Fickian and anomalous release from swellable devices. J Cont Rel 5: 37–42.
19. Bajpai S (2001) Swelling–deswelling behavior of poly(acrylamide-co-maleic acid) hydrogels. J Appl Polym Sci 80: 2782–2789.
20. Donnelly RF, Majithiya R, Thakur RRS, Morrow DIJ, Garland MJ, et al. (2011) Design and physicochemical characterisation of optimised polymeric microneedle arrays prepared by a novel laser-based micromoulding technique. Pharm Res 28: 41–57.
21. Fourtanier A, Berrebi C (1989) Miniature pig as an animal model to study photoaging. Photochem Photobiol 50: 771–784.
22. Woolfson AD, McCafferty DF, McCallion CR, McAdams E, Anderson J (1995) Moisture-activated, electrically conducting bioadhesive hydrogels as interfaces for bioelectrodes: Effect of film hydration on cutaneous adherence in wet environments. J Appl Polym Sci 58: 1291–1296.
23. Donnelly RF, Garland MJ, Morrow DIJ, Migalska K, Thakur RRS, et al. (2010) Optical coherence tomography is a valuable tool in the study of the effects of microneedle geometry on skin penetration characteristics and in-skin dissolution. J Cont Rel 147: 333–341.
24. The International Conference on Harmonisation of Technical Requirements for Registration of Pharmaceuticals for Human Use (ICH) website. Available: http://www.ich.org/. Accessed 2013 Oct 4.
25. McCrudden MTC, Torrisi BM, Al-Zahrani S, McCrudden CM, Donnelly RF et al. (2014) Laser-engineered dissolving microneedle arrays for protein delivery: Potential for enhanced intradermal vaccination. J Pharm Pharmacol doi: 10.1111/jphp.12248.
26. Shevchenko LL (1963) Infrared spectra of salts and complexes of carboxylic acids and some of their derivatives. Russ Chem Rev 32: 201–207.
27. The British Pharmacopoeia 2013 website. Available: http://www.pharmacopoeia.co.uk/2013/. Accessed 2013 Oct 6.
28. Dollery C (1991) Therapeutic Drugs. London: Churchill Livingstone.
29. The National Health Service website. Available: http://www.nhs.uk/Livewell/healthy-living/Pages/height-weight-chart.aspx. Accessed 2013 Oct 5.
30. Nicotinell website. Available: http://www.nicotinell.co.uk/. Accessed 2013 Oct 14.
31. Duragesic website. Available: http://www.duragesic.com/. Accessed 2013 Oct 14.

21

Photoacoustic Tomography of Human Hepatic Malignancies Using Intraoperative Indocyanine Green Fluorescence Imaging

Akinori Miyata[1], Takeaki Ishizawa[1]*, Mako Kamiya[2], Atsushi Shimizu[1], Junichi Kaneko[1], Hideaki Ijichi[3], Junji Shibahara[4], Masashi Fukayama[4], Yutaka Midorikawa[5], Yasuteru Urano[2], Norihiro Kokudo[1]

1 Hepato-Biliary-Pancreatic Surgery Division, Department of Surgery, Graduate School of Medicine, the University of Tokyo, Tokyo, Japan, 2 Laboratory of Chemical Biology and Molecular Imaging, Graduate School of Medicine, the University of Tokyo, Tokyo, Japan, 3 Department of Gastroenterology, Graduate School of Medicine, the University of Tokyo, Tokyo, Japan, 4 Department of Pathology, Graduate School of Medicine, the University of Tokyo, Tokyo, Japan, 5 Genome Science Division, Research Center for Advanced Science & Technology, the University of Tokyo, Tokyo, Japan

Abstract

Recently, fluorescence imaging following the preoperative intravenous injection of indocyanine green has been used in clinical settings to identify hepatic malignancies during surgery. The aim of this study was to evaluate the ability of photoacoustic tomography using indocyanine green as a contrast agent to produce representative fluorescence images of hepatic tumors by visualizing the spatial distribution of indocyanine green on ultrasonographic images. Indocyanine green (0.5 mg/kg, intravenous) was preoperatively administered to 9 patients undergoing hepatectomy. Intraoperatively, photoacoustic tomography was performed on the surface of the resected hepatic specimens (n = 10) under excitation with an 800 nm pulse laser. In 4 hepatocellular carcinoma nodules, photoacoustic imaging identified indocyanine green accumulation in the cancerous tissue. In contrast, in one hepatocellular carcinoma nodule and five adenocarcinoma foci (one intrahepatic cholangiocarcinoma and 4 colorectal liver metastases), photoacoustic imaging delineated indocyanine green accumulation not in the cancerous tissue but rather in the peri-cancerous hepatic parenchyma. Although photoacoustic tomography enabled to visualize spatial distribution of ICG on ultrasonographic images, which was consistent with fluorescence images on cut surfaces of the resected specimens, photoacoustic signals of ICG-containing tissues decreased approximately by 40% even at 4 mm depth from liver surfaces. Photoacoustic tomography using indocyanine green also failed to identify any hepatocellular carcinoma nodules from the body surface of model mice with non-alcoholic steatohepatitis. In conclusion, photoacoustic tomography has a potential to enhance cancer detectability and differential diagnosis by ultrasonographic examinations and intraoperative fluorescence imaging through visualization of stasis of bile-excreting imaging agents in and/or around hepatic tumors. However, further technical advances are needed to improve the visibility of photoacoustic signals emitted from deeply-located lesions.

Editor: Shree Ram Singh, National Cancer Institute, United States of America

Funding: This work was supported by grants from the Takeda Science Foundation, the Ministry of Education, Culture, Sports, Science and Technology of Japan, and the Ministry of Health, Labour and Welfare of Japan. The funders had no role in study design, data collection and analysis, decision to publish, or preparation of the manuscript.

Competing Interests: The authors have declared that no competing interests exist.

* Email: tish-tky@umin.ac.jp

Introduction

In vivo fluorescence imaging using indocyanine green (ICG) has been clinically applied as an intraoperative navigation tool that enables the real-time identification of biological structures, such as the lymphatic system [1,2] and the biliary ducts [3–7], as well as the evaluation of visceral blood perfusion [8–11]. Since 2008, ICG fluorescence imaging has also been used to identify hepatic tumors during open hepatectomy [12–15] and, more recently, laparoscopic hepatectomy [16]. This technique is based on the accumulation of ICG, which is intravenously administered for preoperative liver function testing, in hepatocellular carcinoma (HCC) tissue and in the non-cancerous hepatic parenchyma located around adenocarcinoma foci, such as colorectal liver

metastases (CRLM) and intrahepatic cholangiocarcinoma (ICC) [12]. When fluorescence images of the cut surfaces of resected specimens are obtained, well- to moderately-differentiated HCC shows uniform fluorescence of ICG in the cancerous tissue, while poorly differentiated HCC and adenocarcinoma show rim-type fluorescence around the tumor [17]. Although both types of cancer-associated ICG fluorescence can be detected by commercially-available fluorescence imaging systems as far as the tumors are located beneath the liver surface, there is a need for novel imaging technology that enables the detection of deeply-located hepatic tumors and the visualization of ICG accumulation in and/ or around these lesions on cross-sectional images.

In the last decade, photoacoustic (PA) tomography has been actively developed as a novel optical imaging technology that

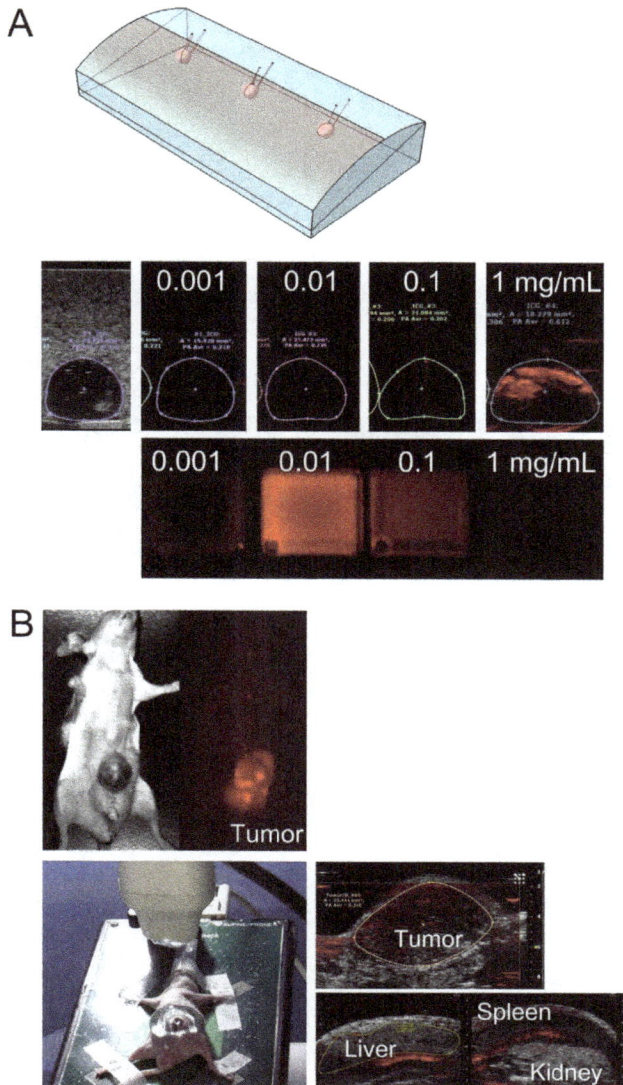

Figure 1. Establishment of PA tomography's ability to visualize ICG-containing tissue. (**A**) Using a human liver tissue-mimicking phantom (top), human plasma containing ICG at concentrations of 0.001, 0.01, 0.1, and 1.0 mg/mL was encapsulated into holes that were 5 mm in diameter and located at a depth of 5 mm from the surface; PA amplitudes were measured using the Vevo LAZR imaging system (middle). Fluorescence images of each ICG-containing plasma sample were also obtained (bottom). (**B**) Fluorescence imaging in a mouse model with subcutaneously implanted well-differentiated human hepatoma cells (HuH-7) identified ICG accumulation in the subcutaneous tumor (left). PA tomography enabled differentiation of tumor-specific PA signals from those of surrounding organs under the conditions of 800-nm excitation light and 54-dB PA gain (right).

enables the real-time visualization of deeply-located biologic structures on ultrasonographic images through the "photoacoustic effect" [18–20]. With this technique, nanosecond laser pulses are transmitted into tissue and absorbed by endogenous chromophores or exogenous molecular imaging agents in targeted structures. The rapid absorption increases focal temperature and produces a thermoelastic expansion that creates acoustic waves. These photoacoustic signals can be detected using ultrasound (US) receivers and used to reconstruct images of the targeted biological

structures according to the absorbed optical energy density. Because ICG has a moderate fluorescence quantum yield, it can be used as a contrast agent in PA imaging in addition to fluorescence imaging [21–23], and its spatial distribution in cancerous and non-cancerous hepatic tissues may be visualized with both modalities. The aim of this study was to evaluate the ability of PA tomography using ICG as a contrast agent to produce representative fluorescence images of hepatic tumors, using both surgically-resected human hepatic samples and a mouse model of HCC (mice with non-alcoholic steatohepatitis [NASH]).

Materials and Methods

This study was conducted with the approval of the Institutional Ethics Review Board of the University of Tokyo Hospital. Written informed consent was obtained from all patients. The animal study was carried out in strict accordance with the recommendations in the Guide for the Care and Use of Laboratory Animals from the National Institutes of Health. The protocol for the animal study was approved by the University of Tokyo's Committee on the Ethics of Animal Experiments. All surgery was performed under isoflurane anesthesia, and all possible efforts were made to minimize suffering.

Establishment of PA tomography's ability to visualize ICG-containing tissue

First, the ability of PA tomography to detect ICG-containing biological material was evaluated using a human liver tissue-mimicking phantom (OST Co., Ltd., Chiba, Japan [24]) with spherical air holes 5 mm in diameter located 5 mm deep to the surface; the model was created with a three-dimensional printer (FASOTEC Co., Ltd., Chiba, Japan). Each hole was filled with human plasma containing ICG at concentrations of 0.001, 0.01, 0.1, and 1.0 mg/mL, and PA images were obtained with the Vevo LAZR imaging system (VisualSonics, Toronto, ON, Canada) as described elsewhere [25,26]. For each ICG solution, the PA signal amplitude was measured and compared with the solution's fluorescence intensity as measured with a Maestro imaging system (CRI, Woburn, Massachusetts, USA) using the near-infrared filter setting (excitation, 730–740 nm; emission, 810 nm long pass) [17].

Next, PA tomography's ability to visualize ICG-containing cancerous tissue was confirmed using a previously-established mouse model with subcutaneously implanted human HuH-7 well-differentiated hepatoma cells (Japanese Collection of Research Bioresources Cell Bank, Osaka, Japan) [27,28]. Photoacoustic imaging of the subcutaneous tumors was performed from the skin surface 48 hours after the intravenous injection of ICG (5 mg/kg) via the tail vein.

Photoacoustic tomography of surgically-resected hepatic tissue in humans

In 9 patients who underwent hepatic resection for malignancies (10 nodules: HCC, n = 5; CRLM, n = 4; and ICC, n = 1), ICG (Diagnogreen, Daiichi Sankyo, Tokyo, Japan) was preoperatively injected (dose, 0.5 mg per kg of body weight; intravenous injection) as part of routine liver function testing performed for surgical planning [12,17]. Intraoperatively, the ICG retained in hepatic tissues was utilized as a contrast agent in PA tomography as well as for fluorescence imaging. Following hepatectomy, PA images of the resected specimens were obtained, and PA signal amplitude was measured with the Vevo LAZR imaging system in the following regions of interest (ROI): cancerous tissue (CA); non-cancerous hepatic tissue around the tumors (Peri), and non-cancerous hepatic tissue 2 mm from the tumors (NC). The

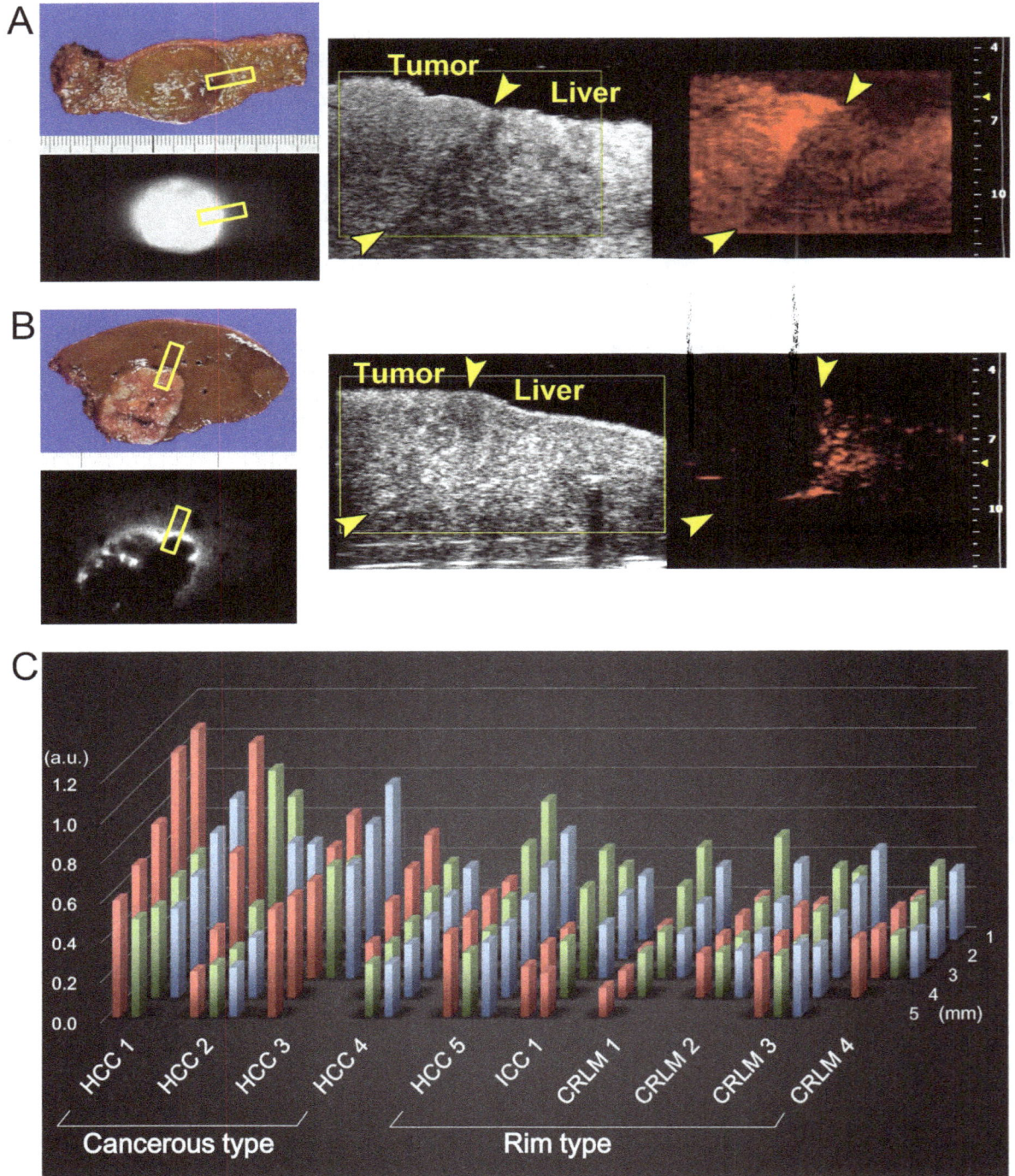

Figure 2. Photoacoustic tomography of surgically-resected hepatic tissue in humans. (**A**) Fluorescence imaging identified uniform fluorescence of ICG on the cut surface of well-differentiated HCC tissue (left). PA tomography from the cut surface of the specimen visualized accumulation of ICG in cancerous tissues on US images (right, please see video S1). (**B**) Fluorescence imaging identified rim-type ICG fluorescence around CRLM lesions on the cut surface of the resected specimen (left). Photoacoustic tomography from the cut surface visualized accumulation of ICG in the peri-cancerous hepatic tissue on US images (right, please see video S2). Yellow squares and arrows in A and B indicate the site where a probe of the imaging system was attached and the boundaries between the tumors and non-cancerous liver parenchyma, respectively. (**C**) Photoacoustic amplitude of each ROI from the resected specimen (red bar indicates cancerous region; green bar, peri-cancerous region; and blue bar, non-cancerous hepatic parenchyma 2 mm from the tumor) according to the depth of the ROI from the sample's surface (depths of 1 to 5 mm). Indocyanine green accumulation was observed in the cancerous tissue in HCC specimens 1–4 (cancerous-type accumulation), while rim-type ICG accumulation was observed in HCC specimen 5, the ICC specimen, and CRLM specimens 1–4.

Table 1. Tumor characteristics and results of fluorescence and PA imaging.

Tumors	Age(y)/Sex	ICG R15 (%)	Interval between ICG injection and surgery (d)	CH/LC	Cancer cell differentiation	Tumor diameter (mm)	Fluorescence patterns	PA patterns
HCC 1	76/F	19.6	40	Yes	Well	24	Cancerous	Cancerous
HCC 2	85/M	1.8	2	No	Moderate	97	Cancerous	Cancerous
HCC 3	69/M	9.8	29	Yes	Moderate	27	Cancerous	Cancerous
HCC 4	80/M	20.7	10	No	Moderate	36	Cancerous	Cancerous
HCC 5	73/F	7.4	14	No	Moderate	23	Rim	Rim
ICC 1	70/F	8.6	8	No	Moderate	59	Rim	Rim
CRLM 1	54/M	9.4	27	No	tub2	15	Rim	Rim
CRLM 2	54/M	9.4	27	No	tub2	16	Rim	Rim
CRLM 3	84/M	8.5	38	No	tub1	20	Rim	Rim
CRLM 4	53/M	1.9	24	No	tub2	17	Rim	Rim

Abbreviations: PA imaging, photoacoustic imaging; ICG R15, preoperative indocyanine green retention rate at 15 minutes; CH/LC, presence of chronic hepatitis or liver cirrhosis; HCC, hepatocellular carcinoma; ICC, intrahepatic cholangiocarcinoma; CRLM, colorectal liver metastasis.

localization of ICG on the resected specimens' cut surfaces was also evaluated by macroscopic fluorescence imaging with a Maestro imaging system followed by pathological examination with fluorescence microscopy [17].

Photoacoustic tomography from the body surface in NASH-HCC model mice

Because direct use of the Vevo LAZR imaging system in patients had not yet been approved, PA tomography's ability to visualize hepatic tumors from the body surface was evaluated in a mouse model. Three male NASH-HCC model mice (STAM, Stelic Institute & Co., Tokyo, Japan) were created by administering low-dose streptozotocin after birth (first hit) followed by a subsequent high-fat diet (second hit) [29]. PA tomography was performed on the living 18-week-old NASH-HCC model mice from the body surface to evaluate the detectability of the hepatic tumors. Following PA imaging, all mice were sacrificed, and their livers were screened for HCC nodules by naked-eye examination and fluorescence imaging with the Maestro imaging system.

Results

Establishment of PA tomography's ability to visualize ICG-containing cancerous tissue

For the plasma encapsulated in the tissue-mimicking phantom, at ICG concentrations of 0.001, 0.01, 0.1, and 1.0 mg/mL, the average PA signal intensity under excitation with 800 nm of light was 0.218, 0.239, 0.202, and 0.612, respectively. In contrast, the fluorescence intensity of the ICG-containing plasma increased with increases in ICG concentration up to 0.01 mg/mL, but then started to decrease; this was most likely due to absorption of near-infrared light by ICG (Fig. 1A).

Photoacoustic tomography's ability to identify hepatic malignancies was evaluated in the mice that had undergone subcutaneous implantation of a well-differentiated human hepatoma cell line (HuH-7). Fluorescence imaging at 48 hours after the intravenous injection of ICG demonstrated ICG accumulation in the implanted tumors. Photoacoustic tomography also enabled identification of tumor-specific ICG signals and their visualization on US images under conditions of 800-nm excitation light and 54-dB PA gain (Fig. 1B).

Photoacoustic tomography of surgically-resected hepatic tissue in humans

Table 1 summarizes tumor-related characteristics and the results of fluorescence imaging and PA tomography using ICG. On ICG fluorescence images, 4 out of 5 HCCs showed uniform fluorescence in the cancerous tissue (cancerous-type fluorescence); in the one remaining HCC lesion and all of the adenocarcinoma lesions (one ICC and 4 CRLM lesions), fluorescence of ICG was detected not in the cancerous tissue but rather in the non-cancerous hepatic tissue surrounding the tumors (rim-type fluorescence). Photoacoustic tomography with ICG reproduced these two fluorescence patterns in all 10 resected hepatic specimens (Fig. 2A and B).

Photoacoustic signal amplitude according to ROI (CA, Peri, and NC) is demonstrated in Fig. 2C. In the CA tissue of HCCs that showed cancerous-type fluorescence and in the Peri tissue of tumors that showed rim-type fluorescence, PA signal amplitude decreased with increases in distance between the liver surface and the ROI: at 4 mm deep to the liver surface, the PA amplitudes ranged from 43% to 83% (median, 61%) of those measured just beneath the liver surface (depth of 1 mm). Thus, ROIs within

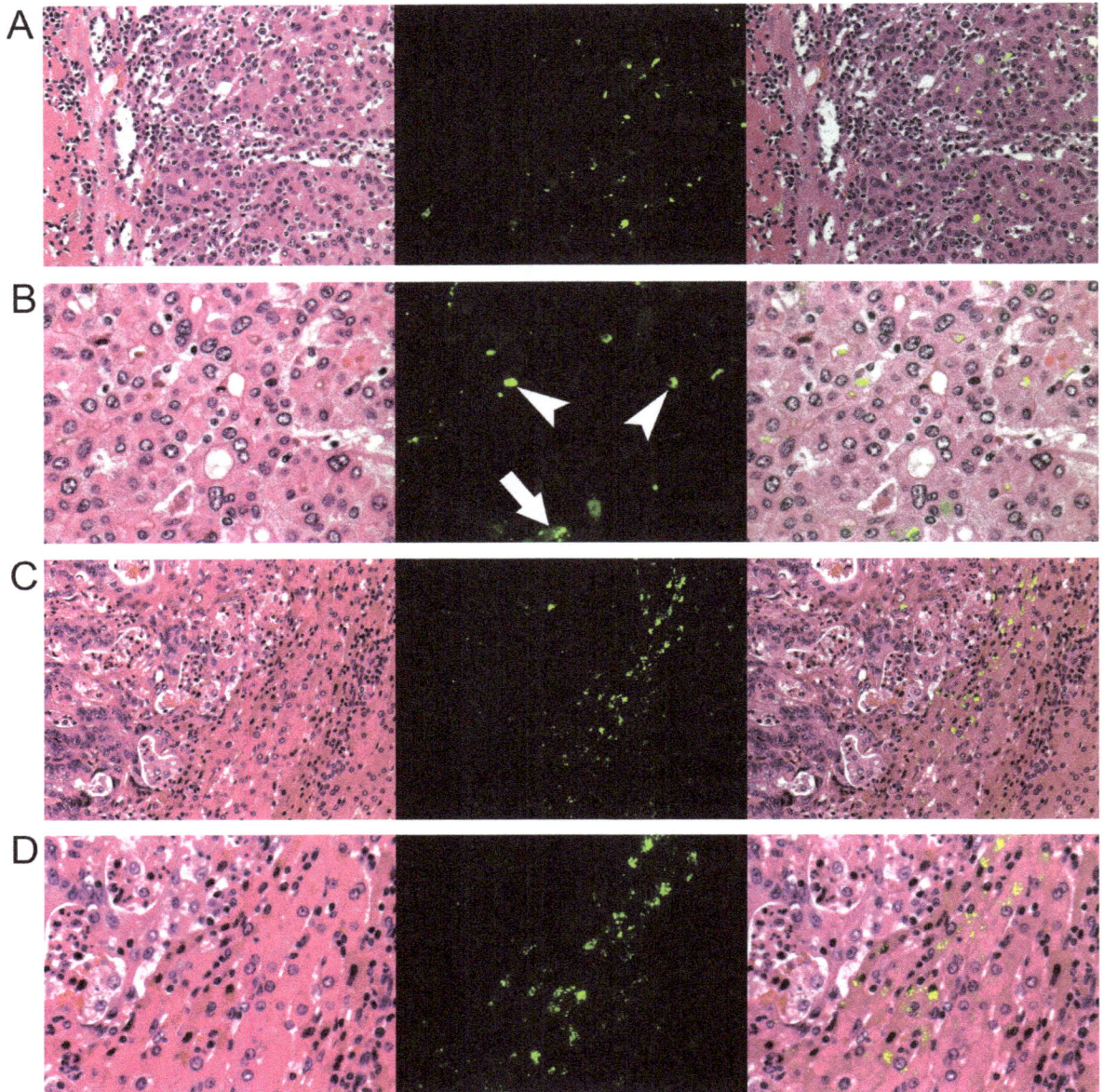

Figure 3. Fluorescence microscopy. Left, hematoxylin-eosin staining; middle, fluorescence images; and right, fusion images of ICG fluorescence, indicated in green, and hematoxylin-eosin staining. (**A**) In well-differentiated HC lesions, ICG fluorescence was identified mainly in the cancerous tissue, as demonstrated in Figure 2A. (**B**) Magnified view of (A). Indocyanine green had accumulated in the pseudoglands (arrowheads) and the cytoplasm of cancer cells (arrow). (**C**) Indocyanine green fluorescence was identified in the peri-cancerous hepatic parenchyma surrounding a CRLM lesion, as demonstrated in Figure 2B. (**D**) Magnified view of (C). Indocyanine green had accumulated in the cytoplasm of relatively small hepatocytes rather than in the intracellular spaces.

3 mm of the liver surface were used for the following analysis of the resected liver specimens to minimize the effect of attenuation on the PA signals.

The ratio of PA signal amplitude in CA tissue relative to that in NC tissue was higher in the 4 tumors showing cancerous-type ICG fluorescence compared with the 6 tumors with rim-type fluorescence (median [range], 1.5 [0.8–1.8] vs. 0.7 [0.5–0.8], $P = 0.01$ [Wilcoxon's rank-sum test]). In contrast, the ratio of PA signal amplitudes in Peri tissue relative to that in NC tissue was lower in the former group.

Fluorescent microscopy revealed the presence of ICG in pseudoglands and cancer cell cytoplasm from HCC tissue showing cancerous-type fluorescence and PA signals (Fig. 3A and B). In contrast, in hepatic tumors showing rim-type fluorescence and PA signals, ICG was identified mainly in the cytoplasm of the hepatocytes surrounding the tumors (Fig. 3C and D).

Photoacoustic tomography from the body surface in NASH-HCC model mice

In the three NASH-HCC model mice, PA tomography was applied to assess hepatic tumor detection from the body surface. Despite the identification of cancerous nodules on US images and spectrum computed tomography, PA tomography was unable to

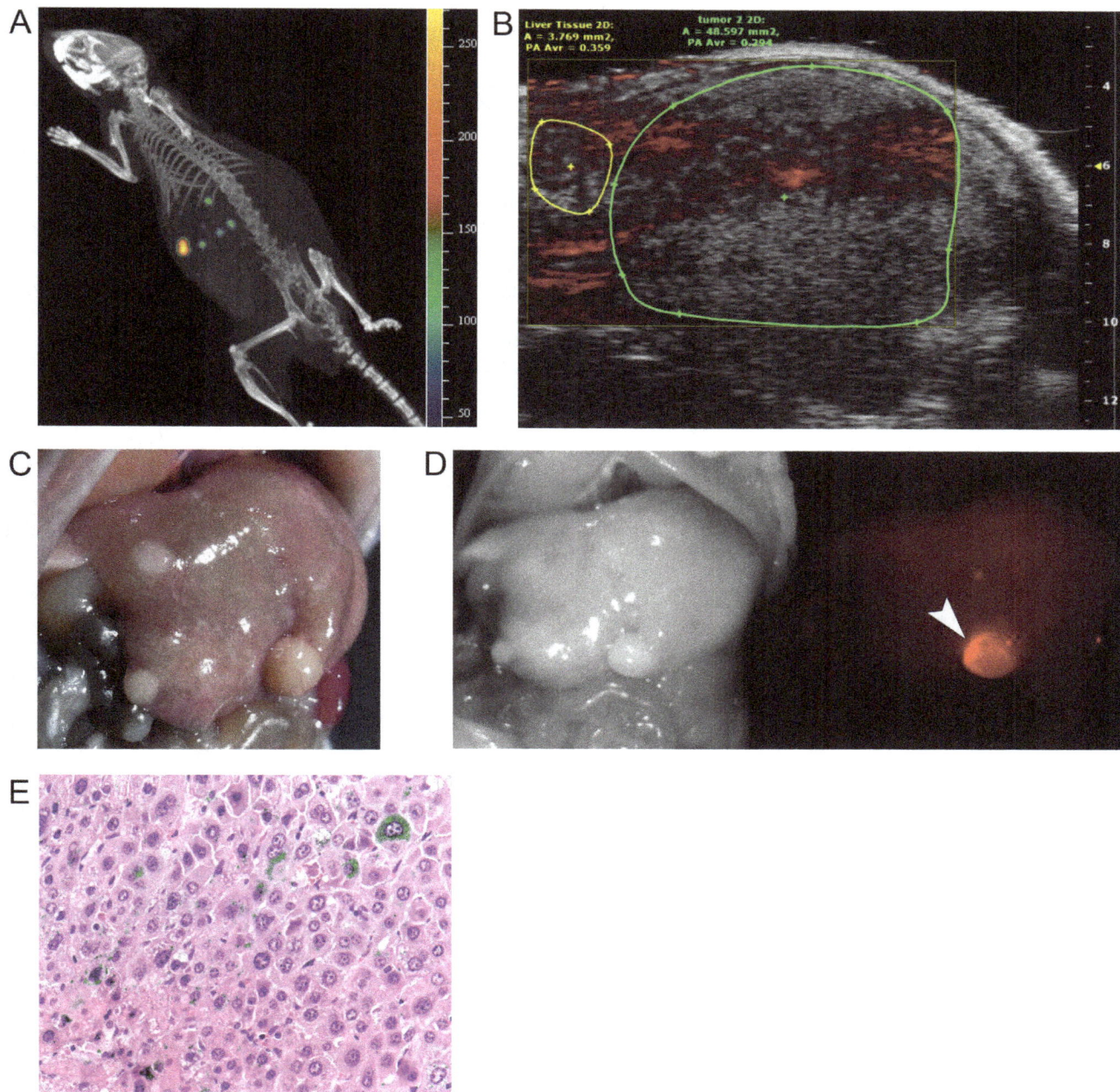

Figure 4. Photoacoustic tomography from the body surface in NASH-HCC model mice. (**A**) Spectrum computed tomography of a living NASH-HCC model mouse identified hepatic tumors with accumulation of ICG that had been intravenously injected 48 hours prior (IVIS Spectrum CT, PerkinElmer, Hopkinton, US; excitation 745 nm, emission 800 nm). (**B**) Photoacoustic tomography failed to visualize any cancer-specific PA signals on US images. (**C, D**) Three liver nodules were macroscopically identified in this mouse (C); one was visualized on fluorescence imaging (D). (**E**) Fluorescence microscopy identified ICG fluorescence (demonstrated in green in this fusion image with hematoxylin-eosin staining) in the cytoplasm of some of the cancerous cells in this NASH-HCC model mouse.

visualize any of these nodules with sufficient signal contrast relative to the background hepatic parenchyma (Fig. 4A and B). On abdominal exploration following sacrifice of the mice, a total of 10 hepatic tumors were macroscopically identified and then microscopically proven to be HCCs that had developed in the NASH livers. Among the 10 HCCs, 4 tumors were visualized by fluorescence imaging of the liver surface (Fig. 4C and D). Fluorescence microscopy demonstrated ICG accumulation in the

cytoplasm of cancerous cells, but ICG-positive cells were infrequent compared with their occurrence in human HCC tissue.

Discussion

In the surgical treatment of hepatic malignancies, US examination has played an indispensable role in the preoperative identification and differential diagnosis of hepatic lesions [30,31]. Recently, intraoperative fluorescence imaging using ICG has begun to be used to detect hepatic tumors on the liver surface prior to hepatectomy and to estimate the histological diagnosis for resected hepatic tumors [12–17]. In the present study, PA tomography enabled clear visualization of the distribution of preoperatively-administered ICG in and/or around hepatic tumors on US images of the surgically-resected specimens. Our results suggest that PA imaging with ICG has the potential to develop into a novel diagnostic tool that can support the localization and differential diagnosis of hepatic tumors established by conventional US examination and intraoperative fluorescence imaging; it does this by enabling the visualization of biliary excretory function in hepatic tumors and non-cancerous hepatic parenchyma.

In the present series, all but one HCC showed cancerous-type ICG fluorescence on the cut surfaces of the resected specimens, while all of the CRLM lesions and the ICC demonstrated rim-type fluorescence. These patterns of ICG accumulation were well reproduced by PA tomography performed from the surface of the resected specimens. In a previous study, the mechanism of cancerous-type fluorescence in HCC was revealed [17]: differentiated HCC cells maintain portal uptake function, but because of biliary excretion disorders caused by functional and/or morphological changes (as suggested by fluorescence microscopy in the present study), ICG accumulates in cancerous tissues. In contrast, ICG accumulation in the non-cancerous hepatic parenchyma around adenocarcinoma lesions has not yet been fully explained. It may be partly due to local biliary congestion resulting from simple compression by the tumors; however, a recent study by van der Vorst and colleagues [15] suggested that the increased presence of immature hepatocytes along with the impaired expression of organic anion transporters could also cause ICG accumulation in peri-cancerous hepatic regions. This theory is supported by the microscopic findings in the present study, in which ICG fluorescence was primarily detected in the cytoplasm of relatively small hepatocytes rather than in the intercellular spaces around these tumors. Visualization of hepatic ICG distribution by PA tomography may be useful not only in the differential diagnosis of hepatic tumors during conventional US examination (by assessing the tumors' bile-producing ability) but also for monitoring the delivery of anticancer agents/sensitizers with biliary excretion properties used for chemotherapy, radiotherapy, and photodynamic treatment.

The major limitation of the current technique used for PA tomography with ICG lies in the small region observable from the liver surface. Although PA signals can be detected from depths of up to 7 cm in theory [32], in our study of resected human hepatic specimens, PA amplitudes markedly decreased with depth of the ROI from the liver surface, decreasing by approximately 40% even at 4 mm in depth. In the mouse models, PA tomography with ICG failed to identify any of the HCC nodules that had developed in the NASH livers. These problems with PA tomography can be primarily attributed to steep attenuation of

the laser pulses used for excitation of ICG and/or attenuation of the PA signals emitted from the targeted regions; these issues can be solved, at least in part, by improving the intensity of the pulse laser and the sensitivity of the detector used in PA imaging systems. Another possible cause of the limited observable range identified in the present study is that the amount of hepatic tumor ICG accumulation was optimal for fluorescence imaging but insufficient for PA tomography, especially in the mouse model, where imaging was performed from the body surface. In the tissue-mimicking phantom plasma samples, PA imaging required at least 10 times the ICG concentration needed for fluorescence imaging, but such a high dosage of intravenous injection of ICG is not realistic (LD_{50} value of ICG is 64.3–72.8 mg/kg in mice) [33]. Novel contrast materials, such as metallic nanoparticles [26] and carbon nanotubes [34], may enable clear visualization of PA signals emitted from deeply-located hepatic tumors through biliary excretion disorders in and around cancerous tissues, if these agents have biliary excretion properties similar to ICG.

In conclusion, PA tomography using ICG is a promising technique that can support US examination of the liver by providing information on biliary excretion disorders in cancerous tissues and peri-cancerous hepatic parenchyma. However, further technical improvement is needed to enable the visualization of deeply-located lesions.

Acknowledgments

The authors acknowledge the significant contributions made by Drs. T. Aoki, Y. Sakamoto, K. Hasegawa, and Y. Sugawara, members of this study group. The authors also thank Summit Pharmaceuticals International Corporation and PRIMETECH Co., Ltd. for arrangement of fluorescence and PA imaging.

Author Contributions

Conceived and designed the experiments: TI. Performed the experiments: AM MK AS JK HI JS. Analyzed the data: TI MF YM YU. Contributed reagents/materials/analysis tools: MK HI YU. Wrote the paper: AM TI NK.

References

1. Ogata F, Azuma R, Kikuchi M, Koshima I, Morimoto Y (2007) Novel lymphography using indocyanine green dye for near-infrared fluorescence labeling. Ann Plast Surg 58: 652–655.
2. Kitai T, Inomoto T, Miwa M, Shikayama T (2005) Fluorescence navigation with indocyanine green for detecting sentinel lymph nodes in breast cancer. Breast Cancer 12: 211–215.
3. Mitsuhashi N, Kimura F, Shimizu H, Imamaki M, Yoshidome H, et al. (2008) Usefulness of intraoperative fluorescence imaging to evaluate local anatomy in hepatobiliary surgery. J Hepatobiliary Pancreat Surg 15: 508–514.
4. Ishizawa T, Tamura S, Masuda K, Aoki T, Hasegawa K, et al. (2009) Intraoperative fluorescent cholangiography using indocyanine green: a biliary road map for safe surgery. J Am Coll Surg 208: e1–e4.

5. Ishizawa T, Bandai Y, Ijichi M, Kaneko J, Hasegawa K, et al. (2010) Fluorescent cholangiography illuminating the biliary tree during laparoscopic cholecystectomy. Br J Surg 97: 1369–1377.
6. Schols RM, Bouvy ND, Masclee AA, van Dam RM, Dejong CH, et al. (2013) Fluorescence cholangiography during laparoscopic cholecystectomy: a feasibility study on early biliary tract delineation. Surg Endosc 2013; 27: 1530–1536.
7. Spinoglio G, Priora F, Bianchi PP, Lucido FS, Licciardello A, et al. (2013) Real-time near-infrared (NIR) fluorescent cholangiography in single-site robotic cholecystectomy (SSRC): a single-institutional prospective study. Surg Endosc 27: 2156–2162.
8. Rubens FD, Ruel M, Fremes SE (2002) A new and simplified method for coronary and graft imaging during CABG. Heart Surg Forum 5: 141–144.

9. Raabe A, Nakaji P, Beck J, Kim LJ, Hsu FP, et al. (2005) Prospective evaluation of surgical microscope-integrated intraoperative near-infrared indocyanine green videoangiography during aneurysm surgery. J Neurosurg 103: 982–989.

10. Kawaguchi Y, Ishizawa T, Miyata Y, Yamashita S, Masuda K, et al. (2013) Portal uptake function in veno-occlusive regions evaluated by real-time fluorescent imaging using indocyanine green. J Hepatol 58: 247–253.

11. Ris F, Hompes R, Cunningham C, Lindsey I, Guy R, et al. (2014) Near-infrared (NIR) perfusion angiography in minimally invasive colorectal surgery. Surg Endosc 28: 2221–2226.

12. Ishizawa T, Fukushima N, Shibahara J, Masuda K, Tamura S, et al. (2009) Real-time identification of liver cancers by using indocyanine green fluorescent imaging. Cancer 115: 2491–2504.

13. Gotoh K, Yamada T, Ishikawa O, Takahashi H, Eguchi H, et al. (2009) A novel image-guided surgery of hepatocellular carcinoma by indocyanine green fluorescence imaging navigation. J Surg Oncol 100: 75–79.

14. Yokoyama N, Otani T, Hashidate H, Maeda C, Katada T, et al. (2012) Real-time detection of hepatic micrometastases from pancreatic cancer by intraoperative fluorescence imaging: Preliminary results of a prospective study. Cancer 118: 2813–2819.

15. van der Vorst JR, Schaafsma BE, Hutteman M, Verbeek FP, Liefers GJ, et al. (2013) Near-infrared fluorescence-guided resection of colorectal liver metastases. Cancer 119 3411–3418.

16. Kudo H, Ishizawa T, Tani K, Harada N, Ichida A, et al. (2014) Visualization of subcapsular hepatic malignancy by indocyanine-green fluorescence imaging during laparoscopic hepatectomy. Surg Endosc 28: 2504–2508.

17. Ishizawa T, Masuda K, Urano Y, Kawaguchi Y, Satou S, et al. (2014) Mechanistic background and clinical applications of indocyanine green fluorescence imaging of hepatocellular carcinoma. Ann Surg Oncol 21: 440–448.

18. Kruger RA (1994) Photoacoustic ultrasound. Med Phys 21: 127–131.

19. Oraevsky AA, Jacques SL, Tittel FK (1997) Measurement of tissue optical properties by time-resolved detection of laser-induced transient stress. Appl Opt 36: 402–415.

20. Wang LV (2009) Multiscale photoacoustic microscopy and computed tomography. Nat Photonics 29: 503–509.

21. Kim C, Song KH, Gao F, Wang LV (2010) Sentinel lymph nodes and lymphatic vessels: noninvasive dual-modality in vivo mapping by using indocyanine green in rats–volumetric spectroscopic photoacoustic imaging and planar fluorescence imaging. Radiology 255: 442–450.

22. Rajian JR, Fabiilli ML, Fowlkes JB, Carson PL, Wang X (2011) Drug delivery monitoring by photoacoustic tomography with an ICG encapsulated double emulsion. Opt Express 19: 14335–14347.

23. Taruttis A, Morscher S, Burton NC, Razansky D, Ntziachristos V (2012) Fast multispectral optoacoustic tomography (MSOT) for dynamic imaging of pharmacokinetics and biodistribution in multiple organs. PLoS One 7: 30491.

24. Chino K, Akagi K, Dohi M, Fukashiro S, Takahashi H (2012) Reliability and validity of quantifying absolute muscle hardness using ultrasound elastography. PLoS One 7: e45764.

25. Needles A, Heinmiller A, Sun J, Theodoropoulos C, Bates D, et al. (2013) Development and initial application of a fully integrated photoacoustic micro-ultrasound system. IEEE Trans Ultrason Ferroelectr Freq Control 60: 888–897.

26. Nam SY, Ricles LM, Suggs LJ, Emelianov SY (2012) In vivo Ultrasound and Photoacoustic Monitoring of Mesenchymal Stem Cells Labeled with Gold Nanotracers. PLoS One 7: e37267.

27. Nakabayashi H, Taketa K, Miyano K, Yamane T, Sato J (1982) Growth of human hepatoma cells lines with differentiated functions in chemically defined medium. Cancer Res 42: 3858–3863.

28. Kaneko J, Inagaki Y, Ishizawa T, Gao J, Tang W, et al. (2014) Photodynamic therapy for human hepatoma-cell-line tumors utilizing biliary excretion properties of indocyanine green. J Gastroenterol 49: 110–116.

29. Fujii M, Shibazaki Y, Wakamatsu K, Honda Y, Kawauchi Y, et al. (2013) A murine model for non-alcoholic steatohepatitis showing evidence of association between diabetes and hepatocellular carcinoma. Med Mol Morphol 46: 141–152.

30. Zhang K, Kokudo N, Hasegawa K, Arita J, Tang W, et al. (2007) Detection of new tumors by intraoperative ultrasonography during repeated hepatic resections for hepatocellular carcinoma. Arch Surg 142: 1170–1175.

31. Takahashi M, Hasegawa K, Arita J, Hata S, Aoki T, et al. (2012) Contrast-enhanced intraoperative ultrasonography using perfluorobutane microbubbles for the enumeration of colorectal liver metastases. Br J Surg 99: 1271–1277.

32. Wang LV, Hu S (2012) Photoacoustic tomography: in vivo imaging from organelles to organs. Science 335: 1458–1462.

33. Drug interview form of diagnogreen for injection. Available: https://www.medicallibrary-dsc.info/di/diagnogreen_for_injection_25mg/pdf/if_dg_inj_1305_08.pdf. Accessed 2013 May 01.

34. De la Zerda A, Zavaleta C, Keren S, Vaithilingam S, Bodapati S, et al. (2008) Carbon nanotubes as photoacoustic molecular imaging agents in living mice. Nat Nanotechnol 3: 557–562.

22

Rational Classification of Portal Vein Thrombosis and Its Clinical Significance

Jingqin Ma[1], **Zhiping Yan**[1]*, **Jianjun Luo**[1], **Qingxin Liu**[1], **Jianhua Wang**[1], **Shijing Qiu**[2]

1 Department of Interventional Radiology, Zhongshan Hospital, Fudan University, Shanghai, China, **2** Bone and Mineral Research Laboratory, Henry Ford Hospital, Detroit, Michigan, United States of America

Abstract

Portal vein thrombosis (PVT) is commonly classified into acute (symptom duration <60 days and absence of portal carvernoma and portal hypertension) and chronic types. However, the rationality of this classification has received little attention. In this study, 60 patients (40 men and 20 women) with PVT were examined using contrast-enhanced computed tomography (CT). The percentage of vein occlusion, including portal vein (PV) and superior mesenteric vein (SMV), was measured on CT image. Of 60 patients, 17 (28.3%) met the criterion of acute PVT. Symptoms occurred more frequently in patients with superior mesenteric vein thrombosis (SMVT) compared to those without SMVT (p<0.001). However, there was no significant difference in PV occlusion between patients with and without symptoms. The frequency of cavernous transformation was significantly higher in patients with complete PVT than those with partial PVT (p<0.001). Complications of portal hypertension were significantly associated with cirrhosis (p<0.001) rather than with the severity of PVT and presence of cavernoma. These results suggest that the severity of PVT is only associated with the formation of portal cavernoma but unrelated to the onset of symptoms and the development of portal hypertension. We classified PVT into complete and partial types, and each was subclassified into with and without portal cavernoma. In conclusion, neither symptom duration nor cavernous transformation can clearly distinguish between acute and chronic PVT. The new classification system can determine the pathological alterations of PVT, patency of portal vein and outcome of treatment in a longitudinal study.

Editor: Erica Villa, University of Modena & Reggio Emilia, Italy

Funding: These authors have no support or funding to report.

Competing Interests: All authors have declared that no competing interests exist.

* Email: yan.zhiping@zs-hospital.sh.cn

Introduction

Portal vein thrombosis (PVT) is still considered as a rare disease since the primary information has been derived from clinical series and case reports [1,2]. Recently, Ogren et al. [3] reported that PVT was found in 254 cases of 23,796 autopsies, suggesting that the prevalence of PVT is about 1% of the general population. The lower finding rate of PVT may be related to the difficulty of diagnosis because a large number of patients remain asymptomatic [4–6]. With development of imaging techniques (contrast enhanced ultrasound, spiral CT-scan and high definition MRI, etc), PVT may no longer be a rare disease as expected before. PVT has been defined as acute and chronic entities [7]. The duration of symptoms and presence of portal cavernoma or complications of portal hypertension have been used to distinguish between acute and chronic PVT. Although not universally accepted, acute PVT is considered as patients with symptoms < 60 days prior to diagnosis and in the absence of portal cavernoma and/or portal hypertension [8,9]. In contrast, chronic PVT is often accompanied with portal cavernoma and portal hypertension, resulting in esophageal varices, ascites and splenomegaly [4,7]. There is perceptible difference in the treatment of acute and

chronic PVT [7,10]. Recanalization of obstructed veins is often the primary treatment option for acute PVT [7,11–13]. Unlike acute PVT, management of complications of portal hypertension is recommended prior to the recanalization of thrombosed veins for patients with chronic PVT [7,14,15].

Nevertheless, there are two reasons to suggest that the classification of acute and chronic PVT is not perfect in clinical practice. First, the duration of symptoms is sometimes not equal to the duration of thrombosis because the thrombus may have been formed long before the onset of symptoms [4,5]. In this case, chronic PVT is likely to be diagnosed as an acute one. Second, the formation of portal cavernoma is often not associated with the time of thrombosis. Portal cavernoma would develop rapidly (usually as early as a few days after thrombus formation) from pre-existing veins, particularly in patients with complete thrombosis [4,7], or not occur long after PVT (e.g. with symptoms >60 days), particularly in patients with partial thrombosis [16,17]. Thus, it is also illogical to use the presence of portal cavernoma as a criterion to distinguish between acute and chronic PVT.

The purposes of this study were to define the rationality of dividing PTV into acute and chronic types and attempted to find out an appropriate classification for PVT.

Table 1. Relationship of recent symptom onset to the severity of PVT and the presence of MVT and cavernoma.

	Symptom (<60 days)	No Symptom	P
	n = 33	n = 21	
PVT			
Partial	22 (66.7)	15 (71.4)	0.772
Complete	11 (33.3)	6 (28.6)	
SMVT			
No	3 (9.09)	12 (57.1)	<0.001
Yes	30 (90.9)	9 (42.9)	
Cavernoma			
No	19 (57.6)	9 (42.9)	0.403
Yes	14 (42.4)	12 (57.1)	

Data expressed as number (percent).

Materials and Methods

Patient selection

Between January 2005 and November 2012, 71 consecutive patients with PVT were recruited in this study. The following patients were excluded from the study: 1) aged >75 years; 2) without thrombus in portal vein; 3) with the conditions of tumorous thrombosis, severe hepatic encephalopathy or cardiopulmonary co-morbidity and 4) previously received intravenous intervention or surgical portosystemic shunt. The patients with missing data or poor quality CT images were also excluded. After screening, 60 patients (40 men and 20 women) were eligible for this study. The average age was 48.0±13.8 years (range: 16–75 years). Twenty four patients suffered from cirrhosis. The written informed consent to participate in our study and publish these case details was obtained from each adult patient as well as from the guardians on behalf of the children. The study was approved by the Institutional Review Board of Shanghai Zhongshan Hospital.

Computed tomography

All recruited patients were examined using contrast-enhanced 64-slices spiral computed tomography (CT). CT images were read by two experienced radiologists to identify the location of thrombus and the presence of portal cavernoma. The degree of vein occlusion, including portal vein (PV), superior mesenteric vein (SMV) and splenic vein (SV), was measured on CT image using an image analysis program (Image J, NIH). The areas of vein lumen and inside thrombus were measured on the cross-sectional image at the level of the maximum thrombosis. The percentage of lumen occlusion was calculated by the area of thrombus dividing by the area of vein lumen. Maximum lumen occlusion was used for the determination of the severity of portal vein thrombosis (PVT), superior mesenteric vein thrombosis (SMVT) and splenic vein thrombosis (SVT). Thrombosis was arbitrarily defined as complete when the vein lumen was occluded for more than 90% [18]. Liver cirrhosis was also diagnosed using CT imaging as reported elsewhere [19].

PVT Classification

Classification of PVT depended on 3 criteria: 1) onset of symptoms such as abdominal pain or distention, diarrhea, nausea, vomiting, anorexia and fever; 2) development of portal cavernoma; 3) presence of complications of portal hypertension including gastroesophageal variceal bleeding, splenomegaly and ascites. PVT was defined as acute if there was a recent episode of symptoms (<60 days) with no evidence of portal cavernoma and complications of portal hypertension. In contrast, chronic PVT was often asymptomatic, in addition to the presence of portal cavernoma and/or complications of portal hypertension.

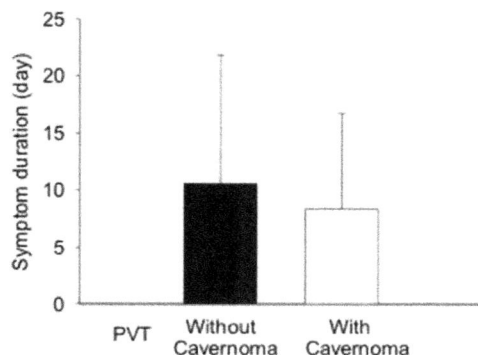

Figure 1. Comparison of symptom duration between PVT patients with and without portal cavernoma. There was no significant difference in symptom duration between two groups.

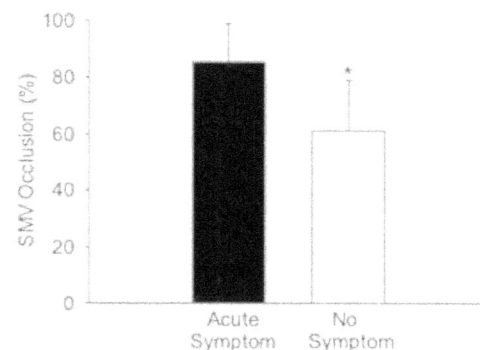

Figure 2. Comparison of superior mesenteric vein (SMV) occlusion between patients with and without recent episode of symptoms. SMV occlusion in patients with symptoms was significantly higher than those without symptom. *p<0.01.

Table 2. Classification of 60 patients with PVT.

	Number	Symptoms	Cavernoma and/or portal
Acute	17	<60 days	No
Chronic	16	<60 days	Yes
	6	≥60 days	Yes
	21	No	Yes

Statistical analysis

Continuous variables were expressed as mean and standard deviation (SD). For continuous variables, the mean values were compared using student t test or one-way ANOVA. Mann-Whitney test or Kruskal–Wallis test was used if the variable was not normally distributed. Categorical variables were compared using Fisher exact test. Logistic analysis was used to assess: 1) the likelihood of symptom onset associated with the presence of SMVT; 2) the likelihood of cavernous transformation associated with the degree of PVT and 3) the risk of complications of portal hypertension associated with cirrhosis. The level of statistical significance was accepted at $p < 0.05$.

Results

Characteristics of patients at diagnosis of PVT

PVT was present in all 60 patients. In these patients, 21 were associated with SMVT, 3 with SVT and 20 suffered thrombosis in both veins.

Of 60 patients, 33 had recent onset of symptoms (symptom duration: 0–37 days prior to diagnosis) and 21 were asymptomatic (Table 1). In these 2 groups, the severity of PVT and the presence of portal cavernoma were not significantly associated with symptom onset (Table 1). There was no significant difference in PV lumen occlusion between patients with and without symptoms. In patients with recent onset of symptoms, there was no significant difference in symptom duration between subjects with and without portal cavernoma (mean duration: 8.40 vs 10.6 days)(Fig 1). However, symptoms occurred significantly more frequent in patients with SMVT than those without SMVT ($p < 0.001$)(Table 1). In patients with SMVT, the SMV lumen occlusion was significantly increased in the subjects with recent symptoms (SMV occlusion 85.5±13.3%) compared to those without symptom (SMV occlusion 65.8±27.9%)($p < 0.05$)(Fig 2). Logistic analysis demonstrated that the likelihood of symptom onset was 13.3 times (Odds ratio = 13.3, 95%CI: 3.07–57.9, $p < 0.001$) higher in patients with SMVT than those without SMVT. According to the criteria of classification, 17 patients (28.3%), who experienced recent onset of symptoms but had no portal cavernoma and

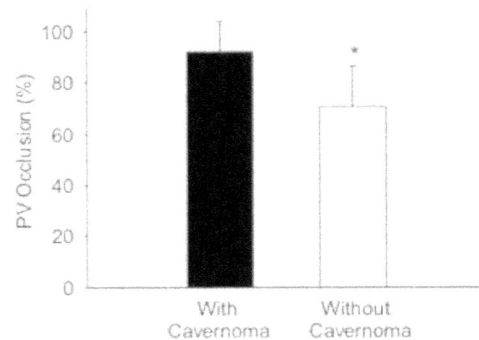

Figure 3. Comparison of portal vein (PV) occlusion between patients with and without cavernoma. PV occlusion in patients with cavernoma was significantly higher than those without cavernoma. *$p < 0.001$.

complication of portal hyertension, were defined as acute PVT and 43 others (71.7%) were defined as chronic PVT (Table 2).

Relationship between severity of PVT and portal cavernoma

The mean occlusion of PV was 81.1±17.1% (range: 8–100%) in 60 patients. Twenty two patients had complete PVT, and 20 (90.9%) of them were associated with portal cavernoma. Conversely, in 38 patients with partial PVT, only 11 (28.9%) were associated with portal cavernoma. The frequency of cavernous transformation was significantly higher in patients with complete PVT than those with partial PVT ($p < 0.001$, Table 3). The PV lumen occlusion was significantly higher in patients with portal cavernoma than those without cavernoma ($p < 0.001$, Fig 3). Logistic analysis demonstrated that the likelihood of cavernous transformation was 24.5 times (Odds ratio = 24.5, 95%CI: 4.89–123, $p < 0.001$) higher in patients with complete PVT than those with partial PVT.

Table 3. Relationship between severity of PVT and cavernous transformation.

	Partial PVT	Complete PVT	P
	n = 38	n = 21	
Cavernoma			
No	27 (71.7)	2 (9.09)	<0.001
Yes	11 (28.9)	20 (90.9)	

Data expressed as number (percent).

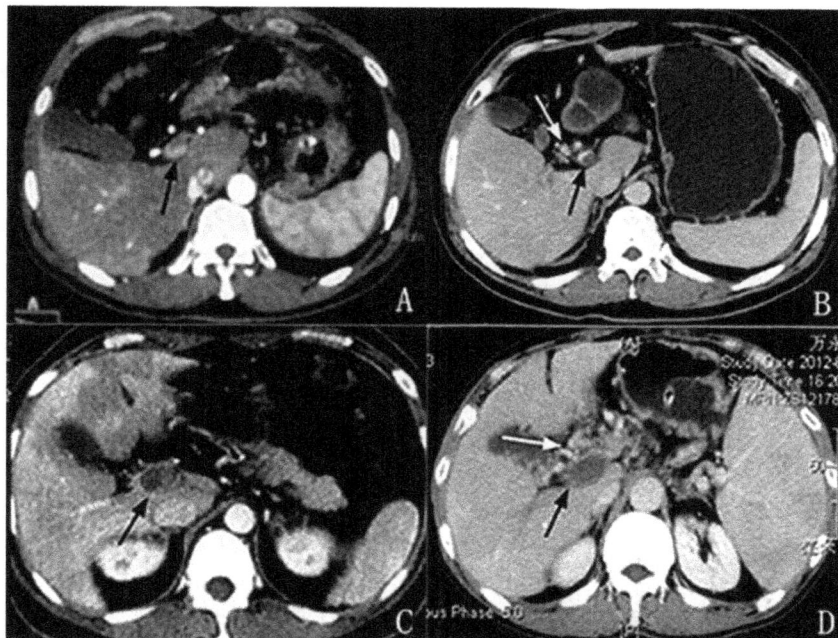

Figure 4. Cross-sectional CT image of portal vein thrombosis and cavernoma: A) partial PVT (black arrow) without cavernoma; B) partial PVT (black arrow) with cavernoma (white arrow); C) complete PVT (black arrow) without carvernoma and D) complete PVT (black arrow) with cavernoma (white arrow).

In this combination between severity of thrombosis and presence of portal cavernoma, four types of PVT were seen (Fig 4): **1) partial PVT without cavernoma (27/60, 45.0%); 2) partial PVT with cavernoma (11/60, 18.3%); 3) complete PVT without cavernoma (2/60, 3.33%) and 4) complete PVT with cavernoma (20/60, 33.3%).**

Relationship between cirrhosis and complications of portal hypertension

Twenty seven patients had complications of portal hypertension, including 26 gastroesophageal variceal bleeding and 1 ascites. Complications were significantly associated with cirrhosis (p< 0.001) rather than the severity of PVT and presence of cavernoma (Table 4). In 27 patients with complications, 19 (70.4%) suffered from cirrhosis. However, in 33 patients without complications only 6 (18.2%) had cirrhosis. The patients with cirrhosis had a 10.7 times (Odds ratio = 10.7, 95%CI: 3.19–35.9, p<0.001) higher risk of complications of portal hypertension compared to those without cirrhosis.

In this study, cirrhosis was diagnosed from liver morphology in CT imaging (Fig 5). The cirrhosis was characterized by surface nodularity and heterogeneity of liver parenchyma. A ratio of transverse caudate lobe width to right lobe width greater than or equal to 0.65 was a positive indicator for the diagnosis of cirrhosis [19]. Splenomegaly was often found in patients with cirrhosis.

Table 4. Relationship of complications of portal hypertension with PVT, cavernoma and cirrhosis.

	Complications	No complications	P
	n = 27	n = 33	
PVT			
Partial	18 (66.7)	20 (60.6)	0.789
Complete	9 (33.3)	13 (39.4)	
Cavernoma			
No	11 (40.7)	18 (54.5)	0.312
Yes	16 (59.3)	15 (45.5)	
Cirrhosis			
No	8 (29.6)	27 (81.8)	<0.001
Yes	19 (70.4)	6 (18.2)	

Data expressed as number (percent).

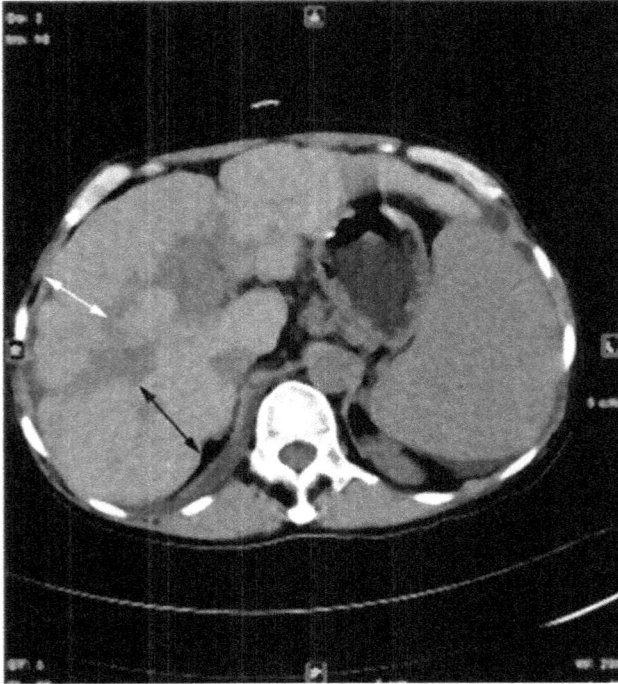

Figure 5. Cirrhotic morphology in CT imaging. Portal venous phase CT scan shows nodularity on the liver surface and heterogeneity of the liver parenchyma. A ratio of transverse caudate lobe width (black arrow) to right lobe width (white arrow) is greater than 0.65. Splenomegaly was present.

Discussion

Acute and chronic PVT, as the name implies, are distinguished by the time of thrombus presence. However, it is difficult to determine the exact time of thrombus formation. Instead, the duration of symptoms and the aftermaths of portal vein occlusion, such as portal cavernoma and portal hypertension, have been used as the criteria to distinguish between acute and chronic PVT [4,7,8,20]. The patients who developed symptoms <60 days and had no evidence of portal cavernoma and portal hypertension can be diagnosed as acute PVT, while the others are considered as chronic PVT [9,21,22]. Based on our results and literature review, we assume that the symptoms are unreliable for the classification of PVT due to the following reasons. First, the symptom onset does not occur at the same time as the initiation of PVT. In other words, the duration of symptoms is not equal to the duration of thrombosis; the former is frequently shorter than the latter. Additionally, many patients with PVT may remain asymptomatic for a long period of time [21]. In our study, 35% (21/60) of patients with PVT were asymptomatic. There is no consensus about the classification of asymptomatic PVT [10,23,24]. Most authors consider asymptomatic PVT as chronic PVT [10,21]. However, there is no evidence to confirm that PVT in asymptomatic patients exists longer than that in patients with symptoms. Last but not least, our results showed that symptom onset was not associated with the severity of PVT but significantly related to the severity of SMVT. The typical presentation of acute PVT is with acute abdomen [22]. It is well known that the symptoms of acute abdomen are associated with bowel ischemia, which is caused by the occlusion of superior mesenteric vein [13,25]. Since the occlusion of portal vein would not directly cause

severe bowel ischemia, the symptom onset seems unlikely to be **the** result of PVT.

When PVT in its acute stage remains unsolved, collateral vessels will appear around portal vein from a few days to weeks and eventually become a spongelike portal cavernoma [26]. The number, size, and location of collaterals are variable among different patients [21,22]. At present, many authors ascertain chronic PVT by the presence of portal cavernoma [6,7,10]. However, the portal cavernoma in some patients does not occur a long time after acute event [16,26,27]. De Gaetano et al. [26] followed up 131 PVT patients up to 6 weeks and found that 56 (42.7%) patients had no portal cavernoma during the whole follow-up period, 66 (50.4%) showed a cavernoma and 9 (6.9%) had no cavernoma at the first examination. In these 9 patients, cavernoma occurred within 6–20 days after thrombus formation. Luca et al. [27] reported that 14% of patients with partial PVT developed to complete PVT in two years, but none of them showed portal cavernoma. Our study demonstrated that the development of portal cavernoma was not correlated with the duration of symptoms. In patients with recent onset of symptoms, 42% were associated with portal cavernoma. The symptom duration for these patients was 2 days shorter than the patients without portal cavernoma, although the statistical significance was not reached. Portal cavernoma may be found very shortly after symptom onset (0–2 days) in some patients. These data suggest that cavernous transformation of portal vein may occur at the early stage of PVT. Accordingly, portal cavernoma is inappropriate to be used for the diagnosis of chronic PVT.

In contrast to symptom onset, cavernous transformation was significantly associated with the severity of PVT. We found that > 90% of patients with complete PVT were accompanied with portal cavernoma, which was remarkably more than 35% in patients with partial PVT. Even in patients with partial PVT, the PV lumen occlusion was significantly higher in subjects with portal cavernoma (PV occlusion = 79.5%) than those without cavernoma (PV occlusion = 68.7%). The likelihood of cavernous transformation in patients with complete PVT (PV occlusion >90%) was 24 times higher than patients with partial PVT (PV occlusion ≤90%).

There are several diverse classifications based on the degree and extension of PVT [28–32] due to their close association with the outcome of treatment [33]. Complete PVT would cause cessation of portal blood flow, resulting in liver to lose about two thirds of its blood supply. However, this condition is usually well tolerated and patients are often asymptomatic [21]. It is probably due to the rapid development of portal cavernoma that is composed of numerous hepatopetal collateral vessels located in the hepatic hilum [34]. These collateral vessels connect the two patent portions proximately and distally to the thrombus and partially supplement the loss of portal vein's contribution to liver blood flow. This compensatory mechanism may make the obstructed portal vein lose its own function and eventually become a thin, fibrotic cord [6,7]. At this stage, portal hypertension may occur [35,36]. The large portal cavernoma may also compress the pliable common bile duct, resulting in the formation of portal biliopathy [37]. Therefore, the changes in thrombus and portal cavernoma should be both examined in the treatment of PVT.

The significant relationship between the severity of PVT and portal cavernoma has made us create a new classification system, in which PVT is classified into 4 types according to the degree of portal vein occlusion and the association with portal cavernoma. Type I is partial PVT without cavernoma, type II is partial PVT associated with cavernoma, type III is complete PVT without cavernoma and type IV is complete PVT associated with cavernoma. In our cohort, 51.6% of PVT patients (complete

33.3% and partial 18.3%) were associated with cavernoma and others (complete 3.33% and partial 45.0%) were not associated with cavernoma, suggesting that cavernous transformation is significantly correlated with the severity of portal vein occlusion. There are **several** advantages of this classification. First, it is easy to do the classification because both PVT and portal cavernoma can be clearly identified by CT or MRI imaging [10,38,39]. Every patient can be clearly classified into a certain type with no ambiguous variable. In addition, the degree of portal vein occlusion can be quantified on CT imaging, which can detect little changes in the severity of PVT. Second, this classification is able to demonstrate the pathological alterations of PVT, patency of portal vein and outcome of treatment. For example, this classification can ascertain whether the partial PVT become worsened, improved or stable with time [27], and can also detect the improvement and recurrence of PVT after anticoagulant and interventional therapies [18,40–43]. Third, optimal treatment can be determined based on this classification, at least during a certain period. For example, cavernoma was once seen as a contraindication of transjugular intrahepatic portosystemic shunt (TIPS) in patients with PVT [44]. With the development of stent design and surgical technique, cavernoma is no longer a contraindication of TIPS, but it does increase the technical difficulty of the procedure [9].

In this study, 27 patients (45%) suffered from complications of portal hypertension, 26 with gastroesophageal variceal bleeding and 1 with severe ascites. The prevalence of complications was 30% in patients without cirrhosis, but increased to 70% in patients with cirrhosis. The risk of complications in patients with cirrhosis was approximately 11 times higher than patients without cirrhosis. Nevertheless, the complications of portal hypertension were not significantly associated with the degree of thrombosis and the presence of portal cavernoma. Likewise, Amarapurkar et al. [45] reported recently that portal vein occlusion is an uncommon cause

of portal hypertension in adults in India. Luca et al. [27] also reported that the progression of partial PVT did not increase the risk of complications resulting from portal hypertension. Liver cirrhosis has been confirmed as a critical factor contributing to the complications of portal hypertension [46]. Ponziani [47] proposed that PVT development is not only a matter of impaired blood flow or pro-coagulation tendency, but also a consequence of the worsening in portal vein outflow due to increased hepatic resistance in cirrhotic liver. Since many cirrhotic patients may have had portal vein hypertension before the occurrence of PVT, the complications in these patients **are** likely to be independent of the severity of PVT.

Our study had some limitations. The major limitation is that this was a cross-sectional retrospective study, which could not ascertain the value of the new classification in the evaluation of PVT progress and treatment outcome. Additionally, the study might not have adequate power to detect significant correlation between the complications of portal hypertension and the severity of PVT and portal cavernoma.

In conclusion, recent onset of symptoms was usually initiated by severe SMVT rather than PVT and portal cavernoma. Neither symptom duration nor cavernous transformation is appropriate to be used as a criterion to distinguish between acute and chronic PVT. It seems rational to classify PVT based on PVT severity and cavernous transformation of portal vein, which is suitable to be used in the longitudinal study to determine the pathological alterations of PVT, patency of portal vein and outcome of treatment.

Author Contributions

Conceived and designed the experiments: ZPY JQM. Performed the experiments: ZPY JJL QXL JQM. Analyzed the data: JQM SJQ JW. Wrote the paper: JQM SJQ.

References

1. Hall TC, Garcea G, Metcalfe M, Bilku D, Dennison AR (2011) Management of acute non-cirrhotic and non-malignant portal vein thrombosis: a systematic review. World J Surg 35: 2510–2520.

2. James AW, Rabl C, Westphalen AC, Fogarty PF, Posselt AM, et al. (2009) Portomesenteric venous thrombosis after laparoscopic surgery: a systematic literature review. Arch Surg 144: 520–526.

3. Ogren M, Bergqvist D, Bjorck M, Acosta S, Eriksson H, et al. (2006) Portal vein thrombosis: prevalence, patient characteristics and lifetime risk: a population study based on 23,796 consecutive autopsies. World J Gastroenterol 12: 2115–2119.

4. Valla DC (2011) Portal vein thrombosis. In: Deleve LD, Garcia-Tsao G, editors. Vascular liver disease: Mechanisms and management. New York, Dordrecht Heidelberg, London: Springer Science+Bussiness Media, LLC. pp.183–196.

5. Amitrano L, Guardascione MA, Scaglione M, Pezzullo L, Sangiuliano N, et al. (2007) Prognostic factors in noncirrhotic patients with splanchnic vein thromboses. Am J Gastroenterol 102: 2464–2470.

6. Hoekstra J, Janssen HL (2009) Vascular liver disorders (II): portal vein thrombosis. Neth J Med 67: 46–53.

7. Condat B, Valla D (2006) Nonmalignant portal vein thrombosis in adults. Nat Clin Pract Gastroenterol Hepatol 3: 505–515.

8. Malkowski P, Pawlak J, Michalowicz B, Szczerban J, Wroblewski T, et al. (2003) Thrombolytic treatment of portal thrombosis. Hepatogastroenterology 50: 2098–2100.

9. Senzolo M, Tibbals J, Cholongitas E, Triantos CK, Burroughs AK, et al. (2006) Transjugular intrahepatic portosystemic shunt for portal vein thrombosis with and without cavernous transformation. Aliment Pharmacol Ther 23: 767–775.

10. Chawla Y, Duseja A, Dhiman RK (2009) Review article: the modern management of portal vein thrombosis. Aliment Pharmacol Ther 30: 881–894.

11. Hollingshead M, Burke CT, Mauro MA, Weeks SM, Dixon RG, et al. (2005) Transcatheter thrombolytic therapy for acute mesenteric and portal vein thrombosis. J Vasc Interv Radiol 16: 651–661.

12. Sheen CL, Lamparelli H, Milne A, Green I, Ramage JK (2000) Clinical features, diagnosis and outcome of acute portal vein thrombosis. QJM 93: 531–534.

13. Kumar S, Sarr MG, Kamath PS (2001) Mesenteric venous thrombosis. N Engl J Med 345: 1683–1688.

14. Boyer TD, Haskal ZJ (2005) American Association for the Study of Liver Diseases Practice Guidelines: the role of transjugular intrahepatic portosystemic shunt creation in the management of portal hypertension. J Vasc Interv Radiol 16: 615–629.

15. Wu J, Li Z, Wang Z, Han X, Ji F, et al. (2013) Surgical and Endovascular Treatment of Severe Complications Secondary to Noncirrhotic Portal Hypertension: Experience of 56 Cases. Ann Vasc Surg.

16. Blum U, Haag K, Rossle M, Ochs A, Gabelmann A, et al. (1995) Noncavernomatous portal vein thrombosis in hepatic cirrhosis: treatment with transjugular intrahepatic portosystemic shunt and local thrombolysis. Radiology 195: 153–157.

17. Belli L, Romani F, Sansalone CV, Aseni P, Rondinara G (1986) Portal thrombosis in cirrhotics. A retrospective analysis. Ann Surg 203: 286–291.

18. Luo J, Yan Z, Wang J, Liu Q, Qu X (2011) Endovascular treatment for nonacute symptomatic portal venous thrombosis through intrahepatic portosystemic shunt approach. J Vasc Interv Radiol 22: 61–69.

19. Brancatelli G, Federle MP, Ambrosini R, Lagalla R, Carriero A, et al. (2007) Cirrhosis: CT and MR imaging evaluation. Eur J Radiol 61: 57–69.

20. Condat B, Pessione F, Helene Denninger M, Hillaire S, Valla D (2000) Recent portal or mesenteric venous thrombosis: increased recognition and frequent recanalization on anticoagulant therapy. Hepatology 32: 466–470.

21. Ponziani FR, Zocco MA, Campanale C, Rinninella E, Tortora A, et al. (2010) Portal vein thrombosis: insight into physiopathology, diagnosis, and treatment. World J Gastroenterol 16: 143–155.

22. Webster GJ, Burroughs AK, Riordan SM (2005) Review article: portal vein thrombosis – new insights into aetiology and management. Aliment Pharmacol Ther 21: 1–9.

23. Parikh S, Shah R, Kapoor P (2010) Portal vein thrombosis. Am J Med 123: 111–119.

24. Primignani M (2010) Portal vein thrombosis, revisited. Dig Liver Dis 42: 163–170.

25. Kim HS, Patra A, Khan J, Arepally A, Streiff MB (2005) Transhepatic catheter-directed thrombectomy and thrombolysis of acute superior mesenteric venous thrombosis. J Vasc Interv Radiol 16: 1685–1691.

26. De Gaetano AM, Lafortune M, Patriquin H, De Franco A, Aubin B, et al. (1995) Cavernous transformation of the portal vein: patterns of intrahepatic and

splanchnic collateral circulation detected with Doppler sonography. AJR Am J Roentgenol 165: 1151–1155.

27. Luca A, Caruso S, Milazzo M, Marrone G, Mamone G, et al. (2012) Natural course of extrahepatic nonmalignant partial portal vein thrombosis in patients with cirrhosis. Radiology 265: 124–132.

28. Nonami T, Yokoyama I, Iwatsuki S, Starzl TE (1992) The incidence of portal vein thrombosis at liver transplantation. Hepatology 16: 1195–1198.

29. Yerdel MA, Gunson B, Mirza D, Karayalcin K, Olliff S, et al. (2000) Portal vein thrombosis in adults undergoing liver transplantation: risk factors, screening, management, and outcome. Transplantation 69: 1873–1881.

30. Bauer J, Johnson S, Durham J, Ludkowski M, Trotter J, et al. (2006) The role of TIPS for portal vein patency in liver transplant patients with portal vein thrombosis. Liver Transpl 12: 1544–1551.

31. Jamieson NV (2000) Changing perspectives in portal vein thrombosis and liver transplantation. Transplantation 69: 1772–1774.

32. Stieber AC, Zetti G, Todo S, Tzakis AG, Fung JJ, et al. (1991) The spectrum of portal vein thrombosis in liver transplantation. Ann Surg 213: 199–206.

33. Qi X, Han G, Wang J, Wu K, Fan D (2010) Degree of portal vein thrombosis. Hepatology 51: 1089–1090.

34. Qi X, Han G, Yin Z, He C, Wang J, et al. (2012) Transjugular intrahepatic portosystemic shunt for portal cavernoma with symptomatic portal hypertension in non-cirrhotic patients. Dig Dis Sci 57: 1072–1082.

35. Valla DC, Condat B (2000) Portal vein thrombosis in adults: pathophysiology, pathogenesis and management. J Hepatol 32: 865–871.

36. Sarin SK, Agarwal SR (2002) Extrahepatic portal vein obstruction. Semin Liver Dis 22: 43–58.

37. Chattopadhyay S, Nundy S (2012) Portal biliopathy. World J Gastroenterol 18: 6177–6182.

38. Lee HK, Park SJ, Yi BH, Yeon EK, Kim JH, et al. (2008) Portal vein thrombosis: CT features. Abdom Imaging 33: 72–79.

39. Qi X, Han G, He C, Yin Z, Guo W, et al. (2012) CT features of non-malignant portal vein thrombosis: a pictorial review. Clin Res Hepatol Gastroenterol 36: 561–568.

40. Spaander MC, Hoekstra J, Hansen BE, Van Buuren HR, Leebeek FW, et al. (2013) Anticoagulant therapy in patients with non-cirrhotic portal vein thrombosis: effect on new thrombotic events and gastrointestinal bleeding. J Thromb Haemost 11: 452–459.

41. Delgado MG, Seijo S, Yepes I, Achecar L, Catalina MV, et al. (2012) Efficacy and safety of anticoagulation on patients with cirrhosis and portal vein thrombosis. Clin Gastroenterol Hepatol 10: 776–783.

42. Luca A, Miraglia R, Caruso S, Milazzo M, Sapere C, et al. (2011) Short- and long-term effects of the transjugular intrahepatic portosystemic shunt on portal vein thrombosis in patients with cirrhosis. Gut 60: 846–852.

43. Plessier A, Darwish-Murad S, Hernandez-Guerra M, Consigny Y, Fabris F, et al. (2010) Acute portal vein thrombosis unrelated to cirrhosis: a prospective multicenter follow-up study. Hepatology 51: 210–218.

44. Walser EM, NcNees SW, DeLa Pena O, Crow WN, Morgan RA, et al. (1998) Portal venous thrombosis: percutaneous therapy and outcome. J Vasc Interv Radiol 9: 119–127.

45. Amarapurkar P, Bhatt N, Patel N, Amarapurkar D (2013) Primary extrahepatic portal vein obstruction in adults: A single center experience. Indian J Gastroenterol.

46. Garcia-Tsao G, Bosch J (2010) Management of varices and variceal hemorrhage in cirrhosis. N Engl J Med 362: 823–832.

47. Ponziani FR, Zocco MA, Garcovich M, D'Aversa F, Roccarina D, et al. (2012) What we should know about portal vein thrombosis in cirrhotic patients: a changing perspective. World J Gastroenterol 18: 5014–5020.

23

A Tri-Modality Image Fusion Method for Target Delineation of Brain Tumors in Radiotherapy

Lu Guo[1], Shuming Shen[1], Eleanor Harris[2], Zheng Wang[3], Wei Jiang[3], Yu Guo[1], Yuanming Feng[1,2]*

1 Department of Biomedical Engineering, Tianjin University, Tianjin, China, **2** Department of Radiation Oncology, East Carolina University, Greenville, North Carolina, United States of America, **3** Department of Radiation Oncology, Tianjin Huanhu Hospital, Tianjin, China

Abstract

Purpose: To develop a tri-modality image fusion method for better target delineation in image-guided radiotherapy for patients with brain tumors.

Methods: A new method of tri-modality image fusion was developed, which can fuse and display all image sets in one panel and one operation. And a feasibility study in gross tumor volume (GTV) delineation using data from three patients with brain tumors was conducted, which included images of simulation CT, MRI, and ^{18}F-fluorodeoxyglucose positron emission tomography (^{18}F-FDG PET) examinations before radiotherapy. Tri-modality image fusion was implemented after image registrations of CT+PET and CT+MRI, and the transparency weight of each modality could be adjusted and set by users. Three radiation oncologists delineated GTVs for all patients using dual-modality (MRI/CT) and tri-modality (MRI/CT/PET) image fusion respectively. Inter-observer variation was assessed by the coefficient of variation (COV), the average distance between surface and centroid (ADSC), and the local standard deviation (SD_{local}). Analysis of COV was also performed to evaluate intra-observer volume variation.

Results: The inter-observer variation analysis showed that, the mean COV was 0.14($\pm$0.09) and 0.07($\pm$0.01) for dual-modality and tri-modality respectively; the standard deviation of ADSC was significantly reduced ($p<0.05$) with tri-modality; SD_{local} averaged over median GTV surface was reduced in patient 2 (from 0.57 cm to 0.39 cm) and patient 3 (from 0.42 cm to 0.36 cm) with the new method. The intra-observer volume variation was also significantly reduced ($p = 0.00$) with the tri-modality method as compared with using the dual-modality method.

Conclusion: With the new tri-modality image fusion method smaller inter- and intra-observer variation in GTV definition for the brain tumors can be achieved, which improves the consistency and accuracy for target delineation in individualized radiotherapy.

Editor: Jian Jian Li, University of California Davis, United States of America

Funding: The authors have no support or funding to report.

Competing Interests: The authors have declared that no competing interests exist.

* Email: fengyu@ecu.edu

Introduction

Accurate target definition plays a crucial role in radiotherapy planning of brain tumors, especially, in the image guided radiotherapy (IGRT) which aims at reducing treatment volume toward target volume while ensuring coverage of target volume in all dimensions [1]. To avoid missing target, the intracranial cancerous tissue involvement must be correctly defined in the gross tumor volume (GTV) delineation. Oftentimes single imaging modality cannot provide sufficient information because of its inherent limitations of discriminating different brain soft-tissues or diseased tissues, and combination of different imaging modalities has to be utilized to get more comprehensive understanding of the disease and fulfill an accurate GTV delineation. Therefore, a proper integration of multiple information resources is necessary for the definition of intracranial tumor extension.

Studies showed that utilization of functional imaging techniques, such as ^{18}F-fluorodeoxyglucose positron emission tomog-

raphy (^{18}F-FDG PET), ^{18}F-fluoromisonidazole PET (^{18}F-FMISO PET), diffusion-weighted MRI (DW-MRI) and dynamic contrast-enhanced MRI (DCE-MRI) in addition to CT provides important value to radiotherapy treatment planning for head and neck squamous cell carcinoma (HNSCC) and early response assessment [2]. And in routine radiotherapy practice delineation of GTV for brain tumors relies upon CT or MRI images, or both. However, there are limitations in visualizing tumor and detecting anaplastic tissue with these two image modalities, which may lead to potential inaccuracy in the lesion definition at different steps of the brain tumor management [3]. For example, the conventional MRI is inefficient for the visualization of gliomatous tissue after therapy [4]. Interpretation of anatomical and functional information from multimodal images opens up new possibilities for optimization of the brain tumor treatment. It was shown that PET/MRI coregistration can significantly improve the sensitivity and specificity of ^{18}F-FDG in evaluating recurrent tumor and treatment-induced changes for brain tumor [5]. And the radiosurgery guided by the combination of MRI or CT and PET stereotactic images was proved to be valuable for treatment [6]. The GTV could be outlined with greater accuracy with the utility of CT, MRI and PET image fusion technique for target delineation in resected high-grade gliomas before radiotherapy [7]. Furthermore, Grosu et al showed that the composite CT, MRI and PET volumes could improve target volume definition and might further reduce inter-observer variability in stereotactic fractionated radiotherapy treatment planning for meningiomas and gliomas [8,9].

The dual-modality image fusion techniques provided in current radiotherapy treatment planning systems (TPS) can fuse and display two image sets in one panel and in one operation. And two fused image pairs will be displayed in two separate panels when using three image sets of different modalities, which is inconvenient for target definition.

A commercial system named Advantage Workstation (GE Healthcare, Milwaukee, WI) is recently available in radiology which can provide PET/CT + MR tri-modality image fusion in one application for optimized brain and body imaging. Although three image sets have been obtained, it displays at most two sets in one panel [10]. And there are not yet validation reports about this tri-modality image fusion technique for radiotherapy treatment planning of patients with brain tumors.

We recently developed a new tri-modality image fusion method which can fuse and display all image sets in one panel and one operation. Its effectiveness for brain tumor GTV delineation was quantitatively evaluated through comparative study with using the current dual-modality image fusion techniques. The method and feasibility study are presented in this report.

Materials and Methods

1. Image data acquisition

Image data of simulation CT, MRI, and ^{18}F-FDG PET-CT prior to radiation therapy from three patients were used in this study with the patients' written consents. The study and consent procedure were specifically approved by the ethics committee of Tianjin Huanhu Hospital and the authors had explicit permission to publish the patient brain images. Among the three patients, one (male, 69 years old) had high-grade glioma and two (one female and one male, 71 and 47 years old, respectively.) had brain metastasis tumors from their non-small cell lung cancer and thyroid carcinoma, respectively. None of these lesions had previously been resected.

CT image sets for radiation treatment planning for the patients was acquired using a Brilliance Big Bore CT (Philips Medical Systems) in supine and head first position. Total number of transverse slices was 224 with slice thickness of 2 mm, and field of view of 242×242 mm^2 and 224×224 mm^2 for the patient with gliomas and brain metastasis respectively.

PET-CT data were obtained with a Biograph64 PET-CT scanner (Siemens Medical Solutions). The applied dose of ^{18}F-FDG was between 246 and 296 MBq for the imaging studies. The patients were positioned supine with head first and 75 transverse images were acquired from a transmission scan of 3 and 4 min duration time for the patient with gliomas and brain metastasis respectively. The slice thickness was 3 mm, and axial field of view was 407×407 mm^2.

MRI data were obtained with a Magnetom Trio Tim scanner (Siemens Medical Solutions). With contrast medium of gadolinium-diethylenetriaminepentacetic acid [Gd-DTPA] (0.1 mmol/kg body weight), the axial, gradient echo T1-weighted sequences were acquired from the foramen magnum to the vertex (repetition time = 250 ms, echo time = 2.46 ms, imaging frequency = 123. 2 Hz, magnetic field strength = 3T, flip angle = 70°). The slice thickness was 2 mm, and field of view was 230×230 mm^2.

2. Image registration

Normally, the rigid bone of skull confines the brain tissue and leads to little significant non-rigid transformation between the different image sets. Therefore, three-dimensional (3D) rigid-body registration is sufficient for aligning those head image sets from different modalities to the same coordinate system. The rigid-body

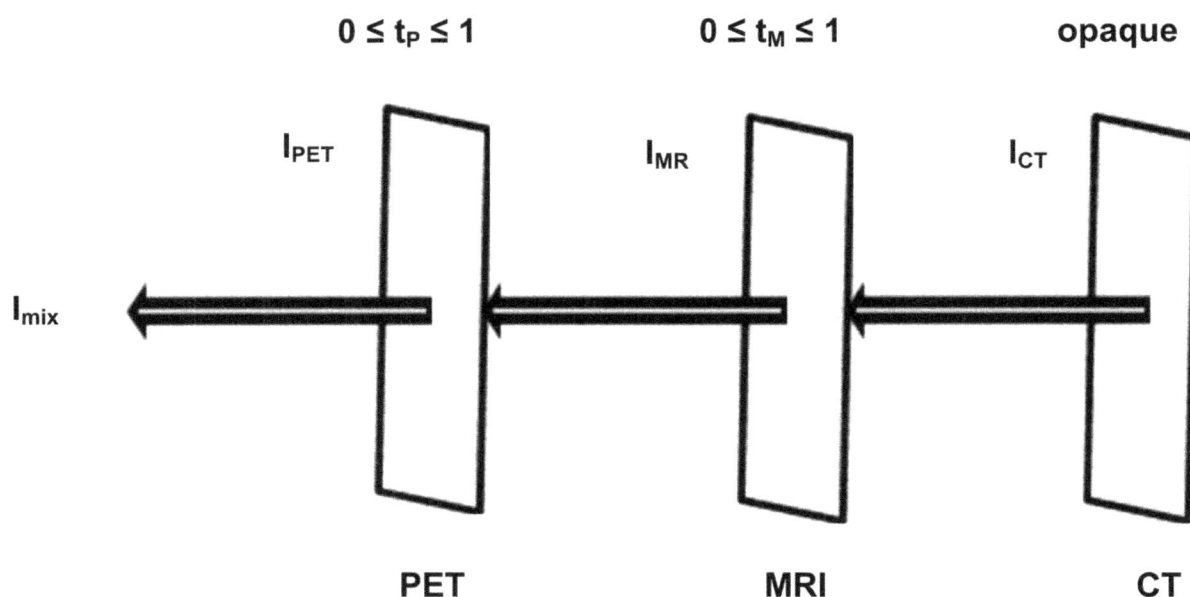

Figure 1. Illustration of tri-modality image fusion. The intensity value of a pixel in the fused image (I_{mix}) is determined based on the corresponding pixel's intensity values in CT, MRI, PET images (I_{CT}, I_{MRI}, I_{PET}).

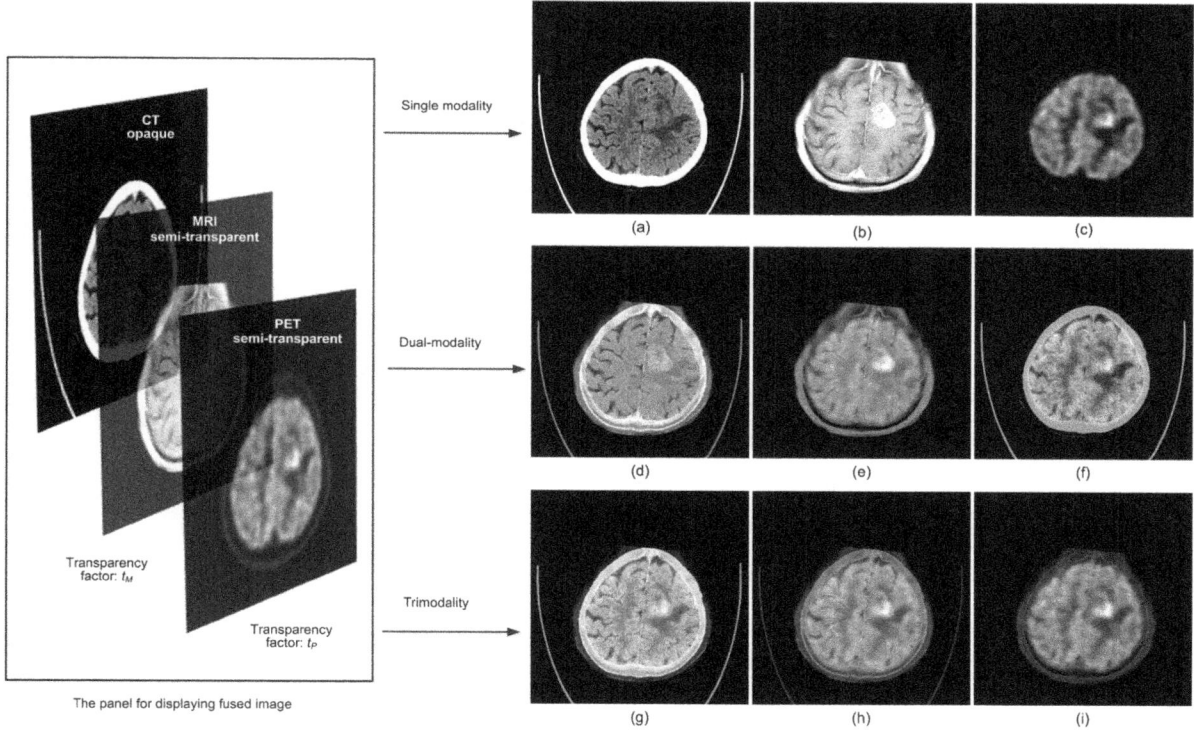

Figure 2. A glioma tumor shown on CT, MRI, and PET images with various t_P and t_M altering in the range of 0 to 1 for patient 1. (a) $t_P = 0$, $t_M = 0$; (b) $t_P = 0$, $t_M = 1$;(c) $t_P = 1$, $t_M = 0$; (d) $t_P = 0$, $t_M = 0.5$; (e) $t_P = 0.5$, $t_M = 1$;(f) $t_P = 0.5$, $t_M = 0$; (g) $t_P = 0.3$, $t_M = 0.3$; (h) $t_P = 0.5$, $t_M = 0.5$; (i) $t_P = 0.7$, $t_M = 0.7$.

registrations of CT+PET and CT+MRI were completed respectively with the automatic image registration tool of MIM 5.2 (MIM Software Inc., Cleveland, OH). Based on the mutual information measure, the software mapped the secondary image sets of PET and MRI to the primary image set of CT respectively. Subsequently, these aligned secondary image sets were imported into an in-house developed software for tri-modality image fusion.

3. New algorithm for tri-modality image fusion

In the study, we set CT image as the primary, background opaque surface and PET/MR images as the foreground semi-transparent surfaces. Based on the transparency model in computer graphics [11,12], we proposed a new algorithm for tri-modality medical image fusion which is illustrated in Figure 1 and expressed with Equation 1.

$$I_{mix} = t_P I_{PET} + (1 - t_P)[t_M I_{MR} + (1 - t_M)I_{CT}] \ 0 \le t_P, t_M \le 1 \quad (1)$$

Here I_{mix} is the intensity value of a pixel in the fused image; I_{PET}, I_{MR}, I_{CT} are the intensity values of the corresponding pixels in PET, MR, and CT images respectively; t_P and t_M are the transparency factor of PET and MR images, respectively, which can be adjusted by the user according to the desired transparency weight of each modality. The display of the fused image would vary along with the change of transparency factor (t_P, t_M). It provides a convenient tool for the user to look for target information over composite images of single modality, dual-modality, or tri-modality in one single panel (Figure 2).

4. GTV delineation

The same group of three radiation oncologists (observers) performed target delineation independently on the composite images of dual-modality image fusion (MRI/CT) and of tri-modality image fusion (MRI/CT/PET), respectively, using the contouring protocol published by Graf et al [13]. The GTVs were first contoured with CT and MRI image sets only and then corrected or re-delineated using the information from PET images. GTV delineation on CT, MRI, and PET was performed according to the following steps: (1) The contrast enhanced T1-weighted MRI images were used to define GTV_{MRI}. (2) CT images were adjusted to bone window and GTV_{MRI} was expand to enclose all tumor manifestation in CT or MRI images to obtain the $GTV_{MRI/CT}$, which was the tumor volume defined with dual-modality image fusion (CT/MRI). (3) Then, the GTV_{PET} was delineated on ^{18}F-FDG PET image set without referencing the $GTV_{MRI/CT}$. The window setting for ^{18}F-FDG-PET was made to optimize alignment between tumor margins on MRI/CT and ^{18}F-FDG-PET in area with tumor-to-normal brain tissue interface. (4) The overlapping region of $GTV_{MRI/CT}$ and GTV_{PET} was defined as GTV_{common} which encompassed the region with pathologic changes shown on all three image modalities (CT, MRI and PET image sets). (5) The volume of $GTV_{MRI/CT}$ located outside the region of enhanced 18F-FDG uptake was re-evaluated by the observers based on the information obtained from CT/MRI/PET image fusion. (6) Thereafter, a part of $GTV_{MRI/CT}$ was added to GTV_{common}. (7) The volume of GTV_{PET} located outside the region with pathologic changes shown on MRI/CT was re-evaluated in the same way. (8) Similarly, a part of GTV_{PET} was added to the GTV_{common}. (9) The final GTV ($GTV_{MRI/CT/PET}$) defined with tri-modality image fusion (CT/MRI/PET) consisted

Table 1. Comparison of GTV volumes defined by each observer with dual-modality image fusion (MRI/CT) and tri-modality (MRI/CT/PET) image fusion.

Patient	$GTV_{MRI/CT}$ (cm³)					$GTV_{MRI/CT/PET}$ (cm³)				
	Obs. 1	Obs. 2	Obs. 3	Mean	COV	Obs. 1	Obs. 2	Obs. 3	Mean	COV
1	19.91	22.72	20.47	21.03	0.07	17.91	19.82	17.69	18.47	0.06
2	14.39	17.01	13.94	15.11	0.11	12.61	14.09	13.27	13.32	0.06
3	2.96	2.92	1.82	2.57	0.25	1.89	1.92	1.64	1.82	0.08

GTV = gross tumor volume; Obs. 1 = observer 1; COV = coefficient of variation.

Table 2. Comparison of ADSC (in cm) for each patient and each observer using dual-modality (MRI/CT) fusion vs. tri-modality (MRI/CT/PET) fusion.

Patient	ADSC with Dual-modality					ADSC with Tri-modality				
	Obs. 1	Obs. 2	Obs. 3	Mean	SD	Obs. 1	Obs. 2	Obs. 3	Mean	SD
1	1.77	1.86	1.79	1.81	0.05	1.73	1.77	1.72	1.74	0.03
2	1.58	1.67	1.58	1.61	0.05	1.51	1.56	1.53	1.53	0.03
3	0.95	0.97	0.85	0.92	0.06	0.83	0.84	0.82	0.83	0.01

ADSC = the average distance between surface and centroid; Obs. 1 = observer 1; SD = standard deviation.

Table 3. SD_{local} (in cm) of GTV shape variation relative to the median GTV shape for each patient at eight quadrants and average over all vertex points on the median GTV.

Modality	Patient	Quadrants No.								Average over GTV
		1	2	3	4	5	6	7	8	
Dual-modality	Patient 1	0.38	0.39	0.56	0.37	0.47	0.45	0.47	0.42	0.44
	Patient 2	0.31	0.46	0.89	0.60	0.42	0.39	0.91	0.56	0.57
	Patient 3	0.50	0.41	0.32	0.39	0.69	0.42	0.27	0.30	0.42
Tri-modality	Patient 1	0.36	0.46	0.71	0.33	0.53	0.47	0.55	0.48	0.50
	Patient 2	0.32	0.35	0.39	0.35	0.33	0.34	0.66	0.44	0.39
	Patient 3	0.37	0.29	0.27	0.35	0.48	0.35	0.38	0.41	0.36

SD_{local} = local standard deviation; GTV = gross tumor volume.

of GTV_{common} and the added parts from $GTV_{MRI/CT}$ and GTV_{PET}. Thus, each observer defined two GTVs ($GTV_{MRI/CT}$ and $GTV_{MRI/CT/PET}$) for the same tumor of each patient in the two composite image sets, respectively.

5. Evaluation of inter-observer variation

5.1 Volume variation. To evaluate the inter-observer variation in the delineations of the GTVs with the schemes of dual-modality image fusion and tri-modality image fusion described in 2.4, GTV volumes of the tumors obtained by each observer were used and the coefficient of variation (COV) of the three volumes defined by the three observers with each scheme for each tumor were calculated and statistically analyzed [14]. COV is defined as the ratio of the standard deviation (SD) to the mean value. And SPSS Statistics 20.0.0. (SPSS Inc., Chicago, IL) was used for a paired sample two-tailed t test on COV to statistically measure the difference between the means for the two schemes. A two-side p value of less than 0.05 was considered to be significant.

5.2 Shape variation. A 3D shape was generated using the marching cubes (MC) algorithm [15] for each GTV involved in this inter-observer variation evaluation. Subsequently, the average distance between surface and centroid (ADSC) was calculated by averaging the distance of each triangle on the surface to its centroid. For each patient and each scheme, the mean and SD of ADSC of the three observers were calculated as a measurement of the inter-observer shape variation. The paired sample two-tailed t test was applied to evaluate the difference between using dual- and tri-modality image fusion methods.

Furthermore, a 3D median surface of GTVs delineated by the three observers was computed using Deurloo's method [16,17] for each patient and each scheme. The median surface was equal to the 50% coverage probability matrix of the three GTVs; in other words, all points in the median surface were determined at least by 50% observers. Afterwards, we calculated the perpendicular distance along the normal vector from each vertex point on the median surface to each GTV surface delineated by the observers. Three distances were obtained for each vertex point constructing the median surface. The standard variation of the three distances represents the local variation on the 3D surface and is called "local standard deviation (SD_{local})" which shows the level of variation in contouring details of GTVs. Subsequently, the median surface was divided into eight regions based on the eight quadrants of a new 3D coordinate system which moved the original point to the mean centroid of three individual GTVs. SD_{local} was averaged at eight regions and all vertex points on the median surface for each patient and each scheme.

6. Evaluation of intra-observer volume variation

The intra-observer variation in GTV volume definition was also investigated. Each GTV was contoured three times by the three observers, respectively. The averaged time interval between these three delineations was about two months. Totally, 54 GTVs were obtained for the analysis. Mean values and SDs of the GTV volumes and the COV were calculated, and the intra-observer variation was statistically analyzed.

Results

1. Inter-observer variation of GTV volumes

The volumes of GTVs for each patient defined by each observer, the mean values of the GTV volumes from the three observers, and the COV with the two schemes are summarized in Table 1. It can be seen that the volumes of GTVs defined with the first scheme varies more than the ones with the second scheme. All the mean values of

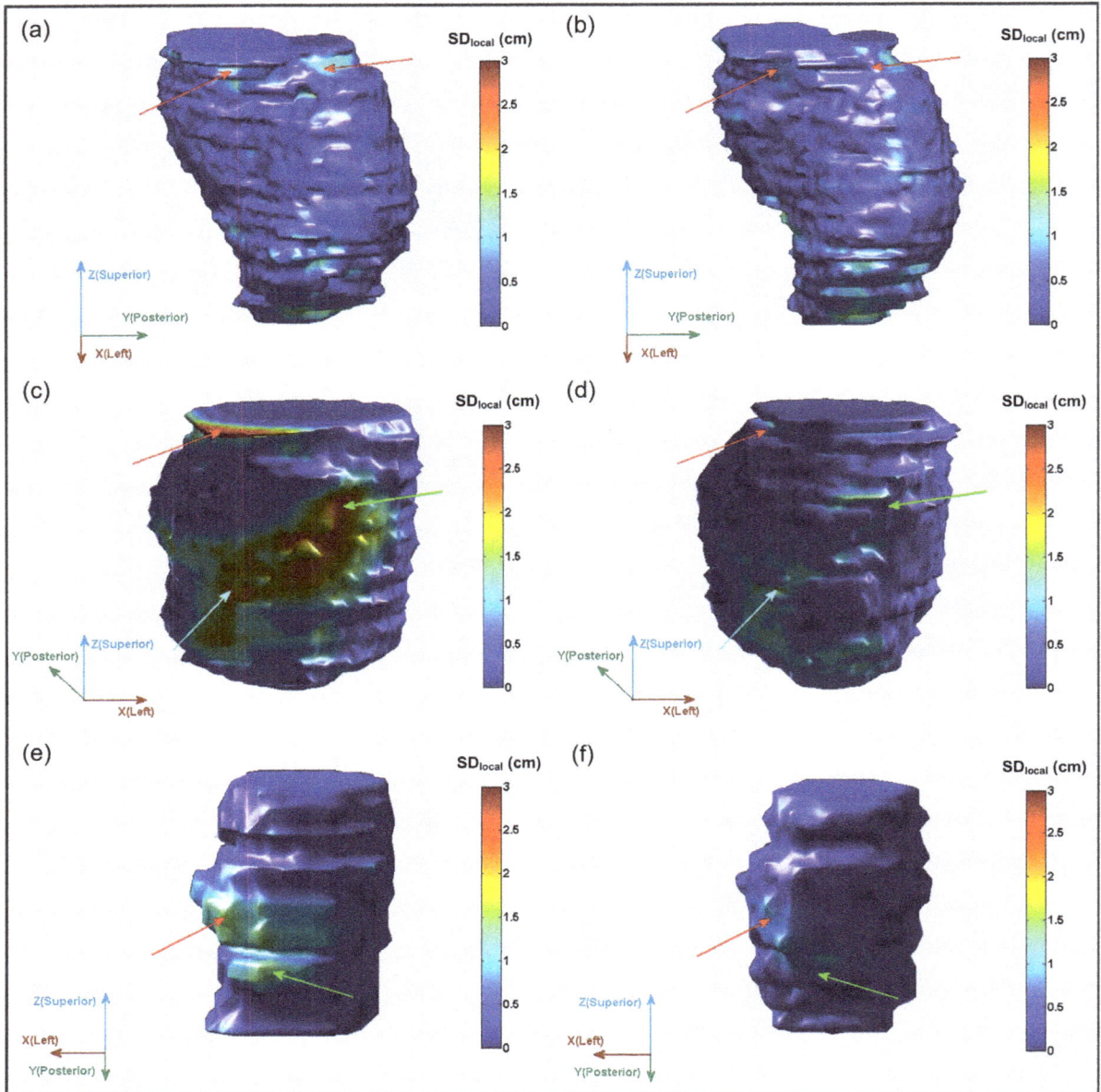

Figure 3. Comparison of the local standard deviation (SD$_{local}$) mapped onto the median surface of GTVs with dual-modality fusion (a, c, e) and GTVs with tri-modality fusion (b, d, f) in color wash (from blue [SD$_{local}$≤0.1 cm] to red [SD$_{local}$≥3 cm]). Red arrows in (a) and (b) point to the same region where SD$_{local}$ is partly reduced with the second scheme for patient 1. Red, green and light blue arrows in (c) and (d) point to the same regions of three quadrants where SD$_{local}$ is largely reduced with the second scheme for patient 2 (ΔSD$_{local}$≥0.2 cm). Red and green arrows in (e) and (f) point to the same regions of two quadrants where SD$_{local}$ is largely reduced with the second scheme for patient 3 (ΔSD$_{local}$≥ 0.2 cm in the area pointed by red arrows).

GTV volumes defined by the three observers are reduced with the second scheme. The mean COV is 0.14(±0.09) and 0.07(±0.01) for the first and second scheme, respectively, but there is no significant difference statistically ($p = 0.30 > 0.05$, 95% confidence interval of the difference is [−0.15, 0.31]), revealing that with the tri-modality image fusion the inter-observer volume variation is not significantly reduced.

2. Inter-observer variation of GTV shapes

The comparison of ADSC between the first and second scheme for each patient and observer is shown in Table 2. For all three cases, the means of ADSC with the second scheme are smaller than the ones with the first scheme. The SDs of ADSC is largely reduced with the second scheme in all cases. And the paired sample two-tailed t test shows that the reduction is statistically significant ($p < 0.05$, 95% confidence interval of the difference is [0.01, 0.05]), demonstrating that 3D shape variation between the GTVs defined by the three observers is significantly reduced with the new tri-modality image fusion method.

The SD$_{local}$ was averaged at eight quadrants and all vertex points on the median surface for each patient and each scheme (Table 3). For patient 1, SD$_{local}$ is partly reduced with the second

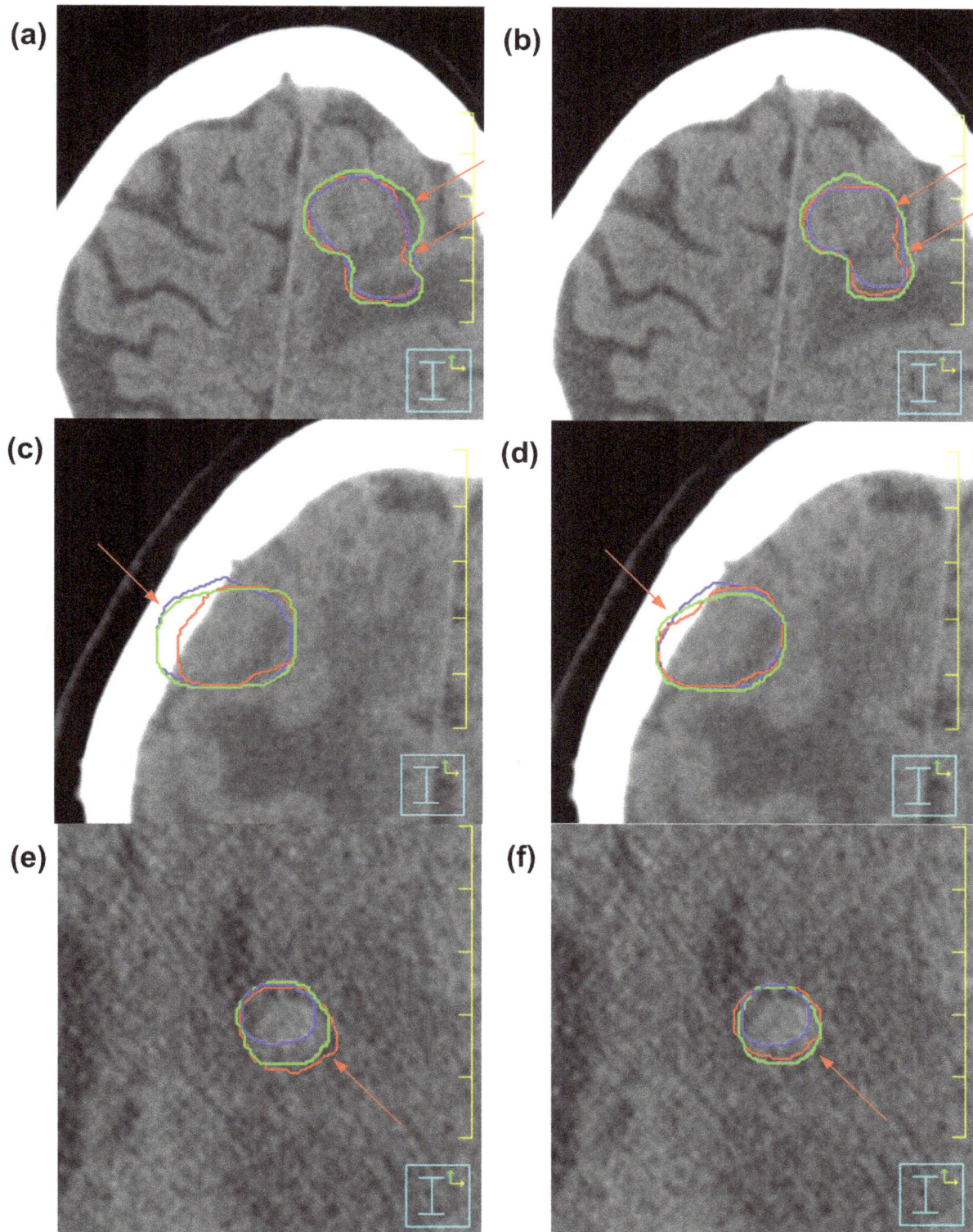

Figure 4. The GTVs delineated on axial slices of patient CT images by the three observers with dual-modality fusion (a, c, e) and tri-modality image fusion (b, d, f) methods, respectively. (a) and (b) are for patient 1; (c) and (d) are for patient 2; (e) and (f) are for patient 3.

scheme at quadrant No. 1 and No. 4. For patient 2, there are large reductions of SD_{local} at seven quadrants, especially at No. 3 ($\Delta SD_{local} = 0.5$ cm), No. 4 ($\Delta SD_{local} = 0.25$ cm), and No. 7 ($\Delta SD_{local} = 0.25$ cm). For patient 3, it is at six quadrants that the SD_{local} is reduced, especially at No. 5 ($\Delta SD_{local} = 0.21$ cm).

Table 4. Intra-observer comparison of GTV volumes obtained with dual-modality image fusion (MRI/CT) and tri-modality (MRI/CT/PET) image fusion.

Observer	Patient	GTV with Dual-modality		GTV with Tri-modality	
		Mean ± SD (cm³)	COV	Mean ± SD (cm³)	COV
Observer 1	Patient 1	21.52±1.48	0.07	17.15±0.68	0.04
	Patient 2	14.05±0.34	0.02	12.44±0.16	0.01
	Patient 3	2.64±0.29	0.11	1.87±0.02	0.01
Observer 2	Patient 1	22.52±1.00	0.04	19.76±0.31	0.02
	Patient 2	16.46±0.51	0.03	14.08±0.13	0.01
	Patient 3	2.79±0.12	0.04	1.94±0.02	0.01
Observer 3	Patient 1	20.28±0.96	0.05	17.55±0.47	0.03
	Patient 2	14.63±0.60	0.04	13.40±0.17	0.01
	Patient 3	1.99±0.16	0.08	1.66±0.02	0.01

GTV = gross tumor volume; COV = coefficient of variation; SD = standard deviation.

The median surfaces of GTVs onto which the SD_{local} was mapped in color for three patients are shown in Figure 3. Up to about 1 cm in SD_{local} has been observed with both schemes (Figure 3a and 3b) for patient 1. Whereas, there are two regions on which the SD_{local} is reduced obviously with the second scheme (the areas pointed with red arrows in Figure 3b). For patient 2, SD_{local} in a large part of areas (quadrant No. 3, No. 4, and No. 7 as indicated by red, green and light blue arrows respectively in Figure 3c) on the median surface of GTVs from the first scheme is larger than 1 cm and the maximum is larger than 3 cm. For the median surface of GTVs from the second scheme (Figure 3d), however, the maximum SD_{local} is 1.64 cm, much smaller than the former. For patient 3, up to 1.5 cm in SD_{local} is observed in two quadrants of the median surface of GTVs from the first scheme (Figure 3e) while the maximum SD_{local} of 1.15 cm over all vertex points on median surface is observed for the GTVs from the second scheme (Figure 3f).

Large reductions of inter-observer contouring variation in GTV delineation are also observed on axial slices of three patient CT images with the assistance of tri-modality image fusion as shown in Figure 4. The axial slices correspond to the same area in median surface as marked by the red arrows in Figure 3.

3. Intra-observer variation of GTV volumes

The mean value and SD of the three repeated GTVs determined by each observer for each patient, the COV with the two schemes are summarized in Table 4. Much smaller SD and COV values are observed with the second scheme than the ones with the first scheme in the results of all three observers' delineation for the patients. The mean of COV for all three observers is significantly reduced, from 0.05 (±0.03) with the first scheme to 0.02 (±0.01) with the second scheme ($p = 0.00$, 95% confidence interval of the difference is [0.01, 0.06]), revealing that the intra-observer volume variation is significantly reduced with the new tri-modality image fusion method.

Discussion

Our study has shown that the tri-modality image fusion method which integrates CT, MRI and ^{18}F-FDG-PET has positive impact on the radiotherapy treatment planning for brain tumors. The volume of GTV contoured for high-grade gliomas and brain metastasis can be reduced as compared with using dual-modality

(CT/MRI) image fusion. The inter-observer variation of GTV shapes (Figure 3, Figure 4 and Table 2) and the intra-observer variation in defining GTV volumes (Table 4) can be significantly reduced.

The interpretation differences between observers, derived from clinical experience, image interpretation skills, compliance to set guidelines, and treatment philosophy [14], were the major component of inter-observer variation in this study. The volume of GTV defined by observer 2 was larger than other two observers' for each patient and scheme (Table 1). The same trend could be found in Table 2 for the parameter of ADSC. Although variation in target definition existed among the observers even with the tri-modality method, the SDs of ADSC were significantly reduced as compared with using dual-modality method. These results indicate that contours can be drawn more consistently with the new tri-modality image fusion method and large reduction of the inter-observer difference can be achieved in GTV definition for brain tumors.

The new method provides convenience to observers in the operation for target delineation due to the adjustable transparency values of foreground images in one single panel, which has not been reported in published studies so far to our knowledge. With our in-house developed software tool, observers are able to view composite images in single modality, dual-modality, or tri-modality mode in one single panel. Observers can change the transparency factors (t_P, t_M) and gain various combinations of tri-modality images' information to facilitate a more comprehensive definition of final $GTV_{MRI/CT/PET}$. And the lessened intra-observer variation of GTV volumes (mean COV is 0.05 and 0.02 for dual- and tri-modality image fusion, respectively) in our study manifests the high reproducibility of results with this software.

Although a relatively small amount of raw data was used in this feasibility study because of the difficulty of getting image data of three modalities for the same tumor site, the results have shown potentials for utilizing three modality image data for the cases for which two image modalities cannot provide sufficient information in target definition for the brain tumors. When the tumor locates close to a critical normal structure or tissue, this method will be helpful for reducing uncertainty in tumor boundary definition and sparing the adjacent normal tissues, especially when high fractional dose and small margins around the tumor are applied.

Conclusion

With the tri-modality (CT/MRI/PET) image fusion method, the inter-observer variation in the delineation of GTV shapes and intra-observer variation in GTV volumes definition for the brain tumors can be reduced. This finding reveals the potential usability of this method for reducing uncertainty in brain tumor boundary delineation in radiotherapy treatment planning.

Author Contributions

Conceived and designed the experiments: YF LG. Performed the experiments: ZW WJ YG. Analyzed the data: LG SS YF. Contributed to the writing of the manuscript: LG YF EH.

References

1. Verellen D, Ridder MD, Storme G (2008) A (short) history of image-guided radiotherapy. Radiother Oncol 86(1): 4–13.
2. Dirix P, Vandecaveye V, De Keyzer F, Stroobants S, Hermans R, et al. (2009) Dose painting in radiotherapy for head and neck squamous cell carcinoma: value of repeated functional imaging with ^{18}F-FDG PET, ^{18}F-Fluoromisonidazole PET, diffusion-weighted MRI, and dynamic contrast-enhanced MRI. J Nucl Med 50(7): 1020–1027.
3. Goldman S (2011) PET for diagnosis and therapy of brain tumors. Médecine Nucléaire 35(5): 347–351.
4. Grosu A-L, Weber WA (2010) PET for radiation treatment planning of brain tumors. Radiother Oncol 96(3): 325–327.
5. Chen W (2007) Clinical applications of PET in brain tumors. J Nucl Med 48(9): 1468–1481.
6. Levivier M, Massager N, Wikler D, Lorenzoni J, Ruiz S, et al. (2004) Use of stereotactic PET images in dosimetry planning of radiosurgery for brain tumors: clinical experience and proposed classification. J Nucl Med 45(7): 1146–1154.
7. Grosu A-L, Weber WA, Riedel E, Jeremic B, Nieder C, et al. (2005) L-(methyl-^{11}C) methionine positron emission tomography for target delineation in resected high-grade gliomas before radiotherapy. Int J Radiat Oncol Biol Phys 63(1): 64–74.
8. Grosu A-L, Lachner R, Wiedenmann N, Stärk S, Thamm R, et al. (2003) Validation of a method for automatic image fusion (BrainLAB System) of CT data and ^{11}C-methionine-PET data for stereotactic radiotherapy using a LINAC: first clinical experience. Int J Radiat Oncol Biol Phys 56(5): 1450–1463.
9. Grosu A-L, Weber WA, Astner ST, Adam M, Krause BJ, et al. (2006) ^{11}C-methionine PET improves the target volume delineation of meningiomas treated with stereotactic fractionated radiotherapy. Int J Radiat Oncol Biol Phys 66(2): 339–344.
10. Veit-Haibach P, Kuhn F, Wiesinger F, Delso G, von Schulthess G (2013) PET–MR imaging using a tri-modality PET/CT–MR system with a dedicated shuttle in clinical routine. Magn Reson Mater Phy 26(1): 25–35.
11. Newell ME, Newell RG, Sancha TL (1972) A solution to the hidden surface problem. Proceedings of the ACM annual conference - Volume 1. Boston, Massachusetts, USA: ACM. 443–450.
12. Rogers DF (1998) Simple transparent models. In: Kane K, Jones EA, editors. Procedural elements for Computer Graphics. 2nd Edition. New York: McGraw-Hill. 498–500.
13. Graf R, Nyuyki F, Steffen IG, Michel R, Fahdt D, et al. (2013) Contribution of ^{68}Ga-DOTATOC PET/CT to target volume delineation of skull base meningiomas treated with stereotactic radiation therapy. Int J Radiat Oncol Biol Phys 85(1): 68–73.
14. Caldwell CB, Mah K, Ung YC, Danjoux CE, Balogh JM, et al. (2001) Observer variation in contouring gross tumor volume in patients with poorly defined non-small-cell lung tumors on CT: the impact of [18]FDG-hybrid PET fusion. Int J Radiat Oncol Biol Phys 51(4): 923–931.
15. Lorensen WE, Cline HE (1987) Marching cubes: A high resolution 3D surface construction algorithm. Siggraph Comput Graph 21: 163–169.
16. Deurloo KEI, Steenbakkers RJHM, Zijp IJ, de Bois JA, Nowak PJCM, et al. (2005) Quantification of shape variation of prostate and seminal vesicles during external beam radiotherapy. Int J Radiat Oncol Biol Phys 61: 228–238.
17. Steenbakkers RJHM, Duppen JC, Fitton I, Deurloo KEI, Zijp IJ, et al. (2006) Reduction of observer variation using matched CT-PET for lung cancer delineation: a three-dimensional analysis. Int J Radiat Oncol Biol Phys 64: 435–448.

24

Implementing Direct Access to Low-Dose Computed Tomography in General Practice—Method, Adaption and Outcome

Louise Mahncke Guldbrandt[1,2]*, Torben Riis Rasmussen[3], Finn Rasmussen[4], Peter Vedsted[1]

1 Research Centre for Cancer Diagnosis in Primary Care, Research Unit for General Practice, Aarhus University, Aarhus, Denmark, **2** Section for General Medical Practice, Department of Public Health, Aarhus University, Aarhus, Denmark, **3** Department of Respiratory Diseases and Allergy, Aarhus University Hospital, Aarhus, Denmark, **4** Department of Radiology, Aarhus University Hospital, Aarhus, Denmark

Abstract

Background: Early detection of lung cancer is crucial as the prognosis depends on the disease stage. Chest radiographs has been the principal diagnostic tool for general practitioners (GPs), but implies a potential risk of false negative results, while computed tomography (CT) has a higher sensitivity. The aim of this study was to describe the implementation of direct access to low-dose CT (LDCT) from general practice.

Methods: We conducted a cohort study nested in a randomised study. A total of 119 general practices with 266 GPs were randomised into two groups. Intervention GPs were offered direct access to chest LDCT combined with a Continuing Medical Education (CME) meeting on lung cancer diagnosis.

Results: During a 19-month period, 648 patients were referred to LDCT (0.18/1000 adults on GP list/month). Half of the patients needed further diagnostic work-up, and 15 (2.3%, 95% CI: 1.3–3.8%) of the patients had lung cancer; 60% (95% CI: 32.3–83.7%) in a localised stage. The GP referral rate was 61% higher for CME participants compared to non-participants.

Conclusion: Of all patients referred to LDCT, 2.3% were diagnosed with lung cancer with a favourable stage distribution. Half of the referred patients needed additional diagnostic work-up. There was an association between participation in CME and use of CT scan. The proportion of cancers diagnosed through the usual fast-track evaluation was 2.2 times higher in the group of CME-participating GPs. The question remains if primary care case-finding with LDCT is a better option for patients having signs and symptoms indicating lung cancer than a screening program. Whether open access to LDCT may provide earlier diagnosis of lung cancer is yet unknown and a randomised trial is required to assess any effect on outcome.

Trial Registration: Clinicaltrials.gov NCT01527214

Editor: Gary Collins, University of Oxford, United Kingdom

Funding: The project was supported by the Committee for Quality Improvement and Continuing Medical Education (KEU) of the Central Denmark Region, the Multi-Practice Committee (MPU) of the Danish College of General Practitioners (DSAM), the Danish Cancer Society, and the Novo Nordisk Foundation. Sponsoring organizations were not involved in any part of the study. The funders had no role in study design, data collection and analysis, decision to publish, or preparation of the manuscript.

Competing Interests: The authors have declared that no competing interests exist.

* Email: louise.mahncke@alm.au.dk

Background

Lung cancer is the leading cause of cancer death among men on a global basis. For women, it is the second leading cause of cancer death [1]. Annually, 4400 patients with lung cancer are diagnosed in Denmark [2]. Disease stage at diagnosis is an important prognostic factor as an advanced stage reduces the opportunity for curative treatment. Therefore, it is crucial to reduce the proportion of lung cancers diagnosed at an advanced stage; in Denmark, advanced-stage cancers account for 70% of all new lung cancers.

In order to reduce the time interval from the first presentation to the healthcare system until treatment, Denmark introduced a fast-track referral program for cancer in 2008 [3,4]. In this program, Danish general practitioners (GPs) can refer patients with "reasonable suspicion" of lung cancer to a fast-track evaluation, a maximum of 72 hours waiting time. Unfortunately, only 25% of Danish lung cancer patients are referred and diagnosed through this fast-track pathway, which is similar to the level of the UK [5–7]. Studies indicate that lung cancer patients have several pre-referral consultations in primary care [8,9]. This could be based on the fact that many lung cancer patients seem to present with unspecific, vague or low-risk-but-not-no-risk symptoms [10]. This implies that GPs needs additional tools than the fast-track in order to ensure early diagnosis of lung cancer. The answer could be direct access to a sensitive diagnostic investigation.

The principal diagnostic tool available for the GPs has for many years been a chest radiograph. However, since about 20% of all lung cancer patients have normal radiographs before diagnosis [11–13], a false negative radiograph may postpone the diagnosis [11]. Thus, an open direct access should perhaps be combined with a technological update in use of Computed Tomography (CT) technology.

In screening trials, low-dose CT is used under the presumptions that 1) lung cancer presents as non-calcified nodules, 2) low-dose CT accurately detects these nodules, and 3) detection of early-stage disease improves prognosis. From screening studies in high risk patients, we already know that approx. 27% of the first-round screened patients needed follow-up scans [14,15]. On the other hand, we do not know the same figures for symptomatic patients visiting their GP. Likewise, we do not know whether the GPs will use direct access to CT when offered the opportunity or (if positive) which patients they will refer. Such data should be available before chest LDCTs are introduced as a routine test for patients with respiratory symptoms.

The aim of this study was to describe the usage and outcome of a technological and organisational upgrade in the form of a brief GP update and implementing direct access to chest CT from general practice for patients with respiratory symptoms. Furthermore, to analyse the association between participating in the update, use of CT scans and referrals for lung cancer suspicion.

Methods

Design

We conducted a cohort study nested in a randomised controlled trial. A random group of GPs were offered a technological upgrade consisting of direct access to chest LDCT combined with a simple Continuing Medical Education (CME) meeting on lung cancer diagnosis.

Setting

The study took place in a large catchment area around Aarhus University Hospital in the Central Denmark Region during 19 months (November 2011 to June 2013).

Denmark has a tax-financed healthcare system with free access to medical advice and treatment in general practices and hospitals. GPs act as gatekeepers to specialized investigations and hospitals referrals.

Before November in 2011, the GPs in the area had three diagnostic work-up possibilities for patients with respiratory symptoms. They could either refer to 1) a chest radiograph 2) the Department of Pulmonary Medicine within normal waiting list or 3) a fast-track pathway. A valid indication for fast track was either an abnormal chest radiograph or certain symptoms (e.g. haemoptysis of >one week's duration or persistent coughing > four weeks). The GPs were not allowed to refer directly to a CT.

Participants

All GPs referring to the Department of Pulmonary Medicine. A total of 266 GPs organised into 119 general practices, were randomised into two groups. The unit of randomisation was the practice address. The randomisation was performed by a Data Manager using Stata 12.0. The 119 practices were allocated a random number between zero and one and then listed from lowest to highest value. The top 60 practice addresses formed the intervention group. In this paper, we include only the intervention group.

Intervention

Six times within an 3-month period, the intervention GPs were informed about the opportunity to refer their patients to a direct chest CT. The letters included information concerning the referral procedures and specific indications for CT requests. These indications embraced a wide range of concerns; the only exception was patients who met the indication for a fast-track referral. The idea was to let the GPs substitute the radiograph with a chest LDCT when wanting to rule out lung cancer.

The GPs were also invited to participate in one of eight offered 1-hour small-group-based CME meetings. The meetings were held during the initial two months. The content of the meeting focused on state-of-the-art knowledge on earlier detection of lung cancer. Algorithms for positive predictive values in primary care were used [10,16]. In addition, participants received information about the CTs, how to use them and how to interpret the reports.

Chest CT, review and lung cancer diagnosis

The Department of Radiology, Aarhus University Hospital, carried out the CTs. Scans were performed on a Brilliance 64 CT Scanner by Philips with a beam collimation of 64×0.625, 2 mm slice thickness, 1 mm increment, 1 pitch and a rotation time of 0.75 s. The effective radiation dose (Monte Carlo simulation program CT-Expo v. 2.1) was 2–3 mSv. Intravenous contrast medium was not administered. The time limit from referral to performed CT was a maximum of two working days.

The CT report was made by three sub-specialised radiologists. The day after the scan, the report combined with the patient's medical history resulted in a recommendation drawn up at a conference between radiologists and chest physicians. This recommendation was forwarded electronically to the GP, who was responsible for informing the patient of the results and referring the patient to further diagnostic work-up if necessary.

If lung nodules (4–10 mm), which could not be categorised as benign, were detected, the GP was responsible for referring the patient to a follow-up program (3, 6 or 12 months after the first scan) based on characteristics of the identified nodules [17]. The follow-up program was decided by the chest physicians.

If the CT scan revealed any suspicion of lung cancer, the patients were referred through the fast track to standard diagnostic work-up at the Department of Pulmonary Medicine by the GP. This included contrast enhanced multi detection CT (including PET/CT if surgery was an option). Furthermore, histologic/cytologic diagnosis was obtained by the least invasive method, which was usually either bronchoscopy with biopsies, fine needle aspiration (FNA) in association with endoscopic ultrasound or endobronchial ultrasound, or transthoracic FNA. The final staging was decided by a multi-disciplinary team based on clinical (cTNM) information. The lung cancers were staged according to the 7th TNM Classification of Malignant Tumors [18]. Early stage cancers were defined as stage I–IIB. Early stage patients were offered surgical resection according to Danish guidelines.

Sample size

The sample size was calculated for the randomised trial and the numbers of GPs needed in the intervention arm was guided by the calculation. In 2008, half of the Danish lung patients waited 34 days or more (the median) from first presentation to primary care until diagnosis of lung cancer [19]. We hoped to be able to show a decrease in the diagnostic interval to a level where only 25% of the patients had to wait for 34 days or more. Thus, the proportion waiting 34 days or more should be halved. With a one-sided alpha of 5% and a power of 80%, we had to include 54 lung cancer patients in each arm with a 1:1 randomisation. It can be assumed that lung cancer patients are randomly distributed among GPs. There could, however, be a higher incidence of cancer in some areas with many smokers and in practices with many elderly patients. To account for an unknown intra-cluster correlation coefficient (ICC), we counted on a design effect of 1.25 [20]. Given the design effect, we had to include a total of 54*2*1.25 = 135 lung cancer patients with questionnaire data and GP involvement in the diagnosis.

Outcome variables

Primary outcomes were characteristics of patients referred and GP variation in use, while secondary outcomes were amount of diagnostic work-up needed and cancer incidence. Finally, we examined the use of the fast-track referral option for suspected lung cancer and the proportion of lung cancer (the positive predictive value (PPV)) in order to evaluate the possible effect of the CME on this aspect.

Data

Based on the GPs' referral notes, we obtained data on the patients symptoms, known diseases and smoking history. We obtained the medical records resulting from completed CT scans, including the consensus evaluation between radiologist and pulmonary physician.

The Danish Lung Cancer Register (DLCR) was used for information on subsequent diagnosis of lung cancer (International Classification of Diseases 10: C34.0-9). The DLCR was established in 2001 as a national data-base. Since 2003, the registered data have covered more than 90% of all lung cancer cases in Denmark [21].

Patients referred to fast-track evaluation for lung cancer are coded DZ 03.1B (lung cancer observation). This code, combined with a unique GP number, gave information about referral to the fast-track pathway.

The Danish Cancer Registry (DCR) was used to obtain information about previous cancer (except non-melanoma skin cancer (C44)). The registry contains information about Danish cancer patients, their date of diagnosis and tumour characteristics. Since 1987, reporting to the DCR has been mandatory [22].

We used the Danish Deprivation Index (DADI) to gather information about deprivation rates in the different GP clinics. The index consists of eight variables resulting in a value number between 10 and 100; the higher the number, the greater the extent of deprivation in the practice population. The variables used are: (i) Proportion of adults aged 20–59 with no employment, (ii) proportion of adults aged 25–59 with no professional education, (iii) proportion of adults aged 25–59 with low income, (iv) proportion of adults aged 18–59 receiving public welfare payments (transfer income or social benefits), (v) proportion of children from parents with no education and no professional skills, (vi) proportion of immigrants, (vii) proportion of adults aged 30+ living alone and (viii) proportion of adults aged 70+ with low income (= the lowest national quartile).

The Health Service Registry was used to gather information about GP list size and age/gender distribution of the patients listed with the GP [23].

The Danish civil registration number, a unique personal identification number, was used to link registers [24].

Statistical analyses

Patient characteristics were described and duration of symptoms was calculated as medians with interquartile intervals (IQI). GP groups were compared using the Wilcoxon's rank-sum test for ordinal or continuous data or Pearsons χ^2 test for unordered or dichotomous categorical data.

Referral rates were calculated based on number of patients referred by the GP per project month per list size (patients aged 25 years and above). We used indirect sex-age standardisation to compare the referral rates between CME-attending GPs and non-attending GPs. We used the CME-attending GPs as the standard population and calculated the referral rates for the patients listed with the GPs in 10-years age groups (25–34, 35–44, etc.). These expected rates were then applied to the non-attending GP list. We calculated the standardized referral rate ratio as number of referrals divided by expected numbers if the age-sex specific rates were the same as those of the standard population. The age-sex referral rate was then obtained by multiplying the referral rate ratio by the crude referral rate of the standard population.

Data were analysed using the statistical software Stata 12.0 (StataCorp LP, TX, USA).

The protocol for the randomised trial and supporting TREND checklist for this study are available as supporting information; see Checklist S1 and Protocol S1.

Ethics

The study was approved by the Danish Data Protection Agency (ref.no: 2011-41-6872) and the Danish Health and Medicines Authority (ref.no: 7-604-04-2/357/KWH). According to the Research Ethics Committee of the Central Denmark Region, the Danish Act on Research Ethics Review of Health Research Projects did not apply to this project (ref.no: 118/2011) as CT is already a widely used technology.

Results

Patients referred

During the study period of 19 months, 649 patients were referred from general practice to direct CT. One patient (0.15%) did not turn up to the scan, resulting in 648 performed CTs. The mean age of scanned patients was 62.1 years (Standard Deviation (SD): 12.3, range: 21–95 years) (Table 1). The mean number of pack years for all smokers (current and former) was 34.5 (SD: 1.4, range: 2–100), and 87 (13.4%, 95% CI: 10.9–16.3%) had never smoked. The most prominent symptom was coughing (78.2%, 95% CI: 74.9–81.4%). The duration of symptoms varied from a median of 1.5 weeks (haemoptysis) to a median of 8.0 weeks (coughing) (Table 2). For 124 (19.1%, 95% CI: 16.2–22.4%) patients, a known lung disease (mostly COPD) was stated in the referral letter (Table 1).

GP participants

A total of 133 GPs had access to direct CT (Figure 1). The possibility was used by 91 (68.4%, 95% CI: 59.8–76.2%) of the GPs (Table 3). The highest absolute number of CT requests from a single GP was 40 (2 per project month), whereas most GPs referred two patients during the study period (median: 2.0, IQI: 0–5) (Table 3).

When we excluded the GPs who did not use the possibility of direct CT, the unadjusted GP referral rate was 0.18 per 1000 patients (≥25 years of age) per month.

There was no difference in GP age, gender, type of clinic (solo or more GPs together), list size or levels of deprivation in relation to the use of CT scans.

In total, 64 (48.1%, 95% CI: 39.4–56.9%) of the GPs participated in the CME meeting. The referral rate to direct CT was statistically significantly higher among GPs working in a clinic with one or more CME-participating GPs. When adjusting for age, gender and list size, the referral rate was 61% higher (95% CI: 54–66%) for GPs working in a clinic with one or more CME-participating GPs than the referral rate for non-participating GPs.

Table 1. Clinical characteristics of the 648 patients referred to direct CT scan from general practice.

	N	(%)[1]	Mean	(95% CI)
Gender:				
Male	314	(48.5)		
Female	334	(51.5)		
Age all	648		62.1	(61.2–63.1)
Age groups:				
20–45 yr	62	(9.6)		
46–65 yr	320	(49.3)		
66–95 yr	266	(41.1)		
Smoking status:				
Never	87	(13.8)		
Current	257	(40.7)		
Former	131	(20.7)		
Missing	157	(24.8)		
Pack years:				
All smokers	133		34.5	(31.6–37.3)
Current	89		38.1	(34.6–41.7)
Former	44		27.1	(23.0–31.2)
Known lung disease:				
All	124	(19.1)		
Previous cancer[2]:				
≥10 years	24	(3.7)		
<10 years	34	(5.2)		

[1]Of all patients.
[2]Listed in DCR before study start (either ≥10 years before study or within 10 years).

The study GPs referred 335 patients to the lung cancer fast-track during the study period, and this resulted in 33 lung cancer diagnoses (PPV 10.2%, 95% CI: 7.2–13.9%). The stage distribution was as follows 8 (23.5%, 95% CI: 10.7–41.2%) were in early stage and 26 (76.5%, 95% CI: 58.8–89.3%) with advanced disease. The unadjusted referral rate to fast-track was 0.13 per 1000 adults listed with the GP per month (95% CI: 0.09–0.20). The referral rate was 0.13 (95% CI: 0.09–0.19) for CME-participating GPs compared with 0.14 (95% CI: 0.09–0.20) for non-participating GPs (p-value: 0.503). The PPV for lung cancer diagnosis as a result of referral to a fast-track lung cancer pathway was 13.3% (95% CI: 8.7–19.1%) for CME-participating GPs and 6.1% (95% CI: 3.0–11.0%) for non-participating GPs (p-value: 0.027), which is equivalent to a 2.2 higher PPV.

Evaluation and conclusions

Of the 648 patients who underwent CT, 234 (36.1%, 95% CI: 32.0–40.0%) patients had a normal scan (Table 4), while lung nodules were found in 147 patients (22.7%, 95% CI: 19.5–26.1%). Cancer suspicion was raised in 84 (13.0%, 95% CI: 10.5–15.8%) of the scans, and suspicion of other lung diseases was raised in 200 (30.9%, 95% CI: 27.3–34.6%). For 301 (46.5%, 95% CI: 42.6–50.4%) patients, no further diagnostic work-up was needed.

A total of 177 (27.3%, 95% CI: 23.9–30.9%) patients received a referral to the Department of Pulmonary Medicine for further diagnostic work-up. Suspicion of disease outside the lungs was raised in 38 (5.9%, 95% CI: 4.2–8.0%) patients (Table 5).

Definitive diagnoses made from baseline scans

Thirty (4.6%, 95% CI: 3.1–6.5%) patients were diagnosed with a severe lung disease (tuberculosis, sarcoidosis or interstitial lung disease). Fifteen (2.3%, 95% CI: 1.3–3.8%) had a non-small cell lung cancer (NSCLC) and none had a small cell lung cancer (SCLC). Stage distribution was as follows: nine (60%, 95% CI: 32.3–83.7%) in early stage and six (40%, 95% CI: 16.3–67.7%) with advanced disease. Six (40.0%, 95% CI: 16.3–67.7%) were stage I tumours. Eight (1.2%) other cancers were diagnosed (three breast cancers, two lymphomas, one rectal cancer, one hepatocellular carcinoma and one mesothelioma).

Discussion

Main results

During the study period, 648 patients were referred to a direct LDCT. The most prominent symptom was coughing with a median duration of two months. Half of the patients needed further diagnostic work-up and 2.3% had lung cancer; 60% in early stage.

Two thirds of the GPs used the direct access to LDCT. CME-participating GPs had a 61% higher CT referral rate than non-participating GPs. CME participation was not associated with increased use of lung cancer fast-track pathways, but was, however, associated with a more than doubled positive predictive value.

Table 2. Symptoms written on referral letters of the 648 patients referred to direct CT scan from general practice.

	N	(%)[1]	Median	(IQI[2], min-max)
Focal symptoms:				
Cough	507	(78.2)		
Duration[3]	309		8	(6–12, 1–104)
Dyspnoea	170	(26, 2)		
Duration[3]	76		8	(5.5–12, 1–103)
Expectoration	165	(25.5)		
Duration[3]	69		8	(4–12, 1–104)
Thorax pain	90	(13.9)		
Duration[3]	46		4.5	(4–12, 1–52)
Haemoptysis	51	(7.9)		
Duration[3]	18		1.5	(1–3, 0–12)
Hoarseness	25	(3.9)		
Duration[3]	10		8	(4–6, 2–40)
General symptoms:				
Fatigue	85	(13.1)		
Duration[3]	42		6	(4–12, –26)
Weight loss	79	(12.2)		
Duration[3]	45		8	(4–12, 1–52)
Impaired general condition	48	(7.4)		
Duration[3]	18		4	(4–6, 2–40)

[1]Of all patients.
[2]Inter quartile interval.
[3]Duration in weeks. Some missing data.

Strength and limitations

A major strength of this study is the well-defined study population of a considerable size of patients. The data obtained from the referral letters and the CT records were complete as were data on GP participation in the CME on lung cancer.

However, a limitation is that we have no knowledge about the kind of diagnostic tool (e.g. plain chest film or fast-track) applied by the GP if (s)he had not had the opportunity of referral to direct CT scan.

The reported results are based on the baseline CT scan. A follow-up study is needed to gain information on lung cancers diagnosed from the repetitive CTs on nodule follow-up indications.

This study was not designed to answer whether a direct LDCT from general practice would reduce the mortality of lung cancer. A high proportion of the lung cancers diagnosed in this study were identified in an early stage, but this is not an advantage in itself. Early-state identification is beneficial only if the frequency of late-stage cancers is reduced, and this will be analysed in a randomised trial including all lung cancers in the study period.

The present study utilised low-dose CT as the diagnostic tool. For lung cancer, CT has a high sensitivity, but a lower specificity. This implies that the method involves risk of patient distress because of a relative high number of false positive scans. Furthermore, a widespread concern is the risk of cancer secondary to radiation from the low-dose CTs and subsequent imaging used to evaluate positive screens. A US study from 2013 addresses this problem in connection to low-dose CT screening studies [25]. Based on epidemiological data on radiation exposure they calculate that if assuming annual low-dose CT from age 55 to

age 74 (20 scans), the lifetime attributable risk of lung cancer mortality is estimated to be 0.07% for males and 0.14 for females. One single low-dose CT utilizes not even half of the total annual radiation exposure from natural and human made sources. In addition, the group of patients referred to a low-dose CT may be among those with a higher risk of having lung cancer or other important diseases and the small radiation dose may contribute only very little to the other risks these patients face.

Generalisability

This Danish single setting with complete inclusion of patients holds the opportunity to generalise the study results to other settings in Denmark, possibly even to other countries in which general practice serves as the first line of healthcare.

Comparison with other studies

In this study, symptomatic patients consulted general practice and the GP referred them to a direct CT scan; 2.3% of the patients were consequently diagnosed with lung cancer. In a US screening study (NLST) (2002–2004) including participants aged 55–74 with at least 30 pack-years [15], 1.1% had lung cancer at baseline. The authors reported 55% stage I cancers compared to 40% in our study. In the screening study, 27.9% of the patients needed follow-up scans. This is comparable to our numbers. Similar results were seen in the Danish randomized lung cancer CT screening trial (DLCST) (2004–2006) [26], which included participants aged 50–70 with at least 20 pack-years; 0.83% of the participants were diagnosed with lung cancers (53% in stage I).

Compared with the screening trials, our study had a wide and GP-based inclusion for referral. By limiting GP access to the CTs

Table 3. The characteristics of the GPs in the intervention group, their use of CT and participation in CME.

	All	CT not used	CT used	p-value	CME participant	Not CME participant	p-value
All GPs, No (%)	133	42 (31.6)	91 (68.4)		64 (48.1)	69 (51.9)	
Gender:							
Female, No (%)	65 (48.9)	18 (27.7)	47 (72.3)	0.358	31 (47.7)	34 (52.3)	1.000
Male, No (%)	68 (51.1)	24 (35.3)	44 (63.7)		33 (48.5)	35 (51.5)	
Age, mean (range)	53.6 (35–68)	54.2 (38–66)	53.4 (35–68)	0.613	54.2 (39–68)	53.1 (35–66)	0.456
Practice type:							
One GP, No (%)	21 (35.0)	11 (52.4)	10 (47.6)	0.090	8 (38.0)	13 (62.0)	0.107
Two or more GPs, No (%)	39 (65.0)	11 (28.2)	28 (71.8)		24 (61.5)	15 (38.5)	
Practice list size/GP Median (range)	1008 (585–2780)	997 (585–1503)	1012 (585–2780)	0.794	1056 (639–2780)	963 (585–1507)	0.080
Number of patients scanned:							
Per GP, Median (IQI)	2 (0–5)	0 (0–0)	3 (2–8)	<0.001	3 (1–9)	1 (0–3)	<0.001
Per practice, Median (IQI)[1]	6 (1–22)	0 (0–3)	17 (4–24)	<0.001	17 (4–23)	3 (0–4)	<0.001
Referral rate[2], Median (IQI)	0.10 (0–0.30)	0 (0–0)	0.18 (0.09–0.45)	<0.001	0.15 (0.05–0.59)	0.05 (0–0.18)	<0.001
DADI[3], Median (IQI)	25.4 (20.5–31.6)	26.5 (19.5–30.8)	25 (20.8–32.0)	0.947	24.1 (19.6–32.8)	26.0 (20.5–30.9)	0.920
CME:							
Participants	64 (48.1)	11 (17.2)	53 (82.8)	<0.001			
Age-sex adjusted referral rate[4]:					1	0.39	

[1]If one GP in a clinic has participated in CME, all GPs in that clinic will count as CME participants.
[2]Referral rate: patient referred/1000 patients in GP list (patients ≥25 years)/project months.
[3]Danish Deprivation Index (min: 10- max: 100).
[4]Referral rate adjusted for age and gender distribution in GP list (patients ≥25 years).

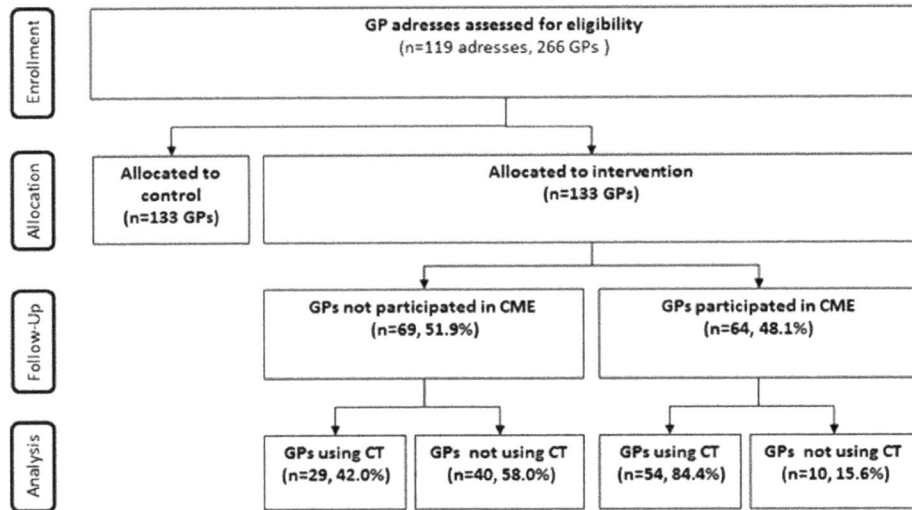

Figure 1. Participants (GPs) flow.

Table 4. The evaluation of the 648 CT scans performed during the study period.

	Number	(%) of all scans
All scans:	648	(100.0)
Evaluation:		
Abnormal scan:	414	(63.9)
Nodules	147	(22.7)
Cancer suspicion:		
All	84	(13.0)
Lung	71	(11.0)
Breast	6	(0.9)
Liver	1	(0.2)
Mesothelioma	3	(0.4)
Renal	2	(0.3)
Occult	1	(0.2)
Lung disease suspicion:		
All	200	(30.9)
Pneumonia	81	(12.5)
Pulmonary fibrosis	69	(10.6)
Emphysema	44	(6.8)
Bronchiectasis	19	(2.9)
Tuberculosis	6	(0.9)
Suspicion of other diseases:		
All	119	(18.4)
Enlarged lymph nodes	52	(8.1)
Liver[1]	32	(4.9)
Bone[2]	21	(3.2)
Biliary[3]	9	(1.4)
Pancreas[4]	5	(0.8)

[1]Lever disease: all focal changes; cysts/metastases observation.
[2]Bone: 13 fracture obs., 1 Mb Bechterew obs., 3 metasteses obs.
[3]Billiary: All cholecystelithiasis obs.
[4]Pancreas: 3 chronic pancreatitis.

Table 5. The conclusion and diagnosis of the 648 CT scans performed during the study period.

	Number	(%) of all scans
All scans:	648	(100.0)
Conclusions:		
No further	301	(46.5)
Pulmonary medicine	177	(27.3)
CT scan (3 month after)	84	(13.0)
CT scan (6 month after)	23	(3.5)
CT scan (12 month after)	51	(7.9)
Other department	38	(5.9)
Treatment by GP	15	(2.3)
Diseases lung:	Number all/new diagnoses[1]	
All	93	(14.4)
Tuberculosis	5/5	(0.8/0.8)
Sarcoidosis	8/7	(1.2/1.1)
Interstitiel	17/17	(2.6/2.6)
Emphysema	44/29	(6.8/4.5)
Bronchiectasis	19/19	(2.9/2.9)
Lung cancer:		
All	15	(2.3)
NSCLC	15	(100.0)[2]
Local	9	(60.0)[2]
Metastatic	6	(40.0)[2]
Other cancer:		
All	8	(1.2)

[1]All lung disease diagnoses were new, except for 15 patients with emphysema and one patient with sarcoidosis (they had the diagnosis before the CT).
[2]Of all lung cancers diagnosed in the study.

with specific criteria (e.g. smokers or age above 50 years), the proportion of lung cancers diagnosed in our study would probably have been higher. However, the non-limited access shows the actual use and outcome when direct access is implemented. The fact that we found 40% stage I cancers in symptomatic patient could be due to an increased awareness of early signs of cancer among GPs in combination with easy access to a direct test.

The frequency of lung cancer was lower among patients referred directly to LDCT than for those referred to the lung cancer fast-track pathway. This indicates that the patients referred to a direct CT are a subgroup of patients with less pronounced symptoms and thus with a lower risk that the symptoms were due to cancer. Patients with "low, but not no risk" may be the ones who most GPs find difficult to handle in primary care. This is also supported by the higher PPV for cancer in the fast-track pathway for CME-participating GPs. We cannot make any causal inference of the associations found as these may be due to comparison of simply two different groups of GPs. However, our results may also indicate an effect of the CME and a changed pattern in use of direct access to CT, which can only be evaluated in an experimental design.

A Danish study found that a strategy with straight-to-test to CT for patients in the lung cancer fast-track was associated with high levels of staff acceptability and a reduction of chest physician time per patient without changing the numbers of performed CTs [27]. This implies that GPs are able to use CTs in a reasonably way.

This is, in this present study, supported by the low overall referral rate.

In terms of variation we found no association between GP characteristics (age, gender, type of clinic, list size or levels of deprivation) and the use of CTs. A review from Scotland concluded that variation in GP referral rates in general is largely unexplained [28]. The study suggests that GPs with an interest or training in a particular field had a higher referral rate in that specialty. This may be the reason for the higher referral rate among GPs who participated in the CME. However, we can make no causal inference as these findings may be related to selection bias.

Conclusion

In a cohort study on direct CT referral from general practice, we found an overall referral rate of 0.10/1000 adults/month. Two-thirds of the GPs used the open access CT option. An association was found between participation in a lung cancer CME and direct referral to CT. An association was also found between GP participation in a CME on lung cancer diagnosis and a higher PPV of lung cancer when referring to the fast-track pathway compared to non-participating GPs.

Among patients referred to a CT, the proportion of lung cancers was 2.3%, 1.2% had other cancers and 14.4% had a non-malignant serious lung disease. The CTs resulted in 53.5% in need of additional diagnostic work-up or follow-up scans. Whether the open access to chest CT will result in earlier diagnosis and better prognosis of lung cancer is yet unknown, and a randomised trial is required to assess any effect on outcome. The results from the randomised trial are under preparation for publication and the authors have planned a two year follow-up on the 648 patients scanned in this study in regard to additional diagnoses as well as further diagnostic procedures. The question remains whether case-finding with LDCT in primary care is a better option for patients having signs and symptoms indicating lung cancer than a screening program. Furthermore, if low-dose CT screening is recommended, a consideration is whether a direct LDCT option from primary care should be implemented as well for patients who are not screened.

References

1. Jemal A, Bray F, Center MM, Ferlay J, Ward E, et al. (2011) Global cancer statistics. CA Cancer J Clin 61: 69–90.
2. Engholm G, Ferlay J, Christensen N, Bray F, Gjerstorff ML, et al. (2010) NORDCAN–a nordic tool for cancer information, planning, quality control and research. Acta Oncol 49: 725–736.
3. Olesen F, Hansen RP, Vedsted P (2009) Delay in diagnosis: The experience in denmark. Br J Cancer 101: S5–S8.
4. Probst HB, Hussain ZB, Andersen O (2012) Cancer patient pathways in denmark as a joint effort between bureaucrats, health professionals and politicians-A national danish project. Health Policy 105: 65–70.
5. Barrett J, Hamilton W (2008) Pathways to the diagnosis of lung cancer in the UK: A cohort study. BMC Fam Pract 9: 31.
6. Elliss-Brookes L, McPhail S, Ives A, Greenslade M, Shelton J, et al. (2012) Routes to diagnosis for cancer - determining the patient journey using multiple routine data sets. Br J Cancer 107: 1220–1226.
7. Neal RD, Allgar VL, Ali N, Leese B, Heywood P, et al. (2007) Stage, survival and delays in lung, colorectal, prostate and ovarian cancer: Comparison between diagnostic routes. Br J Gen Pract 57: 212–219.
8. Lyratzopoulos G, Neal RD, Barbiere JM, Rubin GP, Abel GA (2012) Variation in number of general practitioner consultations before hospital referral for cancer: Findings from the 2010 national cancer patient experience survey in england. Lancet Oncol.
9. Lyratzopoulos G, Abel GA, McPhail S, Neal RD, Rubin GP (2013) Measures of promptness of cancer diagnosis in primary care: Secondary analysis of national audit data on patients with 18 common and rarer cancers. Br J Cancer 108: 686–690. 10.1038/bjc.2013.1 [doi].
10. Hamilton W, Peters TJ, Round A, Sharp D (2005) What are the clinical features of lung cancer before the diagnosis is made? A population based case-control study. Thorax 60: 1059–1065.
11. Bjerager M, Palshof T, Dahl R, Vedsted P, Olesen F (2006) Delay in diagnosis of lung cancer in general practice. Br J Gen Pract 56: 863–868.
12. Quekel LG, Kessels AG, Goei R, van Engelshoven JM (1999) Miss rate of lung cancer on the chest radiograph in clinical practice. Chest 115: 720–724.
13. Stapley S, Sharp D, Hamilton W (2006) Negative chest X-rays in primary care patients with lung cancer. Br J Gen Pract 56: 570–573.
14. Midthun DE, Jett JR (2013) Screening for lung cancer: The US studies. J Surg Oncol.
15. National Lung Screening Trial Research Team, Church TR, Black WC, Aberle DR, Berg CD, et al. (2013) Results of initial low-dose computed tomographic screening for lung cancer. N Engl J Med 368: 1980–1991.
16. Hamilton W (2009) The CAPER studies: Five case-control studies aimed at identifying and quantifying the risk of cancer in symptomatic primary care patients. Br J Cancer 101 Suppl 2: S80–6.: S80–S86.
17. MacMahon H, Austin JH, Gamsu G, Herold CJ, Jett JR, et al. (2005) Guidelines for management of small pulmonary nodules detected on CT scans: A statement from the fleischner society. Radiology 237: 395–400.
18. Goldstraw P, Crowley J, Chansky K, Giroux DJ, Groome PA, et al. (2007) The IASLC lung cancer staging project: Proposals for the revision of the TNM stage groupings in the forthcoming (seventh) edition of the TNM classification of malignant tumours. J Thorac Oncol 2: 706–714.
19. Hansen RP, Vedsted P, Sokolowski I, Sondergaard J, Olesen F (2011) Time intervals from first symptom to treatment of cancer: A cohort study of 2,212 newly diagnosed cancer patients. BMC Health Serv Res 11: 284.
20. Campbell MK, Elbourne DR, Altman DG (2004) CONSORT statement: Extension to cluster randomised trials. BMJ 328: 702–708.
21. Jakobsen E, Palshof T, Osterlind K, Pilegaard H (2009) Data from a national lung cancer registry contributes to improve outcome and quality of surgery: Danish results. Eur J Cardiothorac Surg 35: 348–352.
22. Gjerstorff ML (2011) The danish cancer registry. Scand J Public Health 39: 42–45.
23. Andersen JS, Olivarius Nde F, Krasnik A (2011) The danish national health service register. Scand J Public Health 39: 34–37.
24. Pedersen CB (2011) The danish civil registration system. Scand J Public Health 39: 22–25.
25. Frank L, Christodoulou E, Kazerooni EA (2013) Radiation risk of lung cancer screening. Semin Respir Crit Care Med 34: 738–747. 10.1055/s-0033-1358615 [doi].
26. Pedersen JH, Ashraf H, Dirksen A, Bach K, Hansen H, et al. (2009) The danish randomized lung cancer CT screening trial–overall design and results of the prevalence round. J Thorac Oncol 4: 608–614. 10.1097/JTO.0b013 e3181a0d98f.
27. Guldbrandt LM, Fenger-Gron M, Folkersen BH, Rasmussen TR, Vedsted P (2013) Reduced specialist time with direct computed tomography for suspected lung cancer in primary care. Dan Med J 60: A4738. A4738 [pii].
28. O'Donnell CA (2000) Variation in GP referral rates: What can we learn from the literature? Fam Pract 17: 462–471.

Acknowledgments

We thank the Department of Radiology at Aarhus University Hospital for contribution with the CTs and the Department of Pulmonary Medicine at Aarhus University Hospital for the clinical evaluation of the scans.

Author Contributions

Conceived and designed the experiments: LMG TRR FR PV. Performed the experiments: LMG TRR FR PV. Analyzed the data: LMG PV. Contributed reagents/materials/analysis tools: FR. Wrote the paper: LMG PV FR TRR.

25

Prognostic Significance of Tumor Size of Small Lung Adenocarcinomas Evaluated with Mediastinal Window Settings on Computed Tomography

Yukinori Sakao[1,2]*, Hiroaki Kuroda[1,2], Mingyon Mun[1], Hirofumi Uehara[1], Noriko Motoi[3],
Yuichi Ishikawa[3], Ken Nakagawa[1], Sakae Okumura[1]

1 Department of Thoracic Surgical Oncology, Cancer Institute Hospital, Japanese Foundation for Cancer Research, Tokyo, Japan, 2 Department of Thoracic Surgery, Aichi Cancer Center Hospital, Nagoya, Japan, 3 Department of Pathology, Cancer Institute Hospital, Japanese Foundation for Cancer Research, Tokyo, Japan

Abstract

Background: We aimed to clarify that the size of the lung adenocarcinoma evaluated using mediastinal window on computed tomography is an important and useful modality for predicting invasiveness, lymph node metastasis and prognosis in small adenocarcinoma.

Methods: We evaluated 176 patients with small lung adenocarcinomas (diameter, 1–3 cm) who underwent standard surgical resection. Tumours were examined using computed tomography with thin section conditions (1.25 mm thick on high-resolution computed tomography) with tumour dimensions evaluated under two settings: lung window and mediastinal window. We also determined the patient age, gender, preoperative nodal status, tumour size, tumour disappearance ratio, preoperative serum carcinoembryonic antigen levels and pathological status (lymphatic vessel, vascular vessel or pleural invasion). Recurrence-free survival was used for prognosis.

Results: Lung window, mediastinal window, tumour disappearance ratio and preoperative nodal status were significant predictive factors for recurrence-free survival in univariate analyses. Areas under the receiver operator curves for recurrence were 0.76, 0.73 and 0.65 for mediastinal window, tumour disappearance ratio and lung window, respectively. Lung window, mediastinal window, tumour disappearance ratio, preoperative serum carcinoembryonic antigen levels and preoperative nodal status were significant predictive factors for lymph node metastasis in univariate analyses; areas under the receiver operator curves were 0.61, 0.76, 0.72 and 0.66, for lung window, mediastinal window, tumour disappearance ratio and preoperative serum carcinoembryonic antigen levels, respectively. Lung window, mediastinal window, tumour disappearance ratio, preoperative serum carcinoembryonic antigen levels and preoperative nodal status were significant factors for lymphatic vessel, vascular vessel or pleural invasion in univariate analyses; areas under the receiver operator curves were 0.60, 0.81, 0.81 and 0.65 for lung window, mediastinal window, tumour disappearance ratio and preoperative serum carcinoembryonic antigen levels, respectively.

Conclusions: According to the univariate analyses including a logistic regression and ROCs performed for variables with p-values of <0.05 on univariate analyses, our results suggest that measuring tumour size using mediastinal window on high-resolution computed tomography is a simple and useful preoperative prognosis modality in small adenocarcinoma.

Editor: Prasad S. Adusumilli, Memorial Sloan-Kettering Cancer Center, United States of America

Funding: The authors received no specific funding for this work.

Competing Interests: The authors have declared that no competing interests exist.

* Email: ysakao@aichi-cc.jp

Introduction

We previously reported that the size of lung adenocarcinoma, evaluated using mediastinal window (MD) settings on computed tomography (CT), is a more important predictive prognosis factor than the total tumour size, evaluated using lung window (LD) settings [1] Various studies have documented the correlation between CT findings and the pathological features of lung adenocarcinoma [2–4]. The ground glass opacity (GGO) component is typically recognized as a bronchioloalveolar carcinoma

(BAC) component on microscopic examination, and the BAC is now categorized as an adenocarcinoma in situ that does not affect tumour aggressiveness [5,6]. In contrast, the solid component recognized as invasive lesion being so called scar, which excludes the BAC component in lepidic predominant adenocarcinoma, can be easily defined using MD settings on CT [1,2,5]. Moreover, the solid tumour recognized as a non-lepidic predominant adenocarcinoma, such as acinar, papillary, solid predominant or micropapillary predominant adenocarcinomas, is recognized as invasive adenocarcinoma and shows much more aggressiveness than that by lepidic predominant adenocarcinoma [2,5,7]. Therefore, we have emphasized the importance of determining the size of the solid tumour component in adenocarcinoma using MD settings when evaluating tumour aggressiveness [1,2,5].

This investigation aimed to clarify the importance of the tumour size evaluated by MD settings as a preoperative prognostic predictive factor for anatomical pulmonary resection in patients with small adenocarcinomas (1–3 cm). Furthermore, we would clarify that the preoperative evaluation of tumour diameter by CT with MD settings would enable the prediction of prognosis, lymph node metastasis and tumour invasiveness for patients with clinically early-stage tumours.

Materials and Methods

This was a retrospective study conducted between October 2003 and December 2008 in patients with small lung adenocarcinomas (diameters of ≤3 cm) that underwent standard surgical resections (lobectomy with hilar and mediastinal lymph node dissection) at the Cancer Institute Hospital.

Tumour dimension was evaluated under two different CT imaging conditions: LD [level = −500 Hounsfield unit (HU), width = 1500 HU] and MD (level = 60, width = 350 HU). The CT (multi-detector CT, Toshiba, Japan) images were evaluated for the maximum tumour dimension.

Tumour disappearance ratio (TDR) was defined as 1− MD/ LD.

"For all patients, preoperative staging was assessed using chest CT, CT or ultrasonography for abdominal metastasis, brain CT or magnetic resonance imaging for the brain metastasis and bone scanning for bone metastasis."

Clinical mediastinal and hilar lymph node status was deemed positive if the chest CT findings revealed a lymph node short axis of >1.0 cm. The status of mediastinal, hilar or interlobar nodes was assessed according to the classification for lung cancer in the TNM Classification of Malignant Tumours, Seventh Edition [8]. The CT findings were reviewed by two independent radiologists

We excluded tumours comprising 100% GGO from this study because most of them were believed, on microscopic examination, to be non-invasive or precancerous lesions. The GGO component was defined as hazy and amorphous with increased lung

attenuation, but without obscuration of the underlying vascular markings and bronchial walls. In addition, we excluded a subgroup with BAC or mucinous BAC on microscopic examination that were defined as adenocarcinoma in situ [6]. We also excluded tumours measuring <1 cm because they were few in number and did not undergo standard resections. To select this cohort, the tumour size was used measured by two independent radiologists with CT in LD. Of total 246 patients with small lung adenocarcinomas (diameters of ≤3 cm) who underwent standard surgical resections, 36 were excluded due to lack of thin slice data in CT, 24 were excluded due to adenocarcinoma in situ and 10 were excluded due to size smaller than 1 cm. Therefore, 176 patients were examined in this study.

Patient records were examined for age, gender, preoperative nodal status and tumour size, as evaluated using both MD and LD. Preoperative serum carcinoembryonic antigen (CEA) levels, TDR and pathological status were evaluated using elastic stain, and included lymphatic vessel (ly), vascular vessel (v) and pleural (pl) invasion.

Because individual patients were not identified, our institutional review board (Review Board in Cancer Institute Hospital, Japanese Foundation for Cancer Research) approved this study without the requirement to obtain patient consent. The patient records/information was anonymized and de-identified prior to analysis.

Statistical Analyses

Disease-free survival was assessed. Survival duration was defined as the interval between surgery and either tumour relapse or the most recent follow-up. The Kaplan–Meier method was used to calculate the recurrence-free survival rates. Univariate analyses included a log-rank test, chi-square test and logistic regression. Receiver operating characteristic analyses (ROC) were performed for variables with P-values of <0.05 on univariate analysis using the logistic regression test or the Cox proportional hazards model. All analyses were performed using the JMP 10 software (SAS Institute Incorporated, Cary, North Carolina) and results with P-values of <0.05 were considered statistically significant.

Results

In total, 176 patients were enrolled. This subgroup that excluded BAC and small tumours (<1 cm) comprised 99 females and 77 males, with ages ranging from 34 to 78 (median = 61)

Table 1. Preoperative prognostic factors for disease-free survival with small adenocarcinomas (≤3 cm).

Variables	Odds ratio	95% CI	P value
Gender (female)	0.61	0.34–1.07	.08
Age	0.99	0.97–1.03	.74
LD	1.08	1.02–1.14	.007
MD	1.13	1.08–1.18	<.001
TDR	38.6	7.35–	<.001
CEA	0.33	0.99–1.03	.33
High (>5 ng/ml)/normal)	1.89	0.96–3.72	.066
cN (cN0/cN1-2)	0.23	0.11–0.50	<.001

Logistic regression test (Univariate analyses).
LD: diameter using lung window setting, MD: diameter using mediastinal window setting, RFS: recurrence-free survival, TDR: tumour disappearance ratio (TDR = 1− MD/LD), CEA: carcinoembryonic antigen, cN: preoperative nodal status, CI: confidence interval.

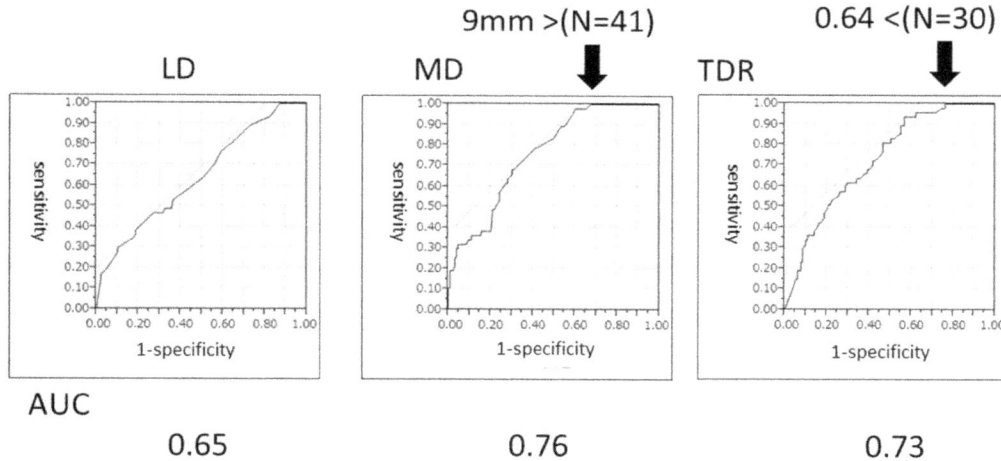

Figure 1. Receiver operating characteristic analyses for recurrence. Tumour dimension was evaluated using lung window (LD) and mediastinal window (MD) settings. TDR: tumour disappearance ratio (TDR $= 1-$ MD/LD). Allow indicated a value at 100% sensitivity.

years. The follow-up periods ranged from 24–84 (median $= 49$) months.

Preoperative prognostic factors for disease-free survival

As shown in Table 1, LD findings, MD findings, TDR and nodal status (cN) were significant prognostic factors for disease-free survival on univariate analyses. The AUCs for recurrence were 0.76, 0.73 and 0.65, for MD, TDR and LD, respectively (Figure 1).The 5-year disease-free survival rates according to MD were 98.1% for $\leq$10 mm (N $= 52$), 71.0% for 11–$\leq$15 mm (N $= 52$) and 49.0% for>15 mm (N $= 72$). (P<0.001) (Figure 2).

Preoperative Factors Associated with Lymph Node Metastasis

As shown in Table 2, LD findings, MD findings, TDR, CEA levels and cN were significant factors associated with lymph node metastasis on univariate analyses. The area under the curves (AUCs) for lymph node metastases were 0.61, 0.76, 0.72 and 0.66 for LD, MD, TDR and CEA, respectively (Figure 3). The incidence of lymph node metastases according to MD were 0% for <10 mm (N $= 52$), 34.6% for>10 mm–15 mm(N $= 52$), 41.2% for>15 mm–20 mm (N $= 34$) and 50.0% for>20 mm (N $= 38$) (Figure 4).

Preoperative factors associated with lymphatic vessel, vascular vessel or pleural invasion in small adenocarcinomas

As shown in Table 3, LD findings, MD findings, TDR, CEA levels and cN were significant factors for lymphatic vessel, vascular vessel or pleural (ly/v/pl) invasion on univariate analyses. The AUCs for ly/v/pl invasion were 0.60, 0.81, 0.81 and 0.65 for LD, MD, TDR and CEA, respectively (Figure 5). The incidence of ly/v/pl invasion according to MD were 0% for $\leq$5 mm (N $= 25$), 25.9% for>5 mm–10 mm (N $= 27$), 41.2% for $\geq$10 mm–15 mm (N $= 52$) and 79.4% for>15 mm(N $= 72$) (Figure 6).

Discussion

Tumour diameter is a major prognostic factor for lung cancer. The most common method for determining tumour size before surgery is by CT using lung window settings [8]. Recently,

attempts were made to classify small peripheral adenocarcinomas into subgroups according to the patterns of tumour growth, which are considered to be associated with the biological characteristics of tumours derived from clinicopathological examination[4,6,9–11]. These subgroups comprise the following: AIS (adenocarcinoma in situ), minimally invasive adenocarcinoma (3-cm lepidic predominant tumour with an invasion of $\leq$5 mm), lepidic predominant, acinar predominant, papillary predominant, micropapillary predominant, solid predominant with mucin production and invasive adenocarcinoma variants.

It has been reported that tumour size was not associated with either indicators of proliferation or tumour invasiveness [1,2,5,9,11]. In fact, histological subgrouping based on growth patterns provides a clear indication of the biological characteristics of peripheral small lung adenocarcinoma than simple lesion size [7,9]. That is, papirally, acinar, micropapillery or solid predom-

Prognosis according to tumor diameter evaluated with MD

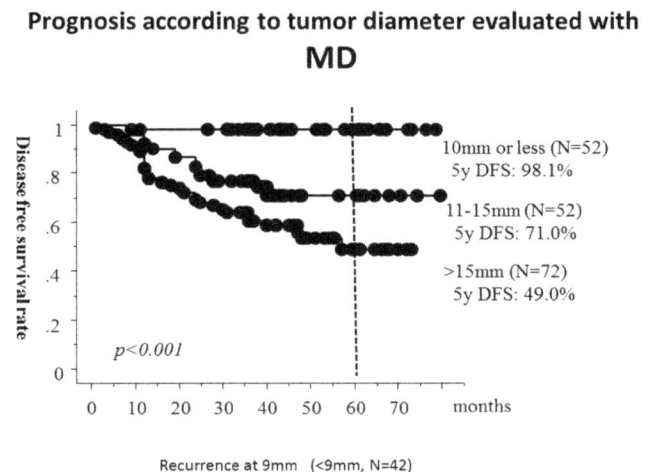

Figure 2. The 5-year disease-free survival curve according to tumour dimension using mediastinal window (MD) settings. Tumour dimension was evaluated using mediastinal window (MD) settings. One case with MD 9 mm showed recurrence and the case is the smallest in MD among all.

Table 2. Preoperative factors associated with lymph node metastasis in small adenocarcinoma (≤3 cm).

Variables	Odds ratio	95% CI	P value
Gender (female)	0.66	0.34–1.28	.22
Age	1.03	0.99–1.03	.86
LD	1.07	1.01–1.15	.03
MD	1.15	1.09–1.21	<.001
TDR	66.7	10.0–	<.001
CEA	1.11	1.01–1.12	.01
High (>5 ng/ml)/normal)	3.0	1.31–6.87	.009
cN (cN0/cN1-2)	30.3	3.76–250	<.001

Logistic regression test (Univariate analyses).
LD: diameter by lung window setting, MD: diameter by mediastinal window setting, TDR: tumour disappearance ratio (TDR = 1− MD/LD), CEA: carcinoembryonic antigen, cN: preoperative nodal status, CI: confidence interval, LN: lymph node.

inant adenocarcinoma have more aggressive character than lepidic predominant adenocarcinoma when tumoue size is limited to 3cm or smaller [7–11].

Furthermore, it has been reported that the larger or more desmoplastic fibrous scars is asosiated with more aggressive tumour invasion and poorer prognoses [7,9–11]. In addition, we previously reported that tumour size, excluding the BAC component (lepidic growth), was an important indicator of tumour invasiveness and that tumour diameter evaluated using MD was associated with the tumour growth pattern (i.e. non-lepidic growth component) and scars [1,2,5]. The solid lesion evaluated with MD in CT is the tumor lesion without lepidic growth adenocarcinoma. As an easy and simple extracting method of the solid area representing an invasive lesion (scar) of the adenocarcinoma or non-lepidic predominant adenocarcinoma (invasive adenocarcinoma), we examined the usefulness of tumour size as evaluated using MD. In other words, using LD to evaluate the total tumour diameter cannot directly detect the solid lesion associated with tumour aggressiveness, but can detect the associated BAC (lepidic growth) component, which is not associated with tumour aggressiveness [1,2,5,14].

In the present study, we confirmed that tumour dimensions determined using MD settings provided additional useful prognostic data that could not be evaluated using LD settings [1,2,5]. Furthermore, tumour size was a significantly better prognostic factor when evaluated using MD instead of LD. The MD were an important predictive factor for prognosis as well as for lymph node involvement and tumour invasiveness in small lung adenocarcinoma (1–3 cm). A new concept −minimally invasive adenocarcinoma (MIA)− has been proposed. This is a small, solitary adenocarcinoma (≤3 cm) with a predominantly lepidic pattern and invasion of ≤5 mm in the greatest dimension in any one focus. Patients with an MIA have a nearly 100% disease-specific survival if it is completely resected. The invasive component to be measured in an MIA is defined as follows: (1) histological subtypes other than a lepidic pattern (i.e., acinar, papillary, micropapillary, and/or solid) or (2) tumor cells infiltrating into myofibroblastic stroma. MIA is excluded if the tumor (1) invades lymphatics, blood vessels, or pleura or (2) has tumor necrosis [6]. Accordin to the present study, when the MD findings were equal or smaller than 5 mm, no patient showed vessel invasion, plural invasion, or tumor relapse. Therefore, MD may be a promising criteria to be

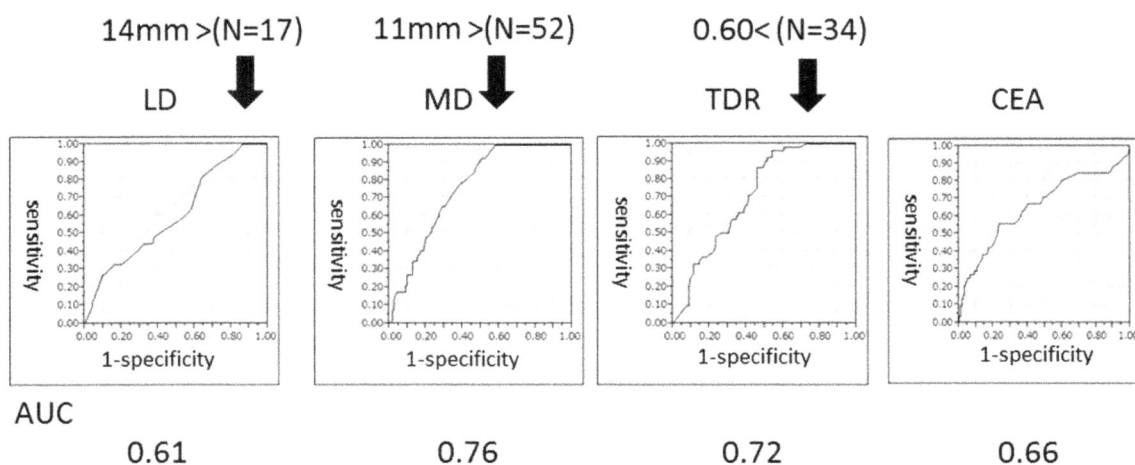

Figure 3. Receiver operating characteristic analyses for lymph node metastasis. Tumour dimension was evaluated using lung window (LD) and mediastinal window (MD) settings. TDR: tumour disappearance ratio (TDR = 1− MD/LD), CEA: carcinoembryonic antigen. Allow indicated a value at 100% sensitivity.

LN metastasis: MD

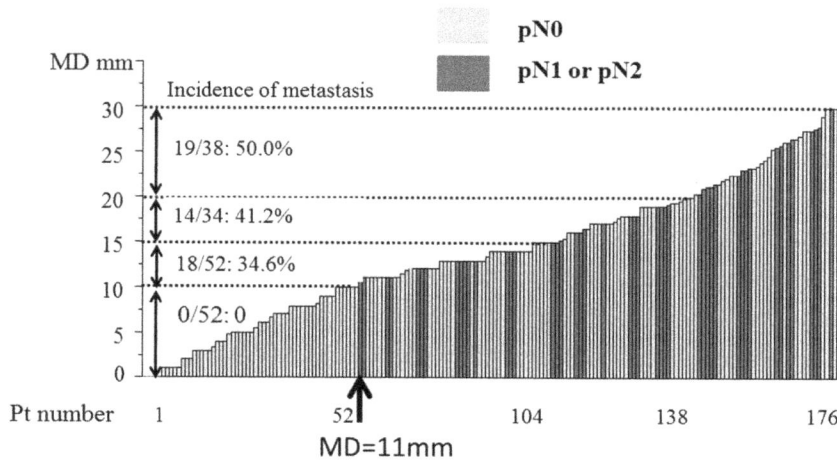

Figure 4. Incidence of lymph node metastasis according to tumour dimension using mediastinal window (MD) settings. Tumour dimension was evaluated using mediastinal window (MD) settings. A black bar showed a patient with lymph node metastasis and a gray bar showed a patient without lymph node metastasis.

used for CT classification as the newly proposed minimally invasive adenocarcinoma.

Tumour markers are used clinically to assist in the diagnosis of patients with non-small-cell lung carcinoma and to monitor progression, recurrence and/or efficiency of treatment. Among these markers, CEA is considered to be the most prevalent marker for the diagnosis and monitoring of lung adenocarcinoma. Serum CEA levels are an important prognostic factor for early-stage adenocarcinoma, such as clinical stage IA tumours [12–14]. In the present study, univariate analysis revealed that CEA levels were correlated with lymph node metastasis and v or pl invasion, with a tendency for predicting postoperative prognosis. However, CEA levels were not a significant prognostic factor for lymph node metastasis following multivariate analyses with MD findings. This may be explained by the high correlation between CEA levels and MD findings. When CEA levels were compared among the tumour size groups, they gradually and significantly increased with tumour stage progression ($P<0.01$). When the mediastinal size

was>20 mm, one-fourth of the patients in this cohort showed serum CEA levels beyond cut off value at 5 ng/ml.

TDR is an established and important prognostic factor. Suzuki et al. reported that radiological non-invasive (neither ly nor v) peripheral lung adenocarcinoma could be defined as an adenocarcinoma of ≤2.0 cm with ≤0.25 consolidation [15]. The results of our study were similar to those of a previous study on TDR [16.17].

The solid type adenocarcinoma on CT was highly associated with non-lepidic predominant adenocarcinoma, such as acinar predominant, papillary predominant and solid predominant with mucin production [2,3,5]. In invasive adenocarcinoma, lepidic predominant adenocarcinomas have a much better prognosis than non-lepidic predominant adenocarcinomas [1,2,5,9–11]. It was therefore suggested that the size of a non-lepidic tumour component evaluated using MD findings on CT was a useful indicator of solid adenocarcinoma aggressiveness.

Table 3. Preoperative factors associated with pleural, lymphatic and vascular invasion in small adenocarcinomas (≤3 cm).

Variables	Odds ratio	95% CI	P value
Gender (female)	0.66	0.36–1.20	.17
Age	1.00	0.97–1.03	.87
LD	1.06	1.00–1.12	.03
MD	1.21	1.14–1.30	<.001
TDR	6.76	3.50–13.2	<.001
CEA	1.23	1.07–1.40	.002
High (>5 ng/ml)/normal)	5.9	2.12–16.3	<.001
cN (cN0/cN1-2)	11.1	1.40–90.9	.03

Logistic regression test (Univariate analyses).
LD: diameter by lung window setting, MD: diameter by mediastinal window setting, TDR: tumour disappearance ratio (TDR = 1 − MD/LD), CEA: carcinoembryonic antigen, cN: preoperative nodal status, CI: confidence interval, ly: lymphatic vessels, v: vascular vessels, pl: pleura.

6mm >(N=25)   0.74 <(N=20)

LD   MD ▼   TDR ▼   CEA

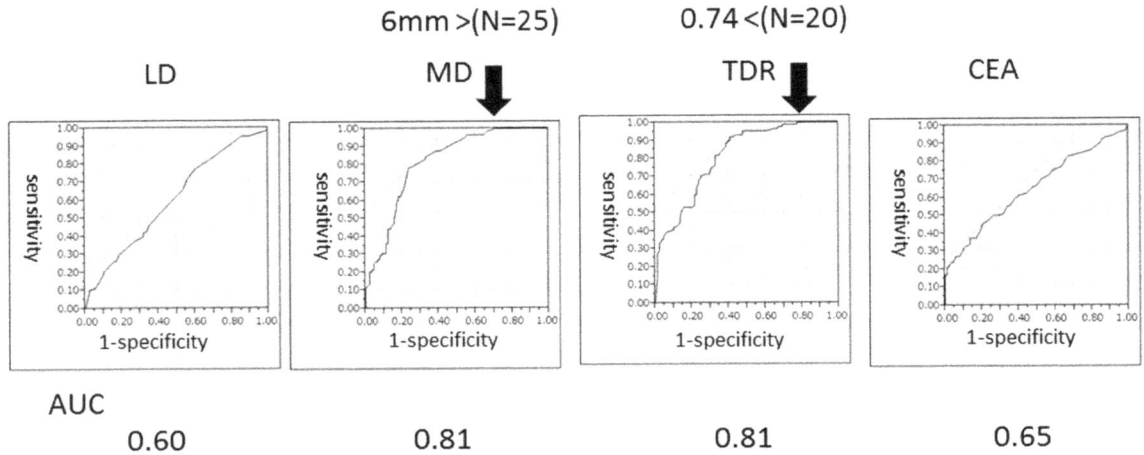

AUC
0.60   0.81   0.81   0.65

Figure 5. Receiver operating characteristic analyses for pleural, lymphatic and vascular invasion. Tumour dimension was evaluated using lung window (LD) and mediastinal window (MD) settings. TDR: tumour disappearance ratio (TDR = 1− MD/LD), CEA: carcinoembryonic antigen. Allow indicated a value at 100% sensitivity.

In this study, the patient population was limited to those with tumour diameters of 1–3 cm. Patients with tumour diameters of < 1 cm were excluded because of the small number of cases and the major bias to perform wedge resection. Another problem was the LD and MD imaging conditions for CT. According to 7th general rule for clinical and pathological record of lung cancer, the recommended LD are a window level of −500 to −700 and a window width of 1000–2000 HU, whereas we used −500 HU and 1500 HU, respectively. The recommended MD are a window level of 30–60 H and a window width of 350–600 HU, while we used 60 HU and 350 HU, respectively.[8]

The differences in these imaging conditions for CT may have affected the MD, LD and TDR results. Furthermore, the solid

component size defined as a lesion without GGO evaluated by LD is a promising method of the solid area representing an invasive lesion (scar) of the adenocarcinoma,

Therefore, further investigations on the optimal CT imaging conditions for assessing the aggressiveness of small adenocarcinomas should be performed in multiple centres with larger sample sizes. The size of the solid lesion (excluding the GGO component) evaluated using LD is also a useful CT-based prognostic factor. Further examination is necessary to clarify the relative utility of both tumour size measured using MD and extracted solid size measured by LD.

In conclusion, our results suggest that measuring tumour size with MD on high-resolution CT is a simple and useful

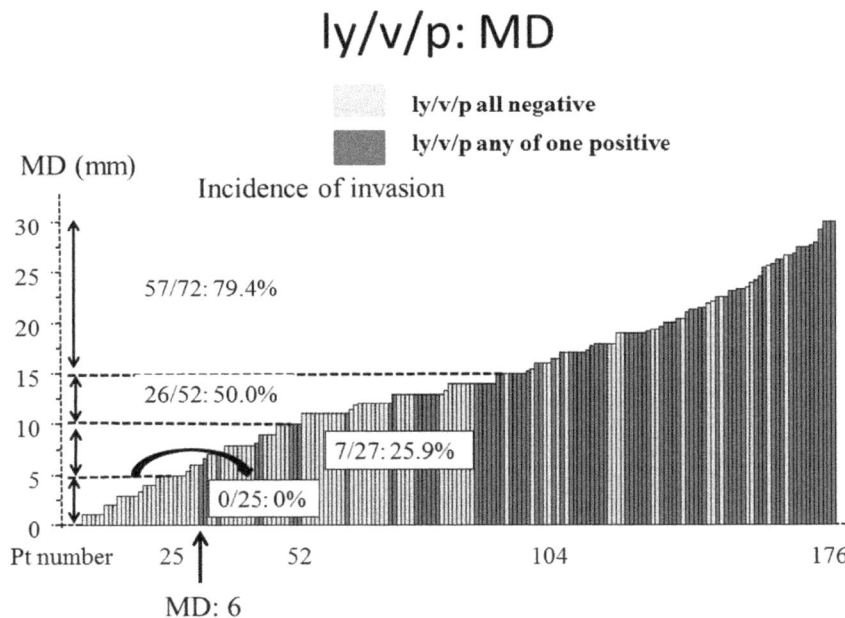

Figure 6. Incidence of lymphatic vessel, vascular vessel or pleural invasion in small adenocarcinomas according to tumour dimension using mediastinal window (MD) settings. A black bar showed a patient with invasion to any of lymphatic vessel, vascular vessel or pleura, and a gray bar showed a patient without any of them.

preoperative modality for predicting invasiveness, lymph node metastasis and prognosis. An increased tumour size with MD correlated with pathological malignant potential reflecting tumour aggressiveness and degree of invasion.

Acknowledgments

CT imaging data and statistical advice were provided by Dr. Kuroda, Dr. Mun and Dr. Uehara. Pathological advice was given by Dr. Ishikawa and Dr. Motoi. Editorial assistance was provided by Dr. Nakagawa and Dr. Okumura.

Author Contributions

Conceived and designed the experiments: SO KN. Analyzed the data: HU HK YS. Contributed reagents/materials/analysis tools: MM YI NM. Wrote the paper: HK YS. Pathological examination and analyses (Chief of the department of pathology): YI. Pathological examination and analyses (Chief of the division of the lung pathology): NM.

References

1. Sakao Y, Nakazono T, Tomimitsu S, Takeda Y, Sakuragi T, et al. (2004) Lung adenocarcinoma can be subtyped according to tumour dimension by computed tomography mediastinal-window setting. Additional size criteria for Clinical T1 adenocarcinoma. Eur J Cardiothorac Surg 26: 1211–1215.

2. Sakao Y, Nakazono T, Sakuragi T, Natsuaki M, Itoh T (2004) Predictive factors for survival in surgically resected clinical IA peripheral adenocarcinoma of the lung. Ann Thorac Surg 77: 1157–1162.

3. Nakazono T, Sakao Y, Yamaguchi K, Imai S, Kumazoe H, et al. (2005) Subtypes of peripheral adenocarcinoma of the lung: differentiation by thin-section CT. Eur Radiol 15: 1563–1568.

4. Bhure UN, Lardinois D, Kalff V, Hany TF, Soltermann A, et al. (2010) Accuracy of CT parameters for assessment of tumour size and aggressiveness in lung adenocarcinoma with bronchoalveolar elements. Br J Radiol 83: 841–849.

5. Sakao Y, Miyamoto H, Sakuraba M, Oh T, Shiomi K, et al. (2007) Prognostic significance of a histologic subtype in small adenocarcinoma of the lung: the impact of non-bronchioloalveolar carcinoma components. Ann Thor Surg 83: 209–214.

6. Travis WD, Brambilla E, Noguchi M, Nicholson AG, Geisinger KR, et al. (2011) International Association for the Study of Lung Cancer/American Thoracic Society/European Respiratory Society International Multidisciplinary Classification of Lung Adenocarcinoma. J Thorac Oncol 6: 244–285.

7. Shimosato Y, Suzuki A, Hashimoto T, Nishiwaki Y, Kodama T, et al. (1980) Prognostic implications of fibrotic focus (scar) in small peripheral lung cancers. Am J Sur g Pathol 4: 365–373.

8. Rusch VW, Asamura H, Watanabe H, Giroux DJ, Rami-Porta R, et al. (2009) The IASLC lung cancer staging project: a proposal for a new international lymph node map in the forthcoming seventh edition of the TNM classification for lung cancer. J Thorac Oncol 4: 568–577.

9. Maeshima AM, Niki T, Maeshima A, Yamada T, Kondo H, et al. (2002) Modified scar grade: a prognostic indicator in small peripheral lung adenocarcinoma. Cancer 95: 2546–54.

10. Borczuk AC, Qian F, Kazeros A, Eleazar J, Assaad A, et al. (2009) Invasive size is an independent predictor of survival in pulmonary adenocarcinoma. Am J Surg Pathol 33: 462–469.

11. Noguchi M, Morikawa A, Kawasaki M, Matsuno Y, Yamada T, et al. (1995) Small adenocarcinoma of the lung. Histologic characteristics and prognosis. Cancer 75: 2844–2852.

12. Kulpa J, Wo'jcik E, Reinfuss M, Kołodziejski L (2002) Carcinoembryonic antigen, squamous cell carcinoma antigen, CYFRA21-1, and neuron-specific enolase in squamous cell lung cancer patients. Clin Chem 48: 1931–1937.

13. Sawabata N, Maeda H, Yokota S, Takeda S, Koma M, et al. (2004) Postoperative serum carcinoembryonic antigen levels in patients with pathologic stage IA nonsmall cell lung carcinoma: subnormal levels as an indicator of favorable prognosis. Cancer 15: 803–809.

14. Sakao Y, Sakuragi T, Natsuaki M, Itoh T (2003) Clinicopathological analysis of prognostic factors in clinical IA peripheral adenocarcinoma of the lung. Ann Thorac Surg 75: 1113–1117.

15. Suzuki K, Koike T, Asakawa T, Kusumoto M, Asamura H, et al. (2011) A prospective radiological study of thin-section computed tomography to predict pathological noninvasiveness in peripheral clinical IA lung cancer (Japan Clinical Oncology Group 0201). J Thorac Oncol 6: 751–756.

16. Okada M, Nishio W, Salkamoto T, Uchino K, Hanioka K, et al. (2004) Correlation between computed tomographic findings, bronchioloalveolar carcinoma component, and biologic behavior of small-sized lung adenocarcinomas. J Thorac Cardiovasc Sur 127: 857–861.

17. Takashima S, Maruyama Y, Hasegawa M, Yamanda T, Honda T, et al. (2002) Prognostic significance of high-resolution CT findings in small peripheral adenocarcinoma of the lung: a retrospective study on 64 patients. Lung Cancer 36: 289–295.

Permissions

All chapters in this book were first published in PLOS ONE, by The Public Library of Science; hereby published with permission under the Creative Commons Attribution License or equivalent. Every chapter published in this book has been scrutinized by our experts. Their significance has been extensively debated. The topics covered herein carry significant findings which will fuel the growth of the discipline. They may even be implemented as practical applications or may be referred to as a beginning point for another development.

The contributors of this book come from diverse backgrounds, making this book a truly international effort. This book will bring forth new frontiers with its revolutionizing research information and detailed analysis of the nascent developments around the world.

We would like to thank all the contributing authors for lending their expertise to make the book truly unique. They have played a crucial role in the development of this book. Without their invaluable contributions this book wouldn't have been possible. They have made vital efforts to compile up to date information on the varied aspects of this subject to make this book a valuable addition to the collection of many professionals and students.

This book was conceptualized with the vision of imparting up-to-date information and advanced data in this field. To ensure the same, a matchless editorial board was set up. Every individual on the board went through rigorous rounds of assessment to prove their worth. After which they invested a large part of their time researching and compiling the most relevant data for our readers.

The editorial board has been involved in producing this book since its inception. They have spent rigorous hours researching and exploring the diverse topics which have resulted in the successful publishing of this book. They have passed on their knowledge of decades through this book. To expedite this challenging task, the publisher supported the team at every step. A small team of assistant editors was also appointed to further simplify the editing procedure and attain best results for the readers.

Apart from the editorial board, the designing team has also invested a significant amount of their time in understanding the subject and creating the most relevant covers. They scrutinized every image to scout for the most suitable representation of the subject and create an appropriate cover for the book.

The publishing team has been an ardent support to the editorial, designing and production team. Their endless efforts to recruit the best for this project, has resulted in the accomplishment of this book. They are a veteran in the field of academics and their pool of knowledge is as vast as their experience in printing. Their expertise and guidance has proved useful at every step. Their uncompromising quality standards have made this book an exceptional effort. Their encouragement from time to time has been an inspiration for everyone.

The publisher and the editorial board hope that this book will prove to be a valuable piece of knowledge for researchers, students, practitioners and scholars across the globe.

List of Contributors

Pietro Emanuele Napoli, Franco Coronella, Giovanni Maria Satta and Maurizio Fossarello
Department of Surgical Sciences, Eye Clinic, University of Cagliari, Cagliari, Italy

Lee R. Ferguson, Sandeep Grover, Sankarathi Balaiya and Kakarla V. Chalam
Department of Ophthalmology, University of Florida College of Medicine, Jacksonville, Florida, United States of America

James M. Dominguez II
Department of Pharmacology and Therapeutics, University of Florida College of Medicine, Gainesville, Florida, United States of America

Kevin Kozak, William Clarke, Ernest Allen and LisaAnn Trembath
Cellectar Biosciences, Inc., Madison, WI, United States of America

Joseph J. Grudzinski and Benjamin Titz
Cellectar Biosciences, Inc., Madison, WI, United States of America
Department of Medical Physics, University of Wisconsin School of Medicine and Public Health, Madison, WI, United States of America

Jamey P. Weichert
Cellectar Biosciences, Inc., Madison, WI, United States of America
Department of Radiology, University of Wisconsin, Madison, WI, United States of America

Michael Stabin
Department of Radiology and Radiological Sciences, Vanderbilt University, Nashville, TN, United States of America

John Marshall
Department of Medicine and Lombardi Comprehensive Cancer Center, Medstar Georgetown University Hospital, Washington, DC, United States of America

Steve Y. Cho
Department of Radiology, Johns Hopkins Hospital, Baltimore, MD, United States of America

Terence Z. Wong
Department of Radiology, Duke University Medical Center, Durham, NC, United States of America

Joanne Mortimer
Department of Medical Oncology and Therapeutics Research, City of Hope, Duarte, CA, United States of America

Jae Joon Hwang, Hyok Park, Chang Seo Park and Ho-Gul Jeong
Department of Oral and Maxillofacial Radiology, Dental Hospital of Yonsei University of College of Dentistry, Seoul, Korea

Kee-Deog Kim
Department of General Dentistry, Dental Hospital of Yonsei University of College of Dentistry, Seoul, Korea

Guoyan Mo
China Key Laboratory of TCM Resource and Prescription, Hubei University of Chinese Medicine, Ministry of Education, Wuhan 430065, China

Qin Ding, Zhongshan Chen, Ming Yan and Yanping Song
Department of Ophthalmology, Wuhan General Hospital of Guangzhou Military Command, Wuhan 430070, China

Yunbo Li
Beijing University of Chinese Medicine Third Affiliated Hospital, Beijing 100029, China

Lijing Bu
Department of Biology, University of New Mexico, Albuquerque, NM, 87131, United States of America

Guohua Yin
Department of Plant Biology and Pathology, Rutgers, The State University of New Jersey, New Brunswick, NJ, 08901, United States of America
Wuhan Sheng Da An Biotech Service Co. Ltd., Wuhan, China

Walter Noordzij, Andor W. Glaudemans, Riemer H. Slart and Rudi A. Dierckx
Department of Nuclear Medicine and Molecular Imaging, University of Groningen, University Medical Center Groningen, Groningen, The Netherlands

André P. van Beek and Anouk N. van der Horst-Schrivers
Department of Endocrinology, University of Groningen, University Medical Center Groningen, Groningen, The Netherlands

René A. Tio
Department of Cardiology, University of Groningen, University Medical Center Groningen, Groningen, The Netherlands

Annemiek M. Walenkamp and Elisabeth G. de Vries
Department of Medical Oncology, University of Groningen, University Medical Center Groningen, Groningen, The Netherlands

Bram van Ginkel
Faculty of Medicine, University of Groningen, University Medical Center Groningen, Groningen, The Netherlands

Shu-Xun Hou, Jia-Liang Zhu, Dong-Feng Ren, Zheng Cao and Jia-Guang Tang
Department of Orthopaedics, The First Affiliated Hospital of General Hospital of Chinese PLA, Beijing, China

Feng Shuang
Department of Orthopaedics, The First Affiliated Hospital of General Hospital of Chinese PLA, Beijing, China
Department of Orthopedics, The 94th Hospital of Chinese PLA, Nanchang, China

Yoshinari Asaoka, Ryosuke Tateishi, Ryo Nakagomi, Mayuko Kondo, Naoto Fujiwara, Tatsuya Minami, Masaya Sato, Koji Uchino, Kenichiro Enooku, Hayato Nakagawa, Yuji Kondo, Haruhiko Yoshida and Kazuhiko Koike
Department of Gastroenterology, Graduate School of Medicine, The University of Tokyo, Tokyo, Japan

Shuichiro Shiina
Department of Gastroenterology, Graduate School of Medicine, Juntendo University, Tokyo, Japan

Masayuki Hata, Kazuaki Miyamoto, Akio Oishi, Yukiko Makiyama, Norimoto Gotoh, Yugo Kimura, Tadamichi Akagi and Nagahisa Yoshimura
Department of Ophthalmology and Visual Sciences, Kyoto University Graduate School of Medicine, Kyoto, Japan

Florian Alten, Christoph R. Clemens and Nicole Eter
Department of Ophthalmology, University of Muenster Medical Center, Muenster, Germany

Jeremias Motte, Carina Ewering and Martin Marziniak
Department of Neurology, University of Muenster Medical Center, Muenster, Germany

Nani Osada
Department of Medical Informatics and Biomathematics, University of Muenster, Muenster, Germany

Ella M. Kadas
Department of Neurology, Charite University Medicine Berlin, Berlin, German

Friedemann Paul
Department of Neurology, Charite University Medicine Berlin, Berlin, German
NeuroCure Clinical Research Center, Berlin, Germany

Synho Do, Sarabjeet Singh, Mannudeep Kalra, Tom Brady, Ellie Shin and Homer Pien
Department of Radiology, Massachusetts General Hospital and Harvard Medical School, Boston, Massachusetts, United States of America

William Clem Karl
Department of Electrical and Computer Engineering, Boston University, Boston, Massachusetts, United States of America

Jieyang Ju, Suicheng Gu, Joseph K. Leader, Shandong Wu and David Gur
Department of Radiology, University of Pittsburgh, Pittsburgh, Pennsylvania, United States of America

Ruosha Li
Department of Biostatistics, University of Pittsburgh, Pittsburgh, Pennsylvania, United States of America

Xiaohua Wang and Yahong Chen
Peking University Third Affiliated Hospital, Beijing, People's Republic of China

Bin Zheng
School of Electrical and Computer Engineering, University of Oklahoma, Norman, Oklahoma, United States of America

Frank Sciurba
Department of Medicine, University of Pittsburgh, Pittsburgh, Pennsylvania, United States of America

Jiantao Pu
Department of Radiology, University of Pittsburgh, Pittsburgh, Pennsylvania, United States of America
Department of Bioengineering, University of Pittsburgh, Pittsburgh, Pennsylvania, United States of America

Kenji Yamaji, Yusuke Suzuki, Hitoshi Suzuki, Kenji Satake, Satoshi Horikoshi and Yasuhiko Tomino
Division of Nephrology, Department of Internal Medicine, Juntendo University School of Medicine, Tokyo, Japan

Jan Novak
Department of Microbiology, University of Alabama at Birmingham, Birmingham, Alabama, United States of America

Jie Tang and Zhen Hong
Department of Neurology, Huashan Hospital, Fudan University, Shanghai, China

Jianhui Fu
Department of Neurology, Huashan Hospital, Fudan University, Shanghai, China
Department of Neurology, Shanghai Pudong Hospital, Fudan University Pudong Medical Center, Shanghai, China

Jinghao Han
Departments of Medicine and Therapeutics, Chinese University of Hong Kong, Prince of Wales Hospital, Hong Kong, China

Mark O. Wielpütz, Marcel Koenigkam-Santos and Michael Puderbach
Department of Diagnostic and Interventional Radiology, University Hospital of Heidelberg, Heidelberg, Germany
Translational Lung Research Center Heidelberg (TLRC), Member of the German Center for Lung Research (DZL), Heidelberg, Germany

Department of Diagnostic and Interventional Radiology with Nuclear Medicine, Thoraxklinik at University of Heidelberg, Heidelberg, Germany
Department of Radiology, German Cancer Research Center (dkfz), Heidelberg, Germany

Diana Bardarova, Hans-Ulrich Kauczor, Monika Eichinger, Bertram J. Jobst and Claus P. Heussel
Department of Diagnostic and Interventional Radiology, University Hospital of Heidelberg, Heidelberg, Germany
Translational Lung Research Center Heidelberg (TLRC), Member of the German Center for Lung Research (DZL), Heidelberg, Germany
Department of Diagnostic and Interventional Radiology with Nuclear Medicine, Thoraxklinik at University of Heidelberg, Heidelberg, Germany

Oliver Weinheimer
Department of Diagnostic and Interventional Radiology, University Hospital of Heidelberg, Heidelberg, Germany
Translational Lung Research Center Heidelberg (TLRC), Member of the German Center for Lung Research (DZL), Heidelberg, Germany

Ralf Eberhardt
Department of Pneumology and Respiratory Critical Care Medicine, Thoraxklinik at University of Heidelberg, Heidelberg, Germany

Katsuharu Yagi, Keiko Watanabe and Masashi Ueda
Graduate School of Medicine, Dentistry, and Pharmaceutical Sciences, Okayama University, Okayama, Japan

Kei Higashikawa
Graduate School of Medicine, Dentistry, and Pharmaceutical Sciences, Okayama University, Okayama, Japan
Japan Society for the Promotion of Science, Tokyo, Japan

Shuichi Enomoto
Graduate School of Medicine, Dentistry, and Pharmaceutical Sciences, Okayama University, Okayama, Japan
Next-generation Imaging Team, RIKEN Center for Life Science Technologies, Kobe, Japan

Shinichiro Kamino and Makoto Hiromura
Next-generation Imaging Team, RIKEN Center for Life Science Technologies, Kobe, Japan

Sara Zarei
Computational Science Research Center, San Diego State University, San Diego, California, United States of America

Ali Mirtar
Electrical and Computer Eng. Dep/University of California San Diego, San Diego, California, United States of America

Forest Rohwer
Department of Biology, San Diego State University, San Diego, California, United States of America

Peter Salamon
Department of Mathematics and Statistics, San Diego State University, San Diego, California, United States of America

Santiago Peña-Zalbidea and Jose María Mateos-Pérez
Unidad de Medicina y Cirugía Experimental, Instituto de Investigación Sanitaria Gregorio Marañón, Madrid, Spain

María Luisa Soto-Montenegro
Unidad de Medicina y Cirugía Experimental, Instituto de Investigación Sanitaria Gregorio Marañón, Madrid, Spain
Centro de Investigación Biomédica en Red de Salud Mental (CIBERSAM), Madrid, Spain

Manuel Desco
Unidad de Medicina y Cirugía Experimental, Instituto de Investigación Sanitaria Gregorio Marañón, Madrid, Spain
Departamento de Bioingeniería e Ingeniería Aerospacial, Universidad Carlos III, Madrid, Spain

Marta Oteo, Eduardo Romero and Miguel Ángel Morcillo
Unidad de Aplicaciones Biomédicas y Farmacocinética, Centro de Investigaciones Energéticas, Medioambientales y Tecnológicas (CIEMAT), Madrid, Spain

Bettina Maiwald, Donald Lobsien, Thomas Kahn and Patrick Stumpp
Department of Diagnostic and Interventional Radiology, University of Leipzig, Leipzig, Germany

Ryan F. Donnelly, Maelíosa T. C. McCrudden, Eneko Larrañeta, Emma McAlister, Aaron J. Courtenay, Mary-Carmel Kearney, Thakur Raghu Raj Singh, Helen O. McCarthy, Victoria L. Kett, Ester Caffarel-Salvador, Sharifa Al-Zahrani and A. David Woolfson
School of Pharmacy, Queen's University Belfast, Belfast, Co. Antrim, United Kingdom

Ahlam Zaid Alkilani
School of Pharmacy, Queen's University Belfast, Belfast, Co. Antrim, United Kingdom
School of Pharmacy, Zarqa University, Zarqa, Jordan

Akinori Miyata, Takeaki Ishizawa, Atsushi Shimizu, Junichi Kaneko and Norihiro Kokudo
Hepato-Biliary-Pancreatic Surgery Division, Department of Surgery, Graduate School of Medicine, the University of Tokyo, Tokyo, Japan

Mako Kamiya and Yasuteru Urano
Laboratory of Chemical Biology and Molecular Imaging, Graduate School of Medicine, the University of Tokyo, Tokyo, Japan

Hideaki Ijichi
Department of Gastroenterology, Graduate School of Medicine, the University of Tokyo, Tokyo, Japan

Junji Shibahara and Masashi Fukayama
Department of Pathology, Graduate School of Medicine, the University of Tokyo, Tokyo, Japan

Yutaka Midorikawa
Genome Science Division, Research Center for Advanced Science & Technology, the University of Tokyo, Tokyo, Japan

Jingqin Ma, Zhiping Yan, Jianjun Luo, Qingxin Liu and Jianhua Wang
Department of Interventional Radiology, Zhongshan Hospital, Fudan University, Shanghai, China

Shijing Qiu
Bone and Mineral Research Laboratory, Henry Ford Hospital, Detroit, Michigan, United States of America

Lu Guo, Shuming Shen and Yu Guo
Department of Biomedical Engineering, Tianjin University, Tianjin, China

Yuanming Feng
Department of Biomedical Engineering, Tianjin University, Tianjin, China
Department of Radiation Oncology, East Carolina University, Greenville, North Carolina, United States of America

Eleanor Harris
Department of Radiation Oncology, East Carolina University, Greenville, North Carolina, United States of America

Zheng Wang and Wei Jiang
Department of Radiation Oncology, Tianjin Huanhu Hospital, Tianjin, China

Peter Vedsted
Research Centre for Cancer Diagnosis in Primary Care, Research Unit for General Practice, Aarhus University, Aarhus, Denmark

Louise Mahncke Guldbrandt
Research Centre for Cancer Diagnosis in Primary Care, Research Unit for General Practice, Aarhus University, Aarhus, Denmark
Section for General Medical Practice, Department of Public Health, Aarhus University, Aarhus, Denmark

Torben Riis Rasmussen
Department of Respiratory Diseases and Allergy, Aarhus University Hospital, Aarhus, Denmark

Finn Rasmussen
Department of Radiology, Aarhus University Hospital, Aarhus, Denmark

Christin Goldschalt, Sara Doll, Brit Ihle and Joachim Kirsch
University of Heidelberg, Institute for Anatomy and Cell Biology, Heidelberg, Germany

Till Sebastian Mutzbauer
University of Heidelberg, Institute for Anatomy and Cell Biology, Heidelberg, Germany
Mutzbauer&Partner, Maxillofacial Surgery and Anesthesiology, Zuerich, Switzerland

Index

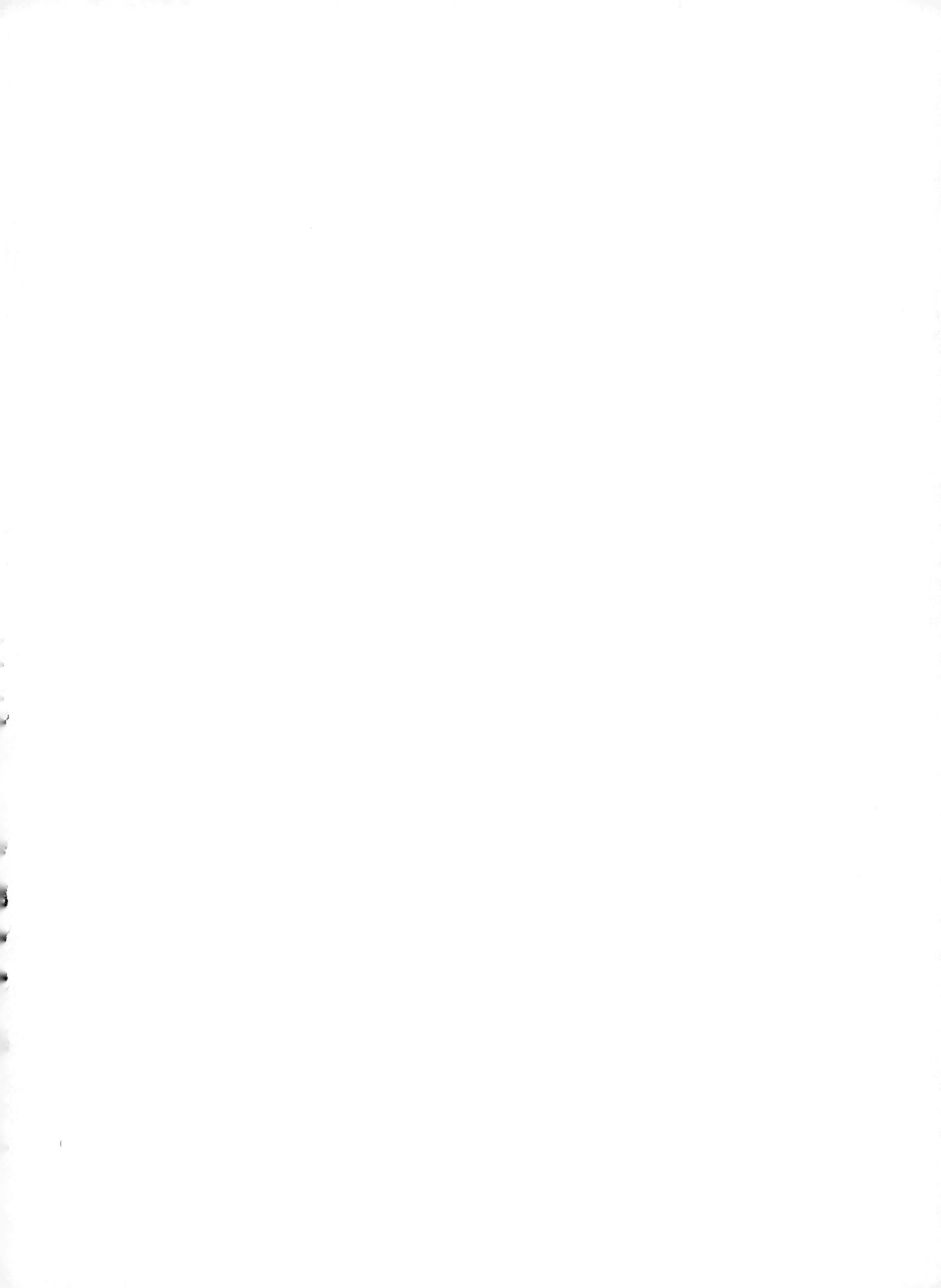

www.ingramcontent.com/pod-product-compliance
Lightning Source LLC
Chambersburg PA
CBHW061249190326
41458CB00011B/3627